An Introduction to Environmental Toxicology

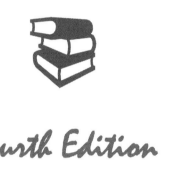

Fourth Edition

Michael H. Dong, MPH, DrPA, PhD

An Introduction to Environmental Toxicology
First (Student) Edition, 2011 (ISBN 978-0-578-09628-5)
Second Edition, 2012 (ISBN 978-1-477-66648-7)
Third Edition, 2014 (ISBN 978-1-494-32408-7)

Copyright © 2011, 2012, 2014, 2018 by Michael H. Dong
ALL RIGHTS RESERVED

No part of this book may be reproduced, stored in a retrieval system, or transmitted, in any form or by any means, electronic, mechanical, photocopying, recording, or otherwise, without the prior written permission of the copyright holder.

Printed by CreateSpace
7290 Investment Drive
North Charleston, South Carolina
USA 29418

ISBN-10: 1979904510
ISBN-13: 978-1-979-90451-3

Dedication

To my family for their appreciation, endurance, and support, which all have made my writing of this edition as well as this book with greater fulfillment and more pleasure.

About the Author

Dr. Michael H. Dong (鄧振麟博士), born in Hong Kong (Special Administrative Region of China), holds a Doctor of Public Administration (Dr.P.A.) degree in (environmental) health policy from the University of Southern California and a Doctor of Philosophy (Ph.D.) degree in environmental epidemiology from the University of Pittsburgh. Dr. Dong has also earned a Master of Public Health (M.P.H.) in environmental/nutritional sciences from the University of California at Los Angeles (UCLA), a B.Sc. in biochemistry from the University of California at Riverside, and a second B.Sc. in forensic science from the California State University at Sacramento (CSUS). For many years until his recent retirement, he was a full member (later an emeritus) of the American College of Nutrition, a full member of the (American) Society of Toxicology, a Certified Nutrition Specialist (CNS), and a Diplomate of the American Board of Toxicology (DABT).

Dr. Dong worked for 25 years as a regulatory toxicologist for the state of California (USA). Prior to his state government employment, Dr. Dong was on military active duty for several years as a U.S. Public Health Service Commissioned Corps officer stationed at the U.S. Food and Drug Administration (at the rank of lieutenant commander). Earlier he served for several years as a U.S. Army Medical Service Corps officer with various assignments working as a nutritional, clinical, or research biochemist (to the rank of captain). Between the two U.S. military services, He worked for a year as an occupational toxicologist as well as an environmental epidemiologist at the U.S. Occupational Safety and Health Administration.

For four years from 2005 to 2009, Michael served as one of the dozen board members of the American Board of Toxicology (ABT) and chaired the ABT certification examination committee during his fourth year of service there. From 2006 to 2008, he served as a voting member of the Scientific Advisory Committee on Alternative Toxicological Methods (SACATM) for the U.S. National Institute of Environmental Health Sciences. Michael also served on the editorial board for the two international journals *Environmental Geochemistry and Health* from 2004 through 2015, and *Human and Ecological Risk Assessment* from 2013 through 2016. And from 2008 through 2014, he was a part-time adjunct lecturer teaching the environmental toxicology course for the Department of Environmental Studies at CSUS.

Michael's academic involvement has included the long series of his online lectures on toxicologic epidemiology, environmental endocrine disruption, and herbal medicine. His published work has extended to such subject matters as physiologically-based pharmacokinetic (PB-PK) modeling and aggregate exposure assessment through probabilistic Monte Carlo simulation, both of which were innovative concepts to environmental health risk assessors at the time and are now widely accepted in the scientific sector. Collectively, Michael's academic and professional trainings all point to his persistent and strong interest in and commitment to promoting environmental and global health. His most recent published work prior to this *Fourth Edition* was titled "The Health Risk Assessment Performed in California for the Herbicide Simazine: A Case Study" (*Hum. Ecol. Risk Assess.* 2015, 21:1496-1517).

Preface

This *Fourth Edition* continues to serve as an introduction to the basic principles, concepts, and issues for/of environmental toxicology intended for undergraduates majoring in environmental toxicology or a related field, as well as for graduate students taking a course in a related field as an elective. It is also intended to serve as supplementary reading for students whose instructors prefer to use their own lecture notes as class materials. This *Fourth Edition* remains as a primer covering lecture materials for a course of 3 to 6 semester units. As before, the 23 chapters have been strategically arranged under four parts to offer students presumably the best flow and mode of comprehension, with each chapter including a set of review questions. Students using this book should have completed a course in general biology and a course in general chemistry.

The *core* content difference between this *Fourth* and the Third as well as the Second Edition is minimal. In addition to the correction of the typos found in the Third Edition, this *Fourth Edition* has made minor refinements but substantial updates on the status and discussion of numerous contemporary issues covered in the book. In particular, this *Fourth Edition* has updated (Chapter 16) the five persistent organic pollutants that the Stockholm Convention has added to its action list since the publication of this book's Third Edition in 2014. It is under this notion that this *Fourth Edition* has continued to include in the back cover the rather encouraging book review conclusion kindly given by Prof. Arthur L. Frank, M.D., Ph.D., professor and former chair of the Department of Environmental & Occupational Health, Drexel University Dornsife School of Public Health (Philadelphia, Pennsylvania, USA).

It is expected that at the end, students can at least tell the commonality and difference between such two closely-related terms as *toxin* and *toxicant*, *human health risk assessment* and *ecological risk assessment*, or *environmental toxicology* and *ecotoxicology*. Students should complete their course as well as the book with the appreciation that acute air pollution episodes such as London fog of 1952 and Meuse Valley of 1930 were environmental tragedies of the past. Today, many environmental toxicologists and health regulatory agencies around the world are more concerned with contemporary issues such as global warming, global infectious diseases (e.g., Ebola, MERS, Zika), electronic waste problems in certain developing countries, plastic marine pollution, and the aftermath of Fukushima nuclear crisis in Japan. An undesired phenomenon happening today is that even some course instructors tend to forget that toxicology in general, and environmental toxicology in particular, should consider adverse health effects caused by harmful biological and physical hazards, not just by toxic chemicals.

As a textbook for a general course in environmental toxicology, it is written primarily *to* students who might not have heard much about the term *toxicology* or *environmental pollution*, and partly *for* those instructors who are overwhelmed by their research agenda or subspecialty interests but otherwise could have written a similar text. This textbook, or reference book to some, takes the position that a student who has completed the course should become familiar with not only the basic concepts and principles for/of environmental toxicology, but also the basic socioeconomic, environmental, regulatory, and global issues pertinent to the *practice* of environmental toxicology.

Toxicology is a study concerning the nature, the adverse effects, the biochemical actions, and the detection (investigation) of all types and forms of toxicants in living systems and the ecosystem, as well as its applications to largely human health issues. Environmental toxicology is that branch of toxicology focusing on the sources and occurrence of (potential) biological, chemical, and physical contaminants in the environment, on their fate and transport in the environment, and on their adverse health effects on population dynamics of affected species. Siding with the theory by some scholars that ecotoxicology is a branch of toxicology different from environmental toxicology, in this book the affected species of greater interest and concern are humans and other mammalians, although some attention is given to other species such as plants and fishes. Regardless, the toxic effects of concern in this book are not limited to the human health kind, but include also those pertaining to other biological in origin and to the ecological in nature.

The book's main objectives, as reflected in its table of contents, are for students as well as other readership to acquire an understanding in four general areas of knowledge pertinent to environmental toxicology: (1) the basic principles for/of environmental toxicology and the major contemporary issues relevant to human and ecosystem health; (2) the occurrence, fate, and transport of major and common pollutants in the environment; (3) the basic biological processes and physiochemical mechanisms through which toxicants exert their effects in humans and other species in the environment; and (4) the concepts and applications for/of both the human health and the ecological risk assessment, including those relevant to health risk perception and communication as they concern the public's awareness pertaining to environmental contamination.

As with the earlier editions, two apologies are due here; and they both have to do with the level at which the readership is targeted. While by certain professional standards this book may not have provided a fully comprehensive index, it has strived to index all the terms, concepts, events, names, and places deemed relevant to most readership. The product of such an effort has been the result of balancing the limited resources, intended readership, and professional judgment as well as personal bias. By personal bias it means that, for instance, in Table 17.2 the mycotoxin *zearalenone* is indexed whereas *palutin* is not. This is because the book takes the position that many students would be interested in the highly estrogenic effects (e.g., infertility, abortion) induced by zearalenone specifically in swine, more so than in the genotoxic effects caused by palutin in various animal species. In any event, part of the title (content) of Table 17.2 is indexed, which lists the major groups and subgroups of mycotoxins including zearalenone and palutin.

The other apology is for the bit of redundancy occurring throughout the book. Most acronyms and certain terms or concepts introduced in a chapter have been redefined or re-decrypted in another chapter. Such redundancy is presumably necessary, as it may be difficult for many readers to sort out materials introduced a while back. Another subtle reason is that some instructors may not utilize all 23 chapters for their course or may not use them in sequence. It is under this notion that the book has opted to apply the present tense in referring to materials *already* covered in an earlier chapter, in the same vein as many news headlines in a full sentence have been so posted online.

Michael H. Dong
January 2018
envs130@gmail.com, USA

Acknowledgments

The author remains truly grateful to Dudley Burton, Ph.D., professor emeritus and former chair of the Department of Environmental Studies, California State University at Sacramento (CSUS) for offering him the great opportunity as an adjunct lecturer to teach the department's course in environmental toxicology.

Special thanks go to all the CSUS students who took the above course, which the author taught for eight years beginning in 2008. In fact, both the development of some of the lecture ideas and the mode of some of the lecture presentations owed much to many of these devoted students, from whose group presentations the author learned a great deal about environmental toxicology.

The author is indebted to many Wikipedia (mostly anonymous) and similar online authors that have so effectively provided him with quick and relevant sources for many of the specifics presented in this book (for this or earlier editions). The author would like to further acknowledge that if it had not been for some of the public domain images and clip arts that he could adopt so freely, he would not have published this *Fourth Edition* as well as this book so affordably and in such a timely and professional manner.

In particular, the two original images in Figure 7.3 (*Internal Anatomy of a Typical Leaf*) and Figure 9.1 (*General Structure of an Animal Cell*) are actually in rather impressive, brilliant colors. They were reproduced necessarily in grayscale for affordable use in this *Fourth Edition*, with kind permission from the National High Magnetic Field Laboratory (NHMFL), Florida State University, USA (*as per email confirmation from Mr. Eric Clark, Coordinator at the Administrative Services, Optical Microscopy Division, NHMFL, on 31 July 2017*).

Last but not least, had the author not been able to utilize freely the freeware version (12.01) of the ACD ChemSketch and the freeware version (4.6) of the FastStone Image Viewer, he would not have been able to provide, respectively, the chemical structures and image resolutions in this *Fourth Edition* in such an effective, affordable, and presentable manner.

Michael H. Dong

CONTENTS

PART I
TOXICOLOGIC CONCEPTS AND ENVIRONMENTAL ISSUES

CHAPTER 1. Scope and Principles for/of Environmental Toxicology   1
  1.1. Introduction   1
      1.1.1. Some Basic Toxicology Terminology   2
      1.1.2. Environmental Toxicology   3
  1.2. Basic Principles for/of Environmental Toxicology   3
      1.2.1. Knowledge on Environmental Exposure/Toxic Dose   4
      1.2.2. Knowledge on Toxic/Undesired Effects   5
      1.2.3. Knowledge on Dose-Response Relationship   5
      1.2.4. Knowledge on Toxicity Testing Methods   6
      1.2.5. Knowledge on (Health) Risk Assessment Framework   7
  1.3. Setting the Proper Perspective   7
      1.3.1. Professional Activities for (Environmental) Toxicologists   7
      1.3.2. Environmental Toxicology *vs*. Ecotoxicology   8
      1.3.3. Epidemiology as Another Very Close Ally   9
      1.3.4. Importance and Scope for/of Environmental Toxicology   10

CHAPTER 2. Environmental Changes and Environmental Health   17
  2.1. Introduction   17
      2.1.1. Knowledge on the Changing World   17
      2.1.2. Impacts of Global Environmental Changes   18
      2.1.3. World's Perspective of Environmental Health   19
  2.2. Major Specific Environmental Changes   19
      2.2.1. Global Climate Changes   19
      2.2.2. Air Pollution   20
      2.2.3. Water Pollution   20
      2.2.4. Soil Contamination   20
      2.2.5. Red Tide Pollution   21
      2.2.6. Electronic Waste Pollution   21
      2.2.7. Deforestation   22
  2.3. Incidence and Spectrum of Environmental Diseases   22

    2.3.1. Incidence and Burden of Environmental Diseases 23
    2.3.2. Spectrum and Nature of Environmental Diseases 24
2.4. Commonly Encountered Environmental Diseases 25
    2.4.1. Cancer 25
    2.4.2. Birth Defects 25
    2.4.3. Reproductive Damage 26
    2.4.4. Respiratory Diseases 26
    2.4.5. Neurological Diseases 27
    2.4.6. Skin Disorders 27
    2.4.7. Diseases Induced by Common Causes/Specific Agents 27

CHAPTER 3. Environmental Pollution and Regulatory Agencies 33
  3.1. Introduction 33
    3.1.1. Impacts of Environmental Pollution 34
    3.1.2. Perceptions of Environmental Pollution 35
  3.2. Concerns with Environmental Pollution 36
    3.2.1. Regulatory Concerns in the United States 37
    3.2.2. Actions on Environmental Pollution Impacts 38
  3.3. Environmental Health Laws and Agencies 40
    3.3.1. Regulatory Agencies in the United States 41
    3.3.2. Environmental Health Laws in the United States 42
    3.3.3. Foreign Environmental Health Laws and Agencies 44

CHAPTER 4. Occurrence and Types of Environmental Toxicants 48
  4.1. Introduction 48
    4.1.1. Contemporary Issues of Environmental Health Concern 48
    4.1.2. Grouping of Environmental Contaminants 49
  4.2. Contemporary Issues: 10 Select Cases 50
    4.2.1. Contaminants in Consumer Products 50
    4.2.2. Contaminants in Food Products 51
    4.2.3. Pollutants in the Open Environment 53
  4.3. Environmental Toxicants of Health Concern 54
    4.3.1. Group I: Individual, Specific Toxicants 55
    4.3.2. Group II: Certain Chemical/Biological Families 57
    4.3.3. Group III: Toxicants of Common/General Concern 59

CHAPTER 5. Fate and Transport of Toxicants in the Environment 66
  5.1. Introduction 66
    5.1.1. Movement in the Environmental Media 66
    5.1.2. Distribution into the Living Organisms 67
  5.2. Fate and Transport of Air Pollutants 67

5.2.1. Local and Long-Range Transport   67
5.2.2. Direct and Indirect Deposition   68
5.2.3. Changes in Chemical/Physical Form   69
5.3. Fate and Transport of Water Contaminants   71
5.3.1. Phase-Transfer and Transport Processes   73
5.3.2. Chemical (Abiotic) Transformation   75
5.3.3. Biological (Biotic) Transformation   75
5.4. Fate and Transport of Soil Contaminants   77
5.4.1. Volatilization from Soils   77
5.4.2. Degradation in Soils   78
5.4.3. Erosion and Runoff from Soils   78
5.4.4. Leaching from Soils   78

PART II
BIOACCUMULATION AND BIODISPOSITION OF TOXICANTS

CHAPTER 6. Bioaccumulation of Persistent Environmental Toxicants   82
6.1. Introduction   82
6.1.1. Relevance of Food Web/Food Chain   82
6.1.2. Relevance to Exposure Hazard Assessment   84
6.2. Bioconcentration and Estimation of Its Potential   84
6.2.1. Bioconcentration in Aquatic Media   84
6.2.2. Bioconcentration Factor (BCF)   85
6.3. Bioaccumulation and Biomagnification   86
6.3.1. Toxic Equivalency in Bioaccumulation   87
6.3.2. Cases of Bioaccumulation and Biomagnification   87
6.3.3. Bioaccumulation of Organochlorines in Seafood   90
6.4. Factors and Conditions Influencing Bioaccumulation   92
6.4.1. Lipophilicity and Bioavailability   93
6.4.2. Metabolic Potential   93
6.4.3. Environmental Mobility   93
6.4.4. A Dynamic Equilibrium Effect   95

CHAPTER 7. Uptake, Distribution, and Excretion of Toxicants   100
7.1. Introduction   100
7.1.1. Localized Effect of Non-Systemic Action   100
7.1.2. Disposition of Systemic Toxicants   100

7.2. Mechanisms of Entry by Toxicants 101
   7.2.1. Structure of Biomembranes 101
   7.2.2. Common Mechanisms of Entry 103
7.3. Uptake and Absorption of Toxicants 103
   7.3.1. Uptake by Plants 104
   7.3.2. Uptake and Absorption by Humans 106
7.4. Distribution and Excretion of Toxicants 107
   7.4.1. Distribution via the Bloodstream 109
   7.4.2. Excretion of Toxicants 109
7.5. Toxicokinetics of Toxicants 112
   7.5.1. Principles and Models/Modeling of Toxicokinetics 112
   7.5.2. Basic Mathematical Concepts 113

CHAPTER 8. Metabolism/Biotransformation of Xenobiotics 117
8.1. Introduction 117
   8.1.1. Metabolism *vs.* Biotransformation 117
   8.1.2. Biotransforming Enzymes and Their General Actions 118
8.2. General Aspects/Processes of Biotransformation 118
   8.2.1. Phase I Enzymatic Reactions 119
   8.2.2. Phase II Enzymatic Reactions 121
8.3. Other Relevant Aspects of Biotransformation 122
   8.3.1. Bioactivation of Xenobiotics 122
   8.3.2. Biotransformation of Endogenous Substances 122
8.4. Characteristics of Cytochrome P450 Enzymes 123
   8.4.1. Families of Cytochrome P450s 123
   8.4.2. Catalytic Activities and Cellular Locations 123
8.5. Characteristics of Other Relevant Enzyme Groups 124
   8.5.1. Enzymes in Phase II Reactions 124
   8.5.2. Antioxidant Enzymes 125
   8.5.3. EROD (7-Ethoxyresorufin-*O*-Deethylase) 126
8.6. Factors/Conditions Affecting Biotransformation 126
   8.6.1. Genetic Polymorphism 127
   8.6.2. Enzyme Inhibitors 128
   8.6.3. Enzyme Inducers 128
   8.6.4. Enzyme Cofactors and Coenzymes 128

CHAPTER 9. Adverse Action/Toxic Response 135
9.1. Introduction 135
   9.1.1. Site and Mechanism of Action 135
   9.1.2. Basic Mechanisms of Action and Toxicodynamics 135
9.2. Primary and Mediated Toxic Actions 136

    9.2.1. Direct Damage to Cell Structures   136
    9.2.2. Reactions Mediated by Free Radicals   137
    9.2.3. Modulation of Receptor Functions   138
    9.2.4. Binding with a Cell's Constituent   140
9.3. Adverse Secondary or Indirect Actions   141
    9.3.1. Allergic Response   141
    9.3.2. Side Effects of Medications   141
    9.3.3. Molecular Complexation   141
    9.3.4. Microbic Invasion   142
9.4. Disruption of Enzymatic Activities   143
    9.4.1. Inhibition of Cofactors or Coenzymes   143
    9.4.2. Inhibition/Inactivation of Active Site   144
9.5. Toxicodynamics of Toxicants   145
    9.5.1. Nonspecific/Exposure-Relevant Adverse Effects   146
    9.5.2. Specific/Mechanism-Based Adverse Effects   147

CHAPTER 10. Factors and Conditions Affecting Toxicity   155
10.1. Introduction   155
    10.1.1. Extrinsic Factors   155
    10.1.2. Intrinsic Cofactors   155
10.2. Environmental Factors   156
    10.2.1. Level of Environmental Exposure   156
    10.2.2. Other Exposure-Related Factors   160
    10.2.3. Nonexposure-Related Factors   161
10.3. Nutritional Factors   163
    10.3.1. Nutritional Status   163
    10.3.2. Macro- and Micro-Nutrients   163
10.4. Physicochemical Factors   166
    10.4.1. Additivity of Toxic Effects   166
    10.4.2. Synergism of Toxic Effects   166
    10.4.3. Potentiation of Toxic Effects   167
    10.4.4. Antagonism of Toxic Effects   167
10.5. Biological Cofactors   168
    10.5.1. Age, Gender, and Health Status   168
    10.5.2. Species, Strain, Race, and Genetics   169

PART III
NATURE AND EFFECTS OF ENVIRONMENTAL TOXICANTS

CHAPTER 11. Air Pollutants – I: Inorganic Gases   177
11.1. Introduction   177
11.1.1. Hazardous Air Pollutants   177
11.1.2. Criteria Inorganic Gaseous Pollutants   177
11.2. Sulfur Dioxide   178
11.2.1. Sources of Pollution   178
11.2.2. Characteristics and Properties   179
11.2.3. Toxic Effects and Advisories   180
11.3. Nitrogen Oxides: Nitrogen Dioxide   182
11.3.1. Sources of Pollution   182
11.3.2. Characteristics and Properties   183
11.3.3. Toxic Effects and Advisories   184
11.4. Tropospheric Ozone   185
11.4.1. Sources of Pollution   186
11.4.2. Characteristics and Properties   186
11.4.3. Toxic Effects and Advisories   187
11.5. Carbon Monoxide   188
11.5.1. Sources of Pollution   188
11.5.2. Characteristics and Properties   189
11.5.3. Toxic Effects and Advisories   190

CHAPTER 12. Air Pollutants – II: Particulate Matter   196
12.1. Introduction   196
12.1.1. Composition of Airborne Particulates   196
12.1.2. Basic Characteristics of Airborne Particulates   197
12.2. Sizes of Particulate Matter   197
12.2.1. Sizes of Regulatory Importance   198
12.2.2. Non-Inhalable Coarse Particles (PM_{10+})   199
12.2.3. Inhalable Coarse Particles ($PM_{2.5-10}$)   201
12.2.4. Fine Particles ($PM_{0.1-2.5}$)   201
12.2.5. Nano- and Ultrafine Particles ($PM_{0.1}$)   202
12.3. Issues on Urban Airborne Particulate Pollution   202
12.3.1. Episodes of Particulate Pollution   203
12.3.2. Monitoring of Particulate Matter   204
12.3.3. Airborne Microbes   205
12.4. Toxic Effects of Airborne Particulates   207
12.4.1. Mechanisms and General Trends   208
12.4.2. Effects on the Respiratory Tract   208
12.4.3. Effects on the Cardiovascular System   209
12.4.4. Other Serious Health Effects   210
12.4.5. Effects/Impacts on the Environment   211

CHAPTER 13. Volatile Organic Compounds   217
   13.1. Introduction   217
      13.1.1. As Precursors of Ozone and Particulate Matter   217
      13.1.2. Sources of Environmental Pollution   218
   13.2. Use Standards and Environmental Health Concerns   218
      13.2.1. Standards for Consumer/Commercial Products   218
      13.2.2. Select Compounds of Environmental Health Concern   219
   13.3. Formaldehyde   220
      13.3.1. Sources and Uses   220
      13.3.2. Exposures and Toxic Effects   222
   13.4. Benzene   223
      13.4.1. Sources and Uses   223
      13.4.2. Exposures and Toxic Effects   224
   13.5. Methyl *tert(iary)*-Butyl Ether   225
      13.5.1. Sources and Uses   225
      13.5.2. Exposures and Toxic Effects   226
   13.6. Methylene Chloride (Dichloromethane)   227
      13.6.1. Sources and Uses   227
      13.6.2. Exposures and Toxic Effects   228
   13.7. Tetrachloroethylene   229
      13.7.1. Sources and Uses   229
      13.7.2. Exposures and Toxic Effects   230
   13.8. Trichloroethylene   230
      13.8.1. Sources and Uses   230
      13.8.2. Exposures and Toxic Effects   231

CHAPTER 14. Toxic and Radioactive Metals   238
   14.1. Introduction   238
      14.1.1. Concepts of Minerals and Heavy Metals   239
      14.1.2. Metals of Environmental Health Concern   239
   14.2. The Three Heavy Metals   239
      14.2.1. Lead   240
      14.2.2. Mercury   241
      14.2.3. Cadmium   242
   14.3. Select Secondary/Pseudo Heavy Metals   244
      14.3.1. Aluminum   245
      14.3.2. Arsenic   246
      14.3.3. Beryllium   247
   14.4. Select Toxic Trace Metals   248
      14.4.1. Chromium   249
      14.4.2. Copper   250

14.4.3. Nickel   252
14.5. Select Radioactive Metals   253
14.5.1. Radium   254
14.5.2. Radon   255

CHAPTER 15. Pesticides and Pesticide Residues   261
15.1. Introduction   261
15.1.1. Health Impacts and Concerns   261
15.1.2. Pesticide Residues as Pollutants   262
15.2. Usage and Classification of Pesticides   262
15.2.1. Statistics on Pesticide Usage   262
15.2.2. Classification of Pesticides   264
15.3. Organochlorine (OC) Pesticides   264
15.3.1. Diphenylethane-Related OCs   265
15.3.2. Cyclodiene-Related OCs   266
15.3.3. Cyclohexane-Related OCs   268
15.4. Organophosphate (OP) Pesticides   269
15.4.1. Delayed Neurotoxic OP Agents   270
15.4.2. Acetylcholinesterase OP Inhibitors   270
15.5. Major Carbamate (CB) Pesticides   271
15.5.1. Carbaryl   271
15.5.2. Propoxur and Some Other CBs   272
15.6. Pyrethrin and Pyrethroid Pesticides   272
15.6.1. Pyrethrins   272
15.6.2. Pyrethroids   273
15.7. Major Phenoxy Pesticides   274
15.7.1. Dichlorophenoxyacetic Acid (2,4-D)   275
15.7.2. Trichlorophenoxyacetic Acid (2,4,5-T)   276
15.8. Major Triazine Pesticides   276
15.8.1. Atrazine   276
15.8.2. Simazine and Propazine   277
15.9. Coumarin and Indandione Pesticides   278
15.9.1. Coumarins   278
15.9.2. Indandiones   278
15.10. Select Novel/Specialty Pesticides   279
15.10.1. Neonicotinoids   279
15.10.2. Glyphosate, Paraquat, and Compound 1080   280

CHAPTER 16. Persistent Toxic Substances   287
16.1. Introduction   287
16.1.1. Chemical *vs.* Environmental Persistence   287

16.1.2. Numerical Persistence Criteria   288
16.1.3. Relevance to Long-Range Transport   289
16.2. The Stockholm Convention of 2001   289
16.2.1. Persistent Pollutants of Global Concerns   290
16.2.2. Stockholm Convention's Aims and Actions   291
16.3. Perfluorooctane Sulfonates/Sulfonyl Fluoride   292
16.3.1. Characteristics, Uses, and Pollution Sources   292
16.3.2. Environmental Health Concerns   294
16.4. Polybrominated Biphenyls   295
16.4.1. Characteristics, Uses, and Pollution Sources   295
16.4.2. Environmental Health Concerns   297
16.5. Polybrominated Diphenyl Ethers   298
16.5.1. Characteristics, Uses, and Pollution Sources   298
16.5.2. Environmental Health Concerns   299
16.6. Polybrominated Cyclododecanes   300
16.6.1. Characteristics, Uses, and Pollution Sources   300
16.6.2. Environmental Health Concerns   301
16.7. Polychlorinated Biphenyls   301
16.7.1. Characteristics, Uses, and Pollution Sources   301
16.7.2. Environmental Health Concerns   302
16.8. Polychlorinated Naphthalenes   303
16.8.1. Characteristics, Uses, and Pollution Sources   304
16.8.2. Environmental Health Concerns   304
16.9. Polychlorinated Butadienes   305
16.9.1. Characteristics, Uses, and Pollution Sources   305
16.9.2. Environmental Health Concerns   306
16.10. Polychlorinated Dioxins/Furans   306
16.10.1. Characteristics, Uses, and Pollution Sources   307
16.10.2. Environmental Health Concerns   307
16.11. Toxic Equivalency Factors   308
16.11.1. WHO's Concept of Toxic Equivalency   308
16.11.2. Application of Toxic Equivalency Factor   310

CHAPTER 17. Biological and Underrated Physical Toxic Agents   318
17.1. Introduction   318
17.1.1. Concepts of Biological Toxic Agents   318
17.1.2. Infection *vs*. Infectious Disease   319
17.2. Pathogenic Microbial Agents   319
17.2.1. Pathogenic Bacteria   320
17.2.2. Pathogenic Viruses   321
17.2.3. Pathogenic Fungi   322

17.2.4. Pathogenic Parasites 323
17.3. Toxins from Microorganisms 324
17.3.1. Toxins from Bacteria 324
17.3.2. Toxins from Fungi 325
17.4. Toxins from Fishes and Plants 329
17.4.1. Toxins from Fishes 329
17.4.2. Toxins from Plants 330
17.5. Venoms from Arthropods 331
17.5.1. Venoms from Arachnids 332
17.5.2. Venoms from Insects 333
17.6. Venoms from Reptiles and Amphibians 334
17.6.1. Venoms from Snakes 334
17.6.2. Venoms from Lizards 335
17.6.3. Venoms from Amphibians 335
17.7. Underrated Harmful Physical Agents/Hazards 336
17.7.1. Traffic Congestion 336
17.7.2. Noise Pollution 337

PART IV
SPECIAL TOPICS, ISSUES, CONSIDERATIONS, AND FOCI

CHAPTER 18. Environmental Mutagenesis/Carcinogenesis 342
18.1. Introduction 342
18.1.1. DNA, RNA, Gene, and Chromosome 342
18.1.2. Characteristics of Tumor and Cancer 344
18.2. Environmental Mutagenesis 345
18.2.1. Concepts of Mutagenesis 345
18.2.2. Point Mutation and Intragenic Mutation 346
18.2.3. Chromosome Aberration 346
18.2.4. Environmental Mutagens 347
18.3. Environmental Carcinogenesis 349
18.3.1. Concepts of Carcinogenesis 350
18.3.2. Mechanism of Carcinogenesis 351
18.3.3. Environmental Carcinogens 353
18.4. DNA Damage and Repair 354
18.4.1. Causes of DNA Damage 356
18.4.2. Mechanisms of DNA Repair 357

CHAPTER 19. Reproductive Toxicity and Endocrine Disruption   362
   19.1. Introduction   362
        19.1.1. Impacts and Causes of Human Birth Defects   363
        19.1.2. Concerns with Human Reproductive Disorders   363
        19.1.3. Concepts of Endocrine Disruption in Humans   364
   19.2. The Endocrine-Reproductive System   365
        19.2.1. The Human Developmental-Reproductive Cycle   365
        19.2.2. The Human Endocrine System   366
        19.2.3. Hormones (The Chemical Messengers)   370
   19.3. Endocrine/Hormonal Disruption   372
        19.3.1. Modes and Mechanisms of Endocrine Disruption   372
        19.3.2. Types of Endocrine Disruptors   373
   19.4. Developmental-Reproductive Effects in Humans   374
        19.4.1. Birth Defects and Environmental Teratogens   374
        19.4.2. Reproductive Effects and Environmental Toxicants   377

CHAPTER 20. Occupational Toxicology/Workplace Hazards   384
   20.1. Introduction   384
        20.1.1. Classic Industrial/Occupational Diseases   384
        20.1.2. Uniqueness of Occupational Toxicology   385
        20.1.3. Occupational Health and Safety Laws   385
   20.2. U.S. Legislation/Agencies for Occupational Health   386
        20.2.1. U.S. Occupational Safety and Health Act   386
        20.2.2. U.S. Occupational Safety and Health Administration   387
        20.2.3. U.S. National Institute for Occupational Safety and Health   388
   20.3. Relevant Concepts for Occupational Toxicology   390
        20.3.1. Exposure Limit Values   390
        20.3.2. Biological Exposure Index Values   391
   20.4. Occupational Toxic Agents/Workplace Hazards   392
        20.4.1. Pesticides   392
        20.4.2. Metals   394
        20.4.3. Organic Solvents   395
        20.4.4. Fibers/Dusts   396
        20.4.5. Other Groups/Kinds of Workplace Hazards   398

CHAPTER 21. Food Toxicants and Toxic Household Substances   404
   21.1. Introduction   404
        21.1.1. Concerns with Food Toxicants   404
        21.1.2. Concerns with Toxic Household Substances   405
   21.2. Toxic Substances in Food Products   405
        21.2.1. Direct Food Additives   406

21.2.2. Indirect Food Additives   410
21.2.3. Food Contaminants   412
21.3. Toxic Substances in Household Products   413
21.3.1. Substances in Personal Care Products   414
21.3.2. Substances in Cleaning Agents   416
21.3.3. Substances in Over-the-Counter Medicines   417
21.3.4. Other Major Relevant Organic Substances   419
21.4. Didactic Cases with Food and Household Products   419
21.4.1. Persistent Toxic Substances in Seafood   420
21.4.2. Lead on Children's Toy Jewelry   420
21.4.3. Triclosan in Antibacterial Products   421
21.4.4. Self-Mitigation and Self-Prevention   422

CHAPTER 22. Human Health Aspects of Ecotoxicology   428
22.1. Introduction   428
22.1.1. Relevance of Aquatic Toxicology   428
22.1.2. Relevance of Wildlife Toxicology   429
22.1.3. Relevance of Hazardous Waste Toxicology   429
22.2. Aquatic Toxicology and Human Health   430
22.2.1. The Basic Aquatic Environment   430
22.2.2. Aquatic Toxicity Tests   431
22.2.3. Regulatory Efforts for Water Quality   433
22.3. Wildlife Toxicology and Human Health   433
22.3.1. Scope and History of Wildlife Toxicology   434
22.3.2. The Basic Wildlife Terrestrial Environment   435
22.3.3. Ecological Risk Assessment   437
22.4. Hazardous Wastes of U.S. and Global Concerns   440
22.4.1. The RCRA Definition and Implications   441
22.4.2. The Superfund Law and Program   442
22.4.3. The United Heckathorn Toxic Site (A Case Study)   443

CHAPTER 23. Environmental Health Risk Assessment   451
23.1. Introduction   451
23.1.1. Health Risk Assessment Activities   451
23.1.2. Subtle Aspects of Health Risk Assessment   453
23.2. Toxicity Assessment   454
23.2.1. Hazard (Endpoint) Identification   455
23.2.2. Animal Toxicity Studies and Test Guidelines   455
23.2.3. Dose-Response Assessment   456
23.3. Human Exposure Assessment   458
23.3.1. Past and Current Perspectives   459

    23.3.2. Direct and Indirect Measurements   460
    23.3.3. Aggregate and Cumulative Exposures   462
23.4. Environmental Health Risk Characterization   463
    23.4.1. Health Risk Measures   464
    23.4.2. Uncertainty and Safety Factors   465
    23.4.3. Health Risk Perception   468
    23.4.4. Health Risk Communication   469

INDEX   476

An Introduction to Environmental Toxicology

Fourth Edition

CHAPTER 1

Scope and Principles for/of Environmental Toxicology

1.1. Introduction

The scope and principles for/of environmental toxicology should begin with the definition of general toxicology, which in its simplest term is *the science of poisons*. The more descriptive definition of general toxicology is that it is *the science studying the nature, the adverse effects, the biochemical actions, and the detection (investigation) of all types and all forms of poisons in living systems and the ecosystem, with a focus being more on human health issues.* Much like medicine, toxicology of all branches is both a science and an art.

The historical development of toxicology dates back to the cave dwellers era, when prehistoric people utilized poisonous plants, animal venoms, and their extracts for execution, hunting, and warfare. By 1500 BC, when the metal mercury was discovered in an Egyptian tomb, medical documents such as the Egyptian *Papyrus Ebers* already revealed that hemlock (a herbal extract used to execute Socrates), certain aconitum species (often used as a Chinese arrow poison), and certain metallic elements (lead, arsenic) were among the highly effective poisons used to kill foes. There were also documentations that the Roman emperor Claudius was poisoned with mushrooms, and that the Egyptian queen Cleopatra VII might have died of a venomous snakebite.

By the late Middle Ages (i.e., around the 14th or 15th century), poisons became widely applied in humankind with greater sophistication. During that period, certain concepts fundamental to toxicology also emerged. Noteworthy about that movement were the contribution of Philippus von Hohenheim, otherwise more commonly known as Paracelsus (circa 1500 AD), and later that of Mathieu Joseph Bonaventure Orfila (circa 1800 AD).

Paracelsus, a German-Swiss physician-alchemist known also as the father of *classic* toxicology, was the first scientist to focus on specific substances as *agents* responsible for the toxicity of a plant or an animal poison. He advanced the notion that the body's response to specific toxic agents depends on the dose received. That notion is now known as the dose-response relationship, one of the basic principles for/of toxicology. Paracelsus is frequently quoted for his famous assertion that *"All substances are poisons; there is none which (that) is not a poison. The right dose differentiates a poison and a remedy."*

Mathieu Orfila, a Spanish-born physician working in a French court, is generally regarded as the father of *modern* toxicology and the founder of clinical or forensic pathology. He was the first forensic toxicologist to apply autopsy materials and chemical analysis systematically as legal proof of poisoning, by way of demonstrating the *adverse effects* of poisons on *specific body tissues* and *organs*.

Modern toxicology is the outgrowth of advances in many related scientific disciplines, including (analytical) chemistry, biochemistry, biology, ecology, epidemiology, medicine, molecular biology, nutritional science, pharmacology, physiology, public health, and more. Since World War II, the production of synthetic fibers, drugs, pesticides, and industrial substances has increased markedly. So has people's knowledge on biochemical materials that sustain biological functions, including especially the hereditary material of life known biochemically as *deoxyribonucleic acid* (which today is commonly known by its acronym DNA). These developments have revolutionized toxicology (and many other life sciences as well) exponentially. Further discussion in this area can be found in numerous places in the literature including Gallo (2001), Lane and Borzelleca (2008), and the U.S. National Institutes of Health (NIH, 2008).

1.1.1. Some Basic Toxicology Terminology

Toxicology is an ever-evolving discipline, and so are the terms it uses in the scientific literature. The terms that it uses for materials causing harmful effects are not always consistent. The most common terms used for these harmful materials include *toxicants, poisons, toxic substances, toxic chemicals, toxic agents, contaminants*, and *pollutants*. Although these terms are used interchangeably in some literature, by definition they differ from one another somewhat. The following are these terms defined largely in accordance with the two dictionaries of toxicology published in the 1990s (i.e., Hodgson *et al.*, 1998; Lewis, 1998).

Toxicants are natural or synthetic materials capable of causing adverse effects on or to living organisms. *Poisons* are toxicants that tend to cause *acute* death or *severe* illness even when exposed to in *trace* amounts. A *toxic substance* is simply any material having toxic properties, short of appreciating its ability to induce adverse effects. Note that gasoline should be referred to more appropriately as a toxic substance in that it contains a mixture of many chemicals, whereas something like cyanide is a discrete *toxic chemical*. Simply put, a *toxic agent*, like a toxic substance, refers to a toxicant using two words instead of one. Yet more importantly, in all cases a toxicant, a toxic substance, or a toxic agent can be *chemical* (e.g., mercury), *physical* (e.g., noise), or *biological* (e.g., snake venom) in nature.

As a legal term (e.g., U.S. Code, 2017), *toxins* are toxicants *produced* by *living cells* or *organisms*, and are capable of causing disease when present in the body tissue of a host organism. Most of them are protein-like materials. For example, botulinum toxin is a neurotoxin (i.e., that acting on the nerve cells) protein produced by the bacterium *Clostridium botulinum* and is perhaps the most potent biological substance known. Note that in toxicology, potency is defined as the ability or capacity to bring about the same toxic effect. By most potent, it means achieving the same lethal (or most severe) effect from the smallest amount of dose. Today, due to modern society's higher expectation for better life, the concern with a toxic substance's potency is no longer in terms of lethal dose or concentration at the 50th percentile (i.e., LD_{50} or LC_{50}, respectively, or more specifically the level required to kill half of the test population). Instead, today's concerns with non-cancer effect or toxicity dose are down to the no observed effect level (NOEL), the no observed *adverse* effect level (NO*A*EL), or NO[A]EL for short. These lower effect levels and other related risk measures, including those for cancer risk, are (further) discussed in Chapter 23.

Xenobiotic is the general term used for a *foreign* substance, usually a chemical, that is found in the body or has been taken into the body. The term is derived from the Greek word *xeno*, which means "foreigner". Xenobiotics may produce beneficial effects (e.g., pharmaceuticals) or may be toxic (e.g., arsenic, lead). They can be natural or synthetic materials, but must be *exogenous* in origin. A *contaminant* or *pollutant* is an undesired xenobiotic or agent (initially) present in a medium that contains a principal component, such as the case of a toxic chemical being the pollutant in the medium air, water, soils, or consumer products like foods.

1.1.2. Environmental Toxicology

As generally accepted (e.g., Hodgson *et al.*, 1998; Lewis, 1998), *environmental toxicology* is that branch of toxicology focusing on three main aspects: (1) the sources of (potential) toxicants in the environment; (2) their fate and transport under various environmental conditions and through food chains; and (3) their adverse effects on population dynamics of affected species. As such, and from a practical perspective, even a brief discussion on the scope and importance for/of environmental toxicology should start with those for/of general toxicology.

Environmental toxicology is best described as an interdisciplinary science currently still at its adolescence. This branch of toxicology is an interdisciplinary science that continues to have a somewhat disputed core of knowledge for some time (and thus the urge for publication of books similar to the present one). As Wright and Welbourn (2002) put it, "*There is still some controversy concerning the stage in a curriculum at which it should be introduced.*"

Siding with the theory advocated by a number of scholars (*see*, e.g., EHA, 2012; WHO, 1986; Wright and Welbourn, 2002) that ecological toxicology (or ecotoxicology for short) is a branch of toxicology different from environmental toxicology, in this book the affected species of greater concern are humans and other mammalians although some attention is given to other species such as plants and fishes. The toxic effects of concern in this book are not limited to the human health kind, but also include those pertaining to other biological in origin or to the ecological in nature. Despite the fact that to some scholars (e.g., WHO, 1986) ecotoxicology is perhaps the closest ally of environmental toxicology, they are indeed two separate branches of toxicology. The distinction between the two branches is discussed in Section (Subsection) 1.3.2 that follows shortly.

1.2. Basic Principles for/of Environmental Toxicology

The basic principles as well as knowledge for/of environmental toxicology are integral to the process what is now known as *health risk assessment/characterization*, where quantitative estimates are determined for the health risk associated with the *environmental* exposure at issue. As reflected in Figure 1.1 below, these principles involve (but are not limited to) the concepts, fundamentals, and understandings of five major subject matters: (1) *toxic dose/environmental exposure*; (2) *toxic/undesired effects*; (3) *dose-response relationship*; (4) *availability of toxicity testing methods*; and (5) *framework of health risk assessment*. Further discussion on these subject matters can be found in EHA (2012), Eaton and Klaassen (2001), NIH (2008), U.S. National Research Council (NRC, 1984, 1994), and the final chapter (Chapter 23) in this book.

4 An Introduction to Environmental Toxicology

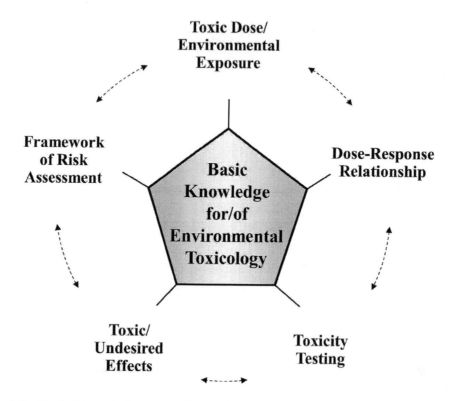

Figure 1.1. Basic Knowledge as well as Principles for/of Environmental Toxicology

1.2.1. Knowledge on Environmental Exposure/Toxic Dose

By definition, *toxic dose* is the amount of a toxicant applied to, or taken by, an organism during a specific time interval. *Exposure*, on the other hand, is the amount that the organism comes in contact with. There are, however, several variables that need to be considered in order to fully characterize the dosing with or exposure to a toxicant. Toxicologically, the most critical variables are the magnitude, the frequency, and the duration of exposure or dosing. Toxic dose can be referred to by its type or form, such as *exposure* or *applied* dose, *absorbed* dose, and (total) *internal* dose. *Dosage* is a dose expressed as some function of the organism and time (e.g., mg of the toxicant per kg of body weight per day).

Dosage is a useful or more practical term in that the clinical and toxic effects of a dose are usually related to age and body size. This explains why there are adult Tylenol® (e.g., 350 mg each) *vs.* children Tylenol® (e.g., 80 mg each) tablets sold over the counter. Another important aspect is the *time* and *duration* over which a dose is given. This is particularly crucial for distinguishing doses that are sufficient to induce a short-term *vs.* a long-term (chronic) effect. For human exposure, the time unit commonly used is 24 hours and hence the usual dosage unit is *the amount* (e.g., mg) *per kg of body weight per day*.

The units for *environmental* exposure are typically expressed as the amount of a *pollutant* (toxicant) in a unit of an environmental medium or component. Examples of this type are mg/L (milligram/liter) for pollutants in liquid or water, mg/g (mg/gram) for pollutants in solid or soil, and mg/m^3 (mg/cubic meter) for pollutants in the atmosphere. Smaller units are frequently encountered when expressing these environmental levels, such as µg/ml, µg/g, or ppm (i.e., *p*arts of the substance *p*er *m*illion parts of the medium's principal component such as air, water, soils, or foods). Likewise, ppb (parts per billion) ≡ µg/L or µg/kg (microgram/kilogram).

1.2.2. Knowledge on Toxic/Undesired Effects

Toxicity is the degree or extent to which an agent can cause an adverse or undesired effect when an organism is exposed to it. The term can also be used as *such an adverse effect* on or to the organism's entire body or its substructures. In relation to *exposure* assessment, (human) adverse effects can be classified as follows: allergic reactions; idiosyncratic reactions (i.e., those highly peculiar to certain individuals); delayed *vs.* immediate toxicity; reversible *vs.* irreversible effects; and localized *vs.* systemic effects (as further discussed in Chapter 9).

Toxic effects are often influenced by the following factors: dosage; age; time and duration of dosing; route of exposure; species; gender; ability to be absorbed (into the host organism's body); nutrition; metabolism; disposition in the body; ability to be excreted (from the host organism's body); presence of other chemicals; and more. The biochemical mechanism in which an (adverse) effect is induced is complicated with many of these influencing factors, of which dosage is the most important or most relevant under normal circumstances (Chapter 10).

Some xenobiotics are themselves toxic. Others must be chemically biotransformed, metabolized, or otherwise broken down within the body before they can induce deleterious effects in a living organism (Chapter 8). Many toxicants available in the body of an organism affect only specific target organs. Others, however, can damage any of the organism's cells, tissues, or organs that they come in contact with. The target cells or organs to be affected by these toxicants may vary depending on the dosage and route of exposure involved. For example, the site of toxic attack may be the *c*entral *n*ervous *s*ystem (CNS) for a toxicant after acute exposure at high levels. Yet the site may well be limited to the liver, the lungs, or the kidneys following chronic exposure to the same toxicant at lower doses or concentrations.

1.2.3. Knowledge on Dose-Response Relationship

Dose-response is defined as the quantitative (or at times, qualitative) relationship *between* the amount of a toxicant taken in or exposed to *and* the incidence or the extent of the toxic response (or of the toxic effect) induced. This relationship, when well founded, can strengthen the hypothesis that the toxicant is responsible for causing the observed effect(s). It will also provide an estimate for the lowest dose that can induce the effect, which is the so-called threshold level or the lowest observed [adverse] effect level (LO[A]EL). By means of its slope, its curve, or the kind, it can also determine the dosage required to reach a certain level of toxic damage (or therapeutic effect). This type of quantitative inference has its limitations in that in most environmental settings, humans and other living organisms are exposed to multiple toxicants, rather than to a particular one for which the relationship is (to be) established.

Toxicants administered or taken in simultaneously may exert their adverse actions independently. Yet in many instances, the presence of one toxicant may drastically affect the host organism's response to another toxicant. The toxicity of a combination of toxicants may be less or more than that predicted from the known effect of each individual toxicant involved. The effect or influence that one toxicant has on the toxicity of another is known as a (bio- or physico-)chemical *interaction* which can fall into one of the following joint effect patterns: *additivity* (additive effect); *antagonism* (reducing or inhibiting the target effect); *potentiation* (enhancing or promoting the effect which otherwise would not have occurred); and *synergism* (resulting in greater than additive effect). Further discussion on these effect patterns is given in Chapter 10.

1.2.4. Knowledge on Toxicity Testing Methods

The investigation into chemical toxicity in general or into chemical interaction in particular is not without difficulty or limitations. Animal studies are rarely conducted to evaluate the toxicity of a target substance in a mixture, or to predict the combined effect of multiple toxicants in a mixture. One reason for not doing so as a common practice is that the toxic effect of the target toxicant could be easily confounded by those of the nontarget substances in the mixture. Another reason is logistic, as many more test animals and dosings would otherwise be required to sort out the various possible combined effect outcomes. Accordingly, the toxicity of a substance is frequently investigated by exposing test animals to the toxicant of concern only, despite the reality that most humans and most other living organisms are exposed to multiple environmental pollutants at or around the same time.

Amidst the limitations noted above, knowledge on toxicity continues to be derived mostly from studies under three categories: (1) epidemiological studies, including routine or clinical observations of people during their normal use of a substance or via accidental exposure; (2) controllable animal studies (i.e., *in vivo*); and (3) even more controllable test tube type assays (i.e., *in vitro*) at the molecular or cellular level using human, animal, or plant tissues. Of the three categories, nowadays the last two are increasingly used for toxicity testing before most any new synthetic product is allowed to be put on the market (*see*, e.g., Section 23.2.2. and Table 23.1). This is especially the case for products such as food additives, pharmaceuticals, pesticides, medical devices, and industrial chemicals made since World War II.

The regulatory requirements of subjecting synthetic products to toxicity testing are crucial in terms of (public) health protection. In the past, a number of notable health tragedies had occurred, mostly in the United States, that were due to the populace's exposure to inadequately tested drugs and other substances. Examples of such health tragedies include: the treatment of syphilis with arsenic in pregnant women until World War II, resulting in severe toxicity; the use of ethylene glycol as the first antibiotic for treatment of Streptococcal infections, leading to over 100 American deaths in 15 states; and the use of thalidomide as an anti-nausea medicine, resulting in thousands of children born with severe birth defects worldwide. It was largely due to these health tragedies that in the United States, the following federal regulatory agencies were established or strengthened to (re-)assure the nation's public health and safety: U.S. Food and Drug Administration (FDA: e.g., for pharmaceuticals, foods, cosmetics, medical devices, vaccines); U.S. Environmental Protection Agency (U.S. EPA: e.g., for agricultural and industrial substances released into the environment); U.S. Consumer Product Safety Commission (CPSC: e.g., for hazardous substances in consumer products, particularly those used in homes); and U.S. Occupational Safety and Health

Administration (OSHA: e.g., for exposure to chemical substances and other toxic agents in workplaces). Further discussion on these agencies is given in Chapter 3.

1.2.5. Knowledge on (Health) Risk Assessment Framework

The analysis of environmental exposure and the evaluation of toxicity test results are all part of the so-called human health or ecological risk assessment activities. In the early years, the risk assessment activities performed by the various federal agencies in the United States were not always consistent or easy to follow. To help resolve these issues, the U.S. National Research Council (NRC, 1983) in the early 1980s published standard terminology for health risk assessment and set forth the basic framework for the process involved. There are essentially four key analytical steps or components in NRC's initial risk assessment paradigm: *hazard identification, dose-response assessment, human exposure assessment*, and *risk characterization* (Chapter 23).

The (by-)products of regulatory risk assessments are generally exposure standards, guidelines, advisories that are set forth by government agencies to protect the public from harmful substances or activities that can cause serious health problems. These exposure standards, guidelines, and advisories provide certain (perceived) acceptable exposure levels for various media (e.g., air, water, soils, foods, medicines, household products) that people come in contact with. In other cases, these standards, guidelines, and advisories may be treated as preventive measures to reduce the exposures of concern (e.g., those measures pertaining to product labeling, personal protective equipment, and medical monitoring or surveillance). Exposure standards differ from exposure guidelines or advisories in that the former tend to be legally acceptable exposure limits or controls, whereas the latter two are recommended or suggested maximum levels.

1.3. Setting the Proper Perspective

In what follows, brief accounts are given on four topics deemed especially relevant in setting a proper perspective for appreciating the role of toxicology in general, and of environmental toxicology in particular. These topics are: (1) professional activities for (environmental) toxicologists; (2) environmental toxicology *vs.* ecotoxicology; (3) epidemiology as another very close ally; and (4) importance and scope of environmental toxicology. There are certainly more topics of this kind than the four discussed below. However, it is this book's position that these other topics are either considered less relevant, or discussed more frequently in other forums (including in other chapters of this book).

1.3.1. Professional Activities for (Environmental) Toxicologists

There are three principal categories of professional activities for (environmental) toxicologists, each of which interacts with or affects the other two (e.g., Eaton and Klaassen, 2001). These three activity categories (in nature) are *descriptive, mechanistic*, and *regulatory*. Although the activities in these three categories have their own distinct characteristics, they each contribute to those in the other two categories. Mechanistic toxicologists have their focus on identifying and understanding the biochemical mechanisms by which chemical, physical, or biological agents exert their adverse effects on living organisms. Descriptive toxicologists are largely analytical, clinical, or forensic scientists whose areas of concern include toxicity testing that provides the needed information for safety evaluation and regulatory requirements. Their work may also provide significant clues to an agent's mechanism of toxicological action. A regulatory toxicologist's main responsibility is to determine, through utilization of the data and information provided by descriptive and mechanistic toxicologists, whether the (environmental) exposure level is sufficiently safe or whether a product poses an acceptable low risk to be used for its intended purpose. It is due to such a regulatory responsibility, or in this sense, that knowledge on the risk assessment framework is almost always a prerequisite for the practice of environmental toxicology.

In practice, toxicologists in each of the three categories may involve themselves in one or more of the numerous toxicology branches whose foci, interests, concerns, and functions are forever evolving and constantly shifting. The more prominent specialties of toxicology include environmental toxicology, occupational toxicology, analytical toxicology, pesticide toxicology, clinical toxicology, molecular and biochemical toxicology, regulatory toxicology, nutritional toxicology, radiation toxicology, epidemiologic toxicology, veterinary toxicology, ecotoxicology, inhalation toxicology, developmental toxicology, immunotoxicology, cardiotoxicology, forensic toxicology, genetic toxicology, and neurotoxicology.

1.3.2. Environmental Toxicology *vs.* Ecotoxicology

Much like ecology *vs.* environmental sciences, to date a small number of scholars still do not care about or appreciate the distinction between ecotoxicology and environmental toxicology despite the fact that many others do. According to Truhaut (1977), ecotoxicology is defined as *"The branch of toxicology concerned with the study of toxic effects, caused by natural or synthetic pollutants, to the constituents of ecosystems, animal (including human), vegetable and microbial, in an integral context."*

Ecotoxicology is allegedly to have its focus on the *integration* of toxicology and ecology or, as Chapman (2002) has suggested it, on *"ecology in the presence of toxicants"*. That branch of toxicology aims to understand, assess, and thereby reduce the adverse effects on natural populations, communities, or ecosystems, whether the stressors (e.g., toxic agents) are natural or anthropogenic in origin. It differs from environmental toxicology in that it attempts to integrate the effects of stressors across *all* levels of a biological organization from the molecular to whole communities and ecosystems, whereas environmental toxicology has a stronger concern with the toxic effects on *individuals* living in a community (Maltby and Naylor, 1990), at least much more so than on the ecosystem.

The publication of Rachel Carson's seminal volume *Silent Spring* (Carlson, 1962) unquestionably catalyzed the separation of environmental toxicology, and later of ecotoxicology, from classical (general) toxicology. The key revolutionary element in Carson's contribution was her extrapolation from adverse effects on single organisms to those at the whole ecosystem and the "balance of nature" (Bazerman *et al.*, 2005). Such a systematic study is distinct from the anthropocentric nature of classical toxicology. On the whole, environmental toxicology is a multidisciplinary science incorporating (likewise) many aspects of (analytical) chemistry, biochemistry, environmental health, epidemiology, molecular biology, physiology, toxicology, and a wealth of other related disciplines to study the (potential) adverse effects of xenobiotics in a community or population. The ultimate goal or objective of this approach is to be able to *anticipate* the effects of environmental contamination so that, should such an incident occur, the most efficient or efficacious action to remediate the detrimental effects can be identified and implemented. As with ecotoxicology, there is a strong (or even a stronger) link between the legislative process on environmental pollution and the practice as well as the development of environmental toxicology.

1.3.3. Epidemiology as Another Very Close Ally

Epidemiology is the branch of medical or public health science concerned with the occurrence, transmission, and control of epidemic diseases in human populations. It also studies the factors that modify, or that are suspected to be capable of modifying, the distribution of a disease. The main purpose of studying disease distribution in a population is for one or both of the following reasons: (1) to determine if there is a health crisis or risk with the disease; and (2) to use the disease distribution observed under some specific conditions as a measure of the association's strength between the disease and a suspected agent, hazard, factor, or condition. Epidemiology students are thereby trained to measure incidence, prevalence, and their interrelation (e.g., Gordis, 1996; Lilienfeld and Stolley, 1994; Rothman and Sander, 1998; Szklo and Nieto, 2000).

Incidence and *prevalence* involve the number of *new* and *existing* cases, respectively, at a specific time point or during a time interval. These rates and other measures of morbidity and mortality are the principal features of descriptive epidemiology, through which an important attempt is to characterize the amount and distribution of disease within a population. Epidemiologists are also given training in analytical methods, in which several study designs are available as practical methodologies to measure associations between exposures and effects. These epidemiological study designs include cohort follow-up, clinical trial, case-control study, cross-sectional study, quasi-experimental analysis, and ecological study. Studies of these types all have human subjects or patients as the observational units (e.g., Gordis, 1996; Lilienfeld and Stolley, 1994; Rothman and Sander, 1998; Szklo and Nieto, 2000).

The selection of hazards or factors for epidemiologic investigation is rarely a random act. It is largely based on some physical or biological, but more typically, chemical and toxicological data as well as understanding. Although the assessment of this type of associations tends to be statistical in nature, the formulation of any of these associations is often based on some biological or toxicological speculation. For example, it might have been that by chance chimney sweeps were seen in the 1770s to associate with higher incidence of cancer of the scrotum. Yet it was largely due to the acceptance of the underlying biological process that more epidemiological studies were conducted to heighten this link.

Naturally, the most convincing evidence for supporting a causal relationship in humans is a well-conducted epidemiological study in which a strong link between exposure and disease in human subjects has been observed, since human data will offer the most direct evidence. Yet well-conducted epidemiological studies are hard to come by, as it is unethical to deliberately subject humans to doses sufficient to cause them bodily harm. For somewhat different objectives, human exposure assessment is covered more fully and more frequently in epidemiology than in toxicology textbooks. Despite this coverage preference, there are several reasons why some epidemiologists, like many toxicologists, do (or did) not find human exposure assessment appealing. These reasons are discussed in Chapter 23 on environmental health risk assessment.

Today's epidemiology is found to play, nevertheless, a greater role in health risk assessment than in early years. Recent advances in epidemiology that are pertinent to health risk assessment include several specialty areas into which general epidemiology at both the basic and the intermediate level have branched out. Coincidentally or not, these specialty areas parallel closely to those of toxicology, such as environmental epidemiology, occupational epidemiology, molecular epidemiology, cardiovascular epidemiology, nutritional epidemiology, reproductive epidemiology, cancer epidemiology, immunoepidemiology, pharmacoepidemiology, neuroepidemiology, and genetic epidemiology. The particular types of diseases that these individual specialties focus on also parallel closely to the various types of adverse effects that health risk assessors attempt to determine during the hazard identification phase. This phase is a key and usually the first component of the human health risk assessment process (Chapter 23).

In particular, environmental epidemiology and occupational epidemiology are the two major branches oriented towards the study of causative exposures, rather than of disease outcomes. Occupational epidemiology is closely related to environmental epidemiology in that many of the environmental contaminants of concern are products or by-products primarily or initially present in a work setting. Accordingly, certain occupational groups are frequently subject to the same or similar types of contaminant insults as the general public are, even though the levels of exposure that each group encounters are likely different. Workers and users will receive the exposure during manufacturing or handling of the products. In contrast, the general public will be exposed to the contaminants that have been emitted (from these products or by-products), spread, or precipitated into the local or global environment.

The exposures to environmental and occupational health hazards are the domain of human health-based risk assessment because they are not only of high concern to the general public or workers, but are also deemed highly preventable via regulatory intervention. It is under this premise that over the years, many countries have enacted numerous health statutes to regulate the exposures to environmental health hazards. In the United States, health statutes in this category are summarized in Chapter 3 (Table 3.2), in part to highlight the legislative side of environmental toxicology. Also note that of all the branches of epidemiology, occupational epidemiology tends to use biomarkers the most for monitoring human exposures. This is because occupational groups are relatively easier to be identified, worked with, and followed up.

1.3.4. Importance and Scope for/of Environmental Toxicology

The significance of treating environmental toxicology as a distinct branch of toxicology is brought out in Sections 1.1.2 and 1.3.2 regarding its distinction from general toxicology and ecotoxicology (respectively). Yet both (sub)sections fall short of spelling out the (subtle) reasons why environmental toxicology is an important study subject on its own. Actually, there are three interrelated aspects pointing to or supporting the importance of environmental toxicology. One aspect and perhaps the most crucial is that, as discussed further in Chapter 2, both the incidence and the spectrum of *environmental* diseases have been expanding markedly, particularly in the industrialized countries since World War II. Coincidentally or not, at about the same time, the use and the production of synthetic materials have increased at a similar pace. Another related aspect is the enormous economic burden incurred from the widespread of environmental diseases that has been taking a substantial toll on human health (and the ecosystem). The third closely related aspect is that, owing to such a huge economic burden, many governments begin to have insufficient resources to improve their people's quality of life, as they can no longer do more with other public health or welfare programs.

The global concerns with these aspects are well reflected in the way in which the World Health Organization (WHO, 2003) looked at environmental health for children in the first year of the World Health Day. As WHO put it well, a child's world centers around the home, the school, and the local community. Yet in real life, these places are often so unhealthy that, especially in the developing and underdeveloped regions, they underlie the majority of deaths as well as a huge burden of diseases among children. WHO went further to condemn and project that over five million children under 15 years of age would die every year from diseases linked to the environments in which they live, learn, and play.

Environmental toxicology is more than about the effects of chemical pollution. Its medical or scientific term covers not only the toxicity and toxicology of environmental pollutants in the air, dust, soil, sediment, water, foods, and other media, but also those of natural toxins in the environment. This definition reasserts the notion that the environmental toxicants of concern are not limited to chemical, but include biological and physical agents (Chapter 17).

The reality is that, in the recent two decades or so between 1997 and 2017, there were at least six environmental pollution episodes reaching global concerns. Five of these concerns involved biological agents as the contaminants, whereas the sixth had to do with persistent toxic chemical substances which are typically treated as a group and thus as a single entity (Chapter 16). The five biological agents of global concern in the recent past were: a mis-folded prion protein; a coronavirus which has a halo or crown-like appearance; a subtype of influenza A virus known as 2009 H1N1; viruses of the *Filoviridae* family causing a hemorrhagic fever disease called Ebola; and a virus of the *Flaviviridae* family causing a mosquito-borne disease called Zika.

A mis-folded (i.e., mis-shaped) form of prion protein has been linked to a variety of diseases in mammals, including notably bovine spongiform encephalopathy (BSE) in cattle. BSE is commonly referred to as mad-cow disease as it causes progressive neurological degeneration predominately in cattle. Similar to BSE in symptoms, Creutzfeldt-Jakob disease (CJD) is a rare brain disorder that occurs in humans. Neither the BSE nor the new variant CJD (*v*CJD) cases were reported in the United States until 2003. Yet between 1986 and 1992, over 180,000 BSE cases among cattle were confirmed in the United Kingdom (WHO, 2002). In more recent years, some BSE cases were also reported in other (predominantly European) countries (e.g., Belgium, Denmark, France, Germany, Ireland, Italy, Spain). In addition, 129 known vCJD (i.e., human) cases were reported between 1996 and 2002, mostly in the United Kingdom. As expected, the main concern with the BSE epidemic in the United Kingdom or other countries is that the infected animals could enter the human food chains. It was due to such public health concerns that immediately following the first case of BSE reported in the United States on 23 December 2003, Japan stopped the $1.4 billion worth of beef imports from the United States until December 2005. A case of BSE found in the United States in April 2012 was the country's fourth but not the world's most recently reported. This fourth American case was discovered in a dairy cow brought to a transfer facility near Hanford, California. More recently in January 2017, Ireland's Department of Agriculture confirmed a BSE case of the atypical (non-classical) type or form that had caused the death of an 18-year-old cow being raised in County Galway.

A coronavirus (CoV) was implicated as the agent responsible for the fatal *s*evere *a*cute *r*espiratory *s*yndrome (SARS) first reported in Asia in February 2003. Within a year, this infectious disease spread to more than two dozen countries in Europe, North America, South America, but predominantly Asia before its global outbreak was contained. The 2003 outbreak involved 8,098 human victims worldwide, of which 774 died. What had made SARS a significant environmental disease was the observation that it tended to spread by close person-to-person contact. The coronavirus was thought to be transmitted readily and easily by respiratory droplets produced from an infected person's cough or sneeze. Some victims were found to have been exposed through foreign travel to other parts of the world with SARS. Air travel(er) thus can be an important transmission vehicle (vector), but is avoidable with effective traveling alerts and regulations. The latest confirmed human cases of SARS were from laboratory-acquired infections reported and contained in China in April 2004 (WHO, 2004). Nonetheless, as of June 2017, nearly 2,000 SARS-like cases have been confirmed by WHO (2017a) since their first documentation in 2012. These SARS-like cases all involved a novel coronavirus, and were referred to by WHO as Middle East respiratory syndrome (MERS) in that they occurred mainly in the Middle East countries. Unlike the SARS cases, the MERS-CoV virus is transmitted from animals (largely camels) to humans.

H1N1 is a new strain (subtype) of influenza A virus. This new strain is specifically called 2009 H1N1 because it was first detected in the United States in April 2009 and declared by WHO two months later as responsible for the flu pandemic initiated in Mexico that year. This disease was more commonly but mistakenly referred to as "*the* swine flu" in that many genes in the two proteins hemagglutinin (H) and neuraminidase (N) in the virus were thought to be very similar to those in influenza viruses commonly observed in pigs. Yet swine flu *per se*, as supposedly found primarily in pigs, can be caused by other related subtypes such as the H1N2, H2N3, H3N1, and H3N2. The 2009 H1N1 flu pandemic was reportedly responsible for over 18,000 human deaths in more than 214 countries (WHO, 2010). While showing some relief of a downward trend in recent years, human infections with H1N1 virus are still ongoing worldwide. In India, for instance, more than 30,000 H1N1-related cases had been reported from the first quarter of 2015, which involved with some 2,000 deaths (Mishra, 2015). H1N1 virus is highly contagious in humans, spreading in the same manner as a common seasonal flu transmits. The symptoms of H1N1 infection include fever, headaches, coughs, sneezes, sore throat, runny or stuffy nose, muscle or joint aches, chills, and fatigue. A number of the infected individuals reportedly had diarrhea and vomiting. Hospitalization and death had occurred as a result of illness associated with this viral infection, primarily in children and adults less than 60 years old and in those with one or more of the underlying medical conditions like asthma, cardiopulmonary disorders, diabetes, and pregnancy (CDC, 2010). A vaccine for this new strain has become available worldwide since October 2009.

Ebola virus disease (EVD), or Ebola for short, is caused by viruses of the *Filoviridae* family. EVD is a type of hemorrhagic fever with a high case fatality rate in humans (up to 90% in past outbreaks). The most recent Ebola outbreak of global concern initiated in West Africa (Guinea, Liberia, and Sierra Leone) in early 2014, and ended about two years later. There were over 28,500 EVD cases reported from this two-year outbreak, along with more than 11,300 deaths (WHO, 2016a). In particular, these statistics included four cases diagnosed in the United States, with three being healthcare workers and the fourth visiting the country from Liberia. The symptoms of Ebola initially include high fever, headaches, chills, and muscle or joint aches. Later, the infected victim may experience internal bleeding resulting in vomiting or coughing blood. The filovirus genus involved has five single-member species, with four known to cause VCD in humans. The viral transmission to humans is initially and mostly from wild animals (e.g., fruit bats, gorillas) and spread in the human population via human-to-human transmission (WHO, 2017b).

Zika virus disease, also known as Zika fever, is caused by a flavivirus that was first identified in monkeys located in Uganda in 1947 and five years later in people living in that country as well as in the United Republic of Tanzania. Zika virus (more technically known as Zikv) is transmitted primarily by *Aedes* mosquitoes, but can be spread through human sexual intercourse and to inborns. The infected victim may experience mild fever, skin rash, conjunctivitis, muscle or joint aches, malaise, and/or headaches. These symptoms normally last for 2 to 10 days. The first large Zika outbreak was reported from the Island of Yap (Micronesia) in 2007. In early 2015, however, an epidemic of Zika fever was found to spread from Brazil to other parts of South and North America, as well as to several islands in the Pacific and Southeast Asia. A year later, WHO (2016b) declared the outbreak a *Public Health Emergency of International Concern* following the scientific consensus that Zika could cause the birth defect microcephaly, in which a baby's head is significantly smaller than expected (Chapter 19). There is now also growing evidence that Zika infection can cause Guillain-Barré syndrome, a rapid-onset muscle weakness condition caused by the body's immune system attacking part of the peripheral nervous system. As of January 2017, more than 100,000 Zika cases have been confirmed in Brazil, with over 2,000 microcephaly cases reported as linked to these cases (PAHO/WHO, 2017).

All in all, the above five global pandemics are agreeably more of a public health issue than one directly related to environmental toxicology or environmental pollution. Yet both the laboratory confirmation of the biological pathogen involved and the development of a high-yield vaccine virus for the H1N1 flu are truly related to toxicity testing, the role of a toxicologist with the proper training.

References

Bazerman C, De los Santos RA, 2005. Measuring Incommensurability: Are Toxicology and Ecotoxicology Bind to What the Other Sees? In *Rhetoric and Incommensurability* (Harris RA, Ed.). West Lafayette, Indiana, USA: Parlor Press, Chapter 10.

Carson R, 1962. *Silent Spring*. Boston, Massachusetts, USA: Houghton Mifflin.

CDC (U.S. Centers for Disease Control and Prevention), 2010. Questions & Answers: 2009 H1N1 Flu ("Swine Flu") and You (webpage dated 10 February 2010). http://www.cdc.gov/h1n1flu/qa.htm (retrieved 3 January 2017).

Chapman PM, 2002. Integrating Toxicology and Ecology: Putting the "Eco" into Ecotoxicology. *Marine Pollut. Bull.* 44:7-15.

Eaton DL, Klaassen CD, 2001. Principles of Toxicology. In *Casarett and Doull's Toxicology: The Basic Science of Poisons* (Klaassen CD, Ed.), 6th Edition. New York, New York, USA: McGraw-Hill, Chapter 2.

EHA (Environmental Health Australia, Ltd.), 2012. Environmental Health Risk Assessment – Guidelines for Assessing Human Health Risks from Environmental Hazards. PO Box 2222, Fortitude Valley BC, Queensland, 4006, Australia.

Gallo MA, 2001. History and Scope of Toxicology. In *Casarett and Doull's Toxicology: The Basic Science of Poisons* (Klaassen CD, Ed.), 6th Edition. New York, New York, USA: McGraw-Hill, Chapter 1.

Gordis L, 1996. *Epidemiology*. Philadelphia, Pennsylvania, USA: Saunders.

Hodgson E, Mailman RB, Chambers JE (Eds.), 1998. *Dictionary of Toxicology*. New York, New York, USA: Grove's Dictionaries Inc.

Lane RW, Borzelleca JF, 2008. Harming and Helping through Time: The History of Toxicology. In *Principles and Methods of Toxicology* (Hayes AW, Ed.), 5th Edition. Boca Raton, Florida, USA: Taylor & Francis Group, Chapter 1.

Lewis RA (Ed.), 1998. *Lewis' Dictionary of Toxicology*. Boca Raton, Florida, USA: Lewis Publishers (CRC Press).

Lilienfeld DE, Stolley PD, 1994. *Foundations of Epidemiology*. New York, New York, USA: Oxford University Press.

Maltby L, Naylor C, 1990. Preliminary Observations on the Ecological Relevance of the Gammarus 'Scope for Growth' Assay: Effect of Zinc on Reproduction. *Functional Ecol.* 4:393-397.

Mishra B, 2015. 2015 Resurgence of Influenza A (H1N1) 09: Smoldering Pandemic in India? *J. Glob. Infect. Dis.* 7:56-59.

NIH (U.S. National Institutes of Health), 2008. *Toxicology Tutor I: Basic Principles Menu*. U.S. National Library of Medicine (Specialized Information Service), Environmental Health and Toxicology (webpage dated 2008). http://sis.nlm.nih.gov/enviro/toxtutor/Tox1/amenu.htm (retrieved 2 March 2009).

NRC (U.S. National Research Council), 1983. *Risk Assessment in the Federal Government. Managing the Process*. Washington DC, USA: National Academy Press.

NRC (U.S. National Research Council), 1994. *Science and Judgment in Risk Assessment*. Washington DC, USA: National Academy Press.

PAHO/WHO (Pan American Health Organization/World Health Organization), 2017. Zika Cases and Congenital Syndrome Associated with Zika Virus Reported by Countries and Territories in the Americas, 2015-2017 (dated 18 January 2017). http://www.paho.org/hq/index.phd?option=com_docmen&task=doc_view&Itemid=270&gid=37706&lan=en (retrieved 4 February 2017).

Rothman KJ, Sander G, 1998. *Modern Epidemiology*. Philadelphia, Pennsylvania, USA: Lippincott-Raven.

Szklo M, Nieto FJ, 2000. *Epidemiology: Beyond the Basics*. Gaithersburg, Maryland, USA: Aspen Publishers.

Truhaut R, 1977. Ecotoxicology: Objectives, Principles and Perspectives. *Ecotoxic. Environ. Safety* 1:151-173.

U.S. Code (United States Code), 2013. Title 18 (Crimes and Criminal Procedure), Chapter 10 (Biological Weapons), Section 178 (Definitions). Office of the Law Revision Counsel, U.S. House of Representative, http://uscode.house.gov/ (still effective as of August 2017).

WHO (World Health Organization), 1986. Environmental Toxicology and Ecotoxicology: Proceedings of the Third International Course. WHO Regional Office for Europe, Copenhagen, Denmark.

WHO (World Health Organization), 2002. Bovine Spongiform Encephalopathy. Fact Sheet No. 113 (Media Centre, revised November 2002). http://www.wiredhealthresources.net/resources/NA/WHO-FS_Bovine-SpongiformEncephalopathy.pdf (retrieved 4 June 2017).

WHO (World Health Organization), 2003. WHD (World Health Day) Brochure, Part II: Introduction. Geneva, Switzerland.

WHO (World Health Organization), 2004. China's Latest SARS Outbreak Has Been Contained, But Biosafety Concerns Remain – Update 7 (dated 18 May 2004). https://www.who.int/csr/don/2004_05_18a/en/ (retrieved 3 January 2017).

WHO (World Health Organization), 2010. Pandemic (H1N1) 2009 – Update 112 (dated 6 August 2010). http://www.who.int/csr/don/2010_08_06/en/ (retrieved 4 January 2017)

WHO (World Health Organization), 2016a. Ebola Situation Report – 16 March 2016. http://www.int/csr disease/ebola/situation-reports/archive/en/ (retrieved 7 June 2017).

WHO (World Health Organization), 2016b. Zika Virus Outbreak Global Response – Interim Report (dated May 2016). Geneva, Switzerland.

WHO (World Health Organization), 2017a. WHO Target Product Profiles for MERS-CoV Vaccines (dated May 2017). http://www.who.int/blueprint/what/research-development/MERS_CoV-TPP_15052017.pdf?ua =1 (retrieved 13 June 2017).

WHO (World Health Organization), 2017b. Ebola Virus Disease – Fact Sheet (updated May 2017). http://www.who.int/mediacentre/factsheets/fs103/en/ (retrieved 24 May 2017).

Wright DA, Welbourn PA, 2002. *Environmental Toxicology*. Cambridge, UK: Cambridge University Press, Chapter 1.

Review Questions

1. What is environmental toxicology? And what is its relationship with general toxicology?
2. Who was Paracelsus? And what was his famous statement (assertion) frequently quoted by today's toxicologists?
3. Who was Mathieu Orfila? And what was his contribution to (classical) toxicology?
4. What are the subtle differences among the terms *toxicant*, *poison*, *contaminant*, *toxic agent*, *pollutant*, *toxic substance*, *toxic chemical*, *toxin*, and *xenobiotic*?
5. What are the three major categories of professional activities for/of (environmental) toxicologists?
6. Why is the term *dosage* a more practical concept than the term *dose*?
7. What are the more prominent factors affecting or influencing the (adverse) effects of an environmental toxicant?
8. What are the three major categories or types of studies from which knowledge on toxicity is constantly obtained?
9. How can chemical interaction affect a dose-response relationship?

16 An Introduction to Environmental Toxicology

10. Name the four basic steps (components) in the health risk assessment paradigm published by the U.S. National Research Council in 1983.
11. Name the five basic principles for/of environmental toxicology.
12. How is ecotoxicology different from environmental toxicology?
13. Why is epidemiology regarded as a very close ally of environmental toxicology?
14. What are the three issues underlying the importance of environmental toxicology?
15. Name the five pandemic infectious diseases discussed in this chapter.
16. Why is knowledge on (health) risk assessment framework an important prerequisite for the practice of environmental toxicology, especially by regulatory toxicologists?

CHAPTER 2

Environmental Changes and Environmental Health

2.1. Introduction

In addition to ecotoxicology (Section 1.3.2) and epidemiology (Section 1.3.3), two allies of environmental toxicology noteworthy are environmental health (science) and environmental sciences, each of which is likewise an interdisciplinary science. Environmental health as a discipline is the branch of public health concerning all aspects of factors and conditions in the environment that may affect human well-being and community health. One of its major study concentrations is on the relationships between people and their environment that promote public health. Environmental sciences, on the other hand, is concerned with the interaction of processes and systems that shapes the natural environment and resources. This latter ally is built on a foundation of biological, physical, chemical, and socioeconomic sciences for the study of environmental processes and systems, as well as for the solution of a wide range of environmental issues including pollution, natural resource, and global climate change. It is largely under this notion that the well-founded Society of Environmental Toxicology and Chemistry (SETAC) has its vision and mission to promote *"the advancement and application of scientific research related to contaminants and other stressors in the environment, the education in the environmental sciences, and the use of science in environmental policy and decision-making."*

Due to space limitation, only global as well as regional environmental changes and environmental diseases are discussed in this chapter. Both aspects are among the three from the two ally disciplines that are regarded as most relevant to the study and the practice of environmental toxicology. The third aspect is environmental pollution, which along with its regulatory burden is discussed in Chapter 3.

2.1.1. Knowledge on the Changing World

The world continues to bring forth significant global as well as local environmental changes every few years, if not every year, due partly to nature's forces and partly to human activities including predominately industrialization and urbanization. As evident from the information given in subsequent chapters, knowledge on this type of changes is a prerequisite for the study and the practice of environmental toxicology. There are at least three fundamental, interrelated aspects of environmental changes that are most relevant to environmental toxicology. One aspect involves a realization of the significant changes that have happened or are happening to or in the global and local environments. Another aspect necessitates an understanding of the impacts that these changes have on humankind and the natural environment. Still another need is for an appreciation of the actions that people, especially environmentalists and regulatory entities, have taken or are about to undertake to cope with these environmental impacts. Whereas this third aspect is discussed as regulatory and environmental concerns in Chapter 3, the first two are the foci of this chapter.

2.1.2. Impacts of Global Environmental Changes

It is important to realize that not all the environmental changes discussed in this chapter (or this book) are necessarily health-related or bad. Some of them can be positive, economic-related, or pertinent to advances in science and technology. For instance, certain food additives (Chapter 21) and almost all pest-killing substances known as pesticides (Chapter 15) are *economic* poisons, without which people would have less healthy foods to consume. The enormous volume of electronic waste (e-waste; Section 2.2.6) which the world needs to cope with today simply reflects the trend that many people are living in a "high-tech" era. The outcome of deforestation is to have more land use. People also tend to improve their environmental conditions from the bad experiences that they have encountered. More bluntly, pollution episodes such as the London fog of 1952 (Section 2.2.2) and the thousands of tons of chemical waste buried in Love Canal (Section 2.2.4) are things no longer occurring in a similar large order of magnitude.

Environmental changes also bring about, nevertheless, dramatic changes in disease pattern. In the first half of 20th century, some infectious diseases such as tuberculosis and pneumonia were leading causes of death in many countries including the United States. Yet since around the mid-1950s, heart disease and cancer have become the top two leading causes of death in the United States (Table 2.1), and have accounted for much of the mortalities in many other countries including even those in the developing regions. The upside of such a new disease pattern is that more chronic (i.e., long-term) diseases prevalent in a country implies that overall its people live longer. This pattern also signifies a more sanitary place for people to live in now than before. The downside is that cancer and other chronic diseases (e.g., cardiovascular diseases) are more complex likely with multiple causes, of which many are considered as environmental in origin. It is this kind of global concerns that has put environmental health into a world perspective.

Table 2.1. Death Cases by Leading Cause and Year in the United States, per 100,000 Population[a]

Cause	2000	2005	2010	2014
All Causes	869.0	815.0	747.0	724.6
Heart disease	257.6	216.8	179.1	167.0
Malignant neoplasm (cancer)	199.6	185.1	172.8	161.2
Chronic lower respiratory diseases	44.2	43.9	42.2	40.5
Unintentional injuries	34.9	39.5	38.0	40.5
Stroke (cerebrovascular disease)	60.9	48.0	39.1	36.5
Alzheimer's disease	18.1	24.0	25.1	25.4
Diabetes mellitus	25.0	24.9	20.8	20.9
Influenza and pneumonia	23.7	21.0	15.1	15.1
Renal (kidney) diseases	13.5	14.7	15.3	13.2
Suicide	10.4	10.9	12.1	13.0

[a]adapted from Table 17 in the U.S. government report *Health, United States, 2015* (NCHS, 2016), with death rates age-adjusted and cause data based on death certificates available to year 2014; renal diseases defined here in Table 2.1 as consisting of nephritis, nephrotic syndrome, and nephrosis.

2.1.3. World's Perspective of Environmental Health

Environmental health as a realm or program activity set out by the World Health Organization (WHO, 2011) is that: *"(It) addresses all the physical, chemical, and biological factors external to a person, and all the related factors impacting behaviours. It encompasses the assessment and control of those environmental factors that can potentially affect health. It is targeted towards preventing disease and creating health-supportive environments. This definition excludes behaviour not related to environment, as well as behaviour related to the social and cultural environment, and genetics."*

Of all age groups, children are uniquely more vulnerable to environmental diseases. One reason for this is that as they grow and develop, there are periods in which the organs and systems in their body are particularly susceptible to the effects of many environmental insults. Another more important reason has to do with the environments that children are in. As noted in Chapter 1, a child's world centers around the home, the school, and the local community. These should be healthy places where the youngsters can thrive, while protected from diseases. Yet to the contrary, these places are often found so unhealthy that they underlie the majority of deaths as well as a huge burden of diseases among children in the developing regions (WHO, 2003).

Fortunately, the suffering of children and adults from most environmental diseases is *not* inevitable. Many of the environmental diseases and deaths can be prevented. Never before has there been such a wide range of tools and strategies to protect people from the hazards lurking in their environments. It is the advance of environmental toxicology that has been ultimately leading to the development of these desperately needed strategies and tools.

2.2. Major Specific Environmental Changes

Amidst urbanization, industrialization, and advances in science or technology, many physical and material changes to the environment have occurred since World War II. The following are the major ones regarded as more relevant to environmental toxicology: changes of global climate (particularly those leading to global warming); increased air and water pollutions; mounting quantities of solid and toxic wastes; destruction of the ozone (O_3) layer by air pollutants; and presence of a growing number of environmental carcinogens and endocrine disruptors. Some of their more relevant, specific, or classic cases are highlighted in the subsections that follow.

2.2.1. Global Climate Changes

In recent years, this type of environmental changes, particularly those leading to global warming, has drawn much public attention (and sometimes or in some places controversies). Studies reviewed by the Intergovernmental Panel on Climate Change (IPCC, 2007) showed that during the 20th century (i.e., 1901 to 2000), the global temperature at the lowest portion of the Earth's atmosphere (i.e., troposphere) increased about 0.5 to 1.0° C (0.9 to 1.8° F). IPCC concluded that most of the increases in the temperatures observed since the 1950s were caused by the increasing levels of greenhouse gases attributed to human activities such as fossil fuel burning and deforestation. Climate changes have reportedly affected the ocean's temperature as well as its productivity and the ecosystems (e.g., Behrenfeld *et al.*, 2006; Sarmiento *et al.*, 2004). It has been suggested (e.g., Lobell *et al.*, 2008) that these changes can have serious implications for agricultural productivity resulting in food shortage. Ozone, water (H_2O) vapor, carbon dioxide (CO_2), nitrous oxide (N_2O), methane (CH_4), and chlorofluorocarbons (CFCs) are the major greenhouse gases that help trap moderate level of atmospheric heat to sustain a habitable temperature of ~15.6° C (~60° F). Without the greenhouse effect (Chapter 5), the Earth would have a practically unlivable temperature of below −19° C (−2° F).

2.2.2. Air Pollution

Air pollution is the presence of contaminants in the atmosphere at such concentrations, durations, and frequencies that they can cause adverse effects on the health of living organisms or their ecosystem. The extent to which air pollution has affected public health can be illustrated by the numerous air pollution-related episodes occurring over the years, dating back to even earlier than December 1952 when the smoggy London experienced 4,000 excess deaths from respiratory and heart problems caused by acid rain and other air pollutants. Similar acute episodes, but less devastating and at times with different kinds of air pollutants, also occurred in other major cities around the world such as Beijing, Los Angeles, New York, and Osaka. Air pollutants of global concern include largely: sulfur oxides (SO_x); nitrogen oxides (NO_x); carbon monoxide (CO); ozone and other photochemical oxidants; different types and sizes of particulates; lead (Pb) and other toxic metals; and *v*olatile *o*rganic *c*ompounds (known more commonly by its acronym VOCs). Major sources of air pollution are fossil fuels combusted for transportation, electricity, heating, and cooking, as well as a variety of industrial and (other) combustion processes.

2.2.3. Water Pollution

Similarly, water pollution is the presence of contaminants in water at such concentrations, durations, and frequencies that they can cause undesired effects on the health of living organisms and the (mainly aquatic) environment. In many developed countries including particularly the United States, most people generally regard water pollution not so much as a health issue, but more as an issue of conservation and preservation of natural beauty and resources. In either case, the major sources of water pollution include inorganic and organic wastes, petroleum compounds, municipal waste, pesticide residues, agricultural runoff, and acid mine drainage. Many industrial processes have the potential to discharge various types of wastes that can cause significant water pollution problems. Water pollution can threaten not only aquatic life, but also human health. Evidence for this kind of human health threats includes the well-watched American film *Erin Brockovich*, which was released in 2000 publicizing specifically how human life was caused by water contamination with the toxic hexavalent metal chromium (denoted by Cr^{6+} or CrVI).

2.2.4. Soil Contamination

For soil contamination, a major concern is the release of an increasing number or volume of toxic substances to the soil which is a relatively stationary medium. One noteworthy aspect is that the release of soil contaminants is not limited to areas adjacent to point sources (e.g., farmlands, industrial facilities). Rather, these soil contaminants can be transported to distant areas away from the point source. One widely known disaster related to land disposal of various hazardous wastes in the American history is that of Love Canal, which initially was an abandoned area near Niagara Falls in the state of New York. The main issue with this environmental tragedy is that a neighborhood developed there in the late 1970s was discovered to have been sitting on top of some 20,000 tons of toxic waste buried more than two decades earlier. This pile of toxic waste contained some 80 different harmful chemical substances, of which about a dozen were known or suspected at the time as human carcinogens.

2.2.5. Red Tide Pollution

Red tide, also known as *harmful algal bloom* (HAB), is a common name given to an environmental phenomenon when algae (e.g., phytoplankton) are present in water bodies in sufficient concentrations that the water there appears murky or discolored to greenish, brownish, or mostly reddish (and hence the term *red tide pollution*). The most important environmental issue with red tides is apparently their toxic and often lethal effects on the coastal species of birds, fish, and marine mammals. For the red tides occurring in the United States, largely in the state of Florida, a potent neurotoxin named *brevetoxin* from the algae species *Karenia brevis* is thought to be responsible for the much intoxication and killing of the coastal creatures. Red tide algae are also linked to skin irritation and burning in people who swim or get splashed in nearby areas with high concentrations of these water plants.

In certain regions, both the frequency and the severity of HAB have been linked to increased nutrient loading from human activities (Lam and Ho, 1989). In particular, the growth of marine phytoplankton (at least when under certain conditions) has been reportedly (e.g., Anderson *et al.*, 2002; Davidson *et al.*, 2014) linked to the availability of nitrates (NO_3^-) and phosphates (PO_4^{3-}), both of which can be abundant in and hence from agricultural runoff.

2.2.6. Electronic Waste Pollution

Electronic waste, nicknamed e-waste, is also known as waste electrical and electronic equipment and products. Technically, it includes the refuses from discarded or end-of-life electrical and electronic products that end up in landfills or incinerators, instead of being reused or recycled. The increasing environmental health concern with e-waste may be justified with the statistics on electronics use. According to a somewhat outdated but still valid white paper report by Cairns (2005), waste electronic equipment has been one of the fastest growing categories of municipal solid waste. Both the rapid growth of the electronics sector and the swift changes in technology indicate that more consumers are replacing more electronic equipment more often than ever before. In that report, the high-end estimates made then were such that in the United States, the cumulative number of obsolete computers alone could well exceed 300 million, along with some 4 billion pounds of plastics, about 1 billion pounds of lead, 2 million pounds of cadmium (Cd), and 4 hundred pounds of mercury (Hg). These computer constituents are all considered toxic to human health and the ecosystem. Most electronic products, including computers, contain carcinogenic or highly toxic substances like polychlorinated biphenyls (PCBs), which were once widely used as coolants and lubricants in transformers, capacitors, and other electronic components. A more recent analysis (Duan *et al.*, 2013) estimated that in the United States 258 million units (or 1.6 million tons) of used electronics (e.g., computers, monitors, televisions, mobile phones) were generated in 2010. And around 171.4 millions (66.4%) of these used units were collected. That analysis further estimated that 8.5% (14.4 millions) of the used electronic products were exported.

2.2.7. Deforestation

For thousands of years, people have been using fire to clear land. Wildfires are therefore a significant force for environmental change. Other means or causes of deforestation include logging, urbanization, mining, and oil exploitation, as well as the conversion of forested lands for agricultural use and cattle-raising (TWI, 1999). The stability of a forest ecosystem can be affected by changes of environmental conditions, including substantial increases in temperatures and atmospheric CO_2 (carbon dioxide) or substantial decreases in deposition rates of nutrients and acidity. Forest ecosystems continue to be threatened by soil acidification and nutrient depletion or nutrient overload (e.g., Matzner, 2004). According to the Food and Agriculture Organization of the United Nations (FAO, 2016), worldwide some 129 million hectares of forestland (an area about the size of South Africa) have been lost since 1990, in spite of the fact that over the past 25 years the rate of net global deforestation has slowed down by more than 5% (from 0.18% to 0.08%). During the ten-year period from 1990 to 2000, the global net annual rate of deforestation reached 36,000 sq. miles (FAO, 2001).

Forests are highly rich sources for foods, fuels, construction materials, fibers, and biological diversity, since much of the Earth's biomass as well as biodiversity above ground is held within its forests (UNEP, 2005). They are also important in water and air filtration, carbon (dioxide) sequestration, and soil stabilization (Williams, 1990, 1994). Since 1990, forests have made up some 31% (approximately 4,000 million hectares) of the world's land areas (FAO, 2016). Two decades ago, it was estimated (Lund and Iremonger, 1998) that roughly 3.7 acres of forestland were needed to supply each person on the planet with enough shelter and fuel.

2.3. Incidence and Spectrum of Environmental Diseases

In public health, environmental diseases are those caused by environmental agents or factors that are not transmitted genetically or, to some scholars, not by infection either. This chapter as well as this book, however, takes on a broader definition to include those communicable diseases (i.e., those caused by infection) occurring at the community level. Pesticides, consumer products, food additives, cigarette smoke, radiation, air pollution, water pollution, and various types of toxic wastes are some of the major sources of environmental contaminants contributing to human diseases in a community. Accordingly, there are numerous types of environmental diseases of public health concern. Although environmental contaminants are found everywhere, the likelihood of people developing a specific environmental disease still depends very much on the type of contaminants present in their own environment and on their genetic susceptibility to such a hazard. Regardless, what seems certain is that environmental diseases thrive in conditions conducive for unhealthy living (e.g., where germs and disease-bearing insects tend to breed, or where drinking water is highly contaminated with agricultural runoff).

As a case in point, one of the Guyana government's nationwide high public health concerns is its two decades old observation of a disproportionately high frequency of numerous communicable diseases including malaria, acute respiratory infections, acute diarrheal disorders, and worm infections (King, 2001). The government concluded that the causes of these diseases (including nervous disorders and hypertension) were largely environmental in nature. It rested its conclusion on the ground that the basic sanitation in many areas in its country was (and still is) lacking or at best most rudimentary, amidst the ongoing problem of over-crowding.

2.3.1. Incidence and Burden of Environmental Diseases

High incidences of environmental diseases have been observed in many developed countries as well. A little more than four decades ago, *Time* (1975) magazine echoed the declaration made by Dr. Irving Selikoff of the New York Mount Sinai School of Medicine, reiterating that "*Environmental disease is becoming the disease of the century.*" Even then, they realized that industrialization along with expanding technology was changing the world radically and exposing humankind to growing amounts of harmful environmental contaminants, of which some were chemicals not available many years ago.

In the industrialized countries, particularly in the United States, the public's growing concern with environmental diseases dates back to the early 1960s, when Rachel Carson (1962) asserted specifically in her once widely read classic book *Silent Spring* that "*The economic costs of environmental disease and disabilities are very significant and they are largely preventable. By taking action to reduce or eliminate exposures to toxic chemicals, the US could save billions of dollars a year in health and related costs and significantly improve public health.*"

Moreover, according to a study (Landrigan *et al.*, 2002) published in the beginning of the 21st century, the annual health-related costs for the four categories of American pediatric diseases under analysis totaled to $55 billion, with $43.4 billion for lead (Pb) poisoning, $9.2 billion for neurobehavioral disorders, $2.0 billion for asthma, and $0.3 billion for childhood cancer. Such findings are not surprising, inasmuch as the U.S. National Health and Nutrition Examination Survey (commonly known by its acronym NHANES) reported that during the years 1991 to 1994, 4.4% of American children aged 1 to 6 years had blood lead levels exceeding the critical level of 10 µg/dL (CDC, 1997). The study estimated that the total of the annual costs for the four categories came to about 2.8% of total U.S. healthcare costs. Four years later, another source (RDHN, 2006) estimated that the annual health-related costs for all environmental diseases in the United States might be as high as $165 billion.

Even at the state level, the total annual cost of asthma alone in California was estimated to be as much as $1.3 billion. That state estimate was given around the same period in 2005 by a group of scientific staff who helped draft the California Senate Bill 600 in an effort to create a chemical monitoring program in the state. According to the bill, for individuals born in the late 1980s with one or more of the 18 most common and major birth defects (Section 2.4.2), the estimated lifetime costs for medical treatment and lost productivity would exceed $1 trillion. The bill's main point of argument was that approximately 85,000 chemical substances were registered for use in the United States, with another some 2,000 being registered each year. Yet over 90% of these substances had never been (fully) tested for their adverse effects on human health.

California is also known to have high incidences of cancer and birth defects. It was due to the public's concerns over these high statistics that in 1986, the state voters passed a law with the intent to keep their consumer products free of toxic substances that have the potential to cause illnesses in the two disease categories. That state law, officially titled *"The Safe Drinking Water and Toxic Enforcement Act of 1986"*, is nicknamed *"Proposition 65"* or *"Prop 65"*. It mandates that anyone in the state must be *informed* about the presence of any substance classified as a toxicant that may cause cancer or reproductive harm (including birth defect).

2.3.2. Spectrum and Nature of Environmental Diseases

Environmental toxicology is an important discipline mostly because there have been growing concerns on environmental diseases which now have been widely recognized and spreading, particularly in the developed and developing countries and since World War II. These environmental diseases can be treated as the trade-offs for accelerating production of chemical substances in the second half of last century. More bluntly, industrial society has since increased human exposure to thousands of chemical substances present in the environment.

Again, environmental diseases and injuries are not caused by chemical substances alone. Some can be induced by biological or physical agents, such as those from venomous snakebites, from dermal contact with poisonous plants, from consumption of poisonous marine animals, from exposure to radiation, and those seen in foodborne outbreaks. Neither are humans the only victims of environmental diseases. Plant diseases can be caused from environmental exposure to biological agents. Many crops are subject to pest infestation for which the treatment is usually with pesticides (Chapter 15). On the other hand, corneal edema and ulcers can be seen in captive marine mammals. According to the *Merck Veterinary Manual* (Kahn, 2008), the causes of these diseases could be (due to) lack of shade, excessive bright light, and nutritional deficiencies. The veterinary manual further specifies that exposure to spills of petroleum hydrocarbons is a major health concern for marine mammals. For one thing, sea otters are especially vulnerable to oil spills owing to their natural grooming habits and their lack of an excessive fat layer. Kidneys, liver, respiratory tract, and gastrointestinal tract are some of the body organs in the exposed marine mammals that can be seriously affected. In these mammals, the body part affected the most is their respiratory tract, as petroleum hydrocarbons are sufficiently volatile.

The toxic effects of environmental exposure, in all settings and for all species including humans, are highly influenced by the route of exposure. Under normal circumstances, the principal sources (and thus routes) of exposure for most animal species including humans are air and water pollutions, followed by ingestion of contaminated foods and direct dermal contact.

In humans, many environmental diseases received first public attention during the late 18th to early 19th century when industrialized changes in agriculture, transportation, and manufacturing had profound socioeconomic and cultural impacts first in Britain and later in the rest of the world. Such public awareness reportedly stemmed from the recognition of occupational illnesses at the time, especially those associated with exposure to highly toxic chemical substances. Substantiating such a connection is the observation that chemical exposures generally are more intense in occupational settings than in the general environment, thereby readily yielding more noticeable illnesses in workplaces. Examples of those early classic occupational diseases included (as further discussed in Chapter 20): *cancer of the scrotal skin* (which in 1775 was linked to soot exposure in chimney sweeps); *silicosis* (a lung disease of miners, grinders, and potters from inhalation of silica dust, dating back to the 1700s); *neurological disorders* (found in workers exposed to lead glazes on pottery, dating back to the 1700s); and certain *bone diseases* (e.g., phossy jaw in workers exposed to white phosphorus in the manufacture of matches, dating back to the 1800s).

2.4. Commonly Encountered Environmental Diseases

In the subsections that follow, brief overviews are presented for the various select groups of environmental diseases that are not only more commonly encountered but also deemed having greater public health concerns, with the specific aim of facilitating the appreciation of the materials covered in other chapters. For the more prominent specific environmental diseases emerging in recent years, they are discussed in the subsequent chapters that address specific causative agents, specific adverse health effects, or both.

2.4.1. Cancer

This group of diseases begins when a cell or a small group of cells in the body multiply more rapidly than at the normal rate. As these cancer cells spread throughout the body, they eventually affect the normal functions of other healthy organs and tissues. It is thought that in most situations, one or more cancer-promoting factors may need to add up before a malignant growth can be developed. Some of these promoting factors include short- or long-term exposure to certain factors, conditions, or agents in the environment, such as cigarette smoke, radiation, alcohol, natural or synthetic chemicals, viruses, or sunlight. People therefore can reduce the risk of getting cancer by limiting their exposure to these harmful agents or factors. More discussion on this group of diseases is given in Chapter 18.

2.4.2. Birth Defects

Diseases under this group are defined as abnormalities of structure, function, or body metabolism present in babies at birth. According to the U.S. Centers for Disease Control and Prevention (CDC, 2008), birth defects affect approximately 3% of babies born in the United States each year (i.e., affecting about 120,000 babies born annually). This group of diseases collectively is one of the leading causes of infant deaths, accounting for some 20% of all infant deaths in the United States. Babies born with birth defects tend to be more susceptible to illness and to long-term disability compared to those born healthy. There are 45 major types of birth defects classified by CDC (2006), of which 18 (e.g., Down syndrome, cleft lip, neural tube defects; *see* Table 19.2) have been determined as more prevalent. Birth defects can occur when pregnant women consume (too much) alcohol or when they are exposed to certain substances (e.g., aspirin, the synthetic estrogen *diethylstilbestrol (DES)*, contents in cigarette smoke, the drug *thalidomide* for morning sickness). These harmful substances can reach the fetus via the placenta. Ionizing radiation is also considered a strong teratogen (i.e., any agent that causes a birth defect). Because of these maternal exposures, some babies are born with one or more body parts, organs, or tissues that have not developed in a normal way. Further discussion on this group of diseases is given in Chapter 19.

2.4.3. Reproductive Damage

Fertility is the ability to conceive and have children. It has estimated that approximately 10% of American couples have infertility problem (NHSR, 2013). Infertility occurs when a woman cannot produce a healthy egg, or when a man cannot produce sufficient sperms. This health condition can be caused from exposure to chemical substances at work, in homes, or elsewhere in the environment, or by infections coming from sexual diseases.

Some natural substances and synthetic pesticides are found structurally so similar to estrogens and androgens that they can actually "mimic" the actions of these important female and male, respectively, sex hormones (Chapter 19). As a result, these endocrine or hormone disruptors may interfere with the development of male and female reproductive organs or with their normal functions (Chapter 19). This type of interference can lead to increased risk of adverse reproductive conditions such as early puberty, low sperm counts, ovarian cysts, and cancer of the breast or the testicle. Certain solvents such as glycol ether can damage male reproductive health and a child's health. Other synthetic substances known as capable of inducing adverse reproductive effects in males include PCBs, lead compounds, and certain pesticides (e.g., 1,2-dibromo-3-chloropropane, Kepone, ethylene dibromide). Male adults therefore should avoid working with or being around these chemicals for at least a few months prior to fathering a child.

2.4.4. Respiratory Diseases

Diseases in this group represent those affecting the respiratory tract (which includes the lungs, bronchial tubes, trachea, and in some literature also the nose and throat). These diseases can be broadly classified as the *obstructive* type (that impeding the airflow; e.g., asthma, bronchiolitis) or the *restrictive* type (that characterized by a loss in lung volume; e.g., pulmonary fibrosis, lung cancer). Causes of these diseases range from infectious agents and environmental exposures, to allergens and genetic origin. Note that the most interaction of humans with the outside world is via their lungs which need to constantly take in the omnipresent air.

According to the American Lung Association (ALA, 2010), around 3.7 million Americans have been diagnosed with a progressive, obstructive pulmonary condition termed *emphysema*. Emphysema is a subtype of *chronic obstructive pulmonary disease* (COPD) that limits the transfer of carbon dioxide (CO_2) and oxygen (O_2) in the lungs due to damage of their air sacs, with symptoms of chest tightness, shortness of breath, loss of appetite, and fatigue. Certain pollutants in the air and the cigarette smoke can affect breathing by damaging sensitive tissues (e.g., the air sacs). Another subgroup of obstructive respiratory diseases is asthma, which affects some 235 million people worldwide (IUATLD, 2011). Some asthma attacks, including those leaving victims breathless and gasping for air, can be triggered by pollutants present in the air or inside the home.

Some other airborne particles can be dangerous in the same way, but ending with different types of pulmonary disorders. These include mineral (e.g., asbestos) or cellulosic (e.g., cotton) fibers and respirable dusts from silica, coal, and iron. These particles can cause scar tissue by damaging sensitive areas of the lungs. This black (as darkened with scars) lung condition is medically termed *pneumoconiosis*. Although the initial symptoms include only inflammation, fibrosis, chest pains, and shortness of breath, the condition can progress to bronchitis, emphysema, or death.

2.4.5. Neurological Diseases

Diseases in this group involve the nervous system which is composed of the brain, the spinal cord, and billions of nerve cells. The brain and the spinal cord as a subsystem is generally referred to as the *c*entral *n*ervous *s*ystem (CNS), from which the nerve cells are responsible for carrying messages and instructions to other parts of the body. When the peripheral nerve cells or the cells in the CNS are damaged by toxicants, so are the neurological pathway and the neural signaling system. An impaired condition of this kind can result in neurological disorders ranging from change in mood or memory to blindness, slurred speech, paralysis, and death. As noted in Chapter 15, certain pesticides are neurotoxic agents of high environmental health concern, particularly those in the organophosphate (OP) family such as parathion and malathion. Most organochlorine pesticides (e.g., dieldrin, lindane) and most pyrethroids (e.g., permethrin) are also neurotoxic agents. So are certain metals (Chapter 14), certain toxins or pathogenic microbial agents (Chapter 17), and numerous various organic solvents (Chapter 20).

2.4.6. Skin Disorders

One commonly encountered noncancerous disorder in this group is dermatitis, which is simply a fancy name for inflamed, irritated skin. This condition can be induced by contact with some pesticides (e.g., propargite) used in farms. Many people also have experienced the oozing bumps and itching caused by poison ivy, poison oak, and poison sumac. Some chemical substances found in paints, cosmetics, and detergents can cause skin rashes and blisters. Too much wind or sun can also make the skin dry and chapped. Certain medications, fabrics, and foods too can cause unusual skin reactions in some people.

2.4.7. Diseases Induced by Common Causes/Specific Agents

In addition to the environmental diseases categorized above by *effect* type, some can be characterized more effectively by concerning the specific or special (groups of) *agents* that induce them. Examples for this latter type of disease concern and hence grouping are briefly discussed below. More examples along with more discussion can be found elsewhere in this book, mainly in Part III (i.e., Chapters 11 through 17).

Some environmental diseases are caused by *neurotoxins* found in seafood, such as *tetrodotoxin* in puffer fish and *ciguatoxin* in oysters and clams (Chapter 17). *Mycotoxins* are toxins produced by fungi which can be found harboring in a variety of plant and crop foods (e.g., legumes, corn, almond nuts). Among the various mycotoxins known to date, *aflatoxins* and particular the *aflatoxin B_1* subtype have been the subject of most intensive investigation worldwide, owing to their acute toxic effects in humans and their potent hepatocarcinogenicity found in rats and certain other laboratory animals (Chapter 17).

Many foreign substances in the body are metabolized (e.g., broken down) into harmless or less harmful compounds by the liver, a topic covered extensively in Chapter 8. Yet some xenobiotics are converted to *free radicals* which are highly reactive and unstable, as by definition they have an unpaired electron. In order to stabilize themselves, these free radicals each will take (hijack) an electron from a nearby molecule which then usually becomes another active free radical. This chain reaction may eventually disrupt the body's normal functions, including having radicals react constantly with lipoproteins in the blood to form plaque-like fatty deposits. These fatty plaques can clog blood vessels to block off blood supply to the heart, causing cardiac attack. Examples of free radicals are *triphenylmethyl radical*, *superoxide radical*, and *hydroxyl radical*, of which the last two are referred to as *reactive oxygen species* (*ROS*) or *oxygen free radicals* in that both are derived from the atom oxygen. Oxygen free radicals are also thought to play a key role in carcinogenesis. In addition to their general endogenous sources (e.g., mitochondria, enzymatic oxidation, peroxisomes), free radicals can be generated from exogenous sources such as (exposure to) heavy metals, industrial solvents, pesticides, tobacco smoke, alcohol, and radiation.

Likewise, adverse effects from environmental exposure to toxic metals are often conveniently treated as a special health concern. *Hexavalent chromium* (denoted by Cr^{6+} or CrVI) is a metal species used (directly or indirectly) in electroplating, textile manufacturing, and paints, and has been found in some drinking water sources. There is mounting evidence that this metal species can cause cancer in laboratory animals if they consume enough drinking water that contains it. The metal's harm to humans was publicized in the movie *Erin Brockovich* released in 2000. The toxic effects inducible by certain metals (e.g., Pb, Hg, Cd) are discussed in Chapter 14.

Some minerals and vitamins essential to human health can be harmful if they overload the body to beyond accommodation. Toxic effects from overdose of this group of substances too are sometimes treated as a special group of environmental diseases for public health concern purposes. This is because their health benefits are oftentimes overrated, leading to their overuse. *Zinc* (Zn), for instance, is a mineral (or more correctly a metallic element) that the human body needs to function properly. However, on rare occasions, some people can be poisoned if there is too much Zn present in their body. Another example is *selenium* (Se), which is an essential trace element; yet at high enough doses it can cause abnormal nails, hair loss, peripheral neuropathy, irritability, dermatitis, and other disorders. *Vitamin A overdose* is more specifically termed *hypervitaminosis A*, which can cause birth defects, liver abnormalities, and osteoporosis; otherwise, it is an essential nutrient known for its role in maintaining or promoting good vision. Still another example is *overdose with vitamin C*, which can cause stomachaches and diarrhea. People in certain health conditions, such as with hemochromatosis or kidney stones, should avoid taking too much of this vitamin which otherwise is known as a highly effective antioxidant capable of reducing oxidative stress (as caused by free radicals).

Persistent organic pollutants (POPs) are among the most prominent pollution-based substances that can cause a wide variety of adverse health effects in humans. They are hydrocarbon (hence by definition *organic*) compounds that persist in the environment likely for years to decades. They are capable of bioaccumulating and biomagnifying manifold in fatty tissues as they move up the food chains (Chapter 6). These environmental pollutants have been associated with many adverse health effects in humans and (other) animals, including reproductive disorders, damage to the nervous system, cancer, interference with the immunological system, and disruption of the endocrine system. There is strong evidence showing long-range transport of certain POPs to remote regions where they have never been used or produced. It was partly due to these findings that in May 2001, at an international conference held in Stockholm, Sweden, over 150 nations including the United States signed a global treaty known as the *Stockholm Convention* (of 2001) *on POPs*. This international treaty has its commitment to reduce or eliminate the global uses, releases, and/or productions of initially *twelve* POPs that are regarded as having the most urgent health concern to the global community.

These so-called "dirty dozen" POPs include: polychlorinated dibenzo-*p(ara)*-dioxins (PCDDs, also nicknamed *dioxins* for short); polychlorinated dibenzofurans (PCDFs, or *furans*); PCBs; and nine organochlorine pesticides (aldrin, chlordane, DDT, dieldrin, endrin, heptachlor, hexachlorobenzene, mirex, and toxaphene). These twelve POPs are also members of the chemical family known as *p*ersistent *o*rgano*c*hlorine compounds (POCs), as they all contain one or more chlorine atoms strongly bonded to their carbons. Many of these chemical compounds have been classified as from possible to likely human carcinogens and are from fairly to highly toxic to several body organs and systems including the liver, kidneys, skin, immunological system, reproductive system, endocrine system, and nervous system. As of 2017, there have been 15 new POPs added to the Stockholm Convention's initial action list (Chapter 16).

References

ALA (American Lung Association), 2010. Chronic Obstructive Pulmonary Disease (COPD) Fact Sheet. 1301 Pennsylvania Avenue NW, Suite 800, Washington DC, USA.

Anderson DM, Glibert PM, Burkholder JM, 2002. Harmful Algal Blooms and Eutrophication: Nutrient Sources, Composition, and Consequences. *Estuaries* 25:704-726.

Behrenfeld MJ, O'Malley RT, Siegel DA, McClain CR, Sarmiento JL, Feldman GC, Milligan AJ, Falkowski PG, Letelier RM, Boss ES, 2006. Climate-Driven Trends in Contemporary Ocean Productivity. *Nature* 444:752-755.

Cairns L, 2005. Electronic Waste: Finding Sustainable Solutions That Work Better for Consumers (A Consumers Union White Paper). Yonkers, New York, USA: Consumers Union.

Carson R, 1962. *Silent Spring*. Boston, Massachusetts, USA: Houghton Mifflin.

CDC (U.S. Centers for Disease Control and Prevention), 1997. Update: Blood Lead Levels – United States, 1991-1994. *MMWR* (CDC Morbidity and Mortality Weekly Report) 46:141-146.

CDC (U.S. Centers for Disease Control and Prevention), 2006. Improved National Prevalence Estimates for 18 Selected Major Birth Defects – United States, 1999-2001. *MMWR* 54:1301-1305.

CDC (U.S. Centers for Disease Control and Prevention), 2008. Update on Overall Prevalence of Major Birth Defects – Atlanta, Georgia, 1978-2005. *MMWR* 57:1-5.

Davidson K, Gowen RJ, Harrison PJ, Fleming LE, Hoagland P, Moschonas G, 2014. Anthropogenic Nutrients and Harmful Algae in Coastal Waters. *J. Environ. Magnt.* 146:206-216.

Duan H, Miller TR, Gregory J, Kirchain R, Linnel J, 2013. Quantitative Characterization of Domestic and Transboundary Flows of Used Electronics – Analysis of Generation, Collection, and Export in the United States. Published jointly by the MIT Materials Systems Laboratory and the National Center for Electronics Recycling under the umbrella of the StEP (Solving the E-Waste Problem) Initiative.

FAO (Food and Agriculture Organization of the United Nations), 2001. Forest Resources Assessment 2000. Main Report FAO Forestry Paper 140. FAO, Rome, Italy.

FAO (Food and Agriculture Organization of the United Nations), 2016. Global Forest Resources Assessment 2015 – How Are the World's Forests Changing? Second Edition. FAO, Rome, Italy.

IPCC (Intergovernmental Panel on Climate Change), 2007. Summary for Policymakers. In *Climate Change 2007: The Physical Science Basis. Contribution of Working Group I to the Fourth Assessment Report of the Intergovernmental Panel on Climate Change* (Solomon S, Qin D, Manning M, Chen Z, Marquis M, Averyt KB, Tignor M, Miller HL, Eds.). New York, New York, USA: Cambridge University Press.

IUATLD (International Union Against Tuberculosis and Lung Disease), 2011. The Global Asthma Report, 2011. 68 Boulevard Saint Michel, 75006 Paris, France (in collaboration with the International Study of Asthma and Allergies in Childhood [ISAAC]).

Kahn CM (Ed.), 2008. *The Merck Veterinary Manual* (Exotic and Laboratory Animals – Marine Mammals: Environmental Diseases), 9th Edition. Whitehouse Station, New Jersey, USA: Merck & Co.

King K, 2001. National Development Strategy – The Problems of the Health Sectors in Guyana. *Staboek News*, 23 September.

Lam CWY, Ho KC, 1989. Red Tides in Tolo Harbor, Hong Kong. In *Red Tides: Biology, Environmental Science and Toxicology* (Okaichi T, Anderson DM, Nemoto T, Eds.). New York, New York: Elsevier.

Landrigan PJ, Schechter CB, Lipton JM, Fahs MC, Schwartz J, 2002. Environmental Pollutants and Disease in American Children: Estimates of Morbidity, Mortality, and Costs for Lead Poisoning, Asthma, Cancer, and Developmental Disabilities. *Environ. Health Perspect.* 110:721-728.

Lobell DB, Burke MB, Tebaldi C, Mastrandrea MD, Falcon WP, Naylor RL, 2008. Prioritizing Climate Change Adaptation Needs for Food Security in 2030. *Science* 319:607-610.

Lund HG, Iremonger S, 1998. Omissions, Commissions, and Decisions – The Need for Integrated Resource Assessments. Proceedings from First International Conference – Geospatial Information in Agriculture and Forestry – Decision Support, Technology, and Applications. 1-3 June 1998, Lake Buena Vista, Florida, USA. ERIM International I:182-189.

Matzner E (Ed.), 2004. *Biogeochemistry of Forested Catchments in a Changing Environment – A German Case Study*. New York, New York, USA: Springer-Verlag.

NCHS (U.S. National Center for Health Statistics), 2016. Health, United States, 2015 – With Special Feature on Racial and Ethnic Health Disparities. NCHS, U.S. Centers for Disease Control and Prevention, Hyattsville, Maryland, USA.

NHSR (National Health Statistics Reports), 2013. Infertility and Impaired Fecundity in the United States, 1982-2010: Data from the National Survey of Family Growth (reported by A. Chandra, C.E. Copen, and E.H. Stephen). No. 67 (August 14). NHSR, U.S. Centers for Disease Control and Prevention, Hyattsville, Maryland, USA.

RDHN (*Rachel's Democracy & Health News*), 2006. Environment, Health, Jobs and Justices – Who Gets to Decide? News No.836, 5 January.

Sarmiento JL, Slater R, Barber R, Bopp L, Doney SC, Hirst AC, Kleypas J, Matear R, Mikolajewicz U, Monfray P, et al., 2004. Response of Ocean Ecosystems to Climate Warming. *Global Biogeochem. Cycles* V18:GB3003 (online journal).

Time, 1975. Disease of the Century. 20 October.

TWI (Third World Institute; Instituto del Tercer Mundo – IteM), 1999. *The World Guide 1999/2000 – An Alternative Reference to the Countries of Our Planet* (1. The Earth and Its Peoples/Deforestation). PO Box 1539, Montevideo 11000, Uruguay.

UNEP (United Nations Environment Programme), 2005. *One Planet Many People: Atlas of Our Changing Environment*. United Nations Avenue, Gigiri, PO Box 30552-00100, Nairobi, Kenya.

WHO (World Health Organization), 2003. WHD (World Health Day) Brochure, Part II: Introduction. Geneva, Switzerland.

WHO (World Health Organization), 2011. Environmental Health (webpage dated 2011). http://www.who.int/topics/environmental_health/en/ (retrieved 15 August 2012).

Williams M, 1990. Forest. In *The Earth as Transformed by Human Action* (Turner BL II, Ed.). New York, New York, USA: Cambridge University Press.

Williams M, 1994. Forest and Tree Cover. In *Changes in Land Use and Land Cover. A Global Perspective* (Meyer WB, Turner BL, II, Eds.). New York, New York, USA: Cambridge University Press.

Review Questions
1. What are the three fundamental, interrelated aspects concerning environmental changes that merit their consideration in studying environmental toxicology?
2. What is greenhouse effect? Name five major greenhouse gases that can cause this effect.
3. How can global warming affect human health, agricultural productivity, and the ocean ecosystems?
4. What may be defined as soil pollution?
5. What happened to London (UK) in December 1952 in relation to environmental health?
6. What was the main issue with the Love Canal tragedy in the United States?
7. Name a metal that was publicized in an American film in 2000 as a water pollutant threatening human health in the United States.
8. Name a neurotoxin found in algae that might have been responsible for the intoxication and killing of coastal birds, fish, and marine mammals.
9. Why is there a global environmental health concern with e-waste?
10. What are some of the environmental health concerns with deforestation?
11. Explain briefly why not all environmental changes should always be regarded as bad or unwelcome.
12. Why are children uniquely more susceptible to environmental diseases?
13. Name two types of classic occupational diseases reported in the 1800s or earlier.
14. What were the four categories of pediatric diseases identified in the early 2000s as responsible for nearly 3% of total healthcare costs in the United States?
15. List two or more environmental factors that (on their own or in combination) may need to add up before a malignant growth can be developed in the (human) body.
16. What are free radicals? What are some of their exogenous sources? And briefly explain why some of them can cause cardiac attack.
17. Briefly characterize the "dirty dozen" POPs (persistent organic pollutants) whose productions and uses are subjected to global elimination or reduction under the Stockholm Convention treaty. As of 2017, how many new POPs have been added to the Convention's initial action list?

18. Match each of the toxic agents in the left column to only one of the diseases or health effects in the right column that the agent can or tend to induce:

    (1) diethylstilbestrol   (a) reproductive effect
    (2) ethylene dibromide   (b) dermatitis
    (3) asbestos   (c) respiratory disease
    (4) DDT   (d) hepatocarcinogenicity
    (5) propargite   (e) birth defect
    (6) aflatoxin B_1 (f) stomach ache
    (7) vitamin C   (g) neurological effect

CHAPTER 3

Environmental Pollution and Regulatory Agencies

3.1. Introduction

As in line with the definitions of air pollution and water pollution given in Chapter 2, environmental pollution simply refers to the presence of one or more contaminants in any component of the (or a certain) environment at such concentrations, durations, and frequencies that they can cause adverse effects on the health of living organisms or their environment. On the other hand, urbanization and industrialization are human-related activities representing two key phenomena in modern time that can bring about serious environmental pollution (as well as environmental changes) whether at the local or global level. The reciprocal interrelationships (of uneven strength) among these phenomena may be summarized schematically as depicted in the upper portion of Figure 3.1 below. Moreover, throughout this chapter as well as this book, the terms *pollution* and *contamination* are treated as synonymous for simplicity sake (as well as to go with the flow).

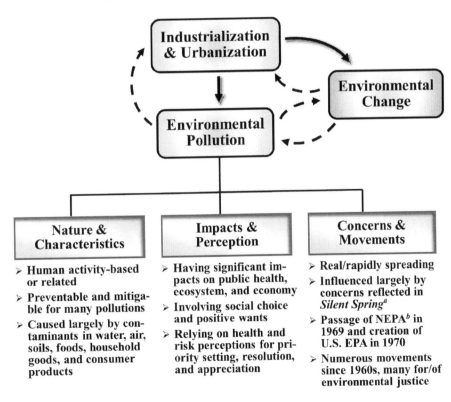

Figure 3.1. Major Characteristics, Impacts, Perceptions, and Concerns of Environmental Pollution Particularly in the United States ([a]Carson [1962]; [b]NEPA ≡ U.S. National Environmental Policy Act)

Implicit in the reciprocal interrelationships depicted in Figure 3.1 above is the general notion that most environmental pollutions are preventable or mitigable conditions, insomuch as the underlying cause for each is almost always linked to one or more human activities. For instance, motor vehicle emission is a human activity-based event that can lead to air pollution. And automobiles are the source contributing up to 90% of the noise pollution in certain parts of the world (e.g., EEA, 2014; Renshaw, 2012). Other human activity-based sources of concern include solid waste disposal facilities, incinerators, large farmlands, and industrial processes, from which many common environmental contaminants involve toxic metals, harmful pesticides, and hazardous chlorinated hydrocarbons. Environmental pollution can also be the consequence of a natural disaster, such as a hurricane which can lead to water pollution from sewage and cause petrochemical spills from ruptured automobiles and boats. Even so, sewage is primarily a human activity-related waste product whereas automobiles and boats are simply human-made conveyances.

3.1.1. Impacts of Environmental Pollution

The impacts of environmental pollution on human health and the ecosystem are profound and real. Environmental pollution along with environmental change has altered the disease pattern in many developed and developing nations over the past 60 years, largely from infectious to chronic diseases being the major causes of death. The growing concern of the *health* impacts of environmental pollution is the focal point of Section 3.2. Yet another even more serious type of impacts is the associated ultimate *economic* loss and burden. This type is far beyond the one incurred for healthcare alone, as can be readily reflected in the monetary example given in Table 3.1 below.

Table 3.1. Estimated Economic Losses Resulting from Pollutions in China around 1992[a]

Impact Factor/Cause Category	Economic Loss (US$ Billion)	Percentage of Total Loss
Water Pollution	4.95	36.1
human health	2.68	(19.5)
industry	1.92	
crop yields	0.19	
livestock	0.10	
fisheries	0.06	
Air Pollution	8.05	58.7
human health	2.80	(20.4)
agriculture	1.00	
household upkeep	1.87	
clothing	0.15	
vehicles	0.15	
buildings	0.13	
acid rain	1.95	
Solid Waste	0.71	5.2
Total	*13.72*	*100.0*

[a]adapted from Xia (1998); 1 US$ ≈ 7.2 ¥ (Chinese *Yuan*, at around the year 1992 currency exchange rate).

As shown in Table 3.1 above, China's total economic loss resulting from environmental pollution around the year 1992 was estimated at about US$13 billion (Xia, 1998). Of this total loss, roughly 59% and 36% were from air pollution and water pollution, respectively, with 40% being for or due to human health regardless of pollution type or source. In essence, the remaining 60% (of the US$13 billion) loss from air, water, and solid waste pollutions combined was for or due to causes and costs other than healthcare-related.

In most instances, such huge economic and health impacts as well as burdens are treated by many scientific and regulatory sectors as highly preventable, though with the understanding that a total elimination of the source(s) is rarely a practical solution. Inasmuch as the causes of environmental pollution are related mostly to human activities, regulatory actions that reflect or involve some form of public decision are generally needed in order to maintain a balance between a community's positive wants and the negative impacts involved. It is the need for such a balance that sets a place for ecological (Chapter 22) and human health (Chapter 23) risk assessment, a scientific paradigm as well as a socioeconomic ideology that has preoccupied, if not masterminded, the field of environmental toxicology since the 1980s.

3.1.2. Perceptions of Environmental Pollution

Ideally, in addition to scientific concerns, the decision for the balance between a community's positive wants and negative impacts should involve cultural, ethical, socioeconomic, and legal considerations. Given the limited resources that governments have, there is a further need to determine whether one pollution source has more or less impacts on human health or the ecosystem than another source has. Regulatory bodies in the position to make such decisions oftentimes need (or opt) to share the complex information on their risk assessment with their stakeholders (i.e., those with an interest in or a concern on the matter). Such sharing is considered highly desirable, if not inevitable, inasmuch as public health activity is a subset of social choice. This subset is a systematic process whereby collective goals are to be pursued and appropriate decisions are to be resolved. In reality, the public's support for any of such decisions comes down largely to a matter of local and individual perception of health risk, since many citizens lack much of the required technical background.

The concept that (health) risk perception is basically a subjective judgmental behavior may be best illustrated starting with the example given by Neely (1994) on traffic accidents. From the 1980s to the 1990s, each year there were roughly 20,000 to 30,000 deaths reported in the United States as from traffic accidents caused by drunk driving. Statistics of this kind were accepted by most Americans with little reactions, at least in terms of prevention and regulatory actions. In contrast, the tampon-toxic shock scare in the early 1980s had received far more public attention, even though the total number of victims did not amount to one weekend's traffic fatalities. The contrast made here bears no accusation that public concerns on drunk driving were low or lacking in those days. Rather, people's dread over a situation or crisis is what has just been contrasted. To many people, dread is an important factor responsible for the development of a person's health risk perception (e.g., Tversky and Kahneman, 1974; U.S. EPA, 2007), as so readily evident in the tampon-toxic shock story.

Toxic shock syndrome (TSS) was not officially recognized as an illness by the U.S. Centers for Disease Control and Prevention (CDC) until the early months of 1980, when the institute received the first 55 cases characterized by a sudden onset of fever, sunburn-like rash, low blood pressure, desquamation (i.e., skin shedding), and abnormalities in three or more major body organs (CDC, 1990). This illness, occurring predominantly in women, was soon confirmed as caused by the bacterium *Streptococcus aureus* and highly correlated with the use of super-absorbent synthetic tampons. The panic over TSS then started creeping rapidly into the minds of many American women within that year which had reportedly the highest as well as the only significant annual incidence of 852 cases and 38 deaths (CDC, 1990). *Streptococcus aureus*, a species commonly colonized in the vagina as well as the nasal and throat passages, is harmless to about 95% of the American population as these people have antibodies to the bacterium's toxin responsible for the toxic shock. For the 5% lacking the antibodies, they are highly susceptible to the fatal disease. Yet apparently, these individuals would have a much higher risk when using super-absorbent synthetic tampons as this type of materials provides an ideal breeding ground for the bacteria.

The fear for TSS among American women, which lingered over to the next couple of years long after the successful recall of the super-absorbent tampons, was apparently not due to the low morbidity and small death toll experienced. Rather, it was largely due to the *dread* that TSS was conceived (perceived) at that time as a highly uncontrollable epidemic sweeping across the nation. That situation was in many ways similar to the more recent situation involving the H1N1 flu pandemic initiated in 2009 (Chapter 1), where CDC released a novel harmless virus for vaccine production (CIDRAP, 2009) even two weeks ahead of the pandemic declaration on 11 June 2009. Such urgency for the vaccine development was based more on the public's concerns over the virus being a new strain with unpredictable epidemic virulence, than on the unimpressive statistic toll experienced with the disease at the time.

The H1N1 pandemic is used as another example here not so much that it fits well the common definition of environmental pollution. It is included here simply because the urgency for the vaccine development and production was based on some form of environmental health risk assessment. Again, as mentioned in Chapter 1, any laboratory confirmation of a viral pathogen or any laboratory development of a high-yield vaccine virus is truly relevant to toxicity testing, the role of a toxicologist with the appropriate training.

3.2. Concerns with Environmental Pollution

In the United States and many other countries, the public's concerns of environmental pollution are real and rapidly spreading. It was back in the 1960s that most scholars and organizations proclaimed the work in *Silent Spring* by Rachel Carson (1962) the starting point of the modern environmental movement. In Carson's book, numerous case studies (or anecdotes as so treated by some people) are included to describe the environmental problems associated with the use of hazardous pesticides and other chemicals in the United States and worldwide. In particular, her book cites several experimental observations purporting to show the link between the spraying of the organochlorine pesticide DDT and the reproductive failure or the survival of several bird species.

Her book also describes in detail the toxic effects that chemical control had placed on all key components of the environment, including air, water, land, wildlife, and humans.

Carson's book was not without serious criticism, as there were enough people appreciating the vital role in which DDT played in controlling malaria transmission by killing the mosquitoes that carried the disease (i.e., the toxin). Yet in numerous places in her book, Carson's concerns and arguments should still be considered fair, objective, and valid. At the least, she did point out explicitly that "*No responsible person contends that insect-borne disease should be ignored. The question that has now urgently presented itself is whether it is either wise or responsible to attack the problem by methods that are rapidly making it worse. The world has heard much of the triumphant war against disease through the control of insect vectors of infection, but it has heard little of the other side of the story.*"

3.2.1. Regulatory Concerns in the United States

The environmental concerns reflected in *Silent Spring* were more than just welcome by the environmental movement community. These concerns were regarded by many sectors as the driving forces behind the creation of both a powerful regulatory agency and the most significant piece of environmental legislation in the American history. It was in late 1969, less than 10 years since the publication of *Silent Spring*, that U.S. Congress presented to the Executive Branch a landmark bill known as the National Environmental Policy Act (NEPA), which was signed into law by then President Richard Nixon on New Year's Day in 1970. NEPA's stated purpose was (and still is) threefold as follows:

- To declare a national policy which will encourage productive and enjoyable harmony between (the people) and (their) environment.

- To promote efforts which will prevent or eliminate damage to the environment and biosphere and stimulate the health and welfare of (the people).

- To enrich (people's) understanding of the ecological systems and natural resources important to the Nation.

Initially and promptly, the U.S. Council of Environmental Quality (CEQ) was formed to fulfill NEPA's statutory intents. Yet the environmental concerns at the time were so intensified by the influence of Carson's work that, before the year 1970 was over, President Nixon was compelled to establish a strong, independent agency by piecing together various programs from several federal agencies. That strong, independent body was named the U.S. Environmental Protection Agency, a federal agency now commonly known by its acronym (U.S.) EPA (and henceforth so used in this book). The intense concerns for environmental issues at the time were evidenced best by the first Earth Day celebration held on 22 April 1970, which brought around 20 million Americans out into the spring sunshine for peaceful grassroots type demonstrations in support of environmental reform (Lewis, 1985). Coincidentally or not, the notion for Earth Day evolved over a period of seven years beginning also in 1962, the year *Silent Spring* was first published.

As Jack Lewis (1985) of U.S. EPA put it well in his article *The Birth of EPA*, "Silent Spring *played in the history of environmentalism roughly the same role that* Uncle Tom's Cabin *played in the abolitionist movement. In fact, EPA today may be said without exaggeration to be the extended shadow of Rachel Carson. The influence of her book has brought together over 14,000 scientists, lawyers, managers, and other employees across the country to fight the good fight for environmental protection.*" At the time of its formation, President Nixon wanted U.S. EPA to be a powerful regulatory agency with the specific responsibility to:

- Establish and enforce environmental protection standards.
- Conduct environmental research.
- Provide assistance to others combating environmental pollution.
- Assist the CEQ (U.S. Council of Environmental Quality) in developing and recommending to the President new policies for environmental protection.

Many of U.S. EPA's early efforts, including the enforcement of Federal Insecticide, Fungicide, and Rodenticide Act (FIFRA) which underwent a significant revision in 1972, are thought to have been related to Carson's work (Hynes, 1989). Some of such early efforts are summarized in *The Birth of EPA*, in which Rachel Carson is specifically described as a person who "*derived her missionary zeal from her fear that fewer species of birds would be singing each spring unless pesticide poisoning was curtailed.*"

It is not surprising that today the concerns with environmental pollution in the United States are far more in scope than dealing with such fundamentals as the creation of U.S. EPA or the passage of NEPA. Nowadays, the concerns and movements on environmental pollution have much to do with, among other things, *environmental justice*. Environmental justice is an idealism centering on the principle that no one sector of the community, including racial, ethnic, national origin, or socioeconomic groups, should be disproportionately impacted by pesticides or other toxic substances. It asserts that anyone whose health or environment may be affected by any chemical exposure shall hold a *stake* in the regulatory process at any level of government. This idealism or ideology is being upheld seriously by U.S. EPA and many state agencies including notably the California Environmental Protection Agency. This type of concerns, along with other aspects of environmental pollution discussed earlier, is summarized schematically in the lower portion of Figure 3.1.

3.2.2. Actions on Environmental Pollution Impacts

Many regulatory and organizational actions have been implemented in the modern past to cope with the health and economic impacts of environmental pollution. Such actions are evident from several environmental legislations enacted and several environmental movements advocated in recent years in the United States and worldwide. These legislations and movements include: the U.S. Clean Air Act; the U.S. Clean Water Act; the FIFRA; the reforestation movement; the anti-red tide movement; the Stockholm Convention on Persistent Organic Pollutants (POPs); and the United Nations' (UN's) establishment of the Intergovernmental Panel on Climate Change (IPCC). Many of these environmental movements and regulatory actions have either caused significant changes to local and global environments or led to new perspectives on environmental regulation, such as the Superfund (law) of 1980 (which was passed under public pressure to provide funding initially for the cleanup of toxic waste buried in Love Canal; *see* Chapter 2 or 22).

In brief but more specifically, the U.S. Clean Air Act of 1970 was amended once more in 1990 to curb three major threats to the nation's natural environment and the health of Americans. The three major threats of air quality concern are acid rain, urban air pollution, and toxic air emissions (e.g., U.S. EPA, 2008a). Similar clean air legislations have been passed in some states and some other countries.

As proclaimed by U.S. EPA (2008b), the U.S. Clean Water Act of 1972 (amended in 1987) is regarded as *"The cornerstone of surface water quality protection in the United States."* This federal statute employs a variety of regulatory and non-regulatory tools to limit direct contaminant discharges into waterways, to finance the municipal wastewater treatment systems, and to manage non-point pollution (e.g., polluted runoff).

The main focus of FIFRA of 1972 was to provide federal control of pesticide distribution, sale, and use in the United States (e.g., U.S. EPA, 2008c). The act gives U.S. EPA the authority not only to assess the consequences of pesticide usage, but also to require certain users (e.g., farmers) to register their pesticides at the time of purchase.

Reforestation movement appeared to have gained serious public attention beginning in the early 1920s (e.g., *The New York Times*, 1922). Yet until more recent years, the American movement of reforestation had been slow compared to those occurring in some developing regions. For instance, it was estimated (FAO, 2010) that during the 20-year period between 1990 and 2010, the United States gained slightly over 900,000 acres of forest each year. In contrast, close to 80 million trees (approximately 20,000 acres) were planted in Indonesia as part of the country's 2007 National Reforestation Movement, all completed within just one week of November with its people from all walks of life (e.g., Reuters.com, 2007).

One prominent American organization with a mission to control and mitigate red tide pollution is Solutions to Avoid Red Tide (also known by its acronym START), which is a member of the Red Tide Alliance. The alliance, which is a partnership located in the state of Florida, consists of the Florida Department of Health in Tallahassee, the Mote Marine Laboratory in Sarasota, and the Florida Fish & Wildlife Research Institute in Saint Petersburg. A similar organization also founded in the United States is the Gulf Coast Preservation Society, with a mission being to restore and protect the rich marine habitat of the Gulf of Mexico. On the other side of the globe, Japan and South Korea had been in the forefront in dispersing clays on a large scale as flocculants to protect aquatic life from red tide pollution (Sengco and Andersen, 2004).

Under the global Stockholm Convention treaty of 2001 on POPs, participating parties are each required to seriously commit to both the development and the implementation of a plan to fulfill their obligations of eliminating or reducing the releases of certain POPs into the environment. It has been projected at an international scientific conference (Dong, 2006), and there is now more evidence emerging (Chapter 16), that their share of the commitment and the number of POPs under consideration continue to expand.

For actions on global climate change, former U.S. Vice-President Al Gore and the UN panel IPCC were awarded the 2007 Nobel Peace Prize for their work on this environmental issue. That award can be regarded as a recognition signifying their many years of efforts in building up and disseminating greater knowledge about human-made climate changes. Al Gore also won an Oscar award in 2007 for his documentary film on global warming. The film, distributed by Paramount Pictures in 2006, was titled *"An Inconvenient Truth"*. Yet despite these high levels of recognition, neither IPCC's work nor Al Gore's on global warming is without merit challenge. There are enough skeptics not convinced that global warming is an environmental issue, particularly in light of the e-mail controversy on climate change. In 2009, hundreds of private e-mail messages and documents were reportedly hacked from a computer server housed at the University of East Anglia in England. The hacked climate e-mails, some of which were sent as far back as in the late 1990s, reportedly caused a stir among skeptics who argued that climate scholars had conspired to deliberately overstate the case for a *human* influence on global warming (Revkin, 2009).

3.3. Environmental Health Laws and Agencies

Treaties, legislations, regulations, and policies pertaining to environmental health and safety are generally enacted or adopted as a result of certain public health concerns or movements. Yet the extent to which the entities are concerned with a particular environmental health issue is influenced largely by their appreciation and perception of environmental health. As noted in Section 2.1.3, the World Health Organization (WHO, 2011) considers environmental health as the realm of concern (or program activity) that *"Addresses all the physical, chemical, and biological factors external to a person, and all the related factors impacting behaviours. It encompasses the assessment and control of those environmental factors that can potentially affect health."* Environmental health legislations thereby refer to the rules of conduct adopted specifically to address (or otherwise to assess and control) the various major aspects of this realm. It should be noted that all laws, including those relevant to environmental health, are with binding legal force and are enforced by appropriate government authorities at the local, national, or international level. Laws are found in treaties, statutes, constitutional provisions, regulations, and court decisions.

More often than not, there are chaos and disorder over the interpretation of certain key legal jargon among toxicologists, especially those not working in a regulatory agency. Therefore, a basic understanding of certain legal terms may become advantageous for health scientists working in or around a regulatory agency. For instance, it is important to note that *statute* is a law created by a legislative body, whether at the regional, federal, state, or local level. It may mean a single or a collection of acts. *Regulation*, on the other hand, is an official rule or order promulgated by government authority. Regulations too have the force of law and are intended to implement a specific statute, oftentimes to direct the conduct of those regulated by the regulating authority.

Another term subject to confusion also requiring clarification is *(agency or organization) policy*, which refers to a deliberate program or course of action intended to guide, influence, or determine certain (agency or organization) decisions, actions, or outcomes. It can also be defined as a statement or an agendum set forth by an (a public) organization to relate its goals and intents to the overall performance of its action or activity. Moreover, the term *order* is an authoritative direction given by a court, another adjudicative entity, or an authority intended to be obeyed. In contrast, the terms *guidelines, guidance*, and in some cases *standard* are advisory in nature and do not have the full force of law. At most, they represent rules or a series of steps to be carried out to implement a policy more efficaciously in an efficient, legal, and/or professional manner.

3.3.1. Regulatory Agencies in the United States

In the United States, environmental health laws at the national level are regulated and enforced by certain federal agencies, which have the added duties to establish and implement their own agency policies and standards relevant to these federal statutes. In the United States, the more prominent federal regulatory agencies implementing environmental health and safety laws include: U.S. EPA (U.S. Environmental Protection Agency); U.S. Food and Drug Administration (FDA); U.S. Occupational Safety and Health Administration (OSHA); U.S. Consumer Product Safety Commission (CPSC); and U.S. Department of Transportation (DOT).

Briefly, U.S. EPA is a non-cabinet regulatory agency charged with safeguarding human health and improving as well as preserving the nation's natural environment. Its areas of environmental health and regulatory concerns include, but are not limited to: air quality and pollution; water quality and pollution; hazardous substances; ecosystems and natural resources; solid and toxic wastes; pesticides; ocean dumping; indoor air; drinking water; oil pollution; and toxic sites. The agency began operation on 2 December 1970, less than a year since the passage of NEPA (U.S. National Environmental Policy Act).

FDA is part of the U.S. Department of Health and Human Services. It is responsible for the safety and health regulations of most types of foods, drugs, cosmetics, food additives, dietary supplements, veterinary products, radiation-emitting devices, medical devices, vaccines, and blood products. The agency's current name was officialized in 1930, with its root dating back to the early 1900s or earlier.

OSHA is an agency of the U.S. Department of Labor. It was created by U.S. Congress under the federal Occupational Safety and Health Act of 1970 (Chapter 20). The agency's mission is to prevent work-related injuries, illnesses, and deaths by promulgating and enforcing standards for workplace safety and health.

CPSC is an independent agency of the U.S. federal government, and was established under the federal Consumer Product Safety Act (CPSA) of 1972. This federal agency is charged with safeguarding consumers (especially children in families) against unreasonable risks of illnesses and injuries associated with products that pose a fire, electrical, chemical, or mechanical hazard or that can cause injury specifically to children.

Beginning operation on 1 April 1967, DOT was established by U.S. Congress as a cabinet department of the Executive Branch. It has the mission to ensure a fast, safe, efficient, accessible, and convenient transportation system for the nation. In terms of environmental health, its areas of regulatory concern include: water shipment of toxic materials (sharing responsibility with U.S. Coast Guard); oil pollution (sharing responsibility with U.S. Coast Guard and U.S. EPA); and transport of hazardous materials in general.

3.3.2. Environmental Health Laws in the United States

Table 3.2 provides a quick overview of the more prominent federal laws dealing with environmental exposures. Also listed in the table are the areas of environmental health and regulatory concerns that each statute covers, as well as the principal federal agency(ies) that is (are) charged with regulating and enforcing the specific statute or its certain aspects.

For the most part, the connection should become clear between each federal statute listed in Table 3.2 and the principal federal agency(ies) charged with enforcing it, once the areas of concern covered by that law have become transparent. One exception is perhaps the connection for the Food Quality Protection Act (FQPA) of 1996, as the law involves the responsibilities of both FDA and U.S. EPA. The law was enacted as an amendment to both FIFRA and the (Federal) Food, Drug, and Cosmetic Act (FD&C Act). This specific amendment calls for stricter safety standards for pesticide residues in foods, particularly for young children under the assumption that this age group tends to be more susceptible to environmental exposure. The FQPA of 1996 requires a complete health risk reassessment of all existing tolerances (i.e., limits) set on the amount of pesticide residues being allowed to remain in or on foods marketed in the United States.

Another connection lacking transparency to some people is that for the Oil Pollution Act (OPA) of 1990, which involves not only U.S. Coast Guard and DOT but also U.S. EPA. This law was enacted in response to the pollution problem caused by the oil tanker *Exxon Valdez*, which on 24 March 1989 spilled over 10 million gallons of crude oil into the water of Prince William Sound (Alaska). The law amended the U.S. Clean Water Act and addressed the wide range of problems associated with the prevention of, response to, and cleanup payment for oil pollution incidents in navigable U.S. waters. Three more federal statutes are likewise noteworthy here. These are the Comprehensive Environmental Response, Compensation, & Liability Act (CERCLA) of 1980, the Bioterrorism Act of 2002, and the FHSA (Federal Hazardous Substances Act) of 1960. From its title, FHSA might not be thought of as primarily for household products and hence not for CPSC alone to regulate and enforce. Yet it is narrower in scope than its title might suggest. The statute is intended primarily for regulation of children's toys and household products.

As further discussed in Chapter 22, CERCLA is more commonly known as Superfund (law). The law was enacted initially in response to the threat of hazardous waste buried the Love Canal toxic site (Section 2.2.4). It allows the federal government to tax on the chemical and petroleum industries for compensation and liability purposes, as reflected in the law's title. Over the first five years after the law's passage, $1.6 billion were collected into a trust fund for use to clean up abandoned or uncontrolled toxic waste sites. The accumulated trust fund is now more known as Superfund, which now becomes CERCLA's nickname. Although Superfund created the U.S. Agency for Toxic Substances and Disease Registry (ATSDR), it empowers U.S. EPA alone to compel the responsible parties to clean up sites that they have contaminated.

Note that the Public Health Security & Bioterrorism Preparedness and Response Act of 2002 (or Bioterrorism Act for short) is not listed in Table 3.2, since it is treated as having less pertinence to factors that are generally addressed under the realm of environmental health. It is nonetheless regarded by some people as the more recent U.S. federal statute on issues relevant to some aspects of environmental health.

Table 3.2. The More Prominent Federal Environmental Health Laws and Regulatory Concerns in the United States[a]

Federal Statute[b]	Areas of Regulatory and Environmental Health Concerns	Agency(ies)[c,d]
(Federal) Food, Drug, & Cosmetic Act (FD&C Act, 1938; amended 2007)	Safety regulation on foods, drugs, cosmetics, medical devices, vaccines, blood products, dietary supplements, color additives, veterinary products, radiation-emitting devices, and more.	FDA
Federal Insecticide, Fungicide & Rodenticide Act (FIFRA, 1947; amended 2007)	Safety regulation on use, sale, and distribution of pesticides	EPA
Federal Hazardous Substances Act (1960; amended 2011)	Safety regulation on household products (especially on product labeling)	CPSC
National Environmental Policy Act (1969; amended 1982)	Promotion of harmony between the people and their environment	EPA
Occupational Safety and Health Act (1970; amended 2004)	Safety standards for toxic agents in (primarily nongovernment) workplaces	OSHA
Poison Prevention Packaging Act (1970; amended 2008)	Child-resistant packaging for toxic household products	CPSC
U.S. Clean Air Act (1970; amended 1990)	Regulation and improvement of nation's air quality	EPA
U.S. Clean Water Act (1972; amended 1987)	Regulation and improvement of nation's water quality	EPA
Consumer Product Safety Act (1972; amended 2011)	Safety regulation on hazardous consumer products	CPSC
Safe Drinking Water Act (1974; amended 1996)	Protection and improvement of nation's drinking water quality	EPA
Hazardous Materials Transportation Act (1975; amended 1990)	Safety regulation on transportation of hazardous and toxic materials in commerce	DOT
Resource Conservation & Recovery Act (1976; amended 1984)	Safety regulation on solid waste disposal, including disposal of hazardous wastes, on *active* sites	EPA
Toxic Substances Control Act (1976; amended 1992)	Safety regulation (including premarket review/approval) on hazardous substances not covered by other statutes,	EPA
Comprehensive Environmental Response, Compensation, & Liability Act (1980; amended 1986; a.k.a. Superfund)	Safety regulation on *inactive* sites contaminated with hazardous wastes	EPA
Oil Pollution Act (1990; amended 2000)	Mitigation and prevention of oil pollution and oil spills	DOT, USCG
Pollution Prevention Act (1990)	Reduction of pollution at and through the source	EPA
Food Quality Protection Act (FQPA, 1996; amended versions of FIFRA and FD&C Act)	Safety regulation on pesticide residues in foods, with a focus on children's exposure	EPA, FDA

[a] see, e.g., Beck et al. (2008) for further discussion, which is the initial source for this table; [b] in parentheses are year of statute's passage and, if any, year of (key or latest) amendment; [c] sole or principal agencies; [d] FDA ≡ U.S. Food and Drug Administration, EPA ≡ U.S. Environmental Protection Agency, CPSC ≡ U.S. Consumer Product Safety Commission, OSHA ≡ U.S. Occupational Safety and Health Administration, DOT ≡ U.S. Department of Transportation, and USCG ≡ U.S. Coast Guard.

3.3.3. Foreign Environmental Health Laws and Agencies

There are likewise numerous environmental health laws and regulatory entities abroad that are equally influential in protecting human health from exposure to environmental contaminants, whether at the global, regional, or national level. A good example is the *Stockholm Convention (on POPs)* treaty, which was adopted in 2001 and put into force in 2004 by more than 150 nations. The aims of this treaty are to schedule and implement worldwide use reduction or elimination of all the POPs put on the Convention's action list, by starting with the twelve that were (and still are) regarded as the worst (and hence the nickname *dirty dozen* given to them).

Another good example is the *Basel Convention on the Control of Transboundary Movements of Hazardous Wastes and Their Disposal*, or Basel Convention for short. This international treaty is regarded as the most comprehensive global environmental agreement on hazardous and other wastes. It represents over 170 parties with the aims of protecting human health and the environment against the harmful effects that may result from improper handling of the wastes at issue, including their disposal, generation, and transboundary movements. The Basel Convention came into force in 1992.

A third example for treaties at the global level is the *Montreal Protocol on Substances That Deplete the Ozone Layer*, or Montreal Protocol for short. This international treaty was adopted to protect ozone (O_3) in the air zone second closest (i.e., the stratosphere layer) to the Earth by phasing out the production of a number of substances (e.g., freons, halons) determined as responsible for ozone depletion. The treaty was opened for signature on 16 September 1987, and put into force on 1 January 1989.

For international health agencies with a regulatory role, among the first coming to the minds of many people is WHO (World Health Organization). Yet legally, WHO may assume only a *coordinating* authority for public health matters within the United Nations system. While the organization's stated mission is "*the attainment by all peoples of the highest possible level of health*", its main activities include: providing leadership on environmental health and other global health matters; shaping health research agenda; setting public health norms and standards; monitoring and assessing health trends; as well as offering technical support to countries in the world.

Another equally influential, equally prominent international organization is the United Nations Environment Programme (UNEP). It serves as the *designated* authority of the United Nations system in tackling and resolving environmental (health) issues at the global and regional levels. Much like WHO, UNEP is not truly a health *regulatory* agency. Regardless, its influential activities do cover a broad range of environmental issues concerning the atmospheric, oceanic, and terrestrial ecosystems, as well as human health.

There are also a number of regulatory authorities abroad at the national or regional level that are as influential and active as those in the United States. These foreign authorities include: the Commission for Environmental Cooperation (CEC); the European Environment Agency (EEA); China's Ministry of Environmental Protection (CMEP); Japan's Ministry of the Environment (JMOE); Australia Department of the Environment and Energy (ADEE); Health Canada; and Germany's Federal Environment Agency (UBA, as from its German name Umwelt Bundesamt). The missions of these foreign entities are similar, all aiming to control and prevent environmental pollution as well as to safeguard public health and preserve the natural environment. As with those agencies in the United States (e.g., U.S. EPA, FDA, CPSC, OSHA), many of these foreign entities are charged with a similar responsibility of enforcing and promoting their own regional or national laws, regulations, and policies that are pertinent to environmental health.

More specifically, CEC was established by Canada, Mexico, and the United States in 1994 under the North American Agreement on Environmental Cooperation, with the aims to address the tri-nation region's environmental issues. The commission was created to foster conservation, protection, and enhancement of the North American environment. In particular, it tracks pollutant releases and supports chemicals management across North America.

EEA is a research arm as well as a monitoring agency of the European Union. Its main task is to provide sound, independent information concerning or relevant to the quality of the natural environment in the region. The agency has 33 countries as its members and another six as cooperating members (as of July 2017). With respect to environmental health, EEA has several functional components addressing issues on air pollution, climate change, industrial pollution, water pollution, noise pollution, and biodiversity in and for the region.

CMEP (China's MEP) is a cabinet-level ministry established in 2008 taking over the responsibilities of China's State Environmental Protection Administration (CSEPA) for the nation's environmental governance. The ministry's regulatory role includes efforts to control and prevent environmental pollution, preserve the nation's natural environment, ensure nuclear safety, and protect public health. Many of these agenda were those of the CSEPA that survived for 20 years.

JMOE is a cabinet-level ministry in Japan. It was upgraded in 2001 from its sub-cabinet level Environmental Agency established in 1971. The then sub-cabinet agency, as well as now JMOE, had many regulatory agenda similar to those of U.S. EPA.

ADEE is a federal level department charged with the responsibility to develop and implement the Australian government's policies and programs pertinent to environment protection and conservation of biodiversity. These environmental agenda are delivered primarily under five major pillars: clear air, clean water, clean land, national heritage, and recently energy efficiency. The recent pillar was cemented to ADEE's ground due to the transfer of the responsibility for energy policy to the department on 19 July 2016. ADEE also has been renamed accordingly as such from its preceding name Department of the Environment.

Health Canada is a federal level department headed by Canada's Minister of Health. Its mission is to help maintain and improve the people's health in the nation. To carry out this responsibility, among other things, the department monitors health and safety risks related to the use and sale of drugs, foods, chemicals, pesticides, radiation, and certain consumer products across the nation and around the world. Through its branches and agencies, the department carries out a number of regulatory programs to protect the people in the nation from harms caused by (use of or exposure to) alcohol, tobacco, hazardous substances, environmental contaminants, pesticides, microbial infections, and unsafe industrial products.

UBA is Germany's central federal authority on all environmental protection-related matters (i.e., the nation's main environmental protection agency). It has two key statutory mandates: (1) the provision of scientific support to the various federal government bodies (e.g., Federal Ministry for the Environment, Federal Ministry of Health); and (2) the implementation of environmental laws (e.g., those pertaining to emissions trading as well as to authorization of chemicals, pharmaceuticals, and pesticides). The German federal agency has the additional responsibility to provide the public with information concerning environmental protection.

References

Beck BD, Calabrese EJ, Slayton TM, Rudel R, 2008. The Use of Toxicology in the Regulatory Process. In *Principles and Methods of Toxicology* (Hayes AW, Ed.), 5th Edition. Boca Raton, Florida, USA: Taylor & Francis Group, Chapter 2.

Carson R, 1962. *Silent Spring*. Boston, Massachusetts, USA: Houghton Mifflin.

CDC (U.S. Centers for Disease Control and Prevention), 1990. Historical Perspectives Reduced Incidence of Menstrual Toxic-Shock Syndrome – United States, 1980-1990. *MMWR* (CDC Morbidity and Mortality Weekly Report) 39:421-423.

CIDRAP (University of Minnesota Center of Infectious Disease Research & Policy), 2009. CDC Releases Viruses for Novel H1N1 Vaccine Development. *CIDRAP News*, 7 May (by Robert Roos, its News Editor).

Dong MH, 2006. Human Health Risk from Consumption of Fish Contaminated with Persistent Organochlorine Compounds (POCs). Planetary lecture presented at the *International Conference on Environmental and Public Health Management: Aquaculture and Environment*, 7-9 December, Croucher Institute for Environmental Sciences, Hong Kong Baptist University, Hong Kong (Special Administrative Region of China).

EEA (European Environment Agency), 2014. Noise in Europe, 2014. EEA Report No. 10/2014. Copenhagen, Denmark.

FAO (Food and Agriculture Organization of the United Nations), 2010. Global Forest Resources Assessment 2010. FAO Forestry Paper 163. Rome, Italy.

Hynes HP, 1989. *The Recurring Silent Spring*. New York, New York, USA: Pergamon Press.

Lewis J, 1985. The Birth of EPA. *EPA Journal*, November Issue. http://www.epagov/history/topics/epa/15c.htm (retrieved 14 August 2012).

Neely WB, 1994. *Introduction to Chemical Exposure and Risk Assessment*. Boca Raton, Florida, USA: CRC Press, Chapter 1.

Renshaw N, 2012. Solutions to Tackle Noise Pollution in Road Transport. Presented at the European Parliament Brussels Meeting on *Addressing the Problem of Noise Pollution in Road Transport*, 21 March 2012.

Reuters.com, 2007. Indonesia Starts Planting 79 Million Trees, https://www.reuters.com/article/environment-indonesia-trees-dc/indonesia-starts-planting-79-million-trees-idUSJAK25378820071128 (retrieved 2 May 2017).

Revkin AC, 2009. Hacked E-Mail Is New Fodder for Climate Dispute. *The New York Times*, 20 November.

Sengco MR, Andersen DM, 2004. Controlling Harmful Algal Blooms through Clay Flocculation. *J. Eukaryol. Microbiol.* 5:169-172.

The New York Times (nytimes.com), 1922. Reforestation Spreading; Conservation Commission Reports 31,994,000 Plantings since 1908, published 29 January.

Tversky A, Kahneman D, 974. Judgment under Uncertainty: Heuristics and Biases. *Science* 185:1124-1131.

U.S. EPA (U.S. Environmental Protection Agency), 2007. Risk Communication in Action: The Risk Communication Workbook. EPA/625/R-05/003.Office of Research and Development,Cincinnati, Ohio, USA.

U.S. EPA (U.S. Environmental Protection Agency), 2008a. Clean Air Act (webpage dated 2008). http://www.epa.gov/air/caa/index.html (retrieved 15 August 2012).

U.S. EPA (U.S. Environmental Protection Agency), 2008b. Clean Water Act (webpage dated 2008). http://www.epa.gov/r5water/cwa.htm (retrieved 15 August 2012).

U.S. EPA (U.S. Environmental Protection Agency), 2008c. Federal Insecticide, Fungicide, and Rodenticide Act (FIFRA) Enforcement (webpage dated 2008). http://www.epa.gov/compliance/civil/fifra/index.html (retrieved 15 August 2012).

WHO (World Health Organization), 2011. Environmental Health (webpage dated 2011). http://www.who.int/topics/environmental_health/en/ (retrieved 15 August 2012).

Xia G, 1998. II. An Estimate of the Economic Consequences of Environmental Pollution in China. In *The Economic Costs of China's Environmental Degradation* (Smil V, Yushi M, Eds.). Cambridge, Massachusetts, USA: American Academy of Arts and Sciences.

Review Questions

1. Briefly describe the nature, characteristics, impacts, and concerns of environmental pollution.
2. What was (and still is) U.S. NEPA's stated purpose?
3. On what date did the *first* Earth Day celebration take place in the United States? And approximately how many Americans participated on that day?
4. From *air* pollution in China in the early 1990s, what impact factor or cause category was responsible for the *second* most economic loss in that nation?
5. What are the three major threats to the nation's environment that the U.S. Clean Air Act has aimed to curb via its amendment passed in 1990?
6. What was the major environmental concern that former U.S. Vice-President Al Gore's documentary film *An Inconvenient Truth* attempted to publicize as a global health problem?
7. What was (and still is) the main focus of the U.S. FIFRA amended in 1972?
8. Name the principal U.S. federal agency(ies) responsible for regulating and enforcing the following federal statutes: a) *Poison Prevention Packaging Act;* b) *Federal Hazardous Substances Act;* c) *Toxic Substances Control Act;* d) *Oil Pollution Act.*
9. What is the basic legal distinction between *law* and *order*, and between *guidance* and *regulation*?
10. Which federal statute in the United States is known as *Superfund (law)*? And how is it related to the missions and functions of U.S. EPA and ATSDR?
11. Name the U.S. federal agency(ies) that is (are) primarily responsible for the health and safety regulations concerning the following: a) blood products; b) radiation-emitting devices; c) oil pollution; d) pesticide residues in food.
12. Name the treaty that is regarded as the most comprehensive global environmental agreement concerning the treatment of hazardous and other wastes.
13. What is the global treaty that is concerned with the worldwide depletion of ozone layer?
14. Name four regulatory agencies abroad for environmental health that are as influential and active as those in the United States.

CHAPTER 4

Occurrence and Types of Environmental Toxicants

4.1. Introduction

In this chapter, brief accounts of 10 environmental contamination events or cases are given to illustrate two points crucial to the practice of environmental toxicology. First, this short list is intended to offer a sense of what the current sensitivity is regarding public and regulatory concerns on environmental health. Second, the list aims to reassure that the *occurrence* of today's environmental health issues rests more on socioeconomic values than on the severity of the health effects involved. Trans fats, for example, are chemically known as unsaturated fatty acids with at least one double bond in the *trans* position. In the United States, the recent federal ban of artificial trans fats in processed foods (Section 4.2.2C) signifies a new perspective from some sectors in the nation concerning environmental health. After all, it is not as if the adverse cardiovascular effects of trans fats were unbeknown to many people until in recent years.

From the first three chapters (particularly Section 2.3.1), it becomes clear that there seem to be countless environmental toxicants of concern regarding their adverse effects on human health and the ecosystem. Many of these toxic agents or substances are characterized in groups systematically in Part III (Chapters 11 through 17), in an effort to offer a fuller understanding of their environmental nature and health effects. In the second half of this chapter, many of them are briefly visited also in groups but in a different perspective for two other reasons. The first reason is that, much like the adverse effects (Chapter 2) that they can cause, further discussion on topics covered in Chapters 5 through 10 cannot be as productive without some knowledge about the general nature and effects of these toxicants. A subtle issue involved here, if not a dilemma, is that neither is it practical to have a fair understanding of the environmental nature and effects of these toxicants unless there is some appreciation of the topics covered in Part II. The other reason is more subtle. The toxicants discussed in this chapter represent those that appear to be of concern more to the general public (e.g., news media, parents) than to other sectors, thereby re-signifying to some extent what the *public's current* sensitivities are like concerning environmental health.

4.1.1. Contemporary Issues of Environmental Health Concern

The five biological agents of recent pandemic concern (i.e., those causing mad-cow disease, SARS/MERS, H1N1 flu, Ebola, Zika) and the notorious group of persistent organic pollutants (POPs) currently subjected to global action are highlighted in Chapters 1 and 2, respectively. Yet there are still many other environmental contaminants (re)emerging within the past decade. Although these other toxicants may not merit as much national or global attention, many can indeed cause a considerable level of harm or threat to human health and the environment. For the reasons given earlier, overviews for 10 select contemporary cases are given later in Section 4.2. This short list of 10, given in Table 4.1 below for a quick preview, has been selected among the many currently considered having high health concerns or causing significant issues on safety regulation in the context of environmental toxicology and environmental health.

Table 4.1. List of 10 Select Contemporary Cases/Events Considered as Significant Issues to Environmental Health and/or Environmental Toxicology

Contaminants in Consumer Products (Section 4.2.1)
    The Ubiquitous Antiseptic Ingredient (Section 4.2.1A)
    Recall of Lead-Containing Toy Jewelry (Section 4.2.1B)
    The Use of Bisphenol A Alternatives (Section 4.2.1C)

Contaminants in Food Products (Section 4.2.2)
    Mercury Level in Tuna (Section 4.2.2A)
    The Unbreakable, Colorful Melamine Dinnerware (Section 4.2.2B)
    Trans Fat Ban in the United States (Section 4.2.2C)

Pollutants in the Open Environment (Section 4.2.3)
    Plastic Marine Pollution (Section 4.2.3A)
    Management of Pharmaceutical Waste (Section 4.2.3B)
    The United Heckathorn Superfund Toxic Site (Section 4.2.3C)
    Electronic Waste (e-Waste) Problems in China (Section 4.2.3D)

4.1.2. Grouping of Environmental Contaminants

Inasmuch as there seem to be countless various contaminants present in the environment, there are bound to be numerous schemes in which these toxicants could or should be grouped for better consideration or analysis. For example, toxicants in the environment can be grouped according to *site of exposure*. To that end, there are indoor air pollutants, ambient air pollutants, drinking water contaminants, pesticide residues in/on foods, food contaminants, soil contaminants, and so forth. Another way is to classify environmental pollutants based on the *type* of health or ecological *effects* that they tend to cause, such as environmental carcinogens, environmental teratogens, environmental endocrine disruptors, and environmental stressors (e.g., water contaminants, air pollutants, traffic congestion, noise pollution). Still another scheme is to categorize them according to their chemical structure, their chemical family, or their physicochemical state, such as toxic metals, pesticides (or their subfamilies insecticides, fungicides, etc.), persistent organochlorine compounds (POCs), and volatile organic compounds (VOCs).

There is simply no definitive or correct way to place environmental contaminants into certain types, groups, or classes. After all, residues of many pesticides that belong to a certain (sub)family (e.g., organochlorines, organophosphates, herbicides; *see*, e.g., Chapter 15) are commonly present in the air, water, soil, or foods. Many of these pesticides also can cause multiple toxic effects in humans or laboratory animals. Still some pesticides are metals, while some others can be both an endocrine disruptor (Chapter 19) and a persistent organic pollutant (Chapter 16).

In any event, the environmental contaminants selected for a brief overview later in Section 4.3 have been categorized according to not only some of the above example schemes but also the ease of their referencing in the literature. Their inclusion for the brief overview, on the other hand, has been made primarily in terms of their availability for environmental exposure and their threats to environmental health. As a result, a few of the select contaminants have a special or specific place all by themselves. Throughout this chapter (as well as this book), the term *contaminant* or *environmental contaminant* is used as defined by the U.S. Agency for Toxic Substances and Disease Registry (ATSDR, 2016): *"A substance (or an agent) that is either present in an environment where it does not belong or is present at levels that might cause harmful (adverse) health effects."* Moreover, in this chapter as well as this book, the words *environment* and *contamination* are defined in their broadest scope and context as can be.

4.2. Contemporary Issues: 10 Select Cases

It should be pointed out that the 10 cases listed in Table 4.1 above and discussed below are not meant to represent or reflect those current issues (e.g., gun control, marijuana cultivation) debatable in nature. They are simply specific contemporary issues, events, or otherwise cases relevant to environmental toxicology or pollution that have occurred within the past decade or so. These select cases tend to have more regional than global ramifications as they all reflect the social, economic, or cultural concerns at the national or local community level. More specifically, for the cases discussed below, all but one currently mean more to American people than to those living in other countries. The tenth case, however, is an issue more to people living in China or some other Asian countries, especially those residing around the e-waste (electronic waste) recycling sites.

4.2.1. Contaminants in Consumer Products

Three sample cases have been specifically selected to represent the contemporary environmental health issues from this product group. The toxicants involved in the three cases are triclosan ($C_{12}H_7Cl_3O_2$), lead (Pb), and bisphenol A ($C_{15}H_{16}O_2$).

A. The Ubiquitous Antiseptic Ingredient

Triclosan is used as an antiseptic (primarily as an antibacterial) agent and thus shows up in hundreds of consumer products, including toothpastes, deodorants, cosmetics, kitchenware, toys, and clothing. Despite the fact that this chemical has been used since the 1970s, environmental health concerns with its overuse have come up only in recent years, when its efficacy in soaps has become questionable for reducing bacterial levels on the hands (e.g., Aiello *et al.*, 2007). There have been many studies linking triclosan to a variety of environmental and health effects ranging from destruction of aquatic ecosystems to skin irritation in humans, antibiotic resistance, and contamination with the carcinogenic dioxins (Glaser, 2004). In particular, a Swedish study detected high levels of triclosan in 3 out of 5 human breast milk samples (Adolfsson-Erici *et al.*, 2002), implicating that this antiseptic agent can be absorbed into the human body and that newborns therefore can easily be exposed to it. The above findings represent merely a rather small portion of the scientific data which the U.S. Food and Drug Administration (FDA, 2016a) used to support its recent ruling that effective 6 September 2017, hand and body soaps can no longer be allowed on the market as over-the-counter (OTC) consumer products if they contain triclosan as an active (antiseptic) ingredient. Nonetheless, as of late 2017, triclosan is still (allowed to be) used in many other consumer products (e.g., toothpastes, acne treatments, soaps used in hospitals and food service settings) that are not specifically listed in the OTC "consumer antiseptic wash" category.

B. Recall of Lead-Containing Toy Jewelry

On 2 June 2016, LaRose Industries recalled the Cra-Z-Jewelz Ultimate Gem Jewelry Machine kits (CPSC, 2016), in which certain components (predominately the slider bracelet) were found to contain lead (Pb) levels up to 10 times higher than the federal limit of 100 ppm for children (Schneiderman, 2016). These toy jewelry kits, reportedly imported from China, were sold at some of the largest retail chains in the United States including K-mart, Target, and Toys-R-Us. At high levels (e.g., from licking), the metal lead can cause a wide array of health effects including kidney damage, neurological disability, premature birth in pregnant women, and death in children (*see* Section 4.3.1H, Section 14.2.1, and Section 21.4.2).

C. The Use of Bisphenol A Alternatives

Bisphenol A (BPA), an organic substance having two hydroxyphenyl groups, is the building block of hard polycarbonate plastics and epoxy resins used in a variety of consumer products including baby bottles and food cans. This organic, first synthesized in 1895 and discovered in 1936 as a synthetic hormone, is now shown capable of mimicking the sex hormone estrogen to interfere with healthy growth and normal body functions. Animal studies have consistently demonstrated that BPA can cause damage to the reproductive, neurological, and immunological systems during critical stages of development, such as during infancy and in the womb (e.g., WGFSM, 2008). One critical health concern with BPA is apparently the findings that, when heating baby bottles to 80° C (176° F) or higher, the chemical was shown to leach out of six major brands available in Canada and the United States (e.g., WGFSM, 2008). In those studies, the synthetic hormone in the leachates was measured at an alarming level range of 4.7 to 8.3 ppb (parts per billion). FDA (2012) thereby has banned BPA in the manufacture of all baby bottles and sippy cups. Many manufacturers are now using bisphenol S (BPS) and bisphenol F (BPF) as alternatives to harden plastics and epoxy resins. Yet there are people in the United States and other countries still eating stuff from plastic containers made with and from food cans lined with BPA. More disturbingly, there is evidence (e.g., Eladak *et al.*, 2015; Qiu *at al.*, 2015; Rochester and Bolden, 2015) showing that BPS and BPF may not be safe alternatives to BPA, as the two BPA analogs are also shown capable of exerting similar adverse reproductive and hormonal effects.

4.2.2. Contaminants in Food Products

Three cases have been specifically selected to represent the contemporary environmental health issues from this product group. The food toxicants involved in the three cases are mercury (Hg), melamine ($C_3H_6N_6$), and trans fats (*trans*-isomer fatty acids).

A. Mercury Level in Tuna

Yellowfin tuna is often sold to consumers in steak form, while being used in small amounts in canned "light" tuna. According to a recent study (Drevnick et al., 2015), mercury (Hg) levels in yellowfin tuna caught in the Pacific Ocean near Hawaii (USA) have been rising at an annual rate of 3.8% since 1998. Although the Hg levels analyzed in that study were found well below the action level of 1 ppm (part per million) set forth by FDA (2000) as unsafe, mercury is nonetheless a toxic metal (Chapter 14) that in the soluble form can accumulate in fatty tissues for a long time. Moreover, young yellowfins are often preyed upon by other pelagic hunters including larger tuna. Under this precaution and after a review of further data on mercury contents in fishes, U.S. EPA and FDA (2017) have continued to jointly advise women of childbearing age to limit their consumption of certain canned tuna (including yellowfin) to no more than 12 ounces (3 servings) per week in spite of the fact that the fish is rich in protein and nutrients.

B. The Unbreakable, Colorful Melamine Dinnerware

Melamine ($C_3H_6N_6$) is an organic base chemical with many industrial applications, insomuch as it is highly fire- and heat-resistant. Widely available in the United States, melamine-based dinner sets come in vibrant colors with trendy designs, and are unbreakable in spite of daily wear and tear. However, melamine tends to absorb heat and radiation and then starts to decompose and leach out, particularly in the presence of highly acidic food items (e.g., tomato sauce). Therefore, the use of melamine-based dinnerware for heating food in the microwave and ovens has become a matter of concern for many people since about a decade ago, shortly after the incident reports were published (e.g., Gossner et al., 2009) linking melamine to renal failure observed in some 300,000 Chinese infants in 2008. The source of the illness was traced to the illegal addition of melamine to infant formula in China. Melamine, owing to its molecular formula, is highly rich in nitrogen (N) and can be utilized to falsify the milk's protein value which is typically measured in terms of N content. Melamine *per se* has low acute toxicity. Yet the organic base can form crystals to give rise to kidney stones when reacting with cyanuric acid ($C_3H_3N_3O_3$), a weak organic acid commonly present in melamine powder. A year prior to these human incident reports, pet food manufactured in the United States using vegetable proteins imported from China were found to have led to the death of a large number of dogs and cats due to renal failure (FDA, 2016b). Further investigation determined that the vegetable proteins (purported to be wheat gluten) were contaminated with melamine.

C. Trans Fat Ban in the United States

Trans fats are made from vegetable oil by adding hydrogen to saturate the unsaturated plant oil in order to increase the shelf life and the flavor stability of foods that are made or cooked with fat. Trans fatty acids can be found commercially in vegetable shortenings and some margarines. According to FDA (2015), artificial trans fats would have to disappear from the American diet by 2018. The federal ban came seven years after lawmakers in the state of California passed a partial ban on use of trans fats. The state law, which was passed in July 2008, specifies that effective New Year's Day in 2010, all restaurants in California can no longer cook foods with trans fats (*The Los*

Angeles Times, 2008). Both the state and the federal ban stemmed from the overwhelming scientific evidence showing that high consumption of trans fats can raise the LDL (low-density lipoprotein) "bad" cholesterol levels in the blood, thereby increasing the risk of coronary heart disease (e.g., FNB, 2005).

4.2.3. Pollutants in the Open Environment
Four cases have been specifically selected to represent the contemporary environmental health issues under this group. The contaminants in these four cases are nonchemical-specific. They include plastics, used pharmaceuticals, pesticides, metals, and organochlorine compounds.

A. Plastic Marine Pollution
As summarized in a Greenpeace report by Allsopp *et al.* (2006), hundreds of thousands of marine creatures (e.g., whales, dolphins, whales, sea turtles) die each year from entanglement with or ingestion of plastic debris present ubiquitously in the seabed, particularly near the coastal regions where large volumes of plastic bags are used and left behind as litter (e.g., Galgani *et al.*, 1995; Thiel *et al.*, 2003). Plastic bags were also blamed to have choked a country's sewer drainage systems during devastating floods, with some eventually ending up as ocean sewage. In response to such environmental concerns, Bandladesh in 2002 became the first nation in the world to ban certain types of thin plastic bags. Shortly after, China, South Africa, Italy, Belgium, and dozens of other nations followed suit, by either instituting a similar ban or imposing a tax on the plastic bags sold (NG News, 2008). In the United States, California reportedly became the nation's first state to ban single-use plastic bags in full force in 2017 (e.g., SDUT, 2016). This state ban, approved by California voters in November 2016, applies to large food retailers, pharmacies, corner markets, and liquor stores (but not restaurants or department stores) across the state.

B. Management of Pharmaceutical Waste
Despite the fact that pharmaceuticals are crucial to the maintenance of human health, they can pollute the environment and public health. A study by the U.S. Geological Survey (USGS, 2002) found that, between 1999 and 2000, many personal care products (e.g., fragrances) and pharmaceuticals (e.g., prescription drugs, OTC medicines, steroids, hormones) were detected in water samples collected from 139 streams in 30 states, though at low levels. Yet it is important to realize that aquatic creatures residing near the contamination sites are likely to be exposed to the waste throughout their entire life cycle even prior to birth. Some pharmaceuticals can be endocrine disruptors, as they have been shown to cause reproductive effects in fishes (Palace *et al.*, 2006; Schultz *et al.*, 2003). At least one study (Brooks *et al.*, 2005) found that certain antidepressants accumulated in fishes living in streams that received a high level of treated urban effluent. To address these concerns, U.S. EPA (2008) filed a proposal in the *Federal Register* to add hazardous waste pharmaceuticals to the federal Universal Waste Rule, which currently includes only batteries, pesticides, and mercury-containing equipment (including lamps) all in the *used* form. The proposed amendment, filed on 2 December 2008, was intended to offer healthcare facility generators (including hospitals/clinics, pharmacies, medical offices, dental offices, and veterinary clinics)

the option to manage all types of pharmaceutical waste as nonhazardous. After several years of facing negative public comments on the 2008 proposal, U.S. EPA (2015) changed its approach to filing another proposal on 25 September 2015 with provisions of sector-specific standards intended *"to ensure the management of hazardous waste pharmaceuticals is safe and workable within the healthcare setting"*.

C. The United Heckathorn Superfund Toxic Site

The United Heckathorn (UH) incident may be described as some deep wounds to a community long waiting to be healed. The U.S. Comprehensive Environmental Response, Compensation, & Liability Act (CERCLA), or commonly known as Superfund (law), was enacted by U.S. Congress on 11 December 1980 initially in response to the appalling tragedy of Love Canal (Sections 2.2.4 and 3.3.2). The act authorizes U.S. EPA to compel responsible parties to clean up toxic waste sites and, where a responsible party cannot be found, to clean up the site on the agency's own effort using a special trust fund nowadays known as Superfund. In 2001, U.S. EPA issued a summary of the first five-year review of its cleanup efforts for the UH toxic site located in Richmond Harbor of Contra Costa County, California. From 1947 to 1966, the UH Superfund toxic site was a place for formulating and packaging pesticides. It now becomes a major source of DDT, dieldrin, and other persistent pesticides polluting the nearby San Francisco Bay. As authorized under CERCLA, in March 1990 U.S. EPA took over from the state of California the investigation and cleanup of this toxic site. In October 2008, U.S. EPA launched and completed its first fish survey around the site to assess the lingering pollution, with a specific intent to update the baseline information for the human health and ecological risks involved. Further elaboration and update on this case are given in Chapter 22 (Section 22.3.2).

D. Electronic Waste (e-Waste) Problems in China

As noted in Chapter 2, e-waste is an emerging major environmental health issue. This is particularly true in China (and other parts in Asia such as India and Malaysia, as well as in many countries in Africa). Over 50 million tons of e-waste are generated worldwide each year, of which over 50% are imported legally or illegally to Asia, mainly to China (Puckett *et al.*, 2002; UNEP, 2005). Most of this e-waste flowing into China ends up in families residing around the recycling sites, where many of these families have members as laborers working to disassemble the waste electronics manually for reclaimable materials. Wearing little protective gear, these workers (and their families) are exposed to a host of toxic chemicals including PCBs (polychlorinated biphenyls), polybrominated diphenyl ethers (PBDEs), toxic metals (e.g., lead, cadmium), and acids. It has been said that Guiyu, a small town located in southern China's Guangdong province, is the e-waste capital of the world. Over 150,000 people there reportedly have become experts at dismantling the world's electronic junk.

4.3. Environmental Toxicants of Health Concern

Highlighted in this section are the issues with environmental toxicants that are deemed to have high health concerns to the public sectors (e.g., parents, news media) while at the same time having high relevance to environmental toxicology. The toxicological profiles highlighted below are comparable to those given in Hodgson *et al.* (1998) and/or at the websites of various health authorities including especially the U.S. National Center for Environmental Health (CDC, 2017) and the U.S. National Library of Medicine (NLM, 2014). Serving as further references where applicable, the one or more chapters in this book that provide elaboration on the specific toxicant(s) are listed in parentheses in the subject heading given for its (their) discussion. The toxicants selected for discussion in this section are divided into three groups, in part to uphold the earlier claim that some of them have a special place of their own: Group I – *Individual, Specific Toxicants*; Group II – *Specific Chemical/Biological Families*; and Group III – *Toxicants of Common/General Concern.*

4.3.1. Group I: Individual, Specific Toxicants

This group includes 11 chemical substances that each appear to have a specific place by themselves in terms of their public health threats or impacts. Of these, three are inorganic gases (carbon dioxide, carbon monoxide, ozone), two are volatile organic compounds (benzene, formaldehyde), and the remaining six are chemical elements all possessing some metallic properties (arsenic, cadmium, chromium, lead, mercury, radon).

A. Arsenic (As; Chapter 14)

This contaminant or toxicant is best characterized as a group of arsenic compounds (commonly referred to as arsenicals), rather than as a single metalloid element. One concern with this group of compounds is that they can come from drinking water and are used in pesticides. Epidemiological studies revealed that the *tri*valent form (As^{3+}) could induce skin cancer. Chromated copper arsenate (CCA) is a wood preservative pesticide containing chromium (Cr), copper (Cu), and As. Since the 1970s, CCA-pressure treated wood has been part of the majority of the American outdoor residential structures, even though it is no longer being produced (but not yet completely eliminated) now for use in decks or playsets in the United States.

B. Benzene (C_6H_6; Chapter 13)

This is an aromatic volatile organic compound (VOC) found largely in crude oil. It is widely used as a constituent of motor fuels and as an intermediate to make other substances that in turn are utilized to make plastics, resins, nylons, and other chemical materials. In homes, benzene may be found in adhesives, gasoline, and tobacco smoke. The VOC has been listed by U.S. EPA as a human carcinogen and a priority toxic pollutant.

C. Cadmium (Cd; Chapter 14)

For a long time, this metal was used as a pigment and for corrosion resistant plating on steel, with its compounds being utilized mainly to stabilize plastics. In recent years, more than 85% of all the cadmium has been used in batteries, especially in the rechargeable nickel-cadmium kind. As with lead, it has no known biological role in higher-order animals. The most dangerous form of occupational exposure to cadmium is inhalation of its fine dust particles and fumes, or ingestion of its soluble compounds. Severe chronic cadmium poisoning can result in renal abnormalities, or in the ill-known *itai-itai* (ouch, ouch) disease (Section 14.2.3).

D. Carbon Dioxide (CO_2)

This is one of the gases readily found in the atmosphere. The gas can be an asphyxiant by replacing an excessive portion of the oxygen in the breathing zone. At high blood concentrations, it can cause unconsciousness or death. When fossil fuels such as propane (which contains mostly carbon) and gasoline react with oxygen, they produce carbon dioxide. Deforestation can increase the atmospheric level of this gas since forests will otherwise break down the gas compound during photosynthesis. It has been speculated that too much carbon dioxide in the air can overwhelm the greenhouse effect to cause global warming.

E. Carbon Monoxide (CO; Chapter 11)

This is a highly acute toxic gas responsible for the most common type of fatal human poisoning in many parts of the world including the United States. It is readily produced by the *incomplete* burning of many common types of fuels (e.g., charcoal, coal, kerosene, natural gas, petroleum oil, wood), and by many common types of equipment powered by internal combustion engines (e.g., automobiles, lawn mowers, portable generators). The gas is included as one of the six *criteria* air pollutants in the United States. Carbon monoxide is known as a silent killer owing to its unique characteristics being not only an acutely fatal but also a totally colorless, odorless, tasteless gas.

F. Chromium (Cr; Chapter 14).

This metal has remarkable magnetic properties and is commonly used in electroplating, paints, and textile manufacturing. It has been found in some drinking water sources. Studies showed that chromium caused cancer in laboratory animals after they had consumed sufficient water containing the metal in its hexavalent form Cr^{6+} (also denoted by CrVI). In contrast, its trivalent form Cr^{3+} (CrIII) in low doses is considered an essential human nutrient, as Cr^{3+} shortage reportedly can cause heart conditions and disruptions of metabolism.

G. Formaldehyde (CH_2O; Chapter 13)

This is a colorless, strong-smelling gas used widely by industry to manufacture building materials as well as many household products (e.g., as an adhesive resin in pressed wood products). Accordingly, it can be found in substantial levels in the indoor and ambient air. This VOC gas is a by-product of combustion and some other natural processes. It is a designated carcinogen in the United States (as well as in many other countries) and can trigger asthma attack.

H. Lead (Pb; Chapter 14)

This is a highly toxic metal used for many years in numerous products found around homes. The metal can cause a wide array of adverse health effects from behavioral problems and learning disabilities to reproductive harms, seizures, and death (e.g., Section 21.4.2). Young children are most at risk, owing to their naïve nature and the fact that many defense mechanisms in their body are still being developed. Major sources of lead exposure for children include: Pb-contaminated dust and toys; deteriorating Pb-based paint (from chewing the paint chips); and Pb-contaminated residential soils. Lead is one of the six *criteria* air pollutants in the United States.

I. Mercury (Hg; Chapter 14)

As with lead, mercury is a highly toxic metal found in the air, water, and soils. The metal exists in several forms: elemental (metallic) mercury (Hg^0), inorganic mercury compounds (e.g., $HgCl_2$), and organic mercury compounds (e.g., CH_3Hg^+). At high levels, exposure to mercury can harm the brain, heart, kidneys, lungs, and immunological system of people at all ages. Exposure to certain forms of the metal at high levels can cause similar biological effects in many (other) animals, especially those consuming fish (which as a group tend to be a rich reservoir for mercury). Severe chronic mercury poisoning can result in the ill-known Minamata disease (Section 14.2.2).

J. Ozone (O_3; Chapter 11)

This gas is an allotrope (i.e., a certain form) of oxygen occurring near the ground level (troposphere) or in the Earth's next upper air layer (stratosphere). Depending on its location in the atmosphere, ozone can be "good" or "bad" to human health and the ecosystem. Tropospheric ozone is a gas pollutant posing a significant health threat, especially to children with asthma. At high levels, the gas will severely damage trees, crops, and other vegetation, in addition to the human body. It is a main component of urban smog. In the stratosphere, ozone plays a key role in keeping the sun's harmful ultraviolet radiation from striking the Earth's surface.

K. Radon (Rn; Chapter 14)

This is a cancer-causing natural radioactive gas that reportedly claims some 20,000 American lives each year. It is the decay product of radium (Ra) formed (likely) somewhat midway via the radioactive decay chain beginning with uranium (U) or thorium (Th). Radon itself undergoes radioactive decay to yield yet another unstable radioactive daughter. The daughter also tends to divide herself into radiation and still another radioactive (grand)daughter. Although radon is no longer utilized in the treatment of various human diseases (e.g., diabetes, cancer, arthritis), it is still being applied to predict earthquakes, in the study of atmospheric transport, and in the exploration for petroleum and uranium. Like thorium, uranium is available in small amounts in most rocks and soils.

4.3.2. Group II: Certain Chemical/Biological Families

This group consists of one biological and five chemical families. Entities in this group include: asbestos; nitrogen oxides (NO_x); persistent organochlorine compounds (POCs); polybrominated diphenyl ethers (PBDEs); sulfur oxides (SO_x); and the one family of biological organisms called *fungi* (or known loosely as molds to many people).

A. Asbestos (Chapter 20)

This is a name given to a family of six naturally occurring fibrous silicate minerals each present in one of two structural forms: the one in serpentine named chrysotile; and the five in amphibole named actinolite, amosite, anthophyllite, crocidolite, and tremolite. Collectively, these six mineral members are used in a variety of building materials for acoustic and thermal insulation and as fire retardants. Higher incidences of lung cancer and mesotheliomas have been associated with occupational exposure to asbestos (e.g., to those entering the air and water from the breakdown of manufactured goods), especially when in combination with cigarette smoking.

B. Molds (Chapter 17)

These microbes are the dominant group of fungi that are found indoors and outdoors in many places. Common genera include *Alternaria, Aspergillus, Cladosporium,* and *Penicillium*. Certain exposed individuals with chronic pulmonary illness (e.g., obstructive lung disease) can develop mold infections in their lungs. These microbes can trigger asthma attack. Areas causing high mold exposure are typically moist or damp surfaces, such as in greenhouses, antique shops, farms, mills, saunas, and constructions.

C. Nitrogen Oxides (NO_x; Chapter 11)

This is the generic term given to a family of highly reactive gases containing the nitrogen (N) and a varying number x of oxygen (O) atoms. The common anthropogenic sources of NO_x include automobile exhausts, electric utilities, and facilities that burn fuels. Some members of nitrogen oxides and sulfur dioxide (SO_2) are known to react with certain atmospheric substances to form acids which fall onto the ground as acid rain, fog, snow, or dry particles. Acid rain has harmful effects on aquatic creatures, plants, and infrastructures (Section 5.2.3C). Nitrogen dioxide (NO_2) and nitric oxide (NO) are the two principal members of NO_x. The health effects of nitrogen dioxide include: eye, nose, and throat irritation; impaired lung function; and increased respiratory infections, especially in young children.

D. Persistent Organochlorine Compounds (POCs; Chapter 16)

These are hydrocarbon (hence *organic*) compounds that each have substituted one or more of their hydrogen (H) atoms for chlorines (Cl). As the carbon-chlorine (C-Cl) bond is chemically highly stable, organochlorines (OCs) are by structure highly persistent even in a very rough environment. The two most prominent POC subfamilies *not* used (to date) as pesticides are *dioxins* and *PCBs*, as briefly discussed below.

Dioxins. This is the general name given to the following two classes of highly toxic and environmentally persistent OCs with chemical structures very similar to one another: polychlorinated dibenzo-*p(ara)*-dioxins (PCDDs); and polychlorinated dibenzofurans (PCDFs). Of the some 200 dioxin congeners (i.e., members), 2,3,7,8-TCDD is the most potent and thus uniquely referred to as *the dioxin*. Most, if not all, dioxin congeners are not intentionally produced but are by-products from industrial or chemical processes such as the chlorine bleaching process at pulp mills and the chlorination at waste or drinking water treatment facilities. Many dioxin congeners are hormone disruptors (Chapter 19). Their extremely low acceptable levels in human fat are currently set at the range of parts per *trillion* (ppt).

Polychlorinated Biphenyls (PCBs). These are some 130 congeners (i.e., structurally similar compounds) that were once manufactured in the United States for a variety of industrial and commercial applications, such as coolants and insulating fluids for electronic transformers and capacitors. (As explained in Table 16.2, up to 209 congeners of PCBs are *theoretically* possible for the PCB family.) As with PCDDs and PCDFs, the most commonly observed health effects of these PCB congeners in humans are skin conditions such as (chlor)acne and rashes. Studies on exposed workers showed changes in blood and urine that could lead to liver damage. Several other occupational studies also implicated that PCBs could cause cancer of the liver in humans.

E. Polybrominated Diphenyl Ethers (PBDEs; Chapter 16)

These congeners are part of the brominated flame retardant family. Many are components of flame retardants used in furniture foam (e.g., *penta*BDE congeners), plastics for television (TV) cabinets (*deca*BDE congeners), and plastics for small appliances and computers (*octa*BDE congeners). Many PBDE congeners are highly persistent, bioaccumulative, and toxic to humans, with an array of adverse health effects including thyroid hormone disruption, fetal malformations, delayed puberty onset, and permanent learning impairment.

F. Sulfur Oxides (SO$_x$; Chapter 11)

Inhaled sulfur dioxide (SO_2), which is the principal member of sulfur oxides (SO_x), readily reacts with the moisture of mucous membranes (e.g., in the respiratory tract) to form the more potent irritant sulfurous acid (H_2SO_3). Sulfur dioxide is produced from the burning of fossil fuels and the smelting of mineral ores that contain sulfur (S). Erupting volcanoes are a significant natural source of sulfur dioxide emissions. When sulfur dioxide combines with water (e.g., with atmospheric water vapor), it forms sulfuric acid (H_2SO_4) which is the principal component of acid rain that can seriously irritate the respiratory tract as well as the eyes in humans and can cause serious damage to plants, aquatic animals, and infrastructures.

4.3.3. Group III: Toxicants of Common/General Concern

Thirteen entities are included in this group. Each entity is a collection of toxicants or toxins grouped together because the public recognize them more as having similar use (household substances, pesticides), similar toxic effects (asthma triggers, environmental endocrine disruptors, free radicals), or similar exposure sources (diesel fuel, drinking water contaminants, food contaminants and additives, particulate matter, plant toxicants, radioactive wastes, terrestrial venoms and poisons, volatile organic compounds).

There are actually some toxicants, such as BPA (bisphenol A), triclosan, and perfluorooctane sulfonate (PFOS), that have been gaining more public attention in recent years. However, to reduce redundancy, they are not included in this or the two preceding subsections. For example, triclosan and BPA are discussed in Sections 4.2.1A and 4.2.1C, respectively, and further discussed in Chapter 21. PFOS and its chemical cousin perfluorooctanoic acid (PFOA) are discussed in Chapter 16, and specifically noted in Section 4.3.3C as among the some 100 water contaminants of high health concern in the United States.

A. Asthma Triggers

Asthma attack can be a fatal or very serious respiratory illness. The agents that can trigger such an attack are usually allergenic in nature, including cockroaches, molds, second-hand smoke, dust mites, paints, warm-blooded pets, perfumes, and many more.

B. Diesel Fuel (Chapter 12)

In many cities, the exhausts from fuel of this type can take on a significant toll of the urban particulate load, insomuch as diesel fuel is widely used nowadays to power delivery trucks, farm rigs, boats, and the kind. The exhaust particulates from such engines burning diesel fuel are usually of *nano*micrometer size. These ultra-tiny particulates are a complex mixture containing over 40 toxic pollutants (e.g., molecules of benzene, arsenic, nitrogen oxides, and formaldehyde).

C. Drinking Water Contaminants

Drinking water, including bottled water, almost always contains at least some small amounts of contaminants. U.S. EPA has set standards for some 100 contaminants in drinking water (*see*, e.g., Section 22.2.2). In addition to the fuel additive methyl *tert(iary)*-butyl ether (MTBE) being a single contaminant entity, the major subgroups or subfamilies of water contaminants on U.S. EPA's list currently include: microbes (e.g., *E. coli*); radionuclides (e.g., radium-226, radon); organic substances (e.g., dioxins, PCBs, pesticides, benzene); inorganics (e.g., Pb, Cr, As); disinfectants (e.g., chlorine); and disinfection by-products (e.g., chlorite). More recently, U.S. EPA (2016) has established health advisories for PFOA and PFOS in drinking water.

D. Environmental Endocrine Disruptors (Chapter 19)

These disruptors are generally defined as exogenous substances that interfere with the secretion, biosynthesis, metabolism, distribution, elimination, or normal function of natural hormones in the body, leading to adverse developmental, reproductive, neurological, immunological, and/or carcinogenic effects in humans and wildlife animals. These xenobiotics include a large number of pesticides, toxic metals, industrial chemical pollutants, foods, fluoride, cosmetics, and more. As specifically defined in Chapter 19, hormones are chemical messengers that a body uses to regulate or influence its many crucial day-to-day biological functions pertinent to the body's development, reproduction, and behavior.

E. Food Contaminants and Additives (Chapter 21)

Contaminants in foods are toxicants inadvertently placed in cooked, processed, or raw foods. These toxicants include: bacterial toxins (e.g., exotoxin of *Clostridium botulinum*); pathogenic microbes; mycotoxins (e.g., aflatoxins from *Aspergillus flavus*); animal toxins; pesticide residues; animal drug residues (e.g., diethylstilbestrol, antibiotics); plant alkaloids; and a variety of industrial chemicals (e.g., PBDEs, PCBs). Substances (mostly antimicrobials and antioxidants) *purposely* added to foods as preservatives are termed *direct additives*, such as butylated hydroxytoluene (BHT) and butylated hydroxyanisole (BHA). Food additives can also be used to change the physical characteristics for processing the food product, or to alter the food's taste or odor (e.g., nitrate).

Due to the recent concerns by some sectors, the adverse health effects of some of these additives have been subjected to further investigation.

F. Free Radicals (Chapters 2, 8, and 9)

As noted in Chapter 2 and further discussed in Chapters 8 and 9, these are strong oxidants that can damage other molecules nearby and the cell structures. Some free radicals tend to react with lipoproteins in the blood to form plaque-like fatty deposits which can end up clogging blood vessels to block off blood supply to the heart, thereby tending to cause cardiac attack. Those derived from the atom oxygen, and thus referred to as reactive oxygen species (ROS) or oxygen free radicals, are thought to also play a key role in carcinogenesis.

G. Household (Toxic) Substances (Chapter 21)

Almost every household uses products or materials that contain hazardous substances in some amount. It is for this very concern that the U.S. Federal Emergency Management Agency (FEMA, 2007) calls for proper storage and handling of these products, as well as for effective reaction during an emergency so to reduce the risk of injury. Statistics (CPSC, 2015) showed that in 2014, emergency rooms in clinics and hospitals across the United States treated 66,800 cases of unintentional pediatric (defined as children <5 years old) poisoning that occurred at home. And the top 10 household products attributing to these cases reportedly included blood pressure medications, pain killers (e.g., acetaminophen), bleach, and laundry packets. On the other hand, a five-year analysis report by U.S. EPA (1989) concluded that the toxic substances in household cleaners were three times more likely to cause cancer compared to ambient air pollution. Although the comparison results from this report are somewhat outdated, what seems more important here is its conclusion that some substances in the household cleaners under analysis were carcinogenic.

H. Particulate Matter (Chapter 12)

This *matter* is also known as particle or particulate pollution which is a complex mixture of very small solid particles and liquid droplets. Particulate matter is made up of hundreds to thousands of tiny molecular components, including acids (e.g., nitrates and sulfates), metals (e.g., Pb, Cd), organic substances, and soil or dust particles. These particulates, with some as tiny as on the *nano*micrometer scale, have been linked to a range of serious respiratory and cardiovascular disorders. As a single entity, it is one of the six designated *criteria* air pollutants in the United States.

I. Pesticides (Chapter 15)

Most of the pesticides available today are substances that are specifically synthesized for use to prevent, destroy, repel, or mitigate one or more types of agricultural and public health pests, which include insects, rodents, weeds, fungi, bacteria, and viruses. Pesticides that are used specifically on insects are often referred to as insecticides; those used specifically on rodents (and some other nuisance animals) are referred to as rodenticides; those used on weeds are referred to as herbicides; and so forth. Many of these substances are acutely highly toxic, carcinogenic, and/or capable of disrupting the endocrine system. Pesticides of the organochlorine family (e.g., aldrin, chlordane, dieldrin, DDT, lindane, mirex, toxaphene) are particularly persistent in the environment. Many of them are members of POPs (persistent organic pollutants), of which many are POCs (persistent organochlorine compounds). Some naturally occurring substances such as certain plant extracts (e.g., pyrethrum, citronella, rotenone) and certain metals (e.g., As, Cu, Hg) also have been used as pesticides.

J. Plant Toxicants (Chapter 17)

These include many types of chemical substances, such as alkaloids, lipids, cardiac glycosides, phenols, and certain drugs of abuse (e.g., nicotine, cocaine, morphine). These toxicants collectively can cause a wide array of health effects including allergic or contact dermatitis, gastrointestinal disturbance, cardiac arrhythmias, hepatocyte (i.e., liver cell) damage, kidney tubular degeneration, seizures, soft tissue calcification, birth defects, abortion, and many more.

K. Radioactive Wastes (Chapters 14 and 22)

Hazardous wastes in this group are generated by processes that produce or use radioactive materials, such as those used for or in national defense, scientific research, nuclear power generation, medicine, and industrial applications. These radioactive wastes can be in gas, liquid, or solid form. The radioactivity in these waste products can remain for a few days (e.g., the radioactive isotope iodine-135) or for as long as thousands of years (e.g., spent or used nuclear fuel). The adverse health effects of radiation can be mild (e.g., reddening of the skin) or with severe consequence (e.g., cancer or early death).

L. Terrestrial Animal Venoms/Poisons (Chapter 17)

These are mostly proteinaceous (protein-like) toxins produced by animals specifically for the poisoning of other species via a mechanism designed to deliver the toxin to their prey or enemy. Examples of this kind include the venoms of bees and wasps (delivered by a sting) and the venoms of snakes (delivered by fangs). Toxic agents in this group are of health concern to people living more in underdeveloped or rural areas than in developed or urban areas.

M. Volatile Organic Compounds (VOCs; Chapter 13)

These hydrocarbon (and hence organic) compounds are readily emitted as gases from thousands of volatile solid and liquid chemical substances: paints; lacquers; paint strippers; cleaning supplies; household products; pesticides; and many more. Collectively, they can cause a wide array of human health effects: irritation of the skin, eyes, nose, throat, and lungs; nausea; loss of coordination; headaches; and damage to the liver, kidneys, or central nervous system. Some VOCs are found to cause cancer in laboratory animals, whereas some others are known (e.g., benzene, vinyl chloride) to cause cancer in humans.

References

Adolfsson-Erici M, Pettersson M, Parkkonen J, Sturve J, 2002. Triclosan, a Commonly Used Bactericide Found in Human Milk and in the Aquatic Environment in Sweden. *Chemosphere* 46:1485-1489.

Aiello AE, Larson EL, Levy SB, 2007. Consumer Antibacterial Soaps: Effective or Just Risky? *Clin. Infect. Dis.* 45:S137-S147.

Allsopp M, Walters A, Santillo D, Johnston P, 2006. Plastic Debris in the World's Oceans. Greenpeace International, Ottho Heldringstraat 5, 1066 AZ Amsterdam, the Netherlands.

ATSDR (U.S. Agency for Toxic Substances and Disease Registry), 2016. ATSDR's Glossary of Terms (webpage last updated 26 January 2016). https://www.atsdr.cdc.gov/glossary.html (retrieved 2 October 2016).

Brooks BW, Chambliss CK, Stanley JK, Ramirez A, Banks KE, Johnson RD, Lewis RJ, 2005. Determination of Select Antidepressants in Fish from an Effluent-Dominated Stream. *Environ. Toxicol. Chem.* 24:464-469.

CDC (U.S. Centers for Disease Control and Prevention), 2017. National Center for Environmental Health A-Z Index (webpage last updated 25 January 2017). https://www.cdc.gov/nceh/az/c.html (retrieved 2 May 2017).

CPSC (U.S. Consumer Product Safety Commission), 2015. Unintentional Pediatric Poisoning Injury Estimates for 2014 (Memorandum prepared by staff members A. Qin and A. Layton, 18 December 2015). Washington DC, USA.

CPSC (U.S. Consumer Product Safety Commission), 2016. LaRose Industries Recalls Cra-Z-Jewelz Ultimate Gem Jewelry Machine due to Violation of Lead Standard. http://www.cpsc.gov/th/recalls/2016/larose-industries-recalls-cra-z-jewelz-ultimate-gem-jewelry-machine (retrieved 11 May 2017).

Drevnick PE, Lamborg CH, Horgan MJ, 2015. Increase in Mercury in Pacific Yellowfin Tuna. *Environ. Toxicol. Chem.* 34:931-934.

Eladak S, Grisin T. Moison D, Guerquin MJ, N'Tumba-Byn T, Pozzi-Gaudin S, Benachi A, Livera G, Rouiller-Fabre V, Habert R, 2015. A New Chapter in the Bisphenol A Story: Bisphenol S and Bisphenol F Are Not Safe Alternatives to This Compound. *Fertil. Steril.* 103:11-21.

FDA (U.S. Food and Drug Administration), 2000. Guidance for Industry: Action Levels for Poisonous or Deleterious Substances in Human Food and Animal Feed. U.S. Department of Health and Human Services, Silver Spring, Maryland, USA.

FDA (U.S. Food and Drug Administration), 2012. Indirect Food Additives: Polymers. *Federal Register* 77:41899-41902.

FDA (U.S. Food and Drug Administration), 2015. Final Determination Regarding Partially Hydrogenated Oils. *Federal Register* 80:34650-34760.

FDA (U.S. Food and Drug Administration), 2016a. Safety and Effectiveness of Consumer Antiseptics: Topical Antimicrobial Drug Products for Over-the-Counter Human Use. *Federal Register* 81:61106-61130.

FDA (U.S. Food and Drug Administration), 2016b. Melamine Pet Food Recall of 2007 (webpage last updated 22 July 2016). http://www.fda.gov/animalveterinary/safetyhealth/recallswithdrawals/ucm129575.htm (retrieved 2 September 2016).

FDA (U.S. Food and Drug Administration), 2017. Advice about Eating Fish, from the Environmental Protection Agency and Food and Drug Administration: Revised Fish Advice; Availability. *Federal Register* 82:6571-6574.

FEMA (U.S. Federal Emergency Management Agency), 2007. Fact Sheet – Household Chemicals. FEMA 567. U.S. Department of Homeland Security, Washington DC, USA.

FNB (Food and Nutrition Board), 2005. *Dietary Reference Intakes for Energy, Carbohydrate, Fiber, Fat, Fatty Acids, Cholesterol, Protein, and Amino Acids (Macronutrients)*. Washington DC, USA: The National Academies Press.

Galgani F, Jaunet S, Campillo A, Guenegen X, His E, 1995. Distribution and Abundance of Debris on the Continental Shelf of the North-Western Mediterranean. *Marine Poll. Bull.* 30:713-717.

Glaser A, 2004. The Ubiquitous Triclosan, a Common Antibacterial Agent Exposed. *Pesticides and You* 24: 12-17.

Gossner CM, Schlundt J, Embarek PB, Hird S, Lo-Fo-Wong D, Beltran JJO, Teoh KN, Tritscher A, 2009. The Melamine Incident: Implications for International Food and Feed Safety. *Environ. Health Perspect.* 117:1803-1808.

Hodgson E, Mailman RB, Chambers JE (Eds.), 1998. *Dictionary of Toxicology*. New York, New York, USA: Grove's Dictionaries Inc.

NG News (NationalGeographic.com News), 2008. Plastic-Bag Bans Gaining Momentum around the World. (reported by J. Roach, 4 April). http://news.nationalgeographic.com/news/2008/04/080404-plastic-bags.html (retrieved 28 October 2016).

NLM (U.S. National Library of Medicine), 2014. Tox Town – Chemicals (webpage last updated 9 December 2014). https://toxtown.nlm.nih.gov/text_version/chemicals.php (retrieved 2 October 2016).

Palace VP, Wautier KG, Evans RE, Blanchfield PJ, Mills KH, Chalanchuk SM, Godard D, McMaster ME, Tetreault GR, Peters LE, *et al.*, 2006. Biochemical and Histopathological Effects in Pearl Dace (*Margariscus margarita*) Chronically Exposed to a Synthetic Estrogen in a Whole Lake Experiment. *Environ. Toxicol. Chem.* 25:1114-1125.

Puckett J, Byster L, Westervelt S, Gutierrez R, Davis S, Hussain A, Dutta M, 2002. Exporting Harms: The High-Tech Trashing of Asia. The Basel Action Network, c/o Asia Pacific Environmental Exchange, 1305 Fourth Avenue, Suite 606, Seattle, Washington, USA.

Qiu W, Zhao Y, Yang M, Farajzadeh M, Pan C, Wayne NL, 2015. Actions of Bisphenol A and Bisphenol S on the Reproductive Neuroendocrine System during Early Development in Zebrafish. *Endocrinology.* 157: 636-647.

Rochester JR, Bolden AL, 2015. Bisphenol S and F: A Systematic Review and Comparison of the Hormonal Activity of Bisphenol A Substitutes. *Environ. Health Perspect.* 123:643-650.

Schneiderman AG, 2016. A.G. Schneiderman Finds Toxic Toys with High Lead Content Sold by K-mart, Target, Toy-R-Us Stores across New York. Press Release Statement, 22 April. Office of the Attorney General, The Capitol, Albany, New York, USA (PDF file retrieved online 11 January 2017).

Schultz IR, Skillman A, Nicolas J-M, Cyr DG, Nagler JJ, 2003. Short-Term Exposure to 17α-Ethynylestradiol Decreases the Fertility of Sexually Maturing Male Rainbow Trout (*Oncorhynchus mykiss*). *Environ. Toxicol. Chem.* 22:1272-1280.

SDUT (*San Diego Union-Tribune*), 2016. Nation's First Statewide Plastic-Bag Ban Now in Effect Across California (reported by J.E. Smith, 11 November).

The Los Angeles Times, 2008. State Bans Trans Fats: Restaurants in California Must Stop Cooking with the Substances, Except in Tiny Amounts, by 2010 (reported by P. McGreevy, 28 July).

Thiel M, Hinojosa I, Vásquez N, Macaya E, 2003. Floating Marine Debris in Coastal Waters of the SE-Pacific (Chile). *Marine Poll. Bull.* 46:224-231.

UNEP (United Nations Environment Programme), 2005. E-Waste, the Hidden Side of IT Equipment's Manufacturing and Use: Environmental Alert Bulletin No. 5. UNEP, P.O. Box 30552, Nairobi, Kenya.

U.S. EPA (U.S. Environmental Protection Agency), 1989. Report to Congress on Indoor Air Quality, Volume II: Assessment and Control of Indoor Air Pollution. EPA 400-1-89-001C. Office of Air and Radiation, Washington DC, USA.

U.S. EPA (U.S. Environmental Protection Agency), 2008. Amendment to the Universal Waste Rule: Addition of Pharmaceuticals. *Federal Register* 73:73520-73544.

U.S. EPA (U.S. Environmental Protection Agency), 2015. Proposed Rule: Management Standards for Hazardous Waste Pharmaceuticals. *Federal Register* 80:58014-58092.

U.S. EPA (U.S. Environmental Protection Agency), 2016. Lifetime Health Advisories and Health Effects Support Documents for Perfluorooctanoic Acid and Perfluorooctane Sulfonate. *Federal Register* 81: 33250-33251.

USGS (U.S. Geological Survey), 2002. Pharmaceuticals, Hormones, and Other Organic Waste-Water Contaminants in U.S. Streams. Fact Sheet FS-027-02. Toxic Substances Hydrology Program, Reston, Virginia, USA.

WGFSM (Work Group for Safe Markets), 2008. Baby's Toxic Bottle: Bisphenol A Leaching from Popular Baby Bottles. WGFSM-Clean Water Fund, 262 Washington Street, No. 301, Boston, Massachusetts, USA.

Review Questions

1. Name an antibacterial ingredient used in hundreds of consumer products (e.g., soaps, shampoos, toothpastes, cosmetics) every day (perhaps until recently) in the United States. And briefly describe its potential adverse health effects to humans.
2. Name one type of debris from entanglement and ingestion of which hundreds of thousands of marine creatures die each year.
3. Name the endocrine-disrupting chemical that was shown in a 2008 report to leach out of popular brands of baby bottles sold in Canada and the United States.
4. What was U.S. EPA's regulatory objective to add pharmaceutical waste to the federal Universal Waste Rule?
5. How does cyanuric acid affect melamine's toxicity in dogs, cats, and humans?
6. How can trans fats biochemically increase the risk of coronary heart disease?
7. Briefly describe three ways in which environmental toxicants may be grouped or classified.
8. Name five agents present in the environment that may trigger an asthma attack.
9. Which gas is commonly nicknamed the silent killer, and why?
10. Briefly describe the characteristics of free radicals and their biochemical actions in the human body.
11. What is airborne particulate matter?
12. Name three chemical families that are commonly referred to as POCs (persistent organochlorine compounds).
13. What are some of the adverse human health effects that plant toxicants can cause?
14. Which chemical family is commonly used as flame retardants in furniture foam and in plastics for television cabinets?
15. How is radon (likely) formed, and what is (are) its major adverse health effect(s)?
16. What are VOCs? And what are some of their adverse health effects on humans?

# CHAPTER 5

Fate and Transport of Toxicants in the Environment

5.1. Introduction

In many scholastic and regulatory sectors, most environmental exposures are treated as preventable and mitigable events, a point made explicitly in Chapters 2 and 3. This notion, or assertion to some people, rests on the argument that there is sufficient knowledge on how toxicants normally move and behave in the environment. In general, when a toxicant is released into the environment, it may move from the point of emission source into or across different environmental media (e.g., air, water, soils, sediments, foods, living organisms) at various locations. The toxicant may move as the original (parent) compound or as a degradate (i.e., breakdown product) with slightly to very different toxicological characteristics. More specifically, the contaminants or their degradates may move within or across various environmental media and undergo biological (biotic) or chemical (abiotic) transformation. These various transport and transformation processes are the subject matters of the present chapter.

Of note here is that there seems to be a lack of general consensus on some of the terms used in describing the behavior and movement of toxicants in the environment. The word *dispersion*, for instance, generally refers to the spread, diffusion, or distribution of materials. However, in air pollution modeling, it is a term referring to specifically the process of spreading out emission over a large area resulting in a lower concentration at the emission source. Yet regardless of how some terms may be used differently in different fields, there are fundamentals about the behavior and movement of materials in the environment that are not subject to much dispute among scholars.

5.1.1. Movement in the Environmental Media

For the most part, a toxicant in the atmosphere or water can move from one location to another by the two common processes known as *advection* and *diffusion*. Advection refers to the process in which a substance in the environment is moved *horizontally* by the mass motion of the medium (mostly air or water). Therefore, the variables that have strong impacts on atmospheric or oceanic advection include predominately the strength and direction of the wind in effect or the characteristics of the eddies in place. Diffusion, on the other hand, refers to the *spontaneous* movement of a substance from an area of high concentration to one of low concentration. The two transport processes can occur at the same time. There have been a number of advection-diffusion equations developed to simulate the concurrent occurrence of the two processes (e.g., Buske *et al.*, 2007, 2012; Jaiswal *et al.*, 2011; Lee *et al.*, 2007; Zhou *et al.*, 2016).

Animal migration, or the so-termed *biotransport* process, is also known capable of transporting environmental toxicants to a location far away (Chapter 6). Leaching, volatilization, and surface runoff are the more prominent phase-transfer processes responsible for transporting soil contaminants from one location to another.

5.1.2. Distribution into the Living Organisms

Pollutants moving in the environment enter terrestrial (or aquatic) plants largely via one of two processes. They can be deposited onto foliage via air (or water) movement, or be taken up by plant roots in contaminated soils. Following uptake by plants, a toxicant can be distributed into the various organs and tissues in the affected botanic organisms (Chapter 7).

In humans and other mammalians, the main portals of entry for environmental toxicants are skin, eyes, lungs, and gastrointestinal tract. Upon absorption, these toxicants may be bound to proteins in the blood. Their rapid transport via the bloodstream or the lymphatic system then follows (Chapter 7). Certain chemical substances (particularly those that are persistent in the environment) may undergo bioconcentration and bioaccumulation upon contact with the body of a biological system. These two biotransfer phenomena, along with biomagnification in a food web, are the topics discussed extensively in Chapter 6.

5.2. Fate and Transport of Air Pollutants

Air pollutants are toxic substances (e.g., chemicals, particulate matter, biological materials) that are introduced into the atmosphere where they can be in the form of solid particles, liquid droplets, or gas molecules. They may be emitted directly from a natural source such as the ashes from volcanic eruptions, or from an anthropogenic source such as nitrogen dioxide (NO_2) from automobile exhausts or sulfur dioxide (SO_2) discharged from factories. Many air pollutants are not emitted directly, however. Instead, they are formed in the atmosphere when other primary pollutants react or interact and thereby are termed *secondary* (i.e., second-generation) pollutants. An example of major secondary air pollutants is ozone (O_3) formed in the troposphere (i.e., the air layer closest to the Earth). Ozone of this type is one of the few key secondary air pollutants that make up photochemical smog. Smog is fog that has become contaminated with smoke. In photochemical smog, the smoke usually comes from such air pollution as motor vehicle exhausts which usually contain high contents of NO_2 and nitric oxide (NO). Not surprisingly, some air pollutants may occur with one portion coming from direct emission and the other (or another) portion coming from reactions or interactions of other primary pollutants. The general sources of air pollutants and their movement schemes are outlined graphically in Figure 5.1.

5.2.1. Local and Long-Range Transport

Many air pollutants, owing to their physicochemical properties, tend to travel short distances within a confined area where meteorological conditions are not as conducive. Yet even for a short distance, the travel could still mean hundreds of miles away, particularly if they travel with the aid of strong wind. In some cases, these air pollutants are so vulnerable to chemical or physical transformation (Section 5.2.3) that they will not be in the air for long. For example, even though elemental mercury (Hg^0) emitted from coal-fired utilities can be transported in the atmosphere for long distances (e.g., thousands of miles), it can be oxidized quickly to divalent mercury (Hg^{2+}). The divalent form of Hg in the gas phase is then removed from the atmosphere within a short distance from the emission source. In general, air pollutants can be removed from the atmosphere by falling onto the ground in precipitation or dust, or simply due to gravity. This type of removal of atmospheric substances is termed *air (atmospheric) deposition*.

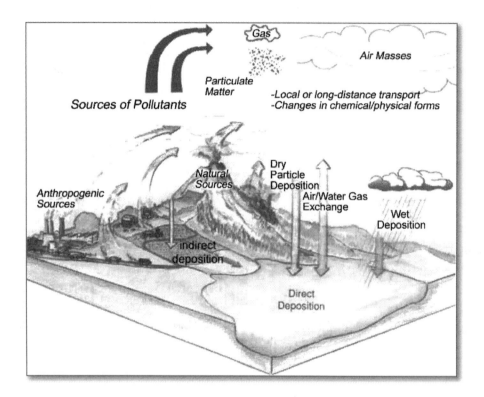

Figure 5.1. A Schematic of the Fate and Transport of Air Pollutants
(*from public domain source: U.S. EPA, 2001*)

Some pollutants from air deposition do not remain deposited on soils or in water for long. They are typically the persistent kind (e.g., PCBs, dioxins, certain forms of mercury). Owing to their chemical stability along with a set of conducive meteorological variables, these substances can be *re-emitted* from the contaminated soil or water. This event then can lead to a pattern known as *the grasshopper effect*, whereby a pollutant is emitted from an original source, transported for some short distances, deposited, and followed by a (large or small) portion of the deposited residues being re-emitted, being re-transported farther, and being re-deposited. The pattern may be repeated almost indefinitely until the pollutant residues reach high elevations or northern climates where cold condensation can and will take effect to retard their hopping (e.g., U.S. EPA, 2001).

5.2.2. Direct and Indirect Deposition

Pollutants from the atmosphere reach a water body generally in one of two modes. They can be deposited directly onto water surface (i.e., direct deposition) or onto land and later be carried away to water bodies through runoff (i.e., indirect deposition). Once these pollutant residues are deposited into the water, they can pose certain undesirable health and environmental threats, such as (threats of) contaminated seafood and unsafe drinking water.

Direct atmospheric deposition *per se* can be divided into two subprocesses: *dry* and *wet* deposition. Dry deposition can be caused by or due to one of several common phenomena in the absence of precipitation. For instance, airborne particles can fall down simply by gravitation or be transported to a surface by another physical force such as random air turbulent motions. A familiar physical phenomenon for this type of deposition is when particles flow too close to a branch of a tree, such as by advection, they may collide and thus be intercepted. Dry deposition is affected by a multiplicity of factors that usually interact in complex ways. The key variables involved are the characteristics of the atmosphere (e.g., temperature, wind speed), the nature of the landing surface (e.g., porosity, pH, aerodynamic roughness), and properties of the depositing species (e.g., shape, diameter, surface charge). Transport of gases through the atmosphere generally depends on turbulent and molecular diffusion. The chemical's solubility and reactivity are additional factors that can affect the capture of gas molecules by the landing surface.

Wet deposition occurs when any form of precipitation (e.g., rain, snow, sleet, cloud, fog) removes the atmospheric particles and delivers them to the Earth's surface. Precipitation occurs when the atmosphere, which basically is a huge volume of gaseous solution, becomes saturated with water vapor to the point that the water molecules condense causing them to precipitate out of this huge tank of gaseous solution and down to the Earth's surface. The water vapor molecules that precipitate out usually carry with them the air pollutant particles. A well-known example is acid rain which is caused by the emissions of mostly sulfur, nitrogen, or carbon compounds that can interact with water molecules in the atmosphere to produce acids. The more accurate term for acid rain is thus *acid deposition*.

5.2.3. Changes in Chemical/Physical Form

Depending on its physicochemical properties, an air pollutant may be subject to one or more chemical and/or physical transformations in the atmosphere. Those crucial phenomena or reactions involving the more prominent air pollutants are highlighted below.

A. Absorption and Release of Solar Radiation

There are gaseous molecules such as water vapor (H_2O) and carbon dioxide (CO_2) in the atmosphere with their atoms being held together loosely enough that they wobble when they absorb heat from the sun. Eventually, these trembling molecules release the absorbed heat in the form of radiant energy which is likely to be absorbed by nearby molecules with similar structural vulnerabilities. This process, which traps heat to near the Earth's surface, leads to the *greenhouse effect* in the same sense that a greenhouse works by keeping heat from the sun. The gaseous molecules responsible for the trapping effect are naturally termed *greenhouse gases*. Without these gases, heat would escape back into space above the troposphere; and then the Earth's average temperature would be below the habitable level. In addition to water vapor and carbon dioxide, the principal greenhouse gases are methane (CH_4), nitrous oxide (N_2O), O_3 (ozone), and chlorofluorocarbons

(CFCs). The principal uses of CFCs are as refrigerants (e.g., freons) in refrigeration units and as propellants in air conditioners, at least in the recent past. Although CFCs in the atmosphere can induce greenhouse effect, they have been found to cause serious depletion of the Earth's ozone shield. It has been said that too much greenhouse effect can lead to global warming.

B. Photochemical Reaction

Photolysis (a.k.a. photodissociation or photodecomposition) is a photochemical reaction occurring frequently in the atmosphere. It is a photoreaction whereby a chemical substance is broken down by a photon (hv), which is an elementary particle as well as the basic unit of all forms of electromagnetic radiation including light. Two of the most relevant photochemical reactions in the troposphere are:

$$O_3 + hv \rightarrow O_2 + O\cdot \tag{5.1}$$

$$NO_2 + hv \rightarrow NO + O\cdot \tag{5.2}$$

In Reaction 5.1, the excited oxygen atom ($O\cdot$) can react with H_2O vapor to produce the hydroxyl radical ($HO\cdot$). This radical is central to atmospheric chemistry in that it acts as an atmospheric detergent to cleanse many hydrocarbon (HC) pollutants by initiating their oxidation in the atmosphere. The oxygen atom ($O\cdot$) produced from Reaction 5.2 (or even from Reaction 5.1), on the other hand, can react with oxygen molecules (O_2) to form O_3; and the other co-product nitric oxide (NO) from Reaction 5.2 can remove O_3 by reacting with the latter to form NO_2 and O_2. The three subsequent or secondary reactions mentioned above are shown below as Reactions 5.3 through 5.5, respectively:

$$O\cdot + H_2O \rightarrow O_2 + HO\cdot \tag{5.3}$$

$$O\cdot + O_2 \rightarrow O_3 \tag{5.4}$$

$$NO + O_3 \rightarrow NO_2 + O_2 \tag{5.5}$$

In the presence of sunlight hv and oxygen, NO_2 can react with many (volatile) organic compounds, but more commonly with acetaldehyde (CH_3CHO) being the organic to produce *peroxyacetylnitrate* (PAN; CH_3CO-OO-NO_2) by first yielding the radical CH_3CO-$OO\cdot$:

$$NO_2 + O_2 + CH_3CHO + hv \rightarrow CH_3CO\text{-}OO\text{-}NO_2 \tag{5.6}$$

Nitrogen dioxide, nitric oxide, ozone, and PAN are the principal substances in photochemical smog. Both ozone and PAN in this type of pollution are secondary (i.e., second-generation), harmful pollutants that can cause breathing difficulties, eye and nose irritation, fatigue, headaches, and aggravation of respiratory problems.

C. Formation of Acid Rain

In addition to being one of the major ingredients in photochemical smog, atmospheric NO_2 can produce nitric acid (HNO_3) when it is oxidized by the hydroxyl radical (HO·) which is readily or easily available (e.g., Reaction 5.3). HNO_3, as produced from NO_2 in Reaction 5.7 below, is one of the acidic components frequently found in acid rain.

$$NO_2 + HO\cdot \rightarrow HNO_3 \tag{5.7}$$

Another acidic component sometimes even more commonly found in acid deposition is sulfuric acid (H_2SO_4). The common route or source of sulfuric acid formation, as shown in Reactions 5.8 through 5.10 below, involves the primary ingredient SO_2 and the three intermediates HO·, bisulfite radical ($HOSO_2\cdot$), and sulfur trioxide (SO_3).

$$SO_2 + HO\cdot \rightarrow HOSO_2\cdot \tag{5.8}$$

$$HOSO_2\cdot + O_2 \rightarrow SO_3 + HO_2\cdot \text{ (perhydroxyl radical)} \tag{5.9}$$

$$SO_3 + H_2O \rightarrow H_2SO_4 \tag{5.10}$$

When the precipitation that falls onto the Earth's surface is acidic, it has harmful effects on humans, plants, aquatic or terrestrial animals, and infrastructures. When reacting with H_2O vapor molecules in the atmosphere, CO_2 (carbon dioxide) too can produce an acidic component of acid rain. This acidic component is carbonic acid (H_2CO_3), which is less acidic than H_2SO_4 or HNO_3.

D. Lightning and Photosynthesis

Motor vehicle exhausts are not the only source of atmospheric NO and NO_2. The nitrogenous oxides can be formed when atmospheric N_2 reacts with atmospheric O_2 in the presence of high temperatures and pressures polarized by lightning strikes. It is the enormous and powerful electric current of lightning that can break N_2 into N atoms which can then react with O_2 to form NO_2 in the air (of which ~80% is N_2 gas).

On the other hand, CO_2 can lower its atmospheric level when pulled for use by plants nearby. Through photosynthesis (Reaction 5.11), plants can use sunlight to convert the captured atmospheric CO_2 molecules into the sugar *carbohydrate* ($C_6H_{12}O_6$) molecules to sustain their life. This explains why and how fruits typically become sweeter when grown under or exposed to more sunlight.

$$6CO_2 + 6H_2O + \text{sunlight } (hv) \rightarrow C_6H_{12}O_6 + 6O_2 \tag{5.11}$$

5.3. Fate and Transport of Water Contaminants

Water contaminants are often studied in terms of organic and inorganic substances. For their fate and transport in aquatic ecosystems, separate discussions on their general physicochemical behaviors in water can be found in the chapter by Lyman (1995). Those discussions provide the foundation for much of the overview given in this section. A modified version of Lyman's discussion on organic compounds is outlined graphically in Figure 5.2 below, only here with a specific focus on POCs (persistent organochlorine compounds). The focus on POCs here is more by preference, as some other organic substances (e.g., those also included in Chapter 16) and some inorganics (e.g., arsenic, cadmium, mercury) are equally very persistent in an aquatic system as well as highly toxic to human health. The reason for the POC preference here is that even though much of what follows applies to these other substances as well, certain physicochemical properties (e.g., lipophilicity) discussed below are more unique to or better known for POCs.

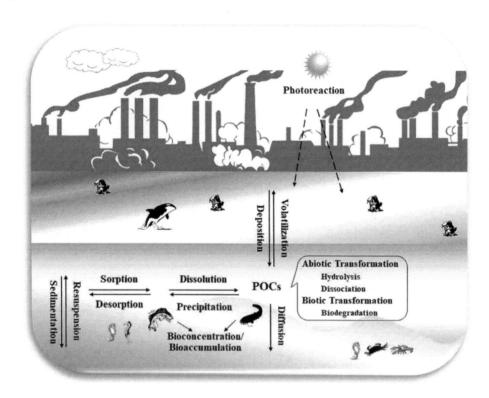

Figure 5.2. A Schematic of the Fate and Transport of Water Contaminants
(*POCs ≡ persistent organochlorine compounds*)

In many situations, whenever a substance manages to get into a water body, initially it will undergo one or more transport or physicochemical phase-transfer processes. For POCs as a group, *dissolution, volatilization,* and *(ad)sorption* appear to be the better-known processes for phase-transfer, whereas *sedimentation* and *diffusion* are the more common processes for transport. Within an aquatic system, POCs can be transformed into different chemical species or forms via one or more of the common abiotic or biotic processes. These transformation processes include, but are not limited to, *dissociation, hydrolysis, oxidation, photolysis,* and *biodegradation*. Each of these transport, phase-transfer, and transformation processes is strongly governed by the substance's physicochemical properties and the conditions of the aquatic system in which the substance is present. The properties and conditions generally considered crucial to the fate and transport of POCs (and many other substances) in aquatic systems are listed in Table 5.1 below.

Table 5.1. Physicochemical Properties and Water Conditions Pertinent to the Fate and Transport of Persistent Organochlorine Compounds in an Aquatic System[a]

Physicochemical Variable	Environmental Variable(s)
Molecular structure	Surface area and depth
Molecular weight	Flow; extent of mixing; bottom scouring
Water solubility	Sedimentation rate
Vapor pressure	Solar irradiation; presence of sensitizer
Henry's law constant (air-water partition)	Population and activity of microbes
Octanol-water partition coefficient (K_{ow})	Concentrations of nutrients and minerals
Light absorption spectrum	Temperature; pH (acidity)
Quantum yield	Nature of suspended particles
Diffusion coefficient	Concentration of suspended particles
Sorption constant for sediments	Water hardness; salinity; ionic strength
Bioconcentration factor	Level of dissolved organic matter
Biodegradation constant	Nature of bottom sediments

[a] see, e.g., Lyman (1995) for further reading, which is also the primary source for this table.

5.3.1. Phase-Transfer and Transport Processes

For POCs (persistent organochlorine compounds) in water, one of the key phase-transfer processes is *dissolution*, which involves a solute (e.g., a POC) being dissolved in a solvent (e.g., water). POCs in general are extremely hydro*phobic* (i.e., lipo*philic*). Dissolution thus is not relevant to most POCs in water unless when bulk quantities of these organic substances are discharged into the water, such as from a chemical spill or an improper waste disposal.

POCs are not completely insoluble in water, however. Although the water solubility of most any POC is extremely low, thus making the substance to behave rather hydrophobically, the total quantity of this substance that is eventually dissolved in the water can still be substantial. This is because in many aquatic systems, water is present in a huge volume compared to the POC content in the same volume, making the ratio of water to substance volume abnormally high (which in turn provides an aquatic system where a substance of very low solubility can still act as fairly soluble). Another reason is that via a reaction as well as a process called sorption (i.e., in the presence of suspended particles acting like a sponge constantly taking up the dissolved POC molecules), the organic's quantity in the water can easily exceed what will be expected from its water solubility. Furthermore, a substance's water solubility will be enhanced by decayed materials or dissolved organic carbon being present in the same water body.

As in accordance with the discussion given by Lyman (1995), the actual rate of dissolution for most any POC will depend on a number of factors including but not limited to:

- Ratio of the local water volume to substance (e.g., POC) volume.
- Degree of mixing in the water.
- Water's temperature (and in certain cases, its pH as well).
- Solubility of the substance (POC) in water.
- Presence of other organic materials affecting the substance's (POC's) water solubility.

One easy and perhaps the most practical approach to estimating a POC's water solubility is through use of its *o*ctanol-*w*ater partition coefficient (K_{ow}) as the predictor. This coefficient is measured as the ratio of a substance's concentration in octanol to its concentration in water at equilibrium and at a specified temperature, with the fatty alcohol octanol ($C_8H_{18}O$) being utilized as a surrogate for fatty tissues and other natural organic matter.

Another crucial phase-transfer for certain POCs is *volatilization* (a.k.a. evaporation) whereby the substance can be transported out of a water surface, across the air-water interface, and into the air directly above the aquatic system, all occurring without the breakdown of the substance into degradates. As to all other chemical groups, volatilization will be most relevant to POCs when the water body in which the organics are present is shallow and clear, and when there is sufficient air movement over the water surface. For this phase-transfer process, it is important for the POC to have a sufficiently high air-water partition coefficient which is often referred to as Henry's law constant for neutral compounds at dilute water concentration. This constant can be estimated from the substance's vapor pressure, molecular weight, and water solubility.

The third crucial phase-transfer process for POCs in water is *sorption* (a.k.a. *adsorption*), a process involving the transfer of a substance from the dissolved state to one in which the substance is attached (i.e., sorbed) to a solid, such as to a sediment. In other words, once the POC is dissolved in an aqueous solution and is relatively nonvolatile, it can be (*ad*)sorbed to a sediment. The sediment can be treated as acting like a sponge or magnet constantly taking up and harboring the molecules dissolved in the water.

The physicochemical basis for sorption of most substances, including POCs, can vary considerably depending on the chemical's properties and the nature of the adsorbent (e.g., a sediment). The general rule is that for low organic carbon sediments, physical adsorption dominates. If the adsorbent has a high organic carbon content, then chemical adsorption dominates. By chemical adsorption, it means that the binding or interaction responsible for sorption is of chemical nature, rather than physical.

The sorption potential K_d is defined as the *ratio* of the amount of the adsorbate sorbed per mass of adsorbent *to* the amount of the adsorbate remaining in the solution at equilibrium (U.S. EPA, 1999). K_d is an important parameter for understanding a substance's *d*istribution between the adsorbent (e.g., soil, sediment) and the surrounding water. For sediments or other adsorbents with a high organic carbon content, a practical value used to describe the sorption potential of a substance (e.g., POC) is its chemical-specific *o*rganic *c*arbon water partition coefficient K_{oc}. This coefficient can be approximated with some accuracy via correlation with the substance's K_{ow} (e.g., Briggs, 1981; Chiou *et al.*, 1983; Doucette, 2003; Karickhoff, 1981).

Once the POC molecules are sorbed to solids suspended in the water column, they will be deposited onto the bottom of the water body when the suspended solids eventually settle onto the bottom, even simply by gravitation. This entire process is termed *sedimentation*. It is not uncommon for bottom sediments to move away horizontally (e.g., via advection) at some appreciable rates. On the other hand, a POC in its undissolved state may be diffused into the sediment directly under the influence of concentration gradient; that is, by moving from areas of high concentration to areas of low concentration. Despite the fact that *diffusion* is a very slow process for most POCs in water, it nonetheless occurs continuously.

It is important to know that, in the three phase-transfer processes discussed above, the chemical movements are bidirectional (i.e., reversible). That is, as depicted in Figure 5.2, for chemical dissolution in water there is *precipitation*, which results in a solute forming a solid phase composed of the solute itself after the substance has exceeded its solubility limit. For volatilization from water, there is *atmospheric deposition*. And for chemical sorption to the sediment, there is *desorption*, which results in the release of the substance's molecules from the sediment.

5.3.2. Chemical (Abiotic) Transformation

In many situations, a POC in water (or in any medium) is not only subject to transport or phase-transfer. It can also undergo transformation into another chemical species or form when reacting with water or other substances in or around the aquatic system. For some POCs with low volatility when they are in clear water, sunlight *photolysis* can be a dominate degradation process. This type of transformation forms oxidation products that are usually more water-soluble while less volatile, typically resulting in reductive dechlorination via cleavage of the carbon-chlorine bond. The process is specific to the wavelength and the sensitizer factors present around the aquatic system. The end results of photolysis frequently involve a variety of reactions of the secondary kind such as dissociation, isomerization, and photoionization (e.g., Lyman, 1995). The aqueous half-lives for photolysis of many POCs are usually shortened when the process is induced with decayed materials in the same aquatic system. This may explain why under certain conditions the potent persistent dioxin 2,3,7,8-TCDD at or near water surface reportedly had a very short half-life of 24 hours in the summer to about 5 days in the winter (Podoll *et al.*, 1986).

One insignificant abiotic transformation process for most POCs but not for the pesticide heptachlor is *hydrolysis*, which involves replacing a chlorine atom by the OH (functional) group from a water molecule. In addition, if a POC acts as an acid or a base, it can undergo *dissociation*. Despite the fact that this chemical reaction does not apply much to most POCs, a few including the wood preservative pentachlorophenol (PCP) are highly susceptible to it.

5.3.3. Biological (Biotic) Transformation

As for most other chemical groups, the other type of transformation for POCs within an aquatic environment is *biotic*. Transformation of this type is commonly referred to as microbiologically-induced degradation, or biodegradation for short. This process is induced largely by microbes with high physiological versatility in sediments that tend to provide a good habitat for benthic biota. Biochemically, biodegradation is a process of electron transfer (that moving an electron from one atom or molecule to another) catalyzed by microbial enzymes. Since many specific enzymes (a group of complex proteins whose general characteristics and functions are given in Chapter 8) are not released outside of microbial cells, water contaminants subject to biodegradation must be brought into these cells first. Oftentimes when a specific organic substance cannot be (readily) utilized as a carbon (i.e., an energy) source by the indigenous microorganisms, it can still be degraded by a similar or the same type of enzymes released by the microbes from metabolizing (breaking down) *other* coexisting chemical substances for energy. This type of biodegradation is termed *co-metabolism*.

Biodegradation is regarded as one of the few crucial processes for many POCs in water, in spite of the fact that it involves a series of slowly occurring metabolic activities with half-lives typically in years. The process is usually slower for more complex structures such as dioxins and PCBs (polychlorinated biphenyls), than for relatively simpler structures such as many OC (organochlorine) pesticides. This kind of structural effect is expected in that a more complex POC structure will involve the cleavage of more carbon-chlorine bonds (with the resultant carbon being used as an energy substrate for microbial growth).

Biodegradation of POCs may be induced in water under *aerobic* (i.e., oxygen-rich) or *anaerobic* (i.e., oxygen-depleted) conditions. In aerobic biodegradation, the microbes utilize oxygen as the ultimate electron acceptor in breaking down the organic, whereas in anaerobic biodegradation they utilize electrophilic substrates such as sulfate and nitrate instead. Still some microbes can utilize both oxygen and inorganic salts as oxidants. The typical end result of biodegradation, regardless of the type of oxidants used, is *either* the conversion of the substance into another form *or* the degradation of the substance into more or less toxic degradates. Rarely would there be a thorough biodegradation leading to the same compound with minor changes in structure.

For POCs (and other substances), historically aerobic biodegradation was treated as the more dominate biotic transformation process compared to the biodegradation under anaerobic conditions. This notion was based on the general observation that more chemical substances are degraded at a higher rate with aerobic microbes, and thus on the misconception that larger volumes are taking place under aerobic conditions. Yet more recently, many types of sediments are known to be good habitats for many more anaerobic than aerobic microbes, and are the places where many POCs can be adsorbed onto. For instance, an extensive collaboration study (Lin *et al.*, 2006) confirmed the existence of a large community of anaerobic bacteria living on rocks about two miles below the Earth's surface, somewhere in a South Africa gold mine. These microbes were found to have been sustained solely by geologically-produced sulfate and hydrogen, with no apparent reliance on substrates (e.g., oxygen) derived from photosynthesis.

For many PCBs and dioxins, the parent compounds can be metabolized aerobically with carbon as an energy substrate for microbial growth. These organics can be degraded by co-metabolism as well. That is, they can be broken down in the presence of one or more other chemical substances serving as the needed substrates for microbial growth. Another way in which these parent compounds can be metabolized is with anaerobic microbes by reductive dechlorination via cleavage of the carbon-chlorine bond. In all instances, for the reasons given earlier, the rate of biodegradation decreases with increasing chlorination; and the process on the whole is very slow, with half-lives typically in years. For example, the half-lives of 2,3,7,8-TCDD in *deep* water range from 2 to 6 years, depending on the aquatic conditions (e.g., aerobic, anaerobic, temperature, pH, in groundwater, in sediments) in which the organic is present (e.g., Chiao *et al.*, 1994; Segstro *et al.*, 1995). Yet in spite of such slowness, biodegradation is the ultimate and, in most situations, the only pathway for complete destruction (degradation) of many POCs.

Because biodegradation of PCP (pentachlorophenol) is relatively rapid and extensive (particularly when this wood preservative is present at low aqueous concentrations), certain indigenous microbes have been utilized on many occasions to bioremediate (i.e., to clean up) this POC contaminant in various groundwater systems (e.g., DoD, 2002; Frick *et al.*, 1988). Studies revealed that with the addition of oxygen and within a month's time, certain indigenous microbes could remove PCP at the relatively low water level of less than 10 mg/L to below or near the U.S. federal drinking water standard of 1 µg/L (Schmidt *et al.*, 1999).

5.4. Fate and Transport of Soil Contaminants

Compared to air and water contaminants, there appear to be fewer health issues and less direct discussion in the environmental toxicology literature concerning soil contaminants or other non-aquatic surface deposits. One reason is that surface contaminants of this type are located in a much more stationary environment and hence in general are deemed less accessible to other ecosystems or to people. It is also for this very reason that this section's focus is on soil contaminants, not including other non-aquatic surface deposits, as terrestrial pollutants of environmental health concern. Overall, the fate and transport mechanisms or processes for soil contaminants in a terrestrial environment involve predominately the following:

- Volatilization (from soils)
- Degradation (in soils)
- Erosion and runoff (from soils)
- Leaching (from soils)

5.4.1. Volatilization from Soils

Volatilization can significantly affect the dissipation of soil (and other non-aquatic surface) contaminants, as this transfer process can discharge them into the atmosphere in substantial quantities. As with water pollutants, volatilization reactions are most significant to contaminants in surface soils that are in (nearly) direct contact with the atmosphere and are contingent on mostly the substance's volatility. This phase-transfer "loss" process is strongly influenced by the soil's pH, organic carbon content, and moist conditions.

Precipitation events (e.g., rain, irrigation) reportedly tend to increase volatilization of certain soil contaminants only. For example, a study showed that volatilization of mercury in soils after a series of rain events was about five orders of magnitude greater than prior to the events (Lindberg *et al.*, 1999). The simulation study by Song and Van Heyst (2005) suggested that soil moisture would enhance the effects of precipitation observed in the mercury experiment mentioned above. However, this does not seem to be the case for some organic substances, such as propargyl bromide (C_3H_3Br) which has been applied as a soil fumigant. This organic was found to evaporate three times *less* from irrigated than non-irrigated soils (Allaire *et al.*, 2004).

5.4.2. Degradation in Soils

In some situations, soils tend to provide a more conducive environment for biodegradation of organic substances than an aquatic system would. Moreover, it seems comparatively easier to artificially stimulate the number and activity of indigenous microbes in contaminated soils than in contaminated water. This type of microbial enhancement has been utilized with some success for the cleanup of organic contaminants in soils, such as the case with the wood preservative PCP noted earlier in relation to its groundwater contamination. Many factors affecting biodegradation of water pollutants apply to that of soil contaminants in the same vein. More specifically, for biodegradation of soil contaminants to be efficacious, elements and factors comparable to those listed in Table 5.1 should be considered. These variables include, but are not limited to: soil conditions (e.g., moisture, pH); suitability for/of microbes; availability of nutrients; and availability of oxygen and other electron acceptors.

Soil contaminants can be degraded via several common abiotic reactions, including photolysis and hydrolysis. For photolysis, the degradation is again most effective when the contaminant is close to the soil surface where it can be exposed to sunlight. For hydrolysis requiring reaction with water, the degradation is most efficacious when the contaminant is in the zone of saturation (i.e., in the area just below the water table).

5.4.3. Erosion and Runoff from Soils

Erosion is the process in which the rocks, soils, or the deposits on their surfaces are being worn away by action of water, ice, wind, or the kind. For instance, high winds can scrub fine contaminant particles bound to soils and discharge them downwind. Water erosion and surface runoff from heavy precipitation events can scrub these fine particles from surface soils as well. Runoff is the water flow that arises when the soil is infiltrated to beyond capacity thereby allowing the excess water to flow over and through the soil. When runoff flows along the ground, it can pick up soil contaminants such as toxic metal or herbicide residues. Surface runoff can be generated by rainfall or frequent heavy irrigation on a large farmland.

With soil contaminants dissolved or suspended in runoff, there likely comes water pollution as well since the contaminant load can reach various receiving aquatic systems (e.g., estuaries, lakes, rivers, streams, oceans). A study (Eckley and Branfireun, 2008) found a significant positive correlation between the mercury levels measured in surface runoff and those measured in the catchment water.

5.4.4. Leaching from Soils

In addition to surface runoff, another major source of water pollution by soil contaminants is leaching. Most chemical substances in soils have the potential or tendency to migrate downward to greater depths with infiltrating water, even down to the groundwater layer. When the soluble contaminant residues are lost (extracted) from a layer of the soil by percolating precipitation, they are carried downward (eluviated) and usually re-deposited (illuviated) in a lower layer. This transport process may eventually allow the contaminant residues to reach beyond the water table down to the groundwater layer. The extent to which a soil contaminant is leached is strongly influenced by a number of relevant physicochemical and environmental parameters: hydraulic loading (e.g., amount of rainfall); water table conditions (e.g., temperature, pH); soil permeability; and the contaminant's tendency to partition between the solid and the aqueous phase (which is mainly a function of the contaminant's solubility as well as its sorption potential binding to organic matters in the soil). Many chemical fertilizers (e.g., ammonium nitrate), pesticides (e.g., atrazine, simazine), and metals (e.g., arsenic, cadmium) in soils are highly susceptible to leaching in this manner.

References

Allaire SE, Yates SR, Ernst FF, 2004. Effect of Soil Moisture and Irrigation on Propargyl Bromide Volatilization and Movement in Soil. *Vadose Zone J.* 3:656-667.

Briggs GG, 1981. Theoretical and Experimental Relationships between Soil Adsorption, Octanol-Water Partition Coefficients, Water Solubilities, Bioconcentration Factors, and the Parachlor. *J. Environ. Agric. Food Chem.* 29:1050-1059.

Buske D, Vilhena MT, Moreira D, Tirabassi T, 2007. Two-Dimensional Steady State Advection-Diffusion Equation – An Analytical Solution. In *Developments in Environmental Science Series 6: Air Pollution Modeling and Its Application XVIII* (Borrego C, Renner E, Eds.). Oxford, UK: Elsevier, pp.802-804.

Buske D, Vilhena MT, Tirabassi T, Bodmann B, 2012. Air Pollution Steady-State Advection-Diffusion Equation: The General Three-Dimensional Solution. *J. Environ. Protect.* 3:1124-1134.

Chiao FF, Currie RC, McKone TE, 1994. Final Draft Report: Intermedia Transfer Factors for Contaminants Found at Hazardous Waste Sites: 2,3,7,8-Tetrachloro-Dibenzo-*p*-Dioxin (TCDD). Risk Science Program, Department of Environmental Toxicology, University of California, Davis, California, USA.

Chiou CT, Porter PE, Schmedding DW, 1983. Partition Equilibria of Non-Ionic Organic Compounds between Soil Organic Matter and Water. *Environ. Sci. Technol.* 17:227-231.

DoD (U.S. Department of Defense), 2002. Building on Cleanup Success, FY02 DERP (Defense Environmental Restoration Program) Annual Report to Congress. Washington DC, USA.

Doucette WJ, 2003. Quantitative Structure-Activity Relationships for Predicting Soil-Sediment Sorption Coefficients for Organic Chemicals. *Environ. Toxicol. Chem.* 22:1771-1788.

Eckley CS, Branfireun B, 2008. Mercury Mobilization in Urban Stormwater Runoff. *Sci. Total Environ.* 403:164-177.

Frick TD, Crawford RL, Martinson M, Chresand T, Bateson G, 1988. Microbiological Cleanup of Groundwater Contaminated by Pentachlorophenol. *Basic Life Sci.* 45:173-191.

Jaiswal DK, Kumar A, Yada RR, 2011. Analytical Solution to the One-Dimensional Advection-Diffusion Equation with Temporally Dependent Coefficients. *J. Water Res. Protect.* 3:76-84.

Karickhoff SW, 1981. Semi-Empirical Estimation of Sorption of Hydrophobic Pollutants on Natural Sediments and Soil. *Chemosphere* 10:833-846.

Lee M-M, Nurser AJG, Coward AC, de Cuevas BA, 2007. Eddy Advective and Diffusive Transports of Heat and Salt in the Southern Ocean. *J. Phys. Oceanogr.* 37:1376-1393.

Lin L-H, Wang P-L, Rumble D, Lippmann-Pipke J, Boice E, Pratt LM, Lollar BS, Broide EL, Hazen TC, Andersen GL, *et al.*, 2006. Long-Term Sustainability of a High-Energy, Low-Diversity Crustal Biome. *Science* 314:479-482.

Lindberg SE, Zhang H, Gustin M, Vette A, Marsik F, Owens J, Casimir A, Ebinghaus R, Edwards G, Fitzgerald C, *et al.*, 1999. Increases in Mercury Emissions from Desert Soils in Response to Rainfall and Irrigation. *J. Geophys. Res.* 104:21879-21888.

Lyman WJ, 1995. Transport and Transformation Processes. In *Fundamentals of Aquatic Toxicology: Effects, Environmental Fate, and Risk Assessment* (Rand GM, Ed.), 2nd Edition. Philadelphia, Pennsylvania, USA: Taylor & Francis, Chapter 15.

Podoll RT, Jaber HM, Mill T, 1986. Tetrachlorodibenzodioxin: Rates of Volatilization and Photolysis in the Environment. *Environ. Sci. Technol.* 20:490-492.

Schmidt LM, Delfino JJ, Preston JF 3rd, St. Laurent G 3rd, 1999. Biodegradation of Low Aqueous Concentration Pentachlorophenol(PCP) Contaminated Groundwater. *Chemosphere* 38:2897-2912.

Segstro MD, Muir DCG, Servos MR, Webster GRB, 1995. Long-Term Fate and Bioavailability of Sediment-Associated Polychlorinated Dibenzo-p-Dioxins in Aquatic Mesocosms. *Environ. Toxicol. Chem.* 14: 1799-1807.

Song X, Van Heyst B, 2005. Volatilization of Mercury from Soils in Response to Simulated Precipitation. *Atmos. Environ.* 39:7494-7505.

U.S. EPA (U.S. Environmental Protection Agency), 1999. Understanding Variation in Partition Coefficient, Kd, Values, Volume I (EPA 402-R-99-004A) & Volume II (EPA 402-R-99-004B). Office of Air and Radiation, Washington DC, USA.

U.S. EPA (U.S. Environmental Protection Agency), 2001. Frequently Asked Questions about Atmospheric Deposition – A Handbook for Watershed Managers. EPA-453/R-01-009. Office of Wetlands, Oceans & Watersheds and Office of Air Quality Planning & Standards, Washington DC, USA.

Zhou JG, Haygarth PM, Withers PJ, Macleod CJ, Falloon PD, Beven KJ, Ockenden MC, Forber KJ, Hollaway MJ, Evans R, *et al.*, 2016. Lattice Boltzmann Method for the Fractional Advection-Diffusion Equation. *Phys. Rev. E.* 93:043310 (online journal).

Review Questions

1. Briefly describe the two principal transport processes whereby a water or an air contaminant generally travels from one location to another in the environment.

2. Name two secondary (i.e., second-generation) air pollutants and describe in general terms how they can occur in the environment.

3. Briefly describe the grasshopper effect in relation to atmospheric deposition of environmental contaminants.

4. Briefly describe the main differences between dry and wet deposition of air pollutants.

5. Briefly explain how acid deposition can be formed.

6. Briefly describe how some air pollutants can cause a greenhouse effect.

7. Give an example to illustrate how hydroxyl radical (HO·) can be formed. And briefly explain why this radical is central to atmospheric chemistry.

8. What is a photon? And why does it play a key role in photochemical smog?

9. Name four principal chemical components (ingredients) in photochemical smog.

10. Name two most toxic acidic components that are likely to be found in acid rain.
11. Name three phase-transfer processes and two transport processes that are common to most water contaminants.
12. Why is it true that dissolution could still lead to a potential water pollution with POCs even though most of these organic substances have very low water solubility?
13. With respect to (ad)sorption of a POC onto sediments with a high organic carbon content, how is its sorption potential K_d related to its *octanol-water* partition coefficient K_{ow}?
14. What may be a common abiotic transformation process for pollutants present on or near a clear water surface?
15. Briefly explain the processes *biodegradation* and *co-metabolism* used in characterizing the biotic transformation of water or soil contaminants. Why is biodegradation not a practical transformation process for air pollutants?
16. Briefly explain why biodegradation is typically slower for dioxins and PCBs than for many organochlorine pesticides.
17. Name a POC that serves as an exception to the rule (or notion) that biodegradation is a very slow process for many POCs.
18. Name the four key processes for transporting soil contaminants in the environment.
19. Name two abiotic reactions through which soil contaminants can be degraded substantially.
20. What may be an explanation that there tends to be less immediate environmental health concerns with soil contaminants than with air and water pollutants?
21. Briefly describe two transport processes whereby soil contaminants can pollute groundwater.

CHAPTER 6

Bioaccumulation of Persistent Environmental Toxicants

6.1. Introduction

In its broadest term, *bioaccumulation* is a construct concerning the accumulation of substances in a biological organism. It involves primarily three interrelated quantitation processes termed *bioconcentration*, *bioaccumulation*, and *biomagnification*. These three processes are highly relevant to the exposure analysis component inherent in ecological (Chapter 22) or human health (Chapter 23) risk assessment. In this chapter, persistent organochlorine compounds (POCs) in aquatic systems are used to illustrate the dynamics and relevance of bioaccumulation of persistent environmental toxicants. Aquatic systems and POCs are utilized in this chapter as the bioaccumulation setting because most POCs have high lipophilicity and the water environment is conducive to bioconcentration as well as bioaccumulation. The significance of lipophilicity and other key factors to bioaccumulation is discussed toward the end of this chapter in Section 6.4.

It should be noted that bioaccumulation is not limited to organochlorine (OC) compounds. For instance, in addition to elemental mercury (Hg^0), the main forms of mercury commonly found in an aquatic system are ionic Hg (e.g., those binding to chloride or organic acids) and organic Hg (e.g., notably the monomethyl mercuric cation). The organic monomethyl mercuric cation CH_3Hg^+ (a.k.a. methylmercury) is highly bioaccumulative, at least much more so than inorganic Hg. This is because its organic methyl (CH_3) group is lipophilic and as such, the cation is better retained by living organisms in a food web.

6.1.1. Relevance of Food Web/Food Chain

The conception of bioaccumulation cannot be fully appreciated without some understanding of the dynamic construct of food web, as the two constructs are closely interrelated. In human health or ecological risk assessment, the bioaccumulation construct that is often abstracted into a model is commonly used to simulate xenobiotic accumulation in a food web in order to give a fuller account of the dietary exposure to the substance at issue. A food web model, on the other hand, offers a practical means to validate the abstracted bioaccumulation model, in that the former model can be applied to systematically characterize the latter and can relate causality to the interconnections observed between the biota and their ecosystem, ecoregion, or even ecozone.

Food webs are each a representation of the feeding relationships between species within an ecosystem, an ecoregion, or as high up as an ecozone. They can be regarded as systematic, graphic descriptions of the prey-predator relationships among species within an ecological community. More specifically, a food web is a series of related food chains which each show a simpler, linear link of prey-predator relationships. Each food web thereby attempts to outline a more complex yet more complete interconnected system of the feeding relationships (i.e., of the related food chains) occurring within a given ecological community.

Organisms in a food chain are grouped into hierarchic positions known as *trophic* levels. The trophic level of an organism is its position in a food chain or, more specifically, its position in the sequence of feedings and food energy transfer within an ecological community. A simple and yet relatively complete food chain is often illustrated by four basic trophic levels as follows: plants → herbivores → carnivores → omnivores. Plants or phytoplankton are *auto*trophs as they produce their own food. As such, they are the primary producers and are on the first (i.e., base) trophic level. Herbivores are their primary consumers and as such are on the second trophic level. Carnivores that consume these herbivores are considered as secondary consumers to the plants and are placed on the third trophic level. There are omnivores such as humans that consume both the herbivores and carnivores. These omnivores are hence called tertiary consumers (to the plants) and are put on the fourth trophic level. Figure 6.1 below shows a simplified food chain (or even a simplified food web) that can be used to characterize the bioaccumulation of POCs involving human exposure.

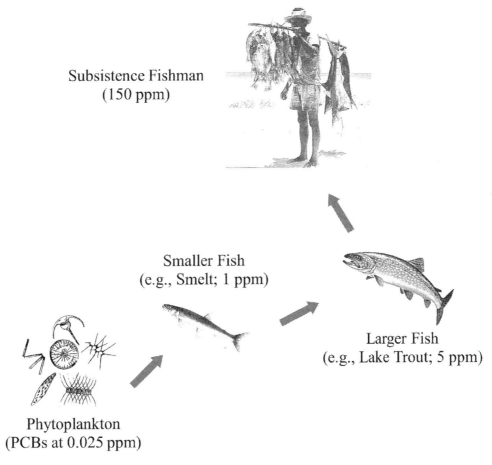

Figure 6.1. A Simplified Aquatic Food Chain for Persistent Bioaccumulative (Toxic) Substances
(*exemplified with PCBs ≡ polychlorinated biphenyls in each body; ppm ≡ parts per million*)

6.1.2. Relevance to Exposure Hazard Assessment

Bioaccumulation is a crucial component of exposure hazard assessment for POCs and other groups of persistent substances. The capability of predicting accurately the bioaccumulation of substances in aquatic systems, which typically involve fish, has thereby become a key element in assessing human health and ecological impacts of environmental pollutants. This notion rests on the argument that the assessment of a more realistic, fuller dietary exposure of humans or piscivorous wildlife to a substance needs to account for the substance's bioaccumulation in the environment (which includes likely an aquatic system).

For non-bioaccumulative substances, human health or ecological risk is related more directly to their external (e.g., environmental) concentrations. In contrast, the risk of bioaccumulative substances (as defined in Section 6.2 below) is related more to their levels in the body tissues of the target organism. This complicates the older, conventional approach to health or ecological risk assessment for bioaccumulative substances, as there is supposedly a need to account for the bioaccumulation of these substances in a food web.

Substances that are lipophilic tend to build up to higher concentrations in humans or other higher-order animals since their bodies have relatively more fatty tissues, a point being made explicitly in the sections that follow. Persistent, bioaccumulative, toxic substances (PBTs) released into an aquatic system thus have the potential to bioaccumulate to the point where these contaminants can adversely affect the health of the aquatic biota or of humans and (other) animals that consume these contaminated creatures.

6.2. Bioconcentration and Estimation of Its Potential

When contaminants are not already degraded in the environment, they are subject to *bioconcentration*. From a health risk assessment perspective, bioconcentration is one of the few most crucial biotransfer processes in the overall fate and transport of persistent toxicants in the environment. This process refers to both the uptake and the retention of a toxicant in an organism's tissue, typically to the extent that its concentration in the host organism's tissue can eventually be much higher than its (source) concentration in the surrounding medium (e.g., water).

6.2.1. Bioconcentration in Aquatic Media

Toxicants such as the lipophilic POCs can be accumulated in fish tissue through direct uptake, with concentrations up to *million* times greater than their concentrations in the surrounding water (i.e., the source). The extent of this type of chemical concentration is commonly measured as an index referred to as *bioconcentration factor* (BCF). This index is expressed as the ratio of the substance's concentration in an organism's tissue (e.g., in mg/kg wet or lipid weight) to its concentration in the surrounding medium (typically in water in mg/L) *at equilibrium*. Many BCF estimations have been based on aquatic measurements since fish and other aquatic creatures generally provide a rich lipophilic microenvironment conducive to bioconcentration.

In the United States, substances are considered to have an alarming potential for bioconcentration if they have a BCF value ≥1,000 or a $\log_{10} K_{ow}$ value >4 (Corl, 2001; U.S. EPA, 1999). These criterion values are below those adopted by Canada (CEPA, 2000) and some other western countries (*see*, e.g., Table 16.1 in Chapter 16).

6.2.2. Bioconcentration Factor (BCF)

For POCs in fish, their BCFs can be approximated from the log of their K_{ow} (*o*ctanol-*w*ater partition coefficient, as briefly described in Chapter 5) using the log-linear regression *$\log_{10}$ (BCF) = [(0.79) x $\log_{10}$ (K_{ow}) – 0.40]* given by van Gestel *et al.* (1985). Similar equations by others (e.g., Veith *et al.*, 1980) may be used, though expectedly ending with somewhat different results. As shown in Table 6.1 below, using the van Gestel equation, a BCF value of over one million has been estimated for the PCB 209 and the *octa*CDD congener (*see* Chapter 16 for their definition and congener nomenclature).

Table 6.1. Bioconcentration Factors (BCFs) Estimated/Projected for Select Persistent Organochlorine Compounds (POCs)[a]

Select POC	$\log_{10} K_{ow}$[b]	BCF (L/kg)[b]
Lindane	3.55[a]	254
PCP (Pentachlorophenol)	4.59[a]	1,683
Dieldrin	4.95[a]	3,240
Heptachlor	4.95[a]	3,240
HCB (Hexachlorobenzene)	5.18[a]	4,923
PCB 28	5.80[b]	15,205
p,p'-DDT	5.90[a]	18,239
2,3,7,8-TCDF	6.10[b]	26,242
Aldrin	6.29[a]	37,077
2,3,7,8-TCDD	6.80[b]	93,756
PCB 138	6.97[c]	127,732
*hexa*CDD (1,2,3,4,7,8-)	7.80[b]	578,096
*octa*CDD (1,2,3,4,6,7,8,9-)	8.20[b][d]	1,196,741
PCB 209	8.27[e]	1,359,252

[a]from approximation with $\log_{10} K_{ow}$ based on the equation $\log_{10}$ (BCF) = [0.79 x $\log_{10}$ (K_{ow}) – 0.40] (van Gestel *et al.*, 1985), using where applicable the midrange of the $\log_{10} K_{ow}$ calculated or measured within 20° – 25°C (68° – 77°F), with the majority at 25°C; K_{ow} ≡ *o*ctanol-*w*ater partition coefficient (*see* text); *see* Table 16.2 for numbering of PCB, PCDD, and PCDF congeners.

[b][a] Montgomery (1993); [b] MacKay *et al.* (1992); [c] Rapaport and Eisenreich (1984); [d] Shiu *et al.* (1988); [e] Hawker and Connell (1988); note that BCF can be expressed as unitless as L (liter of water) ≈ kg (kilogram).

Another quantitative approach widely utilized for approximating BCFs from K_{ow} is via application of the log-log *q*uantitative *s*tructure-*a*ctivity *r*elationship (QSAR) framework. In its simplest term, the QSAR framework is a statistical (primarily regression) model relating the physicochemical properties of a substance (i.e., the predictor variables) to its (biological) activity (i.e., the response variable). Several regulatory agencies including notably U.S. EPA have utilized the K_{ow}-based QSAR model to approximate BCFs for hundreds of substances including many POCs. An extensive review by Cronin *et al.* (2002) was published relating the QSAR framework's applicability as well as its application for BCF approximation.

A BCF value can also be determined directly from a site-specific field study, which must show that the test substance's concentration in water remained constant over the range of the organism's inhabitation and for a duration not less than 4 weeks (to ensure an equilibrium state). Another required condition is that the substance's bioavailability must not be affected by its (gradual) removal from the solution through competing mechanisms. The third, final required condition is that the substance's concentration which the test organism was exposed to must be below the lowest that would cause an adverse effect on the organism.

For BCFs measured in a laboratory setting instead, a total of five conditions should be met. First, the BCF should be calculated from the test substance's concentrations measured in a test solution. Second, the test should be either of sufficient duration to reach steady state or lasting 4 weeks or longer. Third, as for the field data, the substance's concentration which the test organism was exposed to must be below the lowest that would cause harm to the organism. Fourth, the BCF should be calculated on a wet tissue weight basis. Fifth and lastly, the (geometric) mean should be used if more than two BCF estimates are available for the same species.

In many western and European countries, it is recommended that the laboratory studies for BCF estimation be performed using a method consistent to the one specified in the Organization for Economic Cooperation and Development (OECD, 2012) Test Guidelines 305. In many aspects, the OECD guidelines are similar to those provided (updated) by U.S. EPA (2016). Overall, most regulatory entities have agreed that compared to those from laboratory studies, field data generally provide more accurate or more realistic BCF estimates.

6.3. Bioaccumulation and Biomagnification

Bioaccumulation as a biological phenomenon or quantitation process (*vs.* as a construct) refers to *a single* organism's uptake *and* retention of a toxicant from *all sources*, including all sites and routes, not just from one medium (e.g., water, soils) like in the bioconcentration case. When this organism is consumed by its predator, *biomagnification* occurs. This is because the toxicant is now bioaccumulated in the predator's tissue, with its concentration magnifying in a food chain, in the sense that the predator is likely to consume more than one similarly contaminated prey. Bioaccumulation is most relevant to POC type toxicants in that they tend to concentrate in fatty tissues, particularly in species at the top of a food chain. The reality is that in species on higher trophic levels, the fatty tissues tend to be more abundant and more lipophilic.

In short, aquatic systems tend to be contaminated easily and substantially by OCs (organochlorines) which are mostly highly persistent substances. These POCs subsequently can be concentrated and accumulated inside small aquatic biota within the same aquatic environment. As these contaminated creatures fall prey to carnivorous fishes, birds, and large terrestrial or amphibian species nearby, the contaminant's concentrations are progressively magnified in each of the predators in the food web. Therefore, human seafood eaters too may suffer adverse health effects from bioaccumulation and biomagnification of POCs as well as other POPs (persistent organic pollutants).

Moreover, many ecosystems (e.g., plants, soils, or any of their combinations with or without water) are found able to provide a conducive environment for bioconcentration, bioaccumulation, and biomagnification of these persistent substances.

6.3.1. Toxic Equivalency in Bioaccumulation

One reality about bioaccumulation is that an organism can be exposed to the same toxicant multiple times. An axiom to this notion is that insofar as the organism's health is the endpoint at stake, two structurally similar or even two different substances can be treated as the same ones if, for all practical purposes, both exert the same kind of adverse effects of concern in (nearly) all aspects. It is based on this axiom that in the literature, the concentrations of DDT and its two equally persistent metabolites DDD and DDE (Chapter 15) in a sample were typically combined and reported as one total; that is, simply as the concentration of the sum of all DDT-related compounds (as denoted by ΣDDTs) found in the sample. This approach is also frequently applied for reporting the concentrations of all PCB congeners measured in environmental samples.

The above approach is not utilized across the board, however. For reporting the concentrations of all dioxin congeners in a sample, a modification of the above approach is employed instead. This deviation owes to the fact as well as the concern that the dioxin member 2,3,7,8-TCDD (or TCDD for short) is regarded as the most potent of all congeners in the dioxin family. Therefore, for all other congeners in a mixture, their measured amounts usually are each adjusted downward for their potency relative to that of TCDD. For example, suppose a sample was measured to have 1 unit of TCDD and 5 units of 2,3,7,8-TCDF (or TCDF for short), the *overall* or *total* TCDD-equivalent amount of the two dioxins in the sample would be reported as 1.5 units, since the TCDF potency has been determined by the World Health Organization (WHO) as *one-tenth* of that of TCDD (van den Berg *et al.*, 2006). That is, TCDF has been given a (mammalian) toxic equivalency factor (TEF) of 0.1.

There are *theoretically* 75 possible congeners (members) of PCDDs (polychlorinated dibenzo-*para*-dioxins) and 135 possible congeners of PCDFs (polychlorinated dibenzofurans) that can be found in the environment, simply due to the various numbers and positions that the chlorine atoms can be structurally bonded to the carbon atoms in these congeners. Nevertheless, when based on the *number* of chlorine atoms present alone, there are only 29 members currently subject to TEF consideration. These include: 7 congeners of PCDDs; 10 congeners of PCDFs; and 12 dioxin-like congeners of PCBs. These 29 dioxin and dioxin-like congeners, along with their (mammalian) TEFs assigned by WHO, are listed in Table 16.3 (Chapter 16).

6.3.2. Cases of Bioaccumulation and Biomagnification

Bioaccumulations (and hence bioconcentrations as well) of PCBs, DDTs, and many other OCs are real phenomena. These POCs have been found in some remote regions where these substances have never been produced or used (e.g., Cone, 2005; Matthies and Scheringer, 2001). For instance, the Inuit living in the Canadian Arctic have never used PCBs or other OCs. Yet a study on these people living in northern Quebec showed that their whole blood samples had levels of PCBs and PCB metabolites (e.g., OH-PCBs) up to 70 times higher compared to the whole blood samples pooled from the non-Arctic southern part of Canada (Sandau *et al.*, 2000). One likely source of the Inuit's elevated exposure to these substances was from consuming contaminated marine mammals and fish, which are part of their regular high-protein, high-fat diet.

Coincidentally, around that time period, detectable to alarmingly high levels of PCBs, DDTs, and some other OCs were reported in marine mammal samples collected from California USA (Kajiwara *et al.*, 2001), Finland (Koistinen *et al.*, 1997; Kostamo *et al.*, 2002), and Russia (Muir *et al.*, 2003). Those data showed support of the bioaccumulative nature of many of these persistent pollutants, as evident from the study results briefly accounted for below.

The American (California) study was conducted to analyze the contents of PCBs, DDTs, and other persistent substances in the blubber and livers of 31 marine mammals. These mammals included 15 California sea lions, 6 northern elephant seals, and 10 harbor seals that were found stranded along the Pacific coasts off California between 1991 and 1997. Among the substances analyzed, DDTs were found predominate, followed by PCBs. The highest concentrations were found in the blubber of sea lions, with the highest DDT and PCB levels being 2.9 and 1.3 mg/g, lipid weight, respectively.

In the Finnish study by Koistinen *et al.* (1997), the contents of several OCs were measured in seal samples from the Gulf of Finland and in sediments from the gulf or near Gotland, all collected around 1991. The OCs under analysis included PCBs, their structural cousins polychlorinated diphenyl ethers (PCDEs), and dioxins. The sediment samples included one surface core per sampling site. The seal specimens consisted of 14 ringed seals and 6 grey seals that all were found dead and examined for pathology in late 1991. For all the 50 *tetra*- through *deca*-CDE congeners analyzed (i.e., those diphenyls with 4 to 10 chlorines), their levels in seal blubber ranged from <0.3 to 62 ng/g, lipid weight. In ringed seals with good nutritional status, the levels of most PCDE congeners were found higher in the two adult females than in the young. In the sediments, the levels of dioxin congeners expressed as TCDD-equivalent were found higher compared to those of the dioxin-like PCBs (as defined in Section 16.7).

The other Finnish study by Kostamo *et al.* (2002) was conducted in part to analyze changes in the concentrations of OCs in the blubber of Saimaa ringed seals that died between 1981 and 2000 at Lake Hauivesi, Finland. The study found a substantially higher biomagnification of these substances from prey fish to the ringed seal than to the pike. Its conclusion was based on the higher feeding rate and the metabolism differences observed in the ringed seals.

In the Russian study, the contents of PCBs, DDTs, and several other OCs were analyzed in the blubber of harp seals, ringed seals, and bearded seals, as well as in several fishes and invertebrates, all from the White Sea in northwest Russia. Highest concentrations of ΣPCBs and ΣDDTs were found in specimens from two male bearded seals (with mean concentrations of 4.2 ng/kg and 4.0 ng/kg, lipid weight, respectively). Female harp seals had mean ΣPCB and ΣDDT concentrations of 1.1 ng/kg and 0.6 ng/kg, lipid weight, respectively. The male and female adult ringed seals had similar mean concentrations of ΣPCBs found in the harp seals. The blubber concentrations were considerably lower for all other OCs analyzed in all the seal specimens. The predominate OCs found in the fish samples were PCBs and DDT-related compounds, ranging from approximately 16 to 41 ng/kg, wet weight.

There are still more data from more studies emerging that continue to show support for the bioaccumulative nature of POCs. Some of these studies have been conducted even in a somewhat unique or unconventional setting. For example, there are the Portuguese study by Antunes *et al.* (2007) with cultivated seabass samples, the Brazilian study by Bussolaro *et al.* (2012) with freshwater fish samples, the American study by Liebens and Mohrherr (2015) with sediment samples, the Argentinian study by Durante *et al.* (2016) with dolphin samples, and the Chinese study by Han *et al.* (2017) with soil, rice plant, and food animal samples.

The Portuguese study analyzed 33 PCB congeners in diet pellets, in a biotic compartment, and in three different size classes (length ranges) of seabass (*Dicentrarchus labrax*). The test fish were raised in a semi-intensive fish farm located in the south region of Portugal. Bioaccumulation factor (BAF) and biomagnification factor (BMF), along with biota-suspended particulate matter accumulation factor (BSMAF), were determined to compare the behavior and properties of the different PCB congeners. In that study, BMF was defined as the ratio between the concentration of PCBs in fish tissue and in the diet pellets, both on lipid weight basis. And biomagnification was assumed to occur if the calculated BMF value was greater than 1. The study showed that overall, lower chlorinated PCBs had higher calculated BMF values.

The Brazilian study investigated the bioaccumulative nature of POCs in the native freshwater fish *Hypostomus commersoni*. The POCs were analyzed in the liver and muscle samples of 13 specimens collected in a lake located in the city of Ponta Grossa. Among the POCs analyzed, PCBs were found having the highest concentrations, with a total of 427 ng/g dry weight in the liver samples and a total of 69.2 ng/g dry weight in the muscle samples.

In the American study, POCs were analyzed in the sediments of Escarribia Bay and River in northwest Florida, an estuary area historically polluted by unregulated industrial and domestic sewage releases. In the 57 composite sediment samples collected, 12 (21%) had levels of PCBs exceeding the Florida state's threshold effects level (TEL) of 21.6 µg/kg. For DDTs, their levels were found exceeding the state's probable effects level of 4.8 µg/kg in all the samples except one. For dioxins and dioxin-like PCBs, the mean total TEQ was assessed at 2.6 ng/kg, exceeding the TEL set forth by the U.S. National Oceanic and Atmospheric Administration.

The Argentinian study analyzed PCBs and four OC pesticides in the blubber of 12 common dolphins (*Delphinus delphis*) and 3 Fraser's dolphins (*Lagenodelphis hosei*) obtained from South Atlantic between 1999 and 2012. The study's other main objective was to assess these OCs in relation to age, growth (i.e., the total length), and sexual maturity in common dolphins. Although the correlations came out negative, the ΣDDT and ΣPCB levels in the dolphin samples were not inconsequential (i.e., ranging from 1.5 to 9.5 µg/g lipid weight).

In the Chinese study, the levels and the bioaccumulation potential of PBDEs (polybrominated diphenyl ethers) and PCBs were investigated with soil, rice plant, and food animal samples collected from several e-waste recycling sites located in the city of Changzhou. In particular, the levels of ΣPCBs were found significantly higher in soil samples from the e-waste dismantling sites than those from the residential areas, with a range from 120 to 12,120 ng/g wet weight. The BMF values of ΣPBDEs and ΣPCBs were also found higher at the investigated sites compared to the residential areas.

6.3.3. Bioaccumulation of Organochlorines in Seafood

Bioaccumulation of POCs (persistent organochlorine compounds) in seafood is a real concern to human health for a number of reasons. Seafood *per se* is a global commodity of high health value to humans. According to the Food and Agriculture Organization of the United Nations (FAO, 2016), global supply of food fishes from capture fisheries and aquaculture reached 180 million tons in 2014, which is sufficient to provide an apparent consumption of 20 kg (live weight equivalent) per capita for the world population of some 7.5 billion people. Food fishes are a good commodity not simply due to their availability in huge quantities. They are also an important part of a healthy diet. Fishes generally contain little saturated (bad) fats, which are commonly found in red meat. In addition, they provide high quantities of complete proteins, good fats, and other high quality nutrients (e.g., vitamins, minerals). Proteins are the principal component of human muscles, organs, and glands. These highly complex macromolecules, which are each made of chains of amino acids, are in every part of the human body except the bile and urine.

The good fats found in fishes include *Omega*-3 fatty acids, such as ALA (alpha-linolenic acid), DHA (docosahexaenoic acid), DPA (docosapentaenoic acid), and EPA (eicosapentaenoic acid). Note that not all fish species are good dietary sources for these unsaturated fatty acids which are more commonly known by their acronyms. Lake trout, salmon, mackerel, and certain other species are high in DHA and EPA, whereas only a few fish species (e.g., cod) and certain other seafood (e.g., scallops) have comparatively low but still welcome amounts of ALA.

There is a general consensus that overall, *Omega*-3s provide humans with a good range of health benefits, including the potential for lower risks in cancer (e.g., Fabian *et al.*, 2015) and mental disorders (e.g., Sarris *et al.*, 2012). These fatty acids have been shown to reduce mortality rates of coronary heart disease (Djoussé *et al.*, 2012; Kris-Etherton *et al.*, 2002; Zheng *et al.*, 2012), particularly for the fatal cases (Del Gobbo *et al.*, 2016). They also have been linked to lower risks in stroke (Friedland, 2003) and certain cases of Alzheimer's disease (Morris *et al.*, 2003; Ren *et al.*, 2016). In particular, DHA has been found as a critical component for building brain tissue, nerve growth, and retina function (Horrocks and Yeo, 1999; McCann and Ames, 2005). This 22-carbon *Omega*-3 is thus regarded as essential for infant development (Koletzko *et al.*, 2008). The fatty acid is also a key nutrient for normal brain function in adults. Regardless, the above general consensus is not without controversies, as more studies with different experimental designs are rapidly emerging. Another precaution should be made is that certain *Omega*-3s from certain fish oils may not have the same health benefits as directly from certain fish species.

In all cases, despite their high nutritious values, food fishes in many localities over the world are frequently contaminated with persistent toxic organic (and inorganic) compounds. As shown in Table 6.2 below, some POCs were reportedly found to have bioaccumulated in fish tissues from localities inside and outside of the tropical Southeast Asia and Oceania. The data included in the table were compiled in the late 1990s. They showed that for all localities under study, the POC levels monitored in fish tissue far exceeded U.S. EPA's screening values for at least one of the POCs analyzed. The worst case appeared to have been in the Lake Michigan area in the United States, where the residue levels of PCBs came close to the action level of 5.0 ppm (edible weight) set forth by the United States (FDA, 2000) and Canada (CFIA, 2014).

Table 6.2. Mean Tissue Residue Levels of Select Persistent Organochlorine Compounds in Fishes from Select Localities, Reported around the 1990s[a]

Locality	ΣPCBs	ΣDDTs	Aldrin/Dieldrin	Chlordane	HCB
Screening Value[b]	2.5 ppb	14.4 ppb	0.3 ppb	14 ppb	3.1 ppb
Tropical Southeast Asia and Oceania[c]					
Australia	55.0	22.0	10.0	51.0	4.20
India	3.5	15.0	3.1	2.4	0.07
Indonesia	2.6	28.0	1.2	0.5	0.05
Papua, New Guinea	7.5	0.4	1.3	0.4	0.03
Solomon Islands	3.6	4.8	0.3	0.6	0.02
Thailand	1.6	6.2	3.7	2.6	0.24
Vietnam	10.0	26.0	0.3	0.1	0.05
Outside of Southeast Asia and Oceania[d]					
Baffin Island, Canada	165	129	24.4	127	–
Banks Island, Canada	202	128	24.4	115	–
Maryut Lake, Egypt[e]	21.9	39.6	7.8	–	–
Simo River, Finland[e]	241.1	299.2	–	17.0	7.8
Teno River, Finland[e]	15.3	8.4	–	4.5	1.3
Mediterranean coast, Morocco	–	17.4	2.8	–	0.6
Ob River, Russia[e]	2.5	0.9	–	0.7	–
Catalonia rivers, Spain[e]	181	81	–	–	–
Lake Michigan, United States[e]	2,440	1,830	130	320	–

[a] in ppb (parts per billion ≡ ng/g), wet weight; ΣPCBs ≡ all polychlorinated biphenyl congeners; ΣDDTs ≡ all isomers of DDT (dichlorodiphenyltrichloroethane) and its metabolites; HCB ≡ hexachlorobenzene; except PCBs (as discussed in Chapter 16), the other four are organochlorine pesticides (as discussed in Chapter 15).

[b] concentrations exceeding the screening values for subsistence fishers, from Table 5-4 in U.S. EPA (2000), are considered in this book (and by some sectors) as having a potential public health concern.

[c] extracted from tissue residue values compiled by Allsopp and Johnston (2000) for studies reported by other investigators mostly in the 1990s.

[d] extracted from tissue residue values compiled by Allsopp et al. (2000) for studies reported by other investigators mostly in the 1990s.

[e] in freshwater fishes; all others in marine fishes.

Levels of POC residues in fish tissue from studies reported and compiled in the early 2000s are listed in Table 6.3 below. From a public health perspective, the residue levels in this table appear to fare better compared to the values reported around the 1990s (Table 6.2), except in India where the upper-end DDT levels were extremely high. These high-end levels from India exceeded even Australia's legal food standard of 1.0 ppm (FSANZ, 2017). Although the residue data shown in Table 6.3 are limited to what had been gathered to the early 2000s, what has become certain is that fish contamination by POCs is a global phenomenon. In fact, in the early 2000s an extensive collaboration study (Hites et al., 2004) was conducted to monitor the POC residue levels in various salmon species. That study (further discussed in Section 21.4.1) revealed that for many of the POCs analyzed, the residue levels monitored in farmed and wildlife salmons whether purchased or imported from worldwide far exceeded U.S. EPA's screening values (Table 6.3). Overall, Table 6.2 and Table 6.3 reveal that a sufficient number of monitoring sites had residue levels greater than U.S. EPA's screening values by more than 30-fold. For those localities, no more than one or two fishmeals per month thus may become necessary, especially for children and pregnant women, so that their intake of POCs can be kept below the screening levels which are considered by many authorities to be of (potential) public health concern. However, it is unfortunately well taken that such a health advisory may not be practical to people who rely on fish as their main diet.

Table 6.3. Tissue Residue Levels of Select Persistent Organochlorine Compounds in Fishes from Select Localities, Reported around the Early 2000s[a,b]

Locality	ΣPCDDs/Fs	ΣPCBs	ΣDDTs	Aldrin/Dieldrin
Screening Value[c]	*0.03 ppt*	*2.5 ppb*	*14.4 ppb*	*0.3 ppb*
Pearl River Delta, China[a]	–	–	1.5-62	–
Shanghai, Tianjin, China[b]		0.8-11.4	28.9	
Taihu Lake, China[c]	0.5-3.8	1.5-27.6		
Demietta, Egypt[d]	–	–	20-211	
River Ganges, India[e]	–	–	13.6-1,666	3.1-86.1
Central Adriatic Sea, Italy[f]	–	51.4-177.2	5.2-65.6	–
Coastal waters, Korea[g]	–	3.0-96.6	0.8-27.0	–
Portugal[h]	–	–	30.1-109.9	–
Atlantic SW Coast, Spain[i]	0.04-0.19	0.86-23.8	–	–
Baltic sea, Sweden[j]	0.5-33.4	–	–	–
salmons worldwide[k]	65	73	28	6.3

[a] all tissue residue concentrations are in ppb ≡ parts per billion (ng/g) wet weight, except for ΣPCDDs (including PCDFs); ppt ≡ TEQ-based parts per trillion (ng/kg), *see* Section 6.3.1 for concept and application of TEQ.

[b] [a] Kong *et al.* (2005); [b] Yang *et al.* (2006); [c] Zhang and Jiang (2005); [d] El Nemr and Abd-Allah (2004); [e] Kumari *et al.* (2001); [f] Perugini *et al.* (2006), converted from values given on fat weight basis assuming (as by Gall, 2004) a fat content of 10% for Atlantic mackerel; [g] Yim *et al.* (2005); [h] Campos *et al.* (2005); [i] Bordajandi *et al.* (2006); [j] SNFA (2004); [k] Hites *et al.* (2004).

[c] concentrations exceeding the screening values for subsistence fishers, from Table 5-4 in U.S. EPA (2000), are considered in this book (and by some sectors) as having a potential public health concern.

6.4. Factors and Conditions Influencing Bioaccumulation

Both bioaccumulation and bioconcentration begin as soon as a substance enters an organism from the environment where both the substance (e.g., toxicant) and the organism co-exist. This first phase is referred to as the uptake of the substance, which by and in itself is already a complex process. Within the scientific sector, it is a widely applied concept or axiom that substances tend to diffuse passively from an area of high concentration to one of low concentration. The driving force for this passive transport is the natural tendency of molecules proceeding from order (e.g., highly packed places) to chaos (e.g., loosely packed places). Nonetheless, as discussed below, a number of variables or factors can facilitate or hinder this passive process.

6.4.1. Lipophilicity and Bioavailability

Certain substances such as POCs do not mix well with water, as they are lipophilic. Lipophilic substances tend to move out of water and into the cells of a biological organism that they come in contact with, as these cells (particularly their membranes) offer a less lipid-resistant microenvironment. In general, the same factors facilitating the uptake of a toxicant by an organism continue to operate inside that organism, thus minimizing the toxicant's opportunity of returning to the outer microenvironment. Once inside a mammalian organism, toxicants travel rapidly to its body tissues via the bloodstream and the lymphatic system. At any given time, this toxicant's molecules inside the organism are present either as bound or unbound to plasma proteins present in the various tissues. It is the unbound fraction of the toxicant that is generally more biologically active and available, leading to the significant concept of chemical bioavailability.

Different POCs have different specific binding interactions with different plasma proteins. Therefore, the type of plasma proteins, their concentrations, the binding kinetics between them and a POC, and the plasma flow rate involved are variables that all strongly affect the amount of the POC in the bioactive form. Some toxicants are attracted to certain cellular sites and are temporarily or permanently stored in there upon distribution. If uptake proceeds slowly or is discontinued, or if the protein binding is sufficiently weak, the toxicant can eventually be excreted from the organism's body. The uptake and the storage of substances are also influenced by their water solubility. Substances that are highly water-soluble generally do not readily enter the cells of an organism. Therefore, even when water-soluble toxicants somehow find their ways into a biological organism (e.g., by oral intake), they are easily removed from the organism's body unless the cells inside have specific biochemical processes for retaining them.

6.4.2. Metabolic Potential

Another factor or condition affecting bioaccumulation of toxicants is whether a biological organism's body can break down the substance that has entered its cells or tissues. The process as well as the ability for such a biological breakdown is termed *metabolism*, or more specifically *biotransformation* (Chapter 8). This ability varies among species of biological organisms and also depends largely on a substance's physicochemical properties. For example, pyrethrins are insecticides derived from plants of the chrysanthemum species (Chapter 15). They are highly fat-soluble (lipophilic) but are easily degraded. As such, these insecticides do not accumulate in an organism. This is one reason why this chapter has its focus on toxicants that are *persistent* in the aquatic (or any) environment.

6.4.3. Environmental Mobility

Still another crucial condition that influences bioaccumulation is a substance's mobility in the environment. As discussed in Section 6.3.2, it is evident that PCBs and other OCs can reach remote regions. This type of long-range transport is thought to be generally via atmospheric, oceanic, or terrestrial transport. Of the three, terrestrial transport appears less likely as a major mode for long-range mobility, insomuch as soils, plants, surface runoff, leaching, and the kind are fairly stationary objects or processes. Regardless, in the late 1990s a fourth mode for long-range transport was identified and investigated extensively (e.g., Ewald et al., 1998; UNEP, 1998; Wania, 1998). This fourth mode was via animal migration, or technically termed *biotransport*.

In particular, in the study by Ewald et al. (1998), Pacific salmon were observed to deposit eggs in freshwater and then migrate downstream to the ocean to spend the majority of their lifecycle there. Yet prior to migration back upstream to freshwater for spawning, they accumulated lipids for the energy required for migration as well as for gonadal development. The lipids that the salmon accumulated in their body were found to have been contaminated by lipophilic pollutants, such as PCBs and DDTs, (somehow) present in the ocean.

The salmon study concluded that biotransport of environmental pollutants was more significant than other modes of transport for two reasons. First, lakes that were within reach of salmon migration are quantitatively a larger contributor to *local* contaminant loads compared to an ocean, since the latter is a much larger aquatic system yielding proportionately a lower contaminant load. Second, contaminants via biotransport tend to be more biologically active and less vulnerable to environmental degradation, as they are all within an organism's lipid stores and thereby protected from various oxidation processes (e.g., via ultraviolet radiation).

Pacific salmon are not the only biological species known as capable of transporting POCs to remote areas. Wania (1998) had used whales and seabirds to exemplify the ability of migratory animals in transporting POPs (of which many were POCs) to the Arctic. According to his analysis, the annual amounts ranged from grams to kilograms for POPs (particularly PCBs and DDTs) transported by seabirds in and out of the Arctic. With whales, the estimates for the annual amounts transported were in the order of several tons. Those estimates all suggested that the quantities of some POPs transported by migratory animals, especially whales, might be in a similar order of magnitude as the gross rates estimated for atmospheric and oceanic transports.

In an earlier analysis (Comba et al., 1993) around that period, an effort was made to quantify the biotransport of the pesticide mirex ($C_{10}Cl_{12}$, an OC uniquely with no hydrogen atoms) from Lake Ontario to the St. Lawrence River system. The study estimated that for the years 1950 to 1990, nearly 300 kilograms of mirex were transported downstream with water and sediments, and another 60 kilograms by migrating eels. Those estimates suggested that biotransport of the pesticide was of a similar order of magnitude as the transports in abiotic (e.g., air) media. And in another even earlier study, Lum et al. (1987) found that eels in fact transported more mirex out of Lake Ontario than what these aquatic creatures did to suspended particulate matter (as defined in Chapter 12). As still one more evidence for biotransport being a real long-range transport mode, many migrating birds reportedly died in their winter quarters in the warmer (southern) regions. Yet these birds frequently leave behind in their winter quarters a considerable amount of POCs that their bodies had accumulated from their (northern) summer quarters prior to their seasonal migration (UNEP, 1988).

6.4.4. A Dynamic Equilibrium Effect

As a recap and in essence, when a persistent organic substance enters the cells of a biological organism, it is subject to distribution and then to storage, metabolism (biotransformation), and elimination within that organism (Chapter 7). Bioaccumulation thereby results from actually a dynamic equilibrium between an organism's exposure to a substance and its uptake, storage, as well as degradation inside the organism. As expected, persistent lipophilic toxicants such as POCs are the ones posing a great threat of bioaccumulation and biomagnification within an ecosystem. Posing even a greater threat are those toxicants resistant to biotransformation once inside an organism. Owing to their high lipophilicity, many POCs can be stored in fat deposits for years inside an organism. In general, those POCs that tend to move more freely within an organism's body, or to be excreted rapidly from its body, are less likely to be bioaccumulated. All these factors and effects may be used to help explain why the bioaccumulation of POCs was found being more frequent in an old trout than in a young yellow perch from the same lake. After all, by comparison the older fish is a larger, fatter, and longer-lived creature typically with a lower rate of chemical excretion.

References

Allsopp M, Johnston P, 2000. Unseen Poisons in Asia: A Review of Persistent Organic Pollutant Levels in South and Southeast Asia and Oceania. Greenpeace Research Laboratories, Department of Biological Sciences, University of Exeter, Exeter, UK.

Allsopp M, Erry B, Stringer R, Johnston P, Santillo D, 2000. Recipe for Disaster: A Review of Persistent Organic Pollutants in Food. Greenpeace Research Laboratories, Department of Biological Sciences, University of Exeter, Exeter, UK.

Antunes P, Gil O, Reis-Henriques MA, 2007. Evidence for Higher Biomagnification Factors of Lower Chlorinated PCBs in Cultivated Seabass. *Sci. Total Environ.* 377:36-44.

Bordajandi LR, Martin I, Abad E, Rivera J, Gonzalez MJ, 2006. Organochlorine Compounds (PCBs, PCDDs and PCDFs) in Seafish and Seafood from the Spanish Atlantic Southwest Coast. *Chemosphere* 64:1450-1457.

Bussolaro D, Filipak Neto F, Glinksi A, Roche H, Guiloski IC, Mela M, Silva de Assis HC, Oliveira Ribeiro CA, 2012. Bioaccumulation and Related Effects of PCBs and Organochlorinated Pesticides in Freshwater Fish *Hypostomus commersoni*. *J. Environ. Monit.* 14:2154-2163.

Campos A, Lino CM, Cardoso SM, Silveira MIN, 2005. Organochlorine Pesticide Residues in European Sardine, Horse Mackerel and Atlantic Mackerel from Portugal. *Food Addit. Contamin.* 22:642-646.

CEPA (Canadian Environmental Protection Act of 1999), 2000. Persistence and Bioaccumulation Regulations (SOR/2000-107; 29/3/2000). *Canada Gazette* Part II, 134(7):607-612.

CFIA (Canadian Food Inspection Agency), 2014. Canadian Guidelines for Chemical Contaminants and Toxins in Fish and Fish Products (Appendix 3), amended August. Ontario K1A 0Y9, Canada.

Comba ME, Norstrom RJ, MacDonald CR, Kaiser KLE, 1993. A Lake Ontario-Gulf of St. Lawrence Dynamic Mass Budget for Mirex. *Environ. Sci. Technol.* 27:2198-2206.

Cone M, 2005. *Silent Snow: The Slow Poisoning of the Arctic*. New York, New York, USA: Grove Press, Chapter 1.

Corl E, 2001. Bioaccumulation in the Ecological Risk Assessment (ERA) Process (Issue Papers, 7 August). Technical Support, Atlantic Division, Naval Facilities Engineering Command, Norfolk, Virginia, USA.

Cronin MTD, Walker JD, Jaworska JS, Comber MHI, Watts CD, Worth AP, 2002. Use of QSARs in International Decision-Making Frameworks to Predict Ecologic Effects and Environmental Fate of Chemical Substances. *Environ. Health Perspect.* 111:1376-1390.

Del Gobbo, LC, Imamura F, Aslibekyan S, Marklund M, Virtanen, JK, Wennber M, Yakoob MY, Chiuve SE, dela Crus L, Frazier-Wood AC, *et al.*, 2016. ω-3 Polyunsaturated Fatty Acid Biomarkers and Coronary Heart Disease – Polling Projects of 19 Cohort Studies. *JAMA Intl. Med.* 176:1155-1166.

Djoussé L, Akinkuolie AO, Wu JH, Ding EL, Gaziano JM, 2012. Fish Consumption, Omega-3 Fatty Acids and Risk of Heart Failure: A Meta-Analysis. *Clin. Nutri.* 31:846-853.

Durante CA, Santos-Neto EB, Azevedo A, Crespo EA, Lailson-Brito J, 2016. POPs in the South Latin America: Bioaccumulation of DDT, PCB, HCB, HCH and Mirex in Blubber of Common Dolphin (*Delphinus delphis*) and Fraser's Dolphin (*Lagenodelphis hosei*) from Argentina. *Sci. Total Environ.* 572:352-360.

El Nemr A, Abd-Allah AMA, 2004. Organochlorine Contamination in Some Marketable Fish in Egypt. *Chemosphere* 54:1401-1406.

Ewald G, Larsson P, Linge H, Okla L, Szarzi N, 1998. Biotransport of Organic Pollutants to an Inland Alaska Lake by Migrating Sockeye Salmon (*Onchorhynchus nerka*). *Arctic* 51:478-485.

Fabian CJ, Kimler BF, Hursting SD, 2015. Omega-3 Fatty Acids for Breast Cancer Prevention and Survivorship. *Breast Cancer Res.* 17:62 (online journal).

FAO (Food and Agriculture Organization of the United Nations), 2016. The State of World Fisheries and Aquaculture – Contributing to Food Security and Nutrition for All: Part 1. World Review. FAO, Rome, Italy.

FDA (U.S. Food and Drug Administration), 2000. Guidance for Industry: Action Levels for Poisonous or Deleterious Substances in Human Food and Animal Feed. U.S. Department of Health and Human Services, Silver Spring, Maryland, USA.

Friedland RP, 2003. *Editorial*: Fish Consumption and the Risk of Alzheimer Disease: Is It Time to Make Dietary Recommendations? *Arch. Neurol.* 60:923-924.

FSANZ (Food Standards Code Australia New Zealand), 2017. Australia New Zealand Food Standards Code – Schedule 21: Extraneous Residue Limits (This standard commencing on 1 March 2016; last registered version 18 April 2017 as of retrieval date 3 June 2017). Federal Register of Legislation, Office of Parliamentary Counsel, Forrest ACT 2603, Australia.

Gall K, 2004. Seafood Nutrition and Health. New York Seafood Council, 23 Bay Avenue, Hampton Bays, New York, USA.

Han Z-X, Wang N, Zhang H-L, Zhao Y-X, 2017. Bioaccumulation of PBDEs and PCBs in a Small Food Chain at Electronic Waste Recycling Sites. *J. Environ. Forensics* 18:44-49.

Hawker DW, Connell DW, 1988. Octanol-Water Partition Coefficients of Polychlorinated Biphenyl Congeners. *Environ. Sci. Technol.* 22:382-387.

Hites RA, Foran JA, Carpenter DO, Hamilton MC, Knuth BA, Schwager SJ, 2004. Global Assessment of Organic Contaminants in Farmed Salmon. *Science* 303:226-229.

Horrocks LA, Yeo YK, 1999. Health Benefits of Docosahexaenoic Acid (DHA). *Pharmacol. Res.* 40:211-225.

Kajiwara N, Kannan K, Muraoka M, Watanabe M, Takahashi S, Gulland F, Olsen H, Blankenship AL, Jones PD, Tanabe S, Giesy JP, 2001. Organochlorine Pesticides, Polychlorinated Biphenyls, and Butyltin Compounds in Blubber and Livers of Stranded California Sea Lions, Elephant Seals, and Harbor Seals from Coastal California, USA. *Arch. Environ. Contamin. Toxicol.* 41:90-99.

Koistinen J, Stenman O, Haahti H, Suonpera M, Paasivirta J, 1997. Polychlorinated Diphenyl Ethers, Dibenzo-p-Dioxins, Dibenzofurans and Biphenyls in Seals and Sediment from the Gulf of Finland. *Chemosphere* 35:1249-1269.

Koletzko B, Lien E, Agostoni C, Böhles H, Campoy C, Cetin I, Decsi T, Dudenhausen JW, Dupont C, Forsyth S, *et al.*, 2008. The Roles of Long-Chain Polyunsaturated Fatty Acids in Pregnancy, Lactation and Infancy: Review of Current Knowledge and Consensus Recommendations. *J. Perinat. Med.* 26:5-14.

Kong KY, Cheung KC, Wong CK, Wong MH, 2005. The Residual Dynamic of Polycyclic Aromatic Hydrocarbons and Organochlorine Pesticides in Fishponds of the Pearl River Delta, South China. *Water Res.* 39: 1831-1843.

Kostamo A, Hyvarinen H, Pellinen J, Kukkonen JVK, 2002. Organochlorine Concentrations in the Saimaa Ringed Seal (*Phoca hispida saimensis*) from Lake Haukivesi, Finland, 1981 to 2000, and in Its Diet Today. *Environ. Toxicol. Chem.* 21:1368-1375.

Kris-Etherton PM, Harris WS, Appel LJ, 2002. Fish Consumption, Fish Oil, Omega-3 Fatty Acids, and Cardiovascular Disease. *Circulation* 106:2747-2757.

Kumari A, Sinha RK, Gopal K, 2001. Organochlorine Contamination in the Fish of the River Ganges, India. *Aquatic Ecosys. Health & Magnt.* 4:505-510.

Liebens J, Mohrherr CJ, 2015. DDT, Dioxins, and PCBs in Sediments in a Historically Polluted Estuary along the Gulf of Mexico. *Environ. Practice* 17:89-101.

Lum KR, Kaiser KLE, Comba ME, 1987. Export of Mirex from Lake Ontario to the St. Lawrence Estuary. *Sci. Total Environ.* 67:41-51.

MacKay D, Shiu WY, Ma KC, 1992. *Illustrated Handbook of Physical-Chemical Properties and Environmental Fate of Organic Chemicals*. Boca Raton, Florida, USA: Lewis Publishers.

Matthies M, Scheringer M, 2001. *Editorial*: Long-Range Transport in the Environment. *Environ. Sci. Pollut. Res.* 8:149.

McCann JC, Ames BN, 2005. Is Docosahexaenoic Acid, an n-3 Long-Chain Polyunsaturated Fatty Acid, Required for Development of Normal Brain Function? An Overview of Evidence from Cognitive and Behavioral Tests in Humans and Animals. *Am. J. Clin. Nutri.* 82:281-295.

Montgomery JH, 1993. *Agrochemical Desk Reference: Environmental Data*. Chelsea, Michigan, USA: Lewis Publishers.

Morris MC, Evans DA, Bienias JL, Tangney CC, Bennett DA, Wilson RS, Aggarwal N, Schneider J, 2003. Consumption of Fish and n-3 Fatty Acids and Risk of Incident Alzheimer Disease. *Arch. Neurol.* 60:940-946.

Muir D, Savinova T, Savinov V, Alexeeva L, Potelov V, Svetochev V, 2003. Bioaccumulation of PCBs and Chlorinated Pesticides in Seals, Fishes and Invertebrates from the White Sea, Russia. *Sci. Total Environ.* 306:111-131.

OECD (Organization for Economic Cooperation and Development), 2012. OECD Guidelines for Testing of Chemicals – Test No. 305. Bioaccumulation in Fish: Aqueous and Dietary Exposure. Paris, France.

Perugini M, Giammarino A, Olivieri V, Di Nardo W, Amorena M, 2006. Assessment of Edible Marine Species in the Adriatic Sea for Contamination from Polychlorinated Biphenyls and Organochlorine Insecticides. *J. Food Protect.* 69:1144-1149.

Rapaport RA, Eisenreich SJ, 1984. Chromatographic Determination of Octanol-Water Partition Coefficients (K_{ow}'s) for 58 PCB Polychlorinated Biphenyl Congeners. *Environ. Sci. Technol.* 18:163-170.

Ren H, 2016. Omega-3 Polyunsaturated Fatty Acids Promote Amyloid-β Clearance From the Brain through Mediating the Function of the Glymphatic System. *FASEB J.* 31:282-293.

Sandau CD, Ayotte P, Dewailly E, Duffe J, Norstrom RJ, 2000. Analysis of Hydroxylated Metabolites of PCBs (OH-PCBs) and Other Chlorinated Phenolic Compounds in Whole Blood from Canadian Inuit. *Environ. Health Perspect.* 108:611-616.

Sarris J, Mischoulon D, Schweitzer I, 2012. Omega-3 for Bipolar Disorder: Meta-Analyses of Use in Mania and Bipolar Depression. *J. Clin. Psychiatry* 73:81-86.

Shiu WY, Doucette W, Gobas FAPC, Andren A, MacKay D, 1988. Physical-Chemical Properties of Chlorinated Dibenzo-p-Dioxins. *Environ. Sci. Technol.* 22:651-658.

SNFA (Swedish National Food Administration), 2004. Persistent Organic Pollutants in Fatty Fish in Sweden 2000-2003 (Interim Report 5: Study of Dioxin-like PCBs in Fatty Fish from Sweden 2000-2002). SNFA (Toxicology Division), Box 622, SE-751 26, Uppsala, Sweden.

UNEP (United Nations Environment Programme), 1998. Preparation of an International Legally Binding Instrument for Implementing International Action on Certain Persistent Organic Pollutants. UNEP/POPS/INC. 1/6 (dated 30 April), Geneva, Switzerland.

U.S. EPA (U.S. Environmental Protection Agency), 1999. Category for Persistent, Bioaccumulative, and Toxic New Chemical Substances. *Federal Register* 64:60194-60204.

U.S. EPA (U.S. Environmental Protection Agency), 2000. Guidance for Assessing Chemical Contaminant Data for Use in Fish Advisories – Volume 1: Fish Sampling and Analysis, Third Edition. EPA 823-B-00-007. Office of Water, Washington DC, USA.

U.S. EPA (U.S. Environmental Protection Agency), 2016. Ecological Effects Test Guidelines – OCSPP 850.1730: Fish Bioconcentration Factor (BCF). Office of Chemical Safety and Pollution Prevention, Washington DC, USA.

van den Berg M, Birnbaum LS, Denison M, De Vito M, Farland W, Feeley M, Fiedler H, Hakansson H, Hanberg A, Haws L, *et al.*, 2006. The 2005 World Health Organization Re-evaluation of Human and Mammalian Toxic Equivalency Factors for Dioxins and Dioxin-like Compounds. *Toxicol. Sci.* 93:223-241.

van Gestel CAM, Otermann K, Canton JH, 1985. Relation between Water Solubility, Octanol/Water Partition Coefficients, and Bioconcentration of Organic Chemicals in Fish: A Review. *Regul. Toxicol. Pharmacol.* 5:422-431.

Veith GD, Macek KJ, Petrocelli SR, Carroll J, 1980. An Evaluation of Using Partition Coefficients and Water Solubility to Estimate Bioconcentration Factors for Organic Chemicals in Fish. In *Aquatic Toxicology* (Eaton JG, Parrish PR, Hendricks AC, Eds.). ASTM STP 707. American Society for Testing and Materials (ASTM), Philadelphia, Pennsylvania, USA.

Wania F, 1998. The Significance of Long Range Transport of Persistent Organic Pollutants by Migratory Animals. WECC Report 3/98. WECC Wania Environmental Chemists Corp, 289 Simcoe Street, Suite 404, Toronto, Ontario M5G, Canada.

Yang N, Matsuda M, Kawano M, Wakimoto T, 2006. PCBs and Organochlorine Pesticides (OCPs) in Edible Fish and Shellfish from China. *Chemosphere* 63:1342-1352.

Yim UH, Hong SH, Shim WJ, Oh JR, 2005. Levels of Persistent Organochlorine Contaminants in Fish from Korea and Their Potential Health Risk. *Arch. Environ. Contamin. Toxicol.* 48:358-366.

Zhang G, Jiang G, 2005. Polychlorinated Dibenzo-p-Dioxins/Furans and Polychlorinated Biphenyls in Sediments and Aquatic Organisms from the Taihu Lake, China. *Chemosphere* 61:314-322.

Zheng J, Huang T, Yu Y, Hu X, Yang B, Li D, 2012. Fish Consumption and CHD Mortality: An Updated Meta-Analysis of Seventeen Cohort Studies. *Public Health Nutri.* 15:725-737.

Review Questions
1. Give both the broader and the more specific definition for the term *bioaccumulation*.
2. How are the dynamic construct of bioaccumulation and that of food web related to each other in terms of exposure hazard assessment?
3. What is the definition of *bioconcentration* as a quantitation process or biological phenomenon? And how are the biological events involved in this phenomenon typically assessed quantitatively?
4. What are some of the general methods (techniques) employed to measure bioconcentration factors for (persistent) toxic substances?
5. Why does bioconcentration or bioaccumulation appear to be better studied for toxicants in an aquatic environment than in an atmospheric or a terrestrial environment?
6. How are the quantitation processes *biomagnification* and *bioaccumulation* related to each other?
7. What is a toxic equivalency factor (TEF)? And how is it generally used in estimating the total TCDD-equivalent concentration of all the dioxin and dioxin-like congeners in a mixture?
8. Why are people encouraged to include seafood in their diet? And why is it important to study the bioaccumulation of environmental contaminants from this dietary source?
9. Which locality inside or outside of the tropical Southwest Asia and Oceania appeared to have the worst case (i.e., the highest levels) of fish contamination by POCs in the 1990s?
10. Which locality appeared to have the worst case of fish contamination by DDTs in the early 2000s?
11. Briefly describe three basic factors that can strongly affect or influence bioaccumulation of persistent environmental toxicants.
12. How is bioaccumulation relevant to long-range transport of PBTs?
13. Give at least two reasons why migration of contaminated Pacific salmon can be a significant mode for transport of environmental contaminants.
14. Besides salmon, name three species of migratory animals that were studied in the late 1980s through the late 1990s for the biotransport load of POCs.
15. Briefly explain why the accumulation of a PBT is expected to be more in an old trout than in a young yellow perch from the same aquatic environment.

CHAPTER 7

Uptake, Distribution, and Excretion of Toxicants

7.1. Introduction

In this and the three chapters that follow, the focus is on the fate and the transport of environmental toxicants that are entering or have entered the body of a biological organism, particularly that of a human or a physiologically similar mammalian. Within a biological system being the microenvironment, the fate and the transport of toxicants are generally about their uptake by and disposition in the organism's body. The preference in organism species here is with the sense that unlike ecotoxicology, this is where and what the emphasis lies with environmental toxicology. The foci of these four chapters are on systemic effects which are those occurring at sites distant from the toxicant's point of entry.

7.1.1. Localized Effect of Non-Systemic Action

Systemic effects (more on this topic in Section 7.1.2 below and Chapter 9) tend to be more a concern to environmental toxicologists in that, in many environmental settings, the levels of most toxicants are not alarming enough to call for immediate public health or regulatory action. Nevertheless, when toxicants are present in sufficiently high levels within the microenvironment outside of a biological organism, their toxic effects can be localized on the organism's outer structure (e.g., skin, surface of respiratory tract, surface of gastrointestinal tract), not necessarily systemic. For instance, serious localized rash or irritation of the skin (Section 2.4.6) can be induced by contact with certain pesticide residues, such as with those of the acaricide (mite killer) propargite left on treated foliage upon a fieldworker's reentry.

Another example of non-systemic effect is with ozone (O_3), which at atmospheric concentration above 0.1 ppm (parts per million) can irritate the eyes and upper respiratory tract of people exposed to it. As with sulfur dioxide (SO_2), nitrogen dioxide (NO_2), and hydrogen fluoride (HF), ozone is a major and highly phytotoxic air pollutant capable of causing acute, direct damage to a leaf's structural components without entering its stomata (i.e., the openings between the guard cells on a leaf's surface tissue, *see* Figure 7.3). This type of damage frequently results in leaf chlorosis (yellowing) or necrosis (browning and death), largely due to direct oxidative damage (from oxidative stress) to the leaf's cell membrane (e.g., Schraudner *et al.*, 1998).

7.1.2. Disposition of Systemic Toxicants

Following environmental exposure and along with uptake (and absorption), the disposition of a xenobiotic inside the human body may be broadly divided into a series of biochemical events or phases as depicted graphically in Figure 7.1 below. This series of events also applies to plants which can excrete certain wastes (e.g., minerals) via their roots, shoots, or leaves (e.g., Larcher, 2003). In some plant species, certain wastes can be transported to the cytoplasmic sacs called vacuoles on the leaves which are destined to shed. In some other plant species, certain wastes can be actively secreted via the roots into the soil.

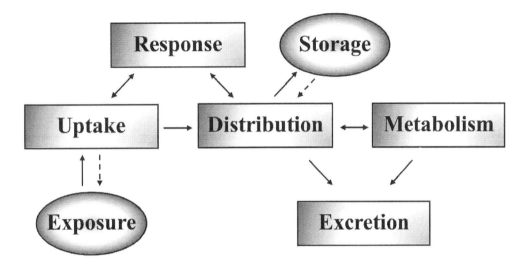

Figure 7.1. Disposition of Xenobiotics inside (and Their Uptake by) a Biological System

Note that in Figure 7.1, those phases in a box are the ones each involving enormous complex and much more dynamic biochemical reactions, whereas the two phases in an eclipse are each requiring relatively fewer, simpler, more static biochemical events. The *uptake*, *distribution*, and *excretion* phases, along with exposure and storage, are discussed in this chapter. Due to their complexities, *metabolism* (largely *biotransformation*) of toxicants and toxic *response* are covered in Chapters 8 and 9, respectively. Also note that the phase (toxic) *response* by the biological organism's body includes as well as reflects the *adverse action* induced by the toxicant.

7.2. Mechanisms of Entry by Toxicants

As alluded to in Figure 7.1, upon exposure all systemic effects begin with the uptake and/or absorption of the xenobiotic by the organism's body. In many instances, the term *uptake* or *intake* is more appropriate than *absorption* when discussing the entry of a xenobiotic into a living organism, in that absorption also connotes the specific process whereby a xenobiotic *actively penetrates* a cell or cellular membrane on the host organism's outer structure. Cell or cellular membranes are also referred to as biological membranes or, in this book, biomembranes for short.

7.2.1. Structure of Biomembranes

Biomembranes, such as those of plasmas, tissues, cells, and cell organelles, are vital to an organism's life. They are those that either protect a cell from the outside environment, or separate the compartments inside a cell in order to safeguard important biological processes and specific events occurring there. These biomembranes, particularly those in a mammalian body, are composed of predominantly proteins and phospholipids, with the lipid portions being arranged as bilayer leaflets embedded with the proteins (Figure 7.2). The phospholipid molecule in each (e.g., outer extracellular fluid) layer has a polar (i.e., water-soluble) head and two much longer nonpolar fatty acid hydrocarbon tails. The two tails are packed together as well as with one or more of those in the opposite (e.g., inner cytoplasm) layer. With such a structural arrangement, biomembranes are generally permeable to certain and largely lipophilic toxicants only, depending on the particular physicochemical properties of the intruders, such as their molecular size, lipid solubility, polarity, and structural similarity to endogenous molecules.

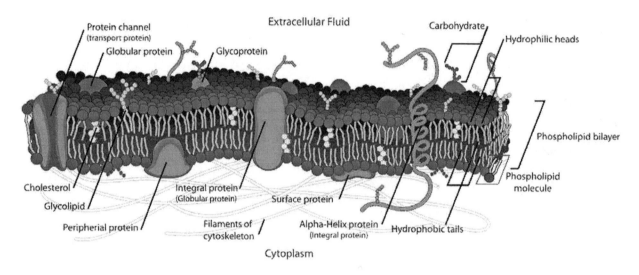

Figure 7.2. General Structure of a Mammalian Biomembrane
(*public domain image from www.freeclipartnow.com*)

The major membrane proteins involved generally fall into two types termed *peripheral proteins* and *integral* (a.k.a. *transmembrane*) *proteins*. The principal function of an integral protein is to transport substances such as ions and macromolecules across the phospholipid bilayer. A peripheral protein, on the other hand, does not interact with the hydrophobic (i.e., nonpolar) core of the bilayer. Instead, it is there to safeguard the membrane surface, regulate cell signaling, and participate in certain other crucial cellular events.

Two major secondary lipids present in a typical biomembrane are glycolipids and steroids. Glycolipids are those that have one or more carbohydrate groups attached. Sphingolipids are the main glycolipids found in many biomembranes and, owing to their backbone molecule sphingosine (an unsaturated amino alcohol), play a key role in signal transmission and cell recognition. The majority of steroids found in a biomembrane are cholesterols which, due to their alcoholic hydroxyl (OH) group, can interact with water and therefore can act as important spacers in the bilayer's hydrophobic core. They are there to prevent crystallization of the fatty acids and to give rigidity as well as stability to the biomembrane.

7.2.2. Common Mechanisms of Entry

There are broadly five common mechanisms of entry enabling or aiding xenobiotics to get into an organism's body or to cross the biomembranes inside. These mechanisms include:

- *Passive diffusion* (a.k.a. *passive transport*) – This refers to the movement of molecules across a biomembrane *without* any expenditure of energy by the cell.

- *Active transport* – This refers to the movement of molecules *against* a concentration gradient or an electrical potential in the direction opposite to passive diffusion, thus *requiring* certain expenditure of energy by the cell.

- *Filtration* – This refers to the movement of molecules across a biomembrane due to hydrostatic pressure (e.g., that generated by the cardiovascular system).

- *Facilitated diffusion* – This refers to the movement of molecules across a biomembrane using *special transport proteins* (primarily integral proteins, *see* Figure 7.2) as carriers that are embedded within the membrane.

- *Endocytosis* – This is the process whereby cells absorb molecules from outside the cell by engulfing these molecules with their membranes. Where the ingested molecules are solids, the process is specifically termed *phagocytosis*; and when liquids are taken in instead, the process is termed *pinocytosis*.

For many xenobiotics, passive transport is the predominate entry mechanism. For a system at a certain constant temperature and for diffusion over unit distance, the rate of passive transport of nonpolar, nonionized lipid-soluble molecules is generally thought to obey closely Fick's law of diffusion as follows:

$$\text{Rate of diffusion} = K \times A \times (C_1 - C_2) \tag{7.1}$$

where K is a rate constant specific to the intruder, A is the surface area in which the diffusion takes place, C_1 is the intruder's concentration outside the membrane, and C_2 is its concentration inside the membrane. Where C_2 is negligible relative to C_1, the quantity $(C_1 - C_2)$ is often treated as C_1.

7.3. Uptake and Absorption of Toxicants

The specific routes and processes involved in the uptake and absorption of toxicants vary considerably across the plant and animal kingdoms. This variation is largely due to the differences in their body structures but also to the ways in which they are exposed to the toxicants. Plants are more dependent on local habitat conditions for their survival, as they are stationary structures. They are included here for discussion not only because the inclusion provides a further appreciation of the numerous and various ways in which toxicants can enter a living organism. It is also because the damage on plants, especially on the consumable kind, has a considerable effect on the health of humans and wildlife.

7.3.1. Uptake by Plants

Plants each typically consist of two main organ systems for uptake of nutrients and other foreign substances: *the shoot* and *the root*. The shoot system includes all parts of a plant above ground, such as leaves, buds, stems, flowers (if any), and fruits (if any). The root system includes those parts below ground, such as roots, tubers, and rhizomes. Plant cells are formed with undifferentiated cells termed *meristems* and then develop into various cell types, which can be broadly grouped into the three general tissue categories: *dermal*, *ground*, and *vascular* (e.g., Purves *et al.*, 1995; Taiz and Zeiger, 2006).

The *dermal* tissues comprise epidermal cells closely packed to shield the outer surface of herbaceous plants (Figure 7.3). These cells secrete a waxy cuticle atop to help reduce water loss from the leaf. Most of the leaf interior between the upper and the lower epidermis are the palisade and the spongy parenchyma cells. The parenchyma (also called mesophyll) cells in these *ground* tissues are the most functional, as they are rich in chloroplast and are actively involved in photosynthesis, storage, and support. The xylem and phloem tubes, along with some other kinds of parenchyma cells, are included in the *vascular* bundles which, located among the spongy mesophyll, are the components responsible for transporting food, water, minerals, hormones, and other materials within a plant as well as its leaf.

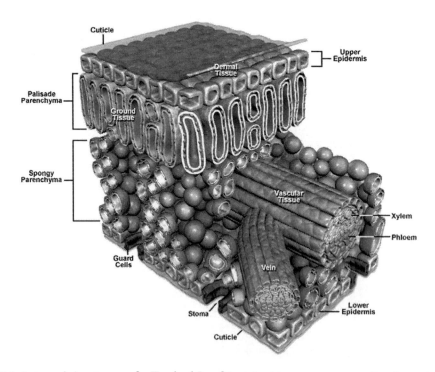

Figure 7.3. Internal Anatomy of a Typical Leaf (*original image: courtesy of and permission from the National High Magnetic Field Laboratory, Florida State University, USA*)

Uptake of environmental toxicants by many terrestrial plants occurs in two common pathways. One pathway is from exposure of their roots to soil contaminants and the other, from exposure of their foliage to pollutants in the air (e.g., Kvesitadze et al., 2006). Indirect damage retarding plant growth can occur when the pollutants cause disturbance of water or nutrient uptake. In particular, when the contaminated soil is acidified by decayed materials or acid rain, the metallic ions (e.g., Pb^{2+}, Cd^{2+}) in the soil become more mobile toward the plant roots. These ions can damage the plant's roots and then its leaves by disrupting its uptake of water and nutrients. Soil acidification can also cause leaching of nutrients, leading to an unhealthy plant suffering from nutrient deficiencies or growth disturbance.

A. Uptake via Plant Leaves

Inasmuch as the amount of a contaminant that enters a plant is what matters the most in terms of plant damage, the stomata at the plant's leaf cells are the most significant structural components. This is because they are the ones mainly responsible for regulating the passage of toxicants into the leaf cells. The extent of such uptake depends on the environmental setting as well as the physicochemical properties of a toxicant along the leaf surface. For example, the flow of a toxicant may be hindered by the leaf's morphology, by the reactions of chemical scavengers occurring within the leaf, or by air movement across the leaf. These factors can affect the polluted air's flux to the leaf surface.

Again, of all the determinants considered, stomatal opening is by far the most crucial in that little or no uptake will occur when the stomata are closed. These surface openings are regulated by a number of factors including meteorological variables (e.g., temperature, light), physicochemical conditions in the guard cells, starch content in the guard cells, and amount of potassium (K^+) ions accumulated in the guard cells (Humble and Raschke, 1971; Jinno and Kuraishi, 1982; Kim and Lee, 2007).

Many toxic substances that enter the leaves of a plant are in solution (e.g., pesticide spray, liquid aerosol), rather than in gas. The permeability of liquids on a leaf surface depends on the moistening of the leaf surface, surface tension of liquid, and morphology of stomata (Kvesitadze et al., 2009). Once inside the leaf cells, toxicants are subject to biochemical reactions that are similar in kind to those observed in a mammalian body (Kvesitadze et al., 2006).

B. Uptake via Plant Roots

Like their leaves, the roots of many terrestrial plants also have stomata serving as passages for soil contaminants. These apertures on plant roots have been found open in all cases to date (e.g., Christodoulakis et al., 2002; Tarkowska and Wacowska, 1987). As water can enter the root via the epidermis, minerals in their inorganic forms can enter the root by being dissolved in water, or by entering on their own as free molecules via predominantly the root hairs. Minerals can enter the root against their concentration gradient (i.e., via active transport). However, most if not all soil contaminants can enter the plant root only through cuticle-free unsuberized cells (Kvesitadze et al., 2009). The ability of plant roots to absorb or extract soil contaminants is most evident from their application for phytoremediation (Kvesitadze et al., 2006; McCutcheon and Schnoor, 2003; Tsao, 2003), a biotechnology relying on the ability of plant roots to remove contaminants (e.g., toxic metals) in soils.

7.3.2. Uptake and Absorption by Humans

As with the above overview for plants due to space limitation, the one for humans in this subsection is necessarily succinct. In general, the main portals for entry of xenobiotics into a human (or most any other mammalian) body are dermal, respiratory, and gastrointestinal (GI). Secondary routes include the eyes, injection, sexual, anal, and wound.

Materials that have just been taken in (or up, depending on one's perspective) via inhalation or ingestion are still treated as outside the body until they penetrate the cellular barriers of the respiratory or GI tract, respectively. More so than the uptake or intake process, absorption varies greatly with the substance and the portal of entry involved.

A. Skin Penetration

Figure 7.4 provides a quick and very simplified schematic overview of the penetration and distribution of xenobiotics via the human skin which is a complex, multilayered structure comprising about 2 m^2 of surface in an average adult. The human skin is a large biomembrane relatively impermeable to most ions and aqueous solutions. This inability is due to the fact that the human skin's outermost layer, termed *epidermis*, has an outermost surface layer of dead, keratinized cells called *stratum corneum* serving as a physical barrier to most chemical penetration. Yet despite such a structural advantage, the molecules of many toxicants can still find their ways deep into the human skin (e.g., organophosphate pesticides in agricultural workers). This is particularly the case when the xenobiotic is a lipid-soluble substance given that biomembranes are composed of largely phospholipids which are highly lipophilic (*see* Section 7.2).

Note that for some substances, their skin permeability reportedly can vary greatly depending on the anatomical site with which they come to contact. For example, it was shwon (Maibach *et al.*, 1971) that for the pesticide parathion, the skin of the human scrotum was 12 times more permeable than the human forearm skin and 6 times more permeable than the human abdomen skin.

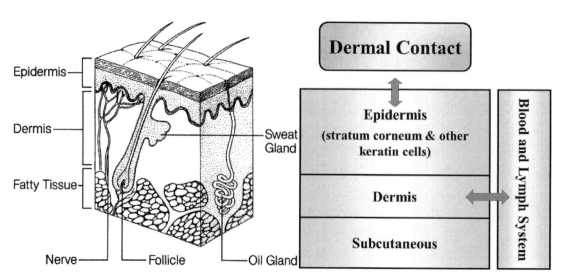

Figure 7.4. Penetration of Xenobiotics through the Human Skin (*skin image per se from public domain at www.freeclipartnow.com*)

B. Respiratory Uptake

Figure 7.5 below provides a quick and simplified schematic overview of the uptake and distribution pathways of toxicants in the human respiratory tract. The main function of this respiratory system is to exchange gases between the bloodstream and the air present in the air sacs termed *alveoli*, which are located in the lowest region of the respiratory tract at the ends of the bronchioles. The respiratory system is an organ in unavoidable contact with air pollutants, inasmuch as an average adult breathes well over 12,000 liters of air per day. This tract is also furnished with several mechanical and immunological mechanisms (e.g., filtration in nasal cavity, sneezing) devoted to keeping itself free from invading particles or microorganisms. In particular, there are small hair-like appendages termed *cilia* located in the primary bronchus that can sweep foreign particles out of the airways, and up to the throat through which the foreign particles may enter the GI.

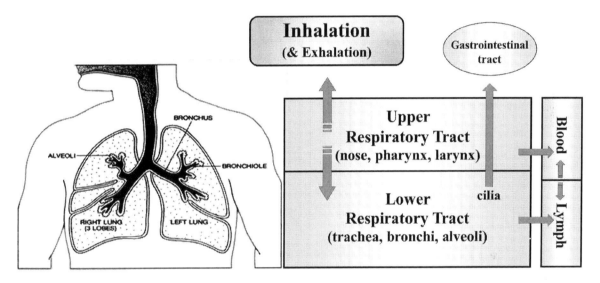

Figure 7.5. Uptake of Xenobiotics through the Human Respiratory Tract (*lung image per se from public domain at www.freeclipartnow.com*)

C. Gastrointestinal (GI) Absorption

Figure 7.6 presents a quick and simplified schematic overview of the absorption of xenobiotics via the human GI tract, which includes the *enterohepatic circulation* (that of bile from the liver to the small intestine) and the *portal venous system* (Figure 7.7). The GI tract may be treated as a long tube running from the mouth to the anus, with its contents external to the rest of the organism's internal body system. Aside from dietary exposure, the oral route of toxicological concern is generally limited to accidental or deliberate ingestion of toxicants.

7.4. Distribution and Excretion of Toxicants

Figures 7.4 through 7.6 present not only a quick and simplified overview of the uptake and absorption of xenobiotics by humans, but also a very brief account of their distribution via the bloodstream and the lymphatic system. Also note that in the human skin, it is the inner layer *dermis* that

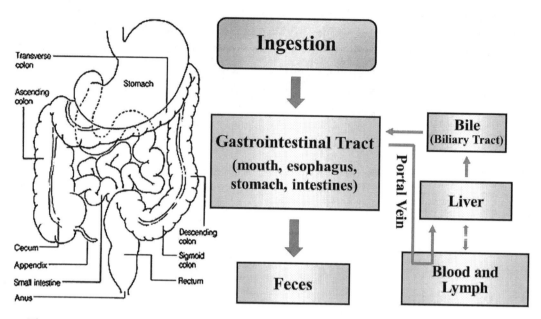

Figure 7.6. Absorption of Xenobiotics through the Human Gastrointestinal (GI) Tract
(*GI tract image per se from public domain at www.freeclipartnow.com*)

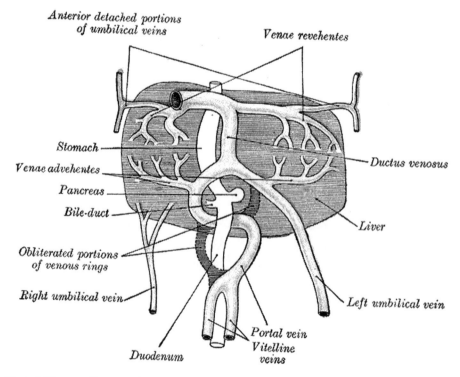

Figure 7.7. Portal Venous System (*image from public domain as published over 100 years ago, downloaded and as per justification at https://en.wikipedia.org/wiki/File:Gray475.png*)

provides maximum opportunity for further distribution of toxicants once they have penetrated the epidermis or the skin appendages (e.g., sweat glands, hair follicles). This opportunity owes to the fact that dermis is where in the skin that harbors most of the blood vessels (and nerve endings). It is also important to note that the *portal venous system* (Figure 7.7) is the component responsible for directing blood from parts (predominately the small intestine) of the GI tract to the liver, where the absorbed toxicant will be *processed* (Chapter 8) prior to their distribution to the cardiovascular system; that is, where the toxicant will undergo the so-termed *first-pass effect* process.

7.4.1. Distribution via the Bloodstream

The body fluids in humans (and certain other mammalians) are composed of three main components: *intracellular fluid*, ~40% of (human) body weight (BW); *interstitial fluid* (a.k.a. *tissue fluid*), ~20% of BW; and *intravascular fluid* (a.k.a. *blood plasma*), ~4% of BW. Of the three, intravascular fluid plays the most significant role in the distribution of absorbed toxicants, as human blood plasma accounts for over 50% of the total blood volume. Lymph is the roughly 10% of the plasma and tissue fluids left behind for taking out the cellular wastes. The transport of toxicants by lymph is comparatively insignificant, given that lymph flow is many times slower compared to blood flow.

Following absorption, toxicants are generally distributed along with plasma proteins. If a toxicant's molecule is bound to a plasma protein, it usually becomes immobilized away from the site of (toxic) action. Toxicants are frequently distributed to the sites of storage (e.g., bones, fats), to the liver or kidneys for metabolic processing, or to the site of action (e.g., binding to the hemoglobin). In particular, lipophilic compounds such as PCBs (polychlorinated biphenyls), dioxins, and DDTs are stored largely in the fats whereas fluoride (F) and lead (Pb), in the bones. It is important to note that whenever there is a large amount of a toxicant stored in one of the depots, it is a potential health hazard. This is because when certain biochemical or physiological disturbance occurs, a large amount of the stored toxicant can be suddenly released to become available for body distribution to the point to *overload* the site of action.

7.4.2. Excretion of Toxicants

Despite the fact that *elimination* of toxicants is the process more for their degradation by metabolism within the body, in general it is used interchangeably with the term *excretion* to describe the chemical disposition phase whereby a substance is *removed* from the body. In any event, this phase is pivotal in determining the potential toxic effects of xenobiotics (or of their metabolites, as defined and discussed in Chapter 8). In a mammalian body, the primary routes of chemical elimination (i.e., excretion) are via urine, feces, and exhaled air. Minor routes include breast milk, tear, saliva, semen, sweat, and hair.

A. Renal Excretion

The main function of a kidney is to remove urea, mineral salts, and waste materials from the blood. Its secondary but still significant functions include: the retention of water, salts, as well as electrolytes (i.e., those substances containing free ions such as potassium ion K^+); the excretion of these substances; and the regulation of blood pressure. The kidney therefore plays a vital role in eliminating toxicants from the body, in keeping the blood clean, and in regulating the amount of fluid in the body. The *nephron*, which is about one million in number in each of the two human kidneys, is the functional unit responsible for renal (i.e., that pertaining to the kidney) excretion. The unit has three main regions central to this primary route of excretion: *the glomerulus*, *the proximal (convoluted) tubule*, and *the distal (convoluted) tubule* (Figure 7.8). The tubular portion closer to the glomerulus is referred to as the *proximal* section.

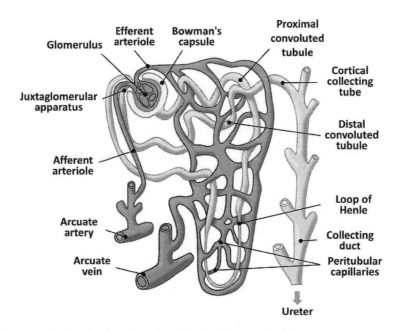

Figure 7.8. Nephron – the Basic Functional Unit of a (Human) Kidney (*original image without labeling downloaded from public domain, as copyright kindly and explicitly waived by author Burton Radons on 16 June 2012 at https://commons.wikimedia.org/wiki/File:Nephron_illustration.svg*)

Urine is composed of water, certain electrolytes, and various waste molecules that are filtered out of the renal blood system. The first phase in urine formation is filtration in the very vascular beginning of the nephron called glomerulus. Roughly 25% of the daily cardiac output passes through the human kidneys, of which about 20% is passively filtered via the numerous relatively large (~70 nm) glomerular pores. Small molecules, whether polar or lipid-soluble, thus readily pass through this sieve-like filter into the nephron tubule. The amount of this filtrate is substantial, about 45 gallons per day in a human adult. The urine, as eliminated, represents only about 1% of the amount of fluid filtrated via the glomerulae into the renal tubules. Molecules too large to pass through or those bound to proteins must be either further altered or eliminated by other mechanisms. Tubular reabsorption is the comparatively less crucial, second phase taking place in the proximal tubule. Nearly all of the water, glucose, K^+, and amino acids lost during the first phase (glomerular filtration) will re-enter the blood from this nephron section by passive diffusion (i.e., to their lower concentrations in the capillaries surrounding the tubule). The urine's pH is one factor that can strongly affect this passive diffusion process as well as urinary excretion.

Another secondary phase, in which solutes may be secreted into the kidney, occurs in the distal tubule. This mechanism permits passive but relies more on active transport of solutes from the peritubular capillaries into the tubular lumen. Solutes actively secreted into this lumen include H^+ and K^+ ions, as well as molecules of some polar and nonpolar substances.

In essence, a toxicant's renal excretion can be approximated as the *sum* of glomerular filtration *and* distal tubular secretion of the toxicant *minus* proximal tubular reabsorption of the toxicant. Small toxicants (both polar and lipid-soluble) are filtered with ease by the glomerulus. In some cases, certain large molecules (including some bound to plasma proteins) can be excreted by passive transfer from the blood and then cross both the capillary cell walls and the nephron tubular membranes to enter into the urine proper.

B. Fecal Excretion

Elimination of toxicants in the feces relies on two physiological processes: *hepatic excretion* involving bile secretion; and *intestinal excretion*. Of the two, the biliary route is the more significant. Bile is a complex fluid flowing through the biliary tract into the small intestine. It contains water, electrolytes, and a host of organic molecules including bile acids, cholesterols, and phospholipids. Many waste products, including bilirubin, are removed from the body by hepatic secretion into the bile and then into the duodenum (i.e., the beginning portion of the small intestine) for excretion in the feces. For certain types of substances (e.g., organic bases, organic acids, neutral compounds), the predominate means of excretion is via special active transport mechanisms. Some metals (e.g., Pb, Hg) are also secreted into the bile. In any case, most substances that tend to be secreted into and through the bile are typically large size ionized molecules such as large-molecular-weight conjugates (e.g., those discussed in Chapter 8).

Note that most of the substances secreted into and from the bile are water-soluble. Therefore, those substances are not likely to be reabsorbed as such from the small intestine back to the liver. Enzymes in the intestinal flora are capable of hydrolyzing some glucuronide and sulfate conjugates (Chapter 8) to produce smaller and less water-soluble substances that can then be reabsorbed along the proximal and distal ileum (i.e., the terminal portion of the small intestine). The process of secretion into the small intestine through the bile, together with reabsorption along the ileum (Figure 7.6) and then back to the liver by the portal circulation (Figure 7.7), is referred to as *enterohepatic circulation*. This process prevents a relatively large amount of the bile acids from leaving the human body. Roughly 95% of the bile acid molecules delivered to the duodenum are reabsorbed into the blood within the ileum, where the venous blood goes straight into the portal vein to allow their repeated passage via the sinusoids (i.e., venous cavities) of the liver. As expected, continuous enterohepatic recycling can occur and therefore can lead to very long half-lives of some lipid-soluble toxicants in (certain part of) the body.

The other key mechanism of fecal elimination is by direct intestinal excretion. Despite the fact that this is not a major pathway of fecal elimination, a considerable number of toxicants can be excreted directly into and out of the intestinal tract and thereby be eliminated directly via this route. Some substances, especially those poorly ionized in the plasma (e.g., weak bases), may passively diffuse via the walls of the capillaries surrounding the intestinal tract and into the intestinal lumen to be eliminated in the feces. Intestinal excretion is not regarded as a major pathway in that it is a slow process compared to hepatic excretion. It is a crucial elimination route only for those toxicants that cannot be easily metabolized or be easily eliminated by other excretion processes.

C. Pulmonary Excretion

The lower respiratory tract, particularly the alveolar region, serves as a significant pathway for excretion of many volatile substances including their gaseous metabolites. As hinted earlier, the main function of alveoli in each lung is for exchange of oxygen (O_2) from the air with carbon dioxide (CO_2) from the blood. This gas(eous) exchange, also known as pulmonary respiration, is maintained predominately by passive diffusion following a concentration gradient. Gaseous substances with a low solubility in the blood are thereby more rapidly eliminated compared to those with a high solubility. Volatile liquid dissolved in the blood are also readily excreted as part of the exhaled air. The amount of a liquid excreted by the alveoli is proportional to its vapor pressure. In reality, exhalation can be an efficient route of excretion for some lipid-soluble toxicants. This is possible in that each alveolus is surrounded by a network of capillaries in a way that the alveolar contents are separated from those in the capillaries only by an extremely thin alveolar membrane. It should be pointed out that some substances can be removed directly by exhalation if they are taken into the respiratory system but have not yet diffused into the alveolar blood.

7.5. Toxicokinetics of Toxicants

For adverse effect as well as the associated toxic response to occur, both the amount and the way in which a toxicant is delivered to the site of (toxic) action is foremost relevant. This type of pursuit is within the realm of toxicokinetics (TK), starting with the notion of reaction kinetics. Reaction kinetics is concerned with the rates and the tendency of chemical processing or, more specifically, with the changes in the reactant concentrations in chemical reactions. In essence, TK is the explanation as well as the study of the kinetics and the quantitative movement of toxicants in a living system. It analyzes the time course of a toxicant *being handled* by the host organism's body. Its focus is on the *quantitative* aspects of toxicant disposition inside an organism's body.

7.5.1. Principles and Models/Modeling of Toxicokinetics

Much like pharmacokinetics (PK) concerning the disposition kinetics of drugs with not much real time physiological data, TK relies heavily on mathematical models for explanation and prediction of a toxicant's disposition kinetics in the body of a biological system. The delivery of a toxicant to the site of action depends on two key disposition processes: *absorption* from the exposure site into the organism's general (cardiac) circulation; and *distribution* via the circulation to the site of action as well as to all other body tissues. Within the distribution process, the toxicant's concentration at the site of action is strongly affected by the rate of elimination (including metabolism and excretion). For simplicity, the toxicant's concentrations in the general circulation, or the *central compartment* in TK modeling jargon, are all that matters under the notion that such time-dependent concentrations can be utilized to reflect those levels at the action site or other tissues of concern or interest. This is why a one-compartment open model (Figure 7.9) is often employed to approximate the disposition kinetics of a substance. If specific interests arise and additional parameter data become available for the disposition kinetics to be represented by further compartments, then two (Figure 7.9) or more anatomic compartments are employed.

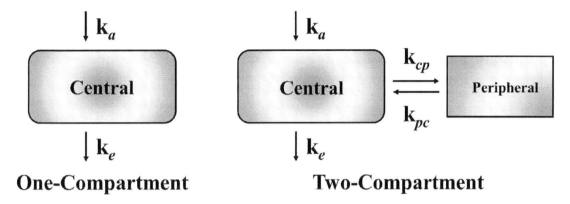

Figure 7.9. Schematic Presentation of One-Compartment and Two-Compartment Open Models (*showing the kinetics parameters to be measured for the time-course disposition of a xenobiotic, where k_a is the absorption rate, k_e is the excretion rate, k_{cp} is the rate for distribution from the central [circulation] to peripheral [e.g., site of action] compartment, and k_{pc} is the rate for distribution from the peripheral to the central compartment*)

One of the more complex compartment models is physiologically-based pharmacokinetics (PB-PK model), or here more appropriately referred to as PB-*T*K model for *t*oxicokinetics. Fundamental to each PB-TK model (e.g., Dong, 1994; Medinsky and Valentine, 2001) is a set of tedious, if not highly complex, mathematical equations that presumably offer a comprehensive time course of the xenobiotic disposition in several pre-selected key anatomic compartments (e.g., lungs, brain, liver, kidneys, muscle). Each of these anatomic regions is to have its own tissue volume, excretion and metabolic rate constants, characteristic blood flow, and tissue-blood partition coefficient that collectively are deemed most responsible for the xenobiotic disposition in that body region. All models used in TK, whether PB-TK or one-compartment, are considered open in the sense that they each allow the toxicant's elimination from the model. Given that the absorption rate of environmental toxicants is usually uncertain, as the *exact* amount of *environmental* exposure rarely becomes known, the rate constant for elimination is relatively more practical and more critical than that for absorption when investigating the time-course disposition of a toxicant.

7.5.2. Basic Mathematical Concepts

The mathematical principles involved in TK analysis are complex and beyond the scope of this introductory text. Accordingly, no attempt is made to describe them in any detail in this chapter. Yet a few basic terms and concepts are thought worth introducing here in an attempt to demonstrate the nature and complexity of the analysis involved. The numerical example in Box 7.1 that follows shortly is for those who are more mathematically inclined. Regardless, it is important to note that, as hinted in the numerical example, knowing the chemical-specific values for some of the kinetics parameters may enable a toxicologist to estimate the amount of a toxicant that a victim has absorbed (i.e., has been exposed to).

A. Volume of Distribution

This parameter is also known as *apparent* volume of distribution (Vd), a term used to quantify the distribution of a toxicant throughout the body after intake or absorption. It is defined as the plasma volume that is apparently required to distribute the absorbed substance to the concentration so measured or projected in the plasma (e.g., in the central compartment). Note that Vd is a hypothetical value, as it does not represent the actual physiological volume of the plasma inside a body. For instance, when a lipophilic toxicant of a known amount enters a body and binds preferentially to the fatty tissues at the expense of the plasma, its measured concentration in the plasma can be very low. This can result in a huge value projected for Vd, which then can be larger than the actual plasma volume in the body. This is unfortunately possible because by definition Vd = [(the total x amount of toxicant in plasma) ÷ (the Cp concentration of toxicant in plasma)]; that is, Vd = x/Cp. In other words, the projected Vd will become larger whenever the measured Cp becomes smaller while x is held constant (e.g., is known as in the case with drug injection).

B. Toxicant Clearance

After intake or absorption, a toxicant is distributed among the body fluids and tissues and then all or a portion of it is eventually cleared or eliminated (mainly by the kidneys and liver). This physiological process, referred to as toxicant or systemic clearance (CL), results in the toxicant's concentration in the plasma decreasing steadily, though at different rates for different substances in different species. More specifically, CL is defined as the plasma *volume* theoretically required for clearing its toxicant within a unit time (e.g., in ml/min), in order to account for the observed rate of a toxicant's systemic elimination from the body. CL thereby expresses the rate or efficiency at which a toxicant is removed from the plasma and not the amount of the toxicant eliminated. Mathematically, it can be expressed as the ratio of elimination rate Ke (e.g., in mg/min) to plasma concentration Cp (e.g., in mg/ml) of the toxicant; that is, CL = Ke/Cp. In most cases especially for a nonvolatile toxicant, its renal elimination is frequently treated as its systemic elimination.

C. Elimination Rate Constant

This rate constant (K) is a chemical-specific parameter used to characterize the *fraction* of a toxicant in the body eliminated per unit time. The value for this *constant* can be approximated by the slope of the line of the log plasma concentration versus time (i.e., plotted against time). It has the following relationship with the two terms discussed above: K = CL/Vd, in units of time^{-1} (e.g., min^{-1}, hr^{-1}). On the other hand, the elimination *rate* Ke of a toxicant is often proportional to its concentration, as elimination is typically a first-order process until such becomes saturated.

D. Area under the Curve

This term (area) refers to the total amount of a toxicant taken in by the host organism's body, irrespective of the rate of absorption. It represents simply that *total* area under the curve (AUC) in a semi-log plot of toxicant concentration in the plasma against time. AUC can be used as a measure of toxicant exposure or the bioavailability of a drug or toxicant absorbed (usually via the oral route). It is mathematically related to the above three parameters K, CL, and Vd as follows: AUC = Cp_0/K = $Cp_0/(CL/Vd)$ = $Cp_0(Vd/CL)$, where Cp_0 is the toxicant's plasma concentration at (or near) time zero serving as the initial point on the curve.

Box 7.1. Numerical Example for Clarification of Basic Disposition Kinetics

> Suppose there are x grams of grapefruit pulp (e.g., a toxicant) in a jar containing 10 ml water (e.g., plasma); and the entire content of the jar is poured into a tank (e.g., an animal body) pre-filled with 990 ml water. The volume of distribution Vd of the pulp in the tank is then 1,000 ml = (x g) ÷ [(x g)/(10 ml + 990 ml)].
>
> If, at each minute, 10 ml of the water containing y mg grapefruit pulp is emptied from the tank, discarded, and replaced with 10 ml of water added into the tank, then the (systemic) clearance CL is 10 ml per min; that is, CL = (Ke/Cp) = (y mg/min ÷ y mg/10 ml) = 10 ml/min.
>
> The elimination rate constant K is CL/Vd = (10 ml/min) ÷ (1,000 ml) = 0.01/min (or at the constant rate of 1% per minute).
>
> Note that for first-order decay reactions, ln ([100%]/[50%]) = K($t_{1/2}$). Therefore, the elimination half-life $t_{1/2}$, which is the time for the pulp concentration in the tank to fall to 50%, is 69.3 min, as $t_{1/2}$ = [(ln 2) ÷ K] = [(0.6931) ÷ (0.01/min)] and ln 2 (i.e., natural log of 2) = 0.6931.

References

Christodoulakis NS, Menti J, Galatis B, 2002, Structure and Development of Stomata on the Primary Root of *Ceratonia siliqua* L. *Ann. Botany* 89:23-29.

Dong MH, 1994. Microcomputer Programs for Physiologically-Based Pharmacokinetic (PB-PK) Modeling. *Comput. Mthds. Programs Biomed.* 45:213-221.

Humble GD, Raschke K, 1971. Stomatal Opening Quantitatively Related to Potassium Transport: Evidence from Electron Probe Analysis. *Plant Physiol.* 48:447-453.

Jinno N, Kuraishi S, 1982. Acid-Induced Stomatal Opening in *Commelina communis* and *Vicia faba*. *Plant Cell Physiol.* 23:1169-1174.

Kim DJ, Lee JS, 2007. Current Theories for Mechanism of Stomatal Opening: Influence of Blue Light; Mesophyll Cells, and Sucrose. *J. Plant Biol.* 50:523-526.

Kvesitadze G, Khatisashvili G, Sadunishvili T, Ramsden JJ, 2006. *Biochemical Mechanisms of Detoxification in Higher Plants: Basis of Phytoremediation*. Berlin, Heidelberg, Germany: Springer-Verlag.

Kvesitadze K, Sadunishvili T, Kvesitadze G, 2009. Mechanisms of Organic Contaminants Uptake and Degradation in Plants. *World Academy of Sci., Engineering & Technol.* 55:458-468.

Larcher W, 2003. *Physiological Plant Ecology: Ecophysiology and Stress Physiology of Functional Groups*, 4th Edition. Berlin, Heidelberg, Germany: Springer-Verlag.

Maibach HJ, Feldmann RJ, Milby TH, Serat WF, 1971. Regional Variation in Percutaneous Penetration in Man. *Arch. Environ. Health* 23:208-211.

McCutcheon SC, Schnoor JL (Eds.), 2003. *Phytoremediation: Transformation and Control of Contaminants*. Hoboken, New Jersey, USA: Wiley/Interscience.

Medinsky MA, Valentine JL, 2001. Toxicokinetics. In *Casarett and Doull's Toxicology: The Basic Science of Poisons* (Klaassen CD, Ed.), 6th Edition. New York, New York, USA: McGraw-Hill, Chapter 7.

Purves WK, Orians GH, Heller HC, 1995. *Life: The Science of Biology*, 4th Edition. Sunderland, Massachusetts, USA: Sinauer Associates.

Schraudner M, Moeder W, Wiese C, van Camp W, Inzé D, Langebartels C, Sandermann H Jr, 1998. Ozone-Induced Oxidative Burst in the Ozone Biomonitor Plant, Tobacco Bel W3. *The Plant J.* 16:235-245.

Taiz L, Zeiger E, 2006. *Plant Physiology*, 4th Edition. Massachusetts, USA: Sinauer Associates.

Tarkowska JA, Wacowska M, 1987. The Significance of the Presence of Stomata on Seedling Roots. *Ann. Botany* 61:305-310.

Tsao D (Ed.), 2003. *Phytoremediation (Advances in Biochemical Engineering/Biotechnology, No. 78)*. Berlin, Heidelberg, Germany: Springer-Verlag.

Review Questions

1. Briefly explain why this chapter has its focus on systemic effects induced by environmental toxicants, rather than on localized effects.
2. Name the major biochemical events involved in the disposition of toxicants inside a biological system.
3. Briefly describe the five common mechanisms of entry enabling or aiding toxicants to get inside an organism's body or to cross the body's biomembranes.
4. What are the two common ways in which terrestrial plants can take up environmental contaminants?
5. Why are biomembranes permeable to only certain (particularly lipophilic) toxicants?
6. Which *structural* component of a plant leaf is most crucial for the uptake of environmental pollutants?
7. How is phytoremediation related to the uptake of toxicants by plant roots?
8. What type of toxicants tends to be absorbed easily by the human skin, and why?
9. Which of the three main human skin layers is most responsible for distributing the absorbed toxicants to the blood, and why?
10. In what way will (or can) inhaled foreign particles be removed from the respiratory tract to enter the gastrointestinal tract?
11. Briefly explain why a toxicant stored in a depot in the human body can become a serious health hazard.
12. What are the primary functions of the portal venous system, and of the enterohepatic circulation?
13. What are the two main *disposition* processes that are primarily responsible for the delivery of a toxicant to the site of (toxic) action?
14. What is likely to be the elimination half-life $t_{1/2}$ if the toxicant clearance is 20 ml/min and the apparent volume of distribution is 2,000 ml?
15. What are the primary routes of chemical elimination in a mammalian body? And why one of them is apparently the most important?
16. Of the three (sub)phases involved in renal excretion (as covered in this chapter), which is the most significant and why?
17. Under what circumstances is intestinal excretion more important than hepatic excretion for fecal elimination of toxicants?
18. What type(s) of toxicants in the blood is (are) eliminated more rapidly and easily via gaseous exchange in the alveolar region?

CHAPTER 8

Metabolism/Biotransformation of Xenobiotics

8.1. Introduction

Contrary to general perception, humans and other mammalians are not physiologically defenseless to the apparently countless environmental toxicants that they may be exposed to. Many environmental toxicants that the human body is exposed to are lipophilic, a biochemical property that enables many of these xenobiotics to penetrate various kinds of biomembranes to some level. In humans, following uptake and absorption, these foreign substances are distributed via the bloodstream and the lymphatic system to various body parts, including the excretory organs where the intruders can be eliminated. While the xenobiotics are in various body tissues and organs, many tend to undergo biotransformation, a process whereby a substance is transformed from one chemical form or species to another by one or more biochemical (re)actions.

Biotransformation of toxicants is commonly thought as synonymous with the biochemical as well as physiological process known as *metabolism* (a.k.a. *metabolic conversions*). Yet metabolism specifically includes other biochemical events basic to cellular *homeostasis,* which is the tendency of a cell to maintain a stable internal environment. Further discussion on this distinction is given in Section 8.1.1 below for a due appreciation of metabolism being one of the three basic attributes that define life. Closely related to this attribute is the set of nutritional factors and conditions that affects the biotransformation and hence the toxicity of toxicants. Biotransformation and metabolic reactions are mostly enzymatic in nature, as virtually all of them are catalyzed by one or more enzymes in the body. Accordingly, a prerequisite to learning chemical biotransformation is some knowledge about the general functions of enzymes. It is for this reason that Section 8.1.2 offers a brief introduction on biotransforming enzymes and their general actions.

8.1.1. Metabolism *vs.* Biotransformation

Biotransformation is for the most part limited to studying the chemical fate of xenobiotics that have entered the body. It is a topic directly and extremely relevant to toxicology. Metabolism, on the other hand, is a broader term used to define the sum total of all biochemical processes and events occurring in living organisms that results in basic life functions such as growth, energy production, and elimination of waste materials. Accordingly, along with growth and reproduction, metabolism is regarded as one of the three main attributes defining an organism's life.

More specifically, metabolism refers to those biochemical reactions that take place in living cells in order for the cells as well as the body to sustain their life by maintaining a homeostatic environment. Such a physiological environment requires a constant energy supply to the body's cells, a constant body temperature, and a constant blood sugar level, among other things. Insofar as cells in the body must perform a vast variety of chemical, mechanical, electrical, and osmotic activities, a continuous supply of energy for such basic cellular functions is indispensable. The two principal sets of metabolic conversions are termed *catabolism* and *anabolism*. Catabolism is the set of metabolic reactions that breaks down large molecules (e.g., the macronutrients proteins, carbohydrates, and lipids) into smaller units to release energy as a by-product. Many times, the term *catabolism* is loosely used interchangeably with *metabolism*. Anabolism, on the other hand, is the set that synthesizes molecules from smaller units, generally powered by the energy released from one or more catabolic reactions.

Metabolism is frequently studied under the two closely related subspecialties *cell* (or *cellular*) *metabolism* and *nutrient* (or *nutritional*) *metabolism*. Cell metabolism is concerned with the sum of biochemical reactions that transpire within cells. In contrast, nutrient metabolism focuses on the molecular fate of nutrients and other dietary substances in the body, including all facets of nutritional biochemistry that have crucial effects on chemical biotransformation (Section 10.3).

8.1.2. Biotransforming Enzymes and Their General Actions

Enzymes are proteins mostly of globular shape and by definition all capable of catalyzing biochemical reactions. They are common targets of drugs and environmental toxicants. Enzymes work by lowering the energy required to activate certain biochemical events. This explains why some reaction rates can be millions of times faster when catalyzed by enzymes than when not, as in the case by the antioxidant enzyme *catalase* (Section 8.5.2). Enzymes are generally highly specific to the reactions that they catalyze since part of their structure is used as the site (in some cases known as receptor) where a specific substrate needs to fit in. For this reason, enzymes are each commonly name after the specific reaction or substrate that they catalyze or interact with. Some enzymes exert their catalytic function to their fullness without any additional component. Many others require binding with non-protein molecules termed *cofactors*. If the cofactor is an *organic* substance, it is more specifically referred to as *coenzyme*. Examples of cofactors and coenzymes in chemical biotransformation are given toward the end of this chapter in Section 8.6.4.

Several groups of enzymes are regarded as particularly important and relevant to toxicologists studying chemical biotransformation. Accordingly, enzymes in these special groups are further characterized in some detail shortly, following Sections 8.2 and 8.3 given on (respectively) the general and other enzymatic processes involved in the biotransformation of xenobiotics.

8.2. General Aspects/Processes of Biotransformation

Upon uptake or absorption, a xenobiotic (e.g., a toxicant) will likely undergo a sequence of biochemical events referred to as *Phase I* (enzymatic) reactions, and then likely followed by one or more *Phase II* (enzymatic) reactions. The typical outcome of a Phase I reaction is a *primary metabolite* that is slightly more polar (i.e., water-soluble) than the parent compound. This change in polarity is accomplished by enzymatically attaching a functional group (e.g., -COOH, -NH$_2$, -OH, -SH) to the parent compound (now termed *primary metabolite*). It is with or onto these functional units that the Phase II enzymes (mostly transferases) and coenzymes (e.g., glucuronic acid) will kick in to conjugate, resulting in a complex called conjugate or *intermediate metabolite*. These conjugates are usually more polar and thus can be more readily excreted from the body.

When the Phase II conjugation is through use of *u*ridine *d*iphosphate glucuronic acid (UDP-glucuronic acid, or glucuronic acid for short) as the coenzyme, and (hence) *U*DP-*g*lucuronyl*t*ransferase (UGT) as the enzyme, it is specifically termed *glucuronidation*. Other Phase II specific conjugations, which are not as predominant, are sulfation, methylation, acetylation, and conjugation with glutathione (GSH) or with certain amino acids (e.g., glycine, glutamine, serine). Some xenobiotics that already contain one or more of the required functional groups will bypass Phase I to directly undergo one or more Phase II reactions. An example is phenol (C_6H_5-OH), which already has one of its carbons on its benzene ring bonded to an OH group.

The main aspects of xenobiotic biotransformation are outlined graphically in Figure 8.1 below, followed by a discussion on their specifics and importance.

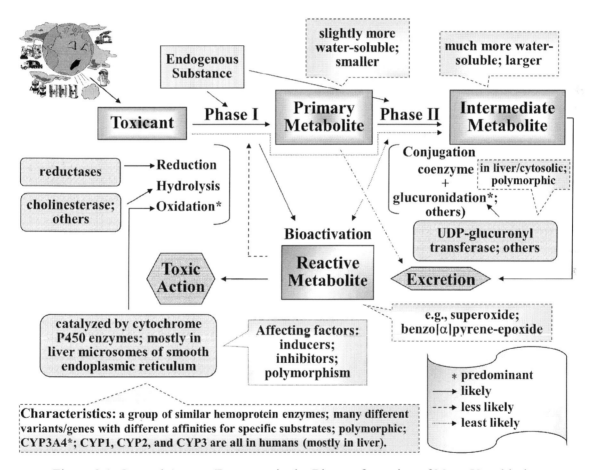

Figure 8.1. General Aspects/Processes in the Biotransformation of Many Xenobiotics

8.2.1. Phase I Enzymatic Reactions

As reflected in Figure 8.1, Phase I (enzymatic) reactions include predominantly *oxidation* and less so *reduction, hydrolysis, hydration, dehydrochlorination* (as well as several others which are even less often). These reactions are catalyzed or mediated by enzymes available much more in the smooth-surfaced endoplasmic reticulum than in the cytosol or other organelles. For enzymes located in the endoplasmic reticulum, they are referred to as the microsomal kind.

A. Oxidation

This reaction group typically involves the *addition* of one oxygen (O_2) molecule, the *removal* of one hydrogen (H) atom, and a *loss* of electrons (thus resulting in an increase in valence as well as in binding capacity). The reactions in this group are mediated predominately by cytochrome P450 enzymes and less so by other *mixed-function oxidases* (MFO), alcohol dehydrogenase, or aldehyde dehydrogenase. The predominant oxidative reaction involved is of the *mono*-oxygenation type (i.e., with the addition of *one* oxygen molecule), as generalized in Reaction 8.1 below:

$$X\text{-}H + O_2 + 2H^+ + 2e^- \rightarrow X\text{-}OH + H_2O \tag{8.1}$$

where X-H is the xenobiotic (i.e., the enzymatic substrate) and X-OH is the resultant primary metabolite product. A closely related enzyme important to this type of oxidation, but not always necessary, is NADPH-cytochrome P450 reductase. This reductase can serve as an important electron (e^-) donor for the cytochrome P450 oxygenase. When a substrate (e.g., a toxicant) binds to the active site (which is around the heme group) of a cytochrome P450, such an enzymatic binding favors the transfer of an e^- from NADP-H (*n*icotinamide *a*denine *d*inucleotide *p*hosphate) through the (action of the) cytochrome reductase or another related reductase (Sligar *et al.*, 1979) to the heme group. The cytochrome P450 reductase contains both the flavin FAD (Section 8.6.4), which can accept e^- from $NADP^+$, and the flavin FMN (Section 8.6.4), which can donate e^- to the cytochrome P450 oxygenase.

Oxidative reactions include numerous specific kinds, such as hydroxylation, dealkylation, deamination, and epoxidation. Hydroxylation adds the functional unit -OH to the parent compound. Oxidative dealkylation involves the removal of an alkyl group, such as the methyl (CH_3) or ethyl (C_2H_5) group, from the parent compound. Oxidative deamination removes an amine (NH_3). Epoxidation requires the interaction with oxygen molecules. The substrate in this last case is often an alkene (i.e., an unsaturated chemical substance with at least one carbon=carbon double bond). The resultant epoxide functional unit consists of a three-member ring with an oxygen atom bonded to two carbon atoms being double bonded to each other. Another common alkene oxidation is dihydroxylation, ending with two carbons on double bond now each attached to the other as well as to an OH group. Of the four oxidative reactions noted above, hydroxylation is the most predominant in Phase I reactions and produces the functional unit (group) -OH that is most ready for Phase II reactions.

B. Reduction

This group chemically has the opposite outcome of oxidation. The reactions in this group each typically involve the *removal* of one oxygen molecule, the *addition* of one hydrogen atom, and a *gain* of e^-. Some representative enzymes are NADPH-cytochrome P450 reductase, nitroreductase, and glutathione (GSH) reductase. An example of this type of reactions is a nitro (NO_2) reduction through which the inexpensive perfume additive *nitrobenzene* (C_6H_5-NO_2) is reduced to the polyurethane precursor *aniline* (C_6H_5-NH_2).

C. Hydrolysis

This reaction group involves the addition of a water (H_2O) molecule to split the substrate (e.g., a toxicant) into two smaller molecular fragments. Some enzymes responsible for Phase I hydrolysis are phosphatases (that removing a phosphate group PO_4^{3-}) and esterases (that splitting esters). Acetylcholinesterase is an esterase, of which highly excessive inhibition in humans (e.g., by organophosphate pesticides) can result in convulsions or death (Chapters 9 and 15).

8.2.2. Phase II Enzymatic Reactions

Biotransformation reactions in this phase are conjugate or synthetic in action. They aim at attaching polar (hydrophilic) or ionizable (that tending to become an ion) groups to the primary metabolites (mainly those from Phase I) to form products that are relatively larger but otherwise more water-soluble and thereby easier to be excreted (e.g., in the urine). The coenzymes or endogenous substances that aid in generating the polar or ionizable groups include: UDP-glucuronic acid (UDPGA); *S-a*denosyl*m*ethionine (SAM); 3'-*p*hospho-*a*denosine-5'-*p*hospho*s*ulfate (PAPS); acetyl coenzyme A (acetyl CoA); certain amino acids (glutamine, glycine, serine); and glutathione (GSH, a *g*lutamine-cysteine-glycine tripeptide containing notably the -*SH* thiol group).

A. Glucuronidation

As noted earlier, this specific type of Phase II reactions is so termed because the enzyme and coenzyme involved are UGT (*U*DP-glucuronosyl*t*ransferase) and UDPGA, respectively. Glucuronidation is the most predominant type of Phase II reactions largely because the functional group for conjugation is -OH, which is readily produced by hydroxylation (the predominant type of oxidation occurring in Phase I reactions). The coenzyme glucuronic acid (UDPGA), first isolated from urine (and hence the name uronic acid), is a highly water-soluble derivative of glucose produced in the liver of humans and most (other) animals.

B. Sulfation, Methylation, Acetylation, and Others

Phase II biotransformation includes other specific types of reactions termed *sulfation, methylation, acetylation, amino acid conjugation,* and *GSH (glutathione) conjugation*. The enzymes involved in sulfation, methylation, and acetylation are *sulfot*ransferase (SULT), *methylt*ransferase (MET), and *N-a*cetyl*t*ransferase (NAT), respectively. The coenzymes required for them are PAPS (3'-phosphoadenosine-5'-phosphosulfate), SAM (S-adenosylmethionine), and acetyl CoA (acetyl coenzyme A), respectively. Members of the *g*lutathione-*S-t*ransferase (GST) family, which collectively are ubiquitously distributed in nature, are responsible for GSH conjugation. For amino acid conjugation, the enzymes involved are not necessarily a transferase. For example, an enzyme named seryl-t(ransfer)RNA synthetase is responsible for mediating the conjugation of the amino acid *serine* with xenobiotics that contain an aromatic hydroxylamine group (Parkinson, 2001).

8.3. Other Relevant Aspects of Biotransformation

As depicted in Figure 8.1, not all Phase I reactions lead to the detoxification of toxicants. Phase I reactions may result in the *(bio)activation* of certain xenobiotics. It is also probable, though not nearly as frequent, to find certain Phase II reactions that can lead to a *reactive* metabolite. Another type of biotransformation involving neither detoxification nor bioactivation is the routine breakdown (more correctly catabolism) of *endogenous* substances.

8.3.1. Bioactivation of Xenobiotics

An example of toxicant bioactivation is the biotransformation of the naturally occurring mycotoxin aflatoxin B_1 to an epoxide metabolite named aflatoxin B_1-2,3-epoxide, which is more reactive than its parent compound with the mutagenicity of causing liver cancer. It was suggested (e.g., Croy *et al.*, 1978; Swenson *et al.*, 1977) that the aflatoxin B_1-DNA adducts found in liver cells was due to the tendency of this epoxide to bind to nuclear DNA. A DNA adduct, which involves a piece of DNA covalently bonded to a foreign molecule, is thought to be a critical intermediate on the pathway of chemical carcinogenesis. After all, it is then a DNA in a damaged or irregular form and thus with a much greater potential for miscarriage of genetic information necessary for cell division and cell growth (Chapter 18).

Benzo[α]pyrene (BαP), frequently found in incomplete burning of cigarette smoke and coal, is another substance that may undergo Phase I reactions to become a reactive epoxide named BαP-7,8-dihydrodiol-9,10-epoxide, which is thought to act as an ultimate carcinogen (e.g., Smart, 2004). The main difference between the two bioactivation mechanisms is that for BαP, it is a two-step epoxidation whereas for aflatoxin B_1, a direct one.

Another pathway is the bioactivation of carbon tetrachloride (CCl_4) to the trichloromethyl free radical $CCl_3 \cdot$ leading to the initiation of lipid peroxidation (Chapter 9) and later to the formation of lipid-protein adducts (Parinandi *et al.*, 1990; Trostchansky and Rubbo, 2007). Lipid peroxidation refers to a biochemical phenomenon in which unsaturated lipids undergo oxidative degradation, as initiated by a free radical (e.g., $CCl_3 \cdot$) stealing electrons from the lipid molecules present on biomembranes nearby.

A third pathway leading to bioactivation of toxicants is *N*-hydroxylation, which is a special kind of hydroxylation involving specifically the oxidation of the nitrogen (N) atom in the NH_2-group of an organic compound. *N*-hydroxylation is the initial step (Morton *et al.*, 1979) in activating the aromatic amine benzidine $(C_6H_4NH_2)_2$, which was linked to bladder cancer and used in high quantities in the past to produce dyes in cloth, paper, and leather.

8.3.2. Biotransformation of Endogenous Substances

Both the Phase I and Phase II reactions can biotransform not only many xenobiotics but also many endogenous substances in the human body. For example, primary bile acids such as cholic acid and chenodeoxycholic acid are synthesized in the human liver by oxidation of cholesterol in multiple steps mediated by several cytochrome P450 enzymes including CYP7A1. Other endogenous substances such as thyroid hormone and bilirubin can undergo the Phase II glucuronidation. And both glucuronidation and sulfation of the sex hormone testosterone have been demonstrated in human livers (e.g., Pacifici *et al.*, 1997). To some scholars, all these reactions involving endogenous substances are of the *metabolic conversion* kind, supposedly not part of the typical *biotransformation* processes.

8.4. Characteristics of Cytochrome P450 Enzymes

As highlighted in Section 8.2.1 as well as in Figure 8.1, the most significant and common enzyme group responsible for Phase I reactions is cytochrome P450 enzymes (a.k.a. P450 enzymes, CYP 450s, or P450s). P450 enzymes are a large and diverse superfamily of hemoproteins found in most tissues of most living organisms. These Phase I enzymes represent most of the monooxygenases known. Note that monooxygenases are generally referred to as *mixed*-function oxidases in that each of the two oxygen (O) atoms in Reaction 8.1 is used for a *different* function. At any rate, in most situations, P450 enzymes play a significant role in the detoxification of xenobiotics. These enzymes derived their popular name P450 from the complex between the ferrous (Fe^{2+}) heme center in their structure and the carbon monoxide (CO) molecule that absorbs light maximally at wavelength 450 nm. Their official as well as technical name now is (or begins with) CYP (standing for *cy*tochrome *P*450).

8.4.1. Families of Cytochrome P450s

There are numerous genetic variants of P450s (i.e., numerous forms with each derived from a specific gene). These variants are commonly termed isoforms and are classified according to the similarities of their amino acid sequences genetically encoded by the DNA in the body. The *family* names for all CYP isoforms (also called CYP iso[en]zymes) are *numbered*, such as CYP*3* or CYP*7*. There are over 70 families used to describe the P450s, of which about 20% have been identified in humans. The CYP families have their own *sub*families each identified by a *letter*, such as CYP2*C* and CYP3*A*. The subfamilies in turn have their specific genes each identified by a *number* again, such as CYP3A*4* and CYP2B*29*. Among the diverse *human* CYP enzyme genes, CYP3A4 is reportedly the most abundant and most important in oxidative reactions (e.g., Eichelbaum and Burk, 2001; Keshava *et al.*, 2004).

8.4.2. Catalytic Activities and Cellular Locations

The catalytic activities of P450s vary considerably in different people as well as in different races. Genetic variation in a population is termed *polymorphism* when both alleles (i.e., variant forms of the same gene pair) exist with a frequency of at least 1 percent. Such a (genetic) polymorphism may have profound clinical consequences, in that people with different CYP genotypes may need to follow different dosage schemes for certain drug treatments. Many P450s *per se* can be *induced* (i.e., with their catalytic activities speeded up) by drugs (e.g., phenobarbital), insecticides (e.g., mirex), and polycyclic aromatic hydrocarbons (e.g., BαP). Yet more importantly, many of the same or other P450s *per se* can be *inhibited* (or slowed down) by drugs (e.g., certain antifungals), substances in tobacco smoke (e.g., BαP), and natural products (e.g., a constituent group of grapefruit juice named furanocoumarins).

124 An Introduction to Environmental Toxicology

Although P450s (and most Phase II and other Phase I enzymes as well) are found in virtually all body tissues in most mammalians, their highest concentrations involved in the biotransformation of xenobiotics are present in the hepatic (i.e., liver) microsomes (i.e., those small vesicles) of the smooth-surfaced endoplasmic reticulum (*see* Figure 9.1 for location of cell organelles), with small quantities contained in the cytosol (i.e., the soluble fraction of the cytoplasm). The mitochondria, lysosomes, and nuclei in the hepatic cell each contain even smaller quantities of this versatile group of biotransforming enzymes.

8.5. Characteristics of Other Relevant Enzyme Groups

Many specific enzyme groups other than cytochrome P450s are also involved in the biotransformation of xenobiotics. Although many of the Phase I enzymes other than cytochrome P450s are not as commonly known in the general discussion of xenobiotic biotransformation, in some cases they are equally important. For example, as with NADPH-dependent cytochrome P450 reductase (Section 8.2.1A), carbonyl reductase belongs to the family of oxidoreductases. This reductase, located primarily in the cytosol, can catalyze the reduction of ketones (e.g., pentoxifylline) to secondary alcohols (Parkinson, 2001). Another example is epoxide hydrolase, which is located largely in the microsomes and cytosol. It belongs to a subcategory of the hydrolytic enzyme group that includes esterases, dehalogenases, and phosphatases. This hydrolase can play the dual role in activating BαP to a tumorigenic epoxide and in detoxifying BαP's other epoxide to a more stable, less toxic product (Parkinson, 2001). Carboxylesterase and (acetyl)cholinesterase are esterases involved in the Phase I hydrolysis. The basic mechanism for the latter's enzymatic inhibition, that can lead to severe health effects, is discussed in Chapters 9 and 15.

Those enzymes that are naturally involved in Phase II reactions, along with antioxidant enzymes and a monooxygenase encoded by the CYP1A1 gene, are regarded as either highly relevant to the biotransformation of xenobiotics or particularly intriguing to environmental toxicologists. Their characteristics are hence specifically highlighted below.

8.5.1. Enzymes in Phase II Reactions

As with cytochrome P450s, and almost an exception among all Phase II enzymes, UGTs (UDP-glucuronyltransferases) are located predominantly in hepatic microsomes. Other Phase II enzymes are primarily cytosolic, as they are not bound to membranes but occur free within the cytoplasm. At least 15 variants of human UGTs have been identified (e.g., Tukey and Strassburg, 2000). Depending on the level involved, a (e.g., hereditary) deficiency in this enzyme can cause hyperbilirubinemia known either as Gilbert's syndrome involving *mild* jaundice or as Crigler-Nijar syndrome involving *severe* jaundice.

Sulfotransferases (SULTs) are widely distributed in tissues, of which at least three isoforms have been identified in humans. Despite the fact that these enzymes usually act as a major detoxification system in the human adult and developing fetus, they are capable of bioactivating precarcinogens to reactive electrophile species which can potentially affect gene expression (Gamage *et al.*, 2006).

Methyltransferases (*N*-MET, *O*-MET, *S*-MET) as a group are commonly found in the cytosol and microsomes but have a relatively minor role in Phase II detoxification. This is because many functional groups (e.g., -*N*H, -*O*H, -*S*H), to which a MET will transfer the methyl unit (CH_3) from its coenzyme SAM (S-adenosylmethionine), are subject to Phase I oxidation first. Two distinct isoforms of *N*-acetyltransferases (NATs), known as NAT1 and NAT2, are found with overlapping substrate specificities in humans (e.g., Payton *et al.*, 2001). The two isozymes are capable of mediating the detoxification of a number of arylamine and hydrazine drugs. A somewhat related form named acyl-CoA amino acid:*N*-acyltransferase is known to catalyze glycine and some other amino acid conjugations.

8.5.2. Antioxidant Enzymes

Antioxidants are molecules or substances capable of preventing or slowing down the oxidative stress to body cells. Oxidation reactions tend to produce free radicals to start a chain reaction by stealing electrons from neighboring molecules which then become free radicals. Antioxidants can either terminate these chain reactions by removing free radical intermediates in the chain or inhibit oxidation reactions by sacrificing (i.e., being oxidized) themselves. This is why they are frequently referred to as *free radical scavengers*. Vitamin E, vitamin C, β-carotene (precursor of vitamin A), and the chemical element selenium (Se) are the most common antioxidants found in human foods. Phytochemicals known to have antioxidant function include: allyl sulfides (e.g., as in garlics, onions); carotenoids (e.g., as in fruits, carrots); flavonoids (e.g., as in fruits, vegetables); and polyphenols (e.g., as in tea, grapes).

Another group of antioxidants are certain enzymes, which are endogenous substances as they are synthesized within the body. Superoxide dismutase (SOD), GSH peroxidase (GPx), and catalase (CAT) are the three mostly investigated antioxidant enzymes. Less popular enzymes with antioxidant activity include GSH reductase, thioredoxin reductase, and heme oxygenase.

As its name implies, SOD (superoxide *di*smutase) has the ability to convert *two* superoxide anion radicals ($O_2^- \cdot$) into one hydrogen peroxide (H_2O_2) and one oxygen ($O \cdot$) ion. However, without the further removal of hydrogen peroxide by GPx or CAT, the dismutation by SOD generally will be of little value since hydrogen peroxide is a strong oxidant. There are three major families of SOD, depending on the metal(s) it has in its reactive center as cofactor(s): the copper (Cu) and zinc (Zn) type; the iron (Fe) or manganese (Mn) type; and the nickel (Ni) type. In humans (and in all other mammals and most chordates), three forms of SOD are present: SOD1 containing Cu and Zn, located in the cytoplasm; SOD2 containing Mn, located in the mitochondria; and SOD3 containing also Cu and Zn, but located outside the cell. The physiological importance of the various forms of SOD is evident from the severe pathologies observed in mice genetically engineered to lack these enzymes. In particular, mice lacking SOD2 were found dead several days after birth, amidst massive oxidative stress (Li *et al.*, 1995). *Drosophila* lacking SOD1 had a dramatically shortened lifespan (Reveillaud *et al*, 1994; Woodruff *et al.*, 2004); and these flies lacking SOD2 died hours after birth (Duttaroy *et al.*, 2003).

CAT (catalase) is found in almost all living aerobic organisms in which it can catalyze the decomposition of hydrogen peroxide (H_2O_2) to water and oxygen (e.g., Chelikani *et al.*, 2004). This antioxidant is a heme-containing redox (*red*uction-*ox*idation) enzyme present in high concentrations in a cellular compartment called peroxisome (Figure 9.1). It has one of the highest turnover rates of all enzymes known. One molecule of CAT is reportedly capable of converting millions of H_2O_2 molecules to water and oxygen per second (e.g., Allaby, 2009). Hydrogen peroxide (H_2O_2) is a harmful by-product of many normal cellular reactions.

A glutathione peroxidase (GPx) can also break down hydrogen peroxide. Glutathione peroxidase is the general name for members in the enzyme family with peroxidase activity. Its main function is to protect living organisms against oxidative stress (and hence damage) by breaking down hydrogen peroxide and by reducing lipid hydroperoxides to their corresponding alcohols. Hydroperoxides are monosubstitution products of hydrogen peroxide, having the basic structure of RO-OH (where R stands for any organyl group). There are several GPx isozymes encoded by various genes, with most containing Se (selenium) as the cofactor. In mammalians, at least five GPx isoforms (as GPx1 through GPx5) have been reported (e.g., Singh *et al.*, 2006). The GPx1 isoform is reportedly the most abundant in mice (de Haan *et al.*, 1998; Potter *et al.*, 2005), and has been linked to an increased risk of cardiovascular events in humans (Blankenberg *et al.*, 2003).

8.5.3. EROD (7-Ethoxyresorufin-*O*-Deethylase)

EROD is a P450-dependent monooxygenase encoded for by the CYP1A1 gene (e.g., Kerzee and Ramos, 2001). These days, EROD is more commonly known as an assay, rather than as an enzyme, used to monitor the induction activity of CYP1A1. The activity of EROD *per se* is widely utilized as a biomarker for exposure of wildlife and fish to polycyclic aromatic hydrocarbons (PAHs) as well as to structurally related or similar compounds such as PCBs (polychlorinated biphenyls) and dioxins. The receptive site in certain cellular proteins is specifically prone to bind with this type of organic substances and is thereby called *a*ryl *h*ydrocarbon (Ah) receptor. Activation of Ah binding with PAH-related compounds, particularly with dioxins, was reported as one of the (first) steps leading to the induction of CYP1A1 in the body (Ma, 2001).

More specifically, when the body is exposed to a PAH type compound, the Ah receptors in its cells will aggressively bind to the xenobiotic's molecules. Such bindings will mediate an elevated level of CYP1A1 in the body. And such a mediation in turn will increase the catalytic activity of CYP1A1 on EROD. A measured increase in EROD activity thereby should reflect an increased exposure to the PAH type compounds in question. The application of EROD activity as an exposure assessment technique in this way has increased in recent years. The increased acceptance of EROD's application to monitor the catalytic activity of CYP1A1 is largely due to the relatively inexpensive and rapid techniques made available for measuring the induction activity involved (e.g., Kennedy and Jones, 1994; Schiwy *et al.*, 2015; Whyte *et al.*, 2000).

8.6. Factors/Conditions Affecting Biotransformation

Many factors and conditions that affect the adverse action of toxicants, which is the topic covered extensively in Chapter 10, are also ones that affect the relative effectiveness and efficiency of xenobiotic biotransformation. These factors and conditions, applying across most species, include:

dose levels; exposure duration; exposure frequency; age; gender; genetic variability; race or strain; nutrition; health status or physiological conditions; and exposure to inducers or inhibitors of Phase I and Phase II enzymes.

As with cytochrome P450s, most other Phase I and most Phase II enzymes are likewise polymorphic although in many cases to a less extent. The activities of these non-P450 enzymes too can be induced or inhibited by certain cofactors, coenzymes, or other substances. In addition to vitamin C, vitamin E, GSH, and Se, several antioxidant enzymes (e.g., SOD, GPx, CAT) discussed in Section 8.5.2 play a key role in the defense against free radical-mediated cellular damage. Certain xenobiotics, such as sodium fluoride (NaF), are found having the ability to induce or inhibit SOD or GPx, depending on the species involved (e.g., Guo *et al.*, 2003; Lawson and Yu, 2003; Sun *et al.*, 1997).

8.6.1. Genetic Polymorphism

As noted in Section 8.4.2, genetic polymorphism in cytochrome P450s comes with profound clinical consequences. To date, the primary concern with polymorphic P450 expression reportedly has been on the development of preclinical drugs (e.g., Pirmohamed and Park, 2003). Such a concern is largely due to the common observation that extensive interindividual variability exists in the biotransformation of drug candidates which are substrates for many of the polymorphic enzymes predominant in Phase I (and at times in Phase II) reactions.

In humans, CYP2D6, CYP2C9, and CYP2C19 polymorphisms reportedly account for the most frequent variations in Phase I metabolism (more accurately, biotransformation) of drugs, as up to 80% of the drugs in use today are metabolized by these three enzymes. Some Africans/African-Americans (~8%), some Caucasians (~7%), and some Asians (~1%) are considered poor metabolizers in that they lack (effective) CYP2D6 in their body (e.g., Abernethy and Flockhart, 2000; Zhou *et al.*, 2009). CYP2C9 is another clinically significant Phase I enzyme because its multiple genetic variants can have variable functional impacts on the efficacy and adverse effects of drugs that the enzyme is responsible for in their elimination from the human body (Zhou *et al.*, 2009). CYP2C19 is responsible for the metabolism of likewise a variety of drugs, particularly those that help reduce gastric acid production (Goldstein and de Morais, 1994).

Genetic polymorphism in Phase II enzymes are also found to give rise to abnormal drug biotransformation and higher susceptibility to carcinogens or other toxicants in various subpopulations. In particular, an epidemiological study (Chen *et al.*, 2006) showed that compared to the 197 controls, 97 lung cancer patients in central south China had higher frequencies of GST_{M1}-null or GST_{T1}-null genotype, or both. Another epidemiological study (Mahmoud *et al.*, 2010) found that the frequency of Egyptian patients carrying the GST_{T1}-null genotype was fourfold higher among those with chronic myeloid leukemia than among those without the disease.

Among the antioxidant enzymes, SOD appears to have been the most investigated to date for its genetic polymorphism effects, particularly those of Mn-SOD in humans. One study (Hsueh *et al.*, 2005) showed that this SOD2 (i.e., Mn-SOD) polymorphism, along with those of NADPH oxidase and endothelial nitric oxide synthase, significantly increased the risk of high blood pressure (i.e., hypertension) in a group of Taiwaneses residing in an area known as hyperendemic of arsenic.

8.6.2. Enzyme Inhibitors

Studies showed that many xenobiotics have the ability to inhibit or retard the catalytic activities of Phase I and Phase II enzymes. Many of these xenobiotics are drugs while some others are phytochemicals and pesticides. These findings have significant clinical implications in that, while nearly all drugs used today are metabolized by Phase I or Phase II enzymes, phytochemicals are treated by many people (patients) as nutrients or drug substitutes.

Although medicinal drugs are normally not regarded as environmental toxicants, they may be treated as factors that can affect significantly the biotransformation of xenobiotics. For instance, patients taking a Phase I enzyme inhibitor drug are expected to have a lower catalytic activity of that enzyme in detoxifying or activating an environmental toxicant of concern in their body. Several chemical inhibitors of GSTs were investigated under this notion for their potential of attenuating or surpassing the resistance of anticancer drugs (Johansson *et al.*, 2007; Mahajan and Atkins, 2005; Mathew *et al.*, 2006; Pratt *et al.*, 1994; Townsend *et al.*, 2003).

Drugs and phytochemicals are not the only groups of substances capable of inhibiting the activities of Phase I and Phase II enzymes. Certain pesticides and their metabolites are notorious inhibitors of a number of these enzymes. The organochlorine pesticide methoxychlor is known to interfere with the catalytic activity of CYP2B6 (Hodgson and Rose, 2007). Examples of Phase I and Phase II enzyme inhibitors, including methoxychlor, are listed in Table 8.1.

8.6.3. Enzyme Inducers

Also included in Table 8.1 are examples of drugs and non-medicinal substances having the ability to *induce* the catalytic activities of Phase I and Phase II enzymes. Among these inducers, the predominate group appears to be drugs again, including the anticonvulsant phenobarbital and antibiotic rifampin, that are actively used today. In the non-drug category, mirex and Kepone represent some of the strong Phase I enzyme inducers. These two organochlorine pesticides are capable of inducing CYP2B1 in mouse hepatic microsomes (Lewandowski *et al.*, 2006).

Inducers of Phase II enzymes apparently have not been investigated to the same extent compared to those of Phase I. Nonetheless, isoflavones in soy, primarily genistein and quercetin, have been under extensive investigation for their potential of inducing Phase II enzyme activities (e.g., Appelt and Reicks, 1999; Froyen *et al.*, 2009; Mikulcik and Fischer, 2001). Sulforaphane, an anticancer as well as an antimicrobial agent, is also considered a strong inducer of Phase II enzymes (e.g., Fahey and Talalay, 1999). This substance is an organosulfur compound extractable from cruciferous vegetables including notably broccoli.

8.6.4. Enzyme Cofactors and Coenzymes

Most enzymes, including most if not all of those in Phase I and Phase II biotransformation, appear in one of two biochemical forms termed *apoenzymes* and *holoenzymes*. Apoenzymes are those not bound to a cofactor and generally not biochemically active, whereas holoenzymes are those bound to one or more cofactors (e.g., Stoker, 2016). In xenobiotic biotransformation, a cofactor is defined as any inorganic or organic substance required to ensure the enzyme's full biochemical capacity. Such a cofactor is referred to as the prosthetic group to the apoenzyme, and is generally *tightly* bound to the enzyme (now called holoenzyme). Many cofactors are metal ions, such as Cu^{2+}, Fe^{2+}, Fe^{3+}, Mg^{2+} (magnesium), and Zn^{2+}.

Table 8.1. Select Inhibitors and Inducers of Phase I and Phase II Enzymes in the Biotransformation of Xenobiotics

Substance	Type/Source	Affected Enzyme(s)[a,b]
I. Enzyme Inhibitors		
dicofenac	anti-inflammatory	UGT[a, b]
disulfiram	antabuse	CYP2E1[c]
ethacrynic acid	diuretic	GST[d]
flavonoids	grapefruit juice	CYP3A4[e]
fluconazole	antifungal	CYP2C19[c]
flunitrazepam	sedative	UGT[b]
fluoxetine	antidepressant	CYP2D6[c], CYP3A4[f]
methoxychlor	organochlorine pesticide	CYP2B6[g]
probenecid	uricosuric	UGT[a]
resveratrol	grape skin, wine	CYP1A1[h], UGT1A1[h]
ritonavir	anti-HIV	CYP3A4[c, f]
safrole	black pepper	CYP1A2[i], CYP2A6[i], CYP2E1[i]
silybin	milk thistle	CYP2C9[j], CYP3A4[j]
silymarin	milk thistle	UGT[k]
TLK99	anti-hematologic	GST[d]
II. Enzyme Inducers		
carbamazepine	anticonvulsant	CYP3A4[c]
ethanol	alcohol	CYP2E1[c]
glucosinolate	cruciferous vegetables	CYP1A2[c, e]
isoflavones	phytochemical	Phase II enzymes[l, m, n]
Kepone (chlordecone)	organochlorine pesticide	CYP2B1[o]
mirex	organochlorine pesticide	CYP2B1[o]
PAHs[b]	charcoal-broiled meat[b]	CYP1A2[c, e]
phenobarbital	anticonvulsant	CYP2B6[c], CYP3A4[c]
phenytoin	anticonvulsant	CYP2B6[c], CYP3A4[c, f]
rifampin	antibiotic	CYP2B6[c], CYP2C19[c], CYP3A4[c]
sulforaphane	cruciferous vegetables	Phase II enzymes[p]

[a] as reported in: [a] Uchaipichat *et al.* (2004); [b] Ghosal *et al.* (2004); [c] Parkinson (2001); [d] Mathew *et al.* (2006); [e] Ensom and Blouin (2006); [f] Zhou (2008); [g] Hodgson and Rose (2007); [h] Leung *et al.* (2009); [i] Ueng *et al.* (2005); [j] Jančová *et al.* (2007); [k] D'Andrea *et al.* (2005); [l] Appelt and Reicks (1999); [m] Froyen *et al.* (2009); [n] Mikulcik and Fischer (2001); [o] Lewandowski *et al.* (2006); [p] Fahey and Talalay (1999).

[b] CYP ≡ cytochrome P450 (Phase I); UGT ≡ UDP-glucuronosyltransferase (Phase II); GST ≡ glutathione S-transferase (Phase II); PAHs ≡ polycyclic aromatic hydrocarbons, which is also contained in tobacco smoke.

If the prosthetic group so required is an *organic* (non-protein) substance, it is more specifically referred to as a *coenzyme* and is generally bound *loosely* to the enzyme. Several common coenzymes such as UDPGA (UDP-glucuronic acid), SAM (S-adenosylmethionine), and PAPS (3'-phospho-adenosine -5'-phosphosulfate) are introduced in Section 8.2.2. Many of the other equally common coenzymes are either vitamins or their derivatives: biotin (a.k.a. vitamin H or vitamin B_7); vitamin C; CoA (coenzyme A) from vitamin B_5; NAD^+ (nicotine adenine dinucleotide) and $NADP^+$ (nicotine adenine dinucleotide phosphate), both from niacin (vitamin B_3); as well as FMN (flavin mononucleotide) and FAD (flavin adenine dinucleotide), both from riboflavin (vitamin B_2). Examples of other coenzymes not vitamin-based and not specific to Phase II enzymes include: heme; ATP (adenosine-5'-triphosphate); CoB (coenzyme B); and GSH (glutathione).

References

Abernethy DR, Flockhart DA, 2000. Molecular Basis of Cardiovascular Drug Metabolism: Implications for Predicting Clinically Important Drug Interactions. *Circulation* 101:1749-1753.

Allaby M, 2009. Catalase. *Oxford Dictionary of Zoology*, 3rd Edition. New York, New York, USA: Oxford University Press.

Appelt LC, Reicks MM, 1999. Soy Induces Phase II Enzymes But Does Not Inhibit Dimethylbenz[a]-anthracene-Induced Carcinogenesis in Female Rats. *J. Nutri.* 129:1820-1826.

Blankenberg S, Rupprecht HJ, Bickel C, Torzewski M, Hafner G, Tiret L, Smieja M, Cambien F, Meyer J, Lackner KJ, 2003. Glutathione Peroxidase 1 Activity and Cardiovascular Events in Patients with Coronary Artery Disease. *NEJM* 349:1605-1613.

Chelikani P, Fita I, Loewen PC, 2004. Diversity of Structures and Properties among Catalases. *Cell. Mol. Life Sci.* 61:192–208.

Chen HC, Cao YF, Hu WX, Liu XF, Liu QX, Zhang J, Liu J, 2006. Genetic Polymorphisms of Phase II Metabolic Enzymes and Lung Cancer Susceptibility in a Population of Central South China. *Dis. Markers* 22: 141-152.

Croy RG, Essigmann JM, Reinhold VN, Wogan GN, 1978. Identification of the Principal Aflatoxin B1-DNA Adduct Formed *in vivo* in Rat Liver. *Proc. Natl. Acad. Sci.* USA 75:1745-1749.

D'Andrea V, Perez LM, Pozzi EJS, 2005. Inhibition of Rat Liver UDP-Glucuronosyltransferase by Silymarin and the Metabolite Silibinin-Glucuronide. *Life Sci.* 77:683-692.

de Haan JB, Bladier C, Griffiths P, Kelner M, O'Shea RD, Cheung NS, Bronson RT, Silvestro MJ, Wild S, Zheng SS, *et al.*, 1998. Mice with a Homozygous Null Mutation for the Most Abundant Glutathione Peroxidase, GPx1, Show Increased Susceptibility to the Oxidative Stress-Inducing Agents Paraquat and Hydrogen Peroxide. *J. Biol. Chem.* 273: 22528-22536.

Duttaroy A, Paul A, Kundu M, Belton A, 2003. A Sod2 Null Mutation Confers Severely Reduced Adult Life Span in *Drosophila*. *Genetics* 165:2295-2299.

Eichelbaum M, Burk O, 2001. CYP3A Genetics in Drug Metabolism. *Natl. Med.* 7:285-287.

Ensom MH, Blouin RA, 2006. Dietary Influences on Drug Disposition. In *Applied Pharmacokinetics and Pharmacodynamics: Principles of Therapeutic Drug Monitoring* (Burton ME, Shaw LM, Schentag JJ, Evans WE, Eds.), 4th Edition. Baltimore, Maryland, USA: Lippincott Williams & Wilkins, Chapter 12.

Fahey JW, Talalay P, 1999. Antioxidant Functions of Sulforaphane: A Potent Inducer of Phase II Detoxication Enzymes. *Food Chem. Toxicol.* 37:973-979.

Froyen EB, Reeves JL, Mitchell AE, Steinberg FM, 2009. Regulation of Phase II Enzymes by Genistein and Daidzein in Male and Female Swiss Webster Mice. *J. Med. Food* 12:1227-1237.

Gamage N, Barnett A, Hempel N, Duggleby RG, Windmill KF, Martin JL, McManus ME, 2006. Human Sulfotransferases and Their Role in Chemical Metabolism. *Toxicol. Sci.* 90:5-22.

Ghosal A, Hapangama N, Yuan Y, Achanfuo-Yeboah J, Iannucci R, Chowdhury S, Alton K, Patrick JE, Zbaida S, 2004. Identification of Human UDP-Glucuronosyltransferase Enzyme(s) Responsible for the Glucuronidation of Ezetimibe (Zetia). *Drug Metab. Disp.* 32:314-320.

Goldstein JA, de Morais SM, 1994. Biochemistry and Molecular Biology of the Human CYP2C Subfamily. *Pharmacogenetics* 4:285-299.

Guo X-Y, Sun G-F, Sun Y-C, 2003. Oxidative Stress from Fluoride-Induced Hepatotoxicity in Rats. *Fluoride* 36:25-29.

Hodgson E, Rose RL, 2007. The Importance of Cytochrome P450 2B6 in the Human Metabolism of Environmental Chemicals. *Pharmacol. Ther.* 113:420-428.

Hsueh Y-M, Lin P, Chen H-W, Shiue H-S, Chung C-J, Tsai C-T, Huang Y-K, Chiou H-Y, Chen C-J, 2005. Genetic Polymorphisms of Oxidative and Antioxidant Enzymes and Arsenic-Related Hypertension. *J. Toxicol. Environ. Health* 68:1471-1484.

Jančová P, Anzenbacherová E, Papoušková B, Lemr K, Lužná P, Veinlichová A, Anzenbacher P, Šimánek V, 2007. Silybin Is Metabolized by Cytochrome P450 2C8 *in vitro*. *Drug Metab. Disp.* 35:2035-2039.

Johansson K, Ahlen K, Rinaldi R, Sahlander K, Siritantikorn A, Morgenstern R, 2007. Microsomal Glutathione Transferase 1 in Anticancer Drug Resistance. *Carcinogenesis* 28:465-470.

Kennedy SW, Jones SP, 1994. Simultaneous Measurement of Cytochrome P4501A Catalytic Activity and Total Protein Concentration with a Fluorescence Plate Reader. *Biochemistry* 222:217-223.

Kerzee JK, Ramos KS, 2001. Constitutive and Inducible Expression of Cyp1a1 and Cyp1b1 in Vascular Smooth Muscle Cells: Role of the Ahr bHLH/PAS Transcription Factor. *Circulation Res.* 89:573-582.

Keshava C, McCanlies EC, Weston A, 2004. CYP3A4 Polymorphisms – Potential Risk Factors for Breast and Prostate Cancer: A HuGE Review. *Am. J. Epid.* 160:825-841.

Lawson P, Yu MH, 2003. Fluoride Inhibition of Superoxide Dismutase (SOD) from the Earthworm *Eisenia fetida*. *Fluoride* 36:143-151.

Leung HY, Yung LH, Shia G, Lua A-L, Leung LK, 2009. The Red Wine Polyphenol Resveratrol Reduces Polycyclic Aromatic Hydrocarbon-Induced DNA Damage in MCF-10A Cells. *Nutri. Toxicol.* 102.1462-1468.

Lewandowski M, Levi P, Hodgson E, 2006. Induction of Cytochrome P-450 Isozymes by Mirex and Chlordecone. *J. Biochem. Toxicol.* 4:195-199.

Li Y, Huang TT, Carlson EJ, Melov S, Ursell PC, Olson JL, Noble LJ, Yoshimura MP, Berger C, Chan PH, *et al.*, 1995. Dilated Cardiomyopathy and Neonatal Lethality in Mutant Mice Lacking Manganese Superoxide Dismutase. *Natl. Genet.* 11:376-381.

Ma Q, 2001. Induction of CYP1A1. The AhR/DRE Paradigm: Transcription, Receptor Regulation, and Expanding Biological Roles. *Curr. Drug Metab.* 2:149-164.

Mahajan S, Atkins WM, 2005. The Chemistry and Biology of Inhibitors and Pro-Drugs Targeted to Glutathione S-Transferases. *Cell. Mol. Life Sci.* 62:1221-1233.

Mahmoud S, Labib DA, Khalifa RH, Abu Khalil RE, Marie MA, 2010. CYP1A1, GSTM1 and GSTT1 Genetic Polymorphism in Egyptian Chronic Myeloid Leukemia Patients. *Res. J. Immunol.* 3:12-21.

Mathew N, Kalyanasundaram M, Balaraman K, 2006. Glutathione S-Transferase (GST) Inhibitors. *Expert Opinion on Therap. Patents* 16:431-444.

Mikulcik EM, Fischer JG, 2001. Possible Mechanism for Protective Effect of the Flavonoid Quercetin. *J. Am. Diet. Assoc.* 101(Suppl):A-35 (Food & Nutrition Conference & Exhibition; Poster Session).

Morton KC, King CM, Baetcke, KP, 1979. Metabolism of Benzidine to N-Hydroxy-N, N'-Diacetylbenzidine and Subsequent Nucleic Acid Binding and Mutagenicity. *Cancer Res.* 39:3107-3113.

Pacifici GM, Gucci A, Giuliani L, 1997. Testosterone Sulphation and Glucuronidation in the Human Liver: Interindividual Variability. *Eur. J. Drug Metab. Pharmacokinet.* 22:253-258.

Parinandi NL, Weis BK, Natarajan V, Schmid HH, 1990. Peroxidative Modification of Phospholipids in Myocardial Membranes. *Arch. Biochem. Biophy.* 280:45-52.

Parkinson A, 2001. Biotransformation of Xenobiotics. In *Casarett and Doull's Toxicology: The Basic Science of Poisons* (Klaassen CD, Ed.), 6th Edition. New York, New York, USA: McGraw-Hill, Chapter 6.

Payton M, Mushtaq A, Yu T-W, Wu L-J, Sinclair J, Sim E, 2001. Eubacterial Arylamine N-Acetyltransferases – Identification and Comparison of 18 Members of the Protein Family with Conserved Active Site Cysteine, Histidine and Aspartate Residues. *Microbiology* 147:1137-1147.

Pirmohamed M, Park BK, 2003. Cytochrome P450 Enzyme Polymorphisms and Adverse Drug Reactions. *Toxicology* 192:23-32.

Potter SM, Mitchell AJ, Cowden WB, Sanni LA, Dinauer M, de Haan JB, Hunt NH, 2005. Phagocyte-Derived Reactive Oxygen Species Do Not Influence the Progression of Murine Blood-Stage Malaria Infections. *Infect. & Immun.* 73:4941-4947.

Pratt WB, Ruddon RW, Ensminger WD, Maybaum J, 1994. *The Anticancer Drugs*. New York, New York, USA: Oxford University Press, p.329.

Reveillaud I, Phillips J, Duyf B, Hilliker A, Kongpachith A, Fleming JE, 1994. Phenotypic Rescue by a Bovine Transgene in a Cu/Zn Superoxide Dismutase-Null Mutant of *Drosophila* Melanogaster. *Mol. Cell. Biol.* 14:1302-1307.

Schiwy A, Brinkmann M, Thiem I, Guder G, Winkens K, Eichbaum K, Nüßber L, Thalmann B, Buchinger S, Reifferscheid G, *et al.*, 2015. Determination of the CYP1A-Inducing Potential of Single Substances, Mixtures and Extracts of Samples in the Micro-EROD Assay with H4IIE Cells. *Nat. Protoc.* 10:1728-1741.

Singh A, Rangasamy T, Thimmulappa RK, Lee H, Osburn WO, Brigelius-Flohé R, Kensler TW, Yamamoto M, Biswal S, 2006. Glutathione Peroxidase 2, the Major Cigarette Smoke-Inducible Isoform of GPX in Lungs, Is Regulated by Nrf2. *Am. J. Respir. Cell Mol. Biol.* 35:639-650.

Sligar S, Cinti DL, Gibson GG, Schenkman JB, 1979. Spin State Control of the Hepatic Cytochrome P-450 Redox Potential. *Biochem. Biophy. Res. Commun.* 90:925-932.

Smart RC, 2004. Chemical Carcinogenesis. In *A Textbook of Modern Toxicology* (Hodgson E, Ed.), 3rd Edition. Hoboken, New York, USA: John Wiley & Sons, Chapter 13.

Stoker HS, 2016. *General, Organic & Biological Chemistry*, 7th Edition. Boston, Massachusetts, USA: Cengage Learning, Chapter 21.

Sun GF, Yu M-H, Ding GY, Shen HY, 1997. Lipid Peroxidation and Changes in Antioxidant Levels in Aluminum Plant Workers. *Environ. Sci.* 5:139-144.

Swenson DH, Lin J-K, Miller EC, Miller JA, 1977. Aflatoxin B1-2,3-Oxide as a Probable Intermediate in the Covalent Binding of Aflatoxins B1 and B2 to Rat Liver DNA and Ribosomal RNA *in vivo*. *Cancer Res.* 37:172-181.

Townsend DM, Kenneth D, Tew KD, 2003. The Role of Glutathione-S-Transferase in Anticancer Drug Resistance. *Oncogene* 22:7369-7375.

Trostchansky A, Rubbo H, 2007. Lipid Nitration and Formation of Lipid-Protein Adducts: Biological Insights. *Amino Acids* 32:517-522.

Tukey RH, Strassburg CP, 2000. Human UDP-Glucuronosyltransferases: Metabolism, Expression, and Disease. *Ann. Rev. Pharmacol. Toxicol.* 40:581-616.

Uchaipichat V, Mackenzie PI, Guo X-H, Gardner-Stephen D, Galetin A, Houston JB, Miners JO, 2004. Human UDP-Glucuronosyltransferases: Isoform Selectivity and Kinetics of 4-Methylumbelliferone and 1-Naphthol Glucuronidation, Effects of Organic Solvents, and Inhibition by Diclofenac and Probenecid. *Drug Metab. & Disp.* 32:412-423.

Ueng YF, Hsieh CH, Don MJ, 2005. Inhibition of Human Cytochrome P450 Enzymes by the Natural Hepatotoxin Safrole. *Food Chem. Toxicol.* 43:707-712.

Whyte JJ, Jung RE, Schmitt CJ, Tillitt DE, 2000. Ethoxyresorufin-O-Deethylase (EROD) Activity in Fish as a Biomarker of Chemical Exposure. *Crit. Rev. Toxicol.* 30:347-570.

Woodruff RC, Phillips JP, Hilliker AJ, 2004. Increased Spontaneous DNA Damage in Cu/Zn Superoxide Dismutase (SOD1) Deficient *Drosophila*. *Genome* 47:1029-1035.

Zhou S-F, 2008. Drugs Behave as Substrates, Inhibitors and Inducers of Human Cytochrome P450 3A4. *Curr. Drug Metab.* 9:310-322.

Zhou S-F, Liu J-P, Chowbay B, 2009. Polymorphism of Human Cytochrome P450 Enzymes and Its Clinical Impact. *Drug Metab. Rev.* 41:89-295.

Review Questions

1. Briefly describe the main differences between metabolism of substances and biotransformation of xenobiotics or drugs.
2. What are the main differences between a primary and an intermediate metabolite produced in xenobiotic biotransformation?
3. What are enzymes? Briefly characterize their general actions and functions.
4. Which of the following is generally regarded as the predominant form of oxidation in Phase I (enzymatic) reactions? a) epoxidation; b) hydroxylation; c) deamination; d) dealkylation.
5. What is a monooxygenation kind of oxidative reactions?
6. How does NADPH-dependent cytochrome P450 reductase biochemically induce the catalytic activity of a cytochrome P450 oxygenase?
7. Which of the following is the most predominant Phase II reactions? a) sulfation; b) glucuronidation; c) conjugation with glutathione; d) conjugation with amino acids; e) methylation.
8. Name three metabolites produced as a result of bioactivation in Phase I or Phase II reactions.
9. Which of the following cytochrome P450 enzymes is the most abundant as well as the most important in humans? a) CYP2B6; b) CYP3A4; c) CYP2C19; d) CYP1A2.
10. Why and how is EROD (7-ethoxyresorufin-*o*-deethylase) typically utilized as a biomarker for exposure of fish to many polycyclic aromatic hydrocarbons?
11. Give three examples of the types of endogenous substances that can undergo chemical biotransformation (i.e., Phase I or Phase II reactions).

12. Which of the following cell organelles in a human liver contains most of the cytochrome P450s? a) mitochondrion; b) lysosome; c) smooth endoplasmic reticulum; d) nucleus.

13. Name the Phase II enzyme in which a deficiency can cause Gilbert's syndrome.

14. Why is genetic polymorphism so important to the development of preclinical drugs, despite the fact that they are generally not regarded as environmental toxicants?

15. What are antioxidants? Name four that are (antioxidant) enzymes.

16. Match the Phase II enzymes (left column) to their generally required coenzyme (right column).

    (1) UGT   (a) SAM
    (2) SULT   (b) acetyl CoA
    (3) MET   (c) PAPS
    (4) NAT   (d) GSH
    (5) GST   (e) glucuronic acid

17. Identify the substances below, if any, that are: (1) Phase I enzyme inhibitors; (2) Phase II enzyme inhibitors; (3) Phase I enzyme inducers; (4) Phase II enzyme inducers.

    (a) methoxychlor   (b) sulforaphane   (c) grapefruit juice
    (d) genistein   (e) safrole   (f) charcoal-broiled meat
    (g) ethanol   (h) TLK99   (i) silymarin
    (j) mirex   (k) Kepone   (l) ritonavir
    (m) resveratrol   (n) glucosinolate   (o) phenobarbital

18. What are the main differences between enzyme cofactors and coenzymes, and between apoenzymes and holoenzymes?

19. Name one coenzyme that is derived from vitamin B_2, and two that are not vitamin-based.

20. Why are coenzymes referred to (or defined) as organic prosthetic compounds yet not supposed to be proteins?

CHAPTER 9

Adverse Action/Toxic Response

9.1. Introduction

Depending on the toxicological properties and the environmental level involved, a living organism's exposure to a toxicant may or may not result in an adverse health effect. Certain defense mechanisms in the organism's body also may or may not launch. For instance, most airborne particles larger than 15 micrometers (μm) in diameter are filtered by the human nasal hairs. If the particles are of the size and shape capable of passing through the nasal septum and deposit in sufficient amounts at a site where tonsils and adenoids are located nearby, immunological defense may kick in to protect against the particles filtered at that point. Immunological response is also a common mode whereby the body protects its cells and organs against microbes of certain pathogenic properties. Still another mode of defense against certain toxicants that have entered the body is via the detoxification processes involved in the biotransformation of xenobiotics (Chapter 8).

9.1.1. Site and Mechanism of Action

In humans and most other mammalians, many individuals respond to toxicants somewhat differently. The way in which an individual responds to a toxicant is affected by many factors or co-factors, but largely by those from within the four categories discussed in Chapter 10. Although some toxicants can damage any cell or tissue in the body that they come in contact with, many affect specific tissues or organs. Toxic damage can result from adverse biochemical, cellular, or macromolecular changes. The site where such changes occur is termed *site of (toxic) action*; and the specific biochemical interaction whereby a toxicant induces its (adverse) effect is termed its *mechanism of (adverse) action*, or the affected site's *(toxic) response*.

This chapter follows the more conventional terminology that mechanism of action is a specific biochemical event underlying a mode of (toxic) action. For example, Carls and Meador (2009) treated baseline toxicity (e.g., narcosis) as a *mode* of toxic action (just like teratogenesis, endocrine disruption, and cytotoxicity), rather than as a mechanism of toxic action. Their argument was that such an action term lacks a *specific* receptor or platform. Yet some other scholars (e.g., Barron *et al.*, 2004) seemed to have used the two terms interchangeably.

9.1.2. Basic Mechanisms of Action and Toxicodynamics

There are more mechanisms of (toxic) action than can be covered in one chapter or even one book. However, many that are particularly relevant or challenging to environmental toxicologists may fall under six general categories as follows: (1) direct damage to cell structures; (2) toxic reactions mediated by free radicals; (3) modulation of receptor functions; (4) binding with a cell's constituent; (5) adverse secondary or indirect actions; and (6) disruption of enzymatic activities. In this chapter, the first four mechanism categories are further subsumed into one broader group to simplify as well as to facilitate the discussion, with the last two being on their own due to their complexities and the unique cellular or molecular platform that they operate on.

Collectively, these three newer general groups of common mechanisms of action can induce, directly or indirectly, many types of adverse effects briefly introduced in Chapter 2. The broader spectrum of these toxic effects is discussed toward the end of this chapter in Section 9.5 under the heading on toxicodynamics (TD). The discussion is given in an effort to offer a fuller appreciation of the mechanisms of action discussed below in Section 9.2 through Section 9.4. As further defined in Section 9.5, TD is about what toxicants can do to the body and thus interrelated closely with toxicokinetics (TK), as the latter is concerned with the quantitative aspects of a toxicant's disposition kinetics (Chapter 7). To put it another way, how a toxic response takes its course is also contingent on the amount and the way in which a toxicant is delivered to the site of action.

9.2. Primary and Mediated Toxic Actions

Based on the conventional definition noted earlier, this chapter may not be correct to include *direct damage* as a mechanism of action category without qualification. The justification or qualification needed here is that whenever direct damage is considered, a specific biochemical site, receptor, or mechanism of action is almost always implicated, such as in direct DNA damage, direct oxidative damage, direct bacterial damage, direct UV (ultraviolet radiation) damage, and so forth. It is under this notion that the term *direct damage* is treated here as a mechanism (*vs.* mode) category that (environmental) toxicologists should be familiar and content with.

Also included in this first broader group are free radical-mediated actions. An appreciation for this type of toxic actions is warranted in that reactive oxygen species (ROS) and the kind are inevitably and constantly produced during normal cellular metabolic processes. These free radicals are associated with many diseases, including cancer.

There is likewise a need to appreciate the modulation of receptor functions given that, in biochemistry and toxicology, receptors are protein molecules ubiquitously embedded in a cell's plasma membrane and within its cytoplasm. These proteinaceous receptors are usually attached by one or more specific kinds of signaling molecules (e.g., hormones, neurotransmitters). If the functions of these receptors are compromised, so are those of the signaling molecules, toxicants, and drugs. The fourth and last mechanism category included in this first, broader group is binding with a cell's constituent. As evident from the discussion presented later in Section 9.2.4, the binding of a toxicant such as carbon monoxide (CO) to a cell's major constituent such as hemoglobin (Hb) can be acutely and extremely fatal.

9.2.1. Direct Damage to Cell Structures

The consequence of direct damage to cell structures can be readily seen on a plant's leaf surface. Many pollutants are phytotoxic, such as sulfur dioxide (SO_2), nitrogen dioxide (NO_2), ozone (O_3), and especially hydrogen fluoride (HF). At sufficiently high levels, pollutants of this kind can directly cause leaf injuries leading to chlorosis or necrosis easily visible. Chlorosis is a condition in which leaves do not produce sufficient chlorophyll for their green appearance and thereby turn pale, yellow, or yellowish white. The cells in an affected leaf then have little or no ability to produce carbohydrates via photosynthesis to sustain their lives. Necrosis is the condition in which death of plant tissues occurs, with the affected area generally turning black or brown. Herbicides are phytotoxic by design, since their only purpose is to get rid of unwanted plants.

As evident from several historical acute air pollution episodes, such as Donora smog of 1948 and London fog of 1952 (Chapter 12), certain air pollutants can also exert direct damage on the surface linings of the human respiratory tract. On the other hand, the highly reactive free radicals (e.g., superoxide radical $O_2\cdot$) can react with protein or lipid molecules on a cell's membrane nearby to directly damage the structures there.

9.2.2. Reactions Mediated by Free Radicals

Actions via this type of biochemical mechanism can result in oxidative stress and eventually damage of cellular components. One major serious consequence is lipid peroxidation, which refers to a more specific reaction process whereby highly reactive free radicals "steal" electrons from the biomembrane *lipid* molecules nearby. These lipid molecules generally are each of a polyunsaturated fatty acid (PURA) moiety. A general scheme involving PURA peroxidation is given below in Reactions 9.1a through 9.1c:

$$\text{PURA-H} + X\cdot \rightarrow \text{PURA}\cdot + X\text{-H} \tag{9.1a}$$

$$\text{PURA}\cdot + O_2 \rightarrow \text{PURA-OO}\cdot \tag{9.1b}$$

$$\text{PURA-OO}\cdot + \text{PURA-H} \rightarrow \text{PURA}\cdot + \text{PURA-OOH} \tag{9.1c}$$

where $X\cdot$ is an energetic one-electron oxidant (e.g., hydroxyl radical $HO\cdot$) and the lipid peroxyl radical PURA-OO· is the chain-carrying culprit (Wagner *et al.*, 1994).

Another chain reaction of this kind, which may occur inside or outside of a living organism, involves a highly reactive hydroxyl radical $HO\cdot$ generated by the Fenton reaction (Reaction 9.2) in which only the inorganic reagents iron (Fe) and hydrogen peroxide (H_2O_2) are required.

$$Fe^{2+} + H_2O_2 \rightarrow Fe^{3+} + HO\cdot + OH^- \tag{9.2a}$$

$$Fe^{3+} + H_2O_2 \rightarrow Fe^{2+} + HO_2\cdot + H^+ \tag{9.2b}$$

Note that the highly reactive perhydroxyl radical ($HO_2\cdot$) generated from Reaction 9.2b can be utilized to oxidize organic contaminants in water or soils as a bioremediation stimulating or pretreatment agent (e.g., Crawford *et al.*, 2004). Studies suggested that antioxidants such as uric acid ($C_5H_4N_4O_3$) could readily suppress the oxidative activity of hydroxyl radical generation by the

Fenton reaction (Howell and Wyngaarden, 1960; Simic and Jovanovic, 1989). Uric acid is produced when purines found in certain foods (e.g., liver, dried beans) and certain drinks (e.g., beer, wine) are broken down completely.

Another notorious adverse reaction mediated by a free radical, but not involving a chain propagation, is the one by trichloromethyl free radical ($CCl_3\cdot$). This free radical, which can be generated from the dehydrogenation of carbon tetrachloride (CCl_4), has been shown to cause serious hepatic (i.e., liver) injuries in several animal studies (Williams and Burk, 1990).

9.2.3. Modulation of Receptor Functions

Receptors of toxicological concerns are protein molecules located primarily at the following three cellular sites: on the plasma membrane separating its interior from its outside environment; inside the cytoplasm of a cell; or on the nuclear envelope (membrane) separating its nucleoplasm (that containing the nucleolus, chromatin, etc.) from its cytoplasm (*see* Figure 9.1). In many instances, the functions of a receptor can be either blocked or activated by one or more certain kinds of endogenous or exogenous molecules referred to as ligands that bind to the receptor's proteinaceous structure. Upon binding, a series of signaling activities occurs in accordance with the receptor's structural characteristics. Unlike enzymes with their substrates, protein receptors by definition do *not catalyze* chemical changes in their ligands.

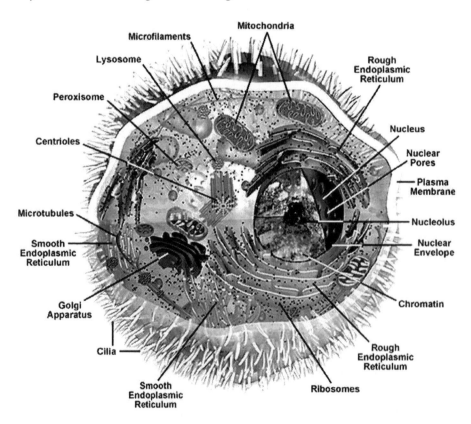

Figure 9.1. General Structure of an Animal Cell (*original image: courtesy of and permission from the National High Magnetic Field Laboratory, Florida State University, USA*)

Intracellular receptors represent the most important class. They include those that respond to steroid hormones (largely found in the cytoplasm's liquid component technically termed cytosol) and thyroid hormones (primarily found in the nucleoplasm). Once activated by ligands (e.g., toxicants), these receptors may be capable of entering the cell nucleus where they can alter gene expression (*see* the aryl hydrocarbon receptor example in Figure 9.2 as well as its discussion toward the end of this subsection).

Receptors located within a cell's plasma membrane (a.k.a. biomembrane) include peripheral, but mostly integral, proteins (as illustrated in Figure 7.2). Integral protein receptors consist of largely those for hormonal functions and neurotransmission; and they mostly fall into one of the two structural categories termed *ionotropic* and *metabotropic*. Ionotropic type transmembrane protein receptors are ligand-gated ion channels capable of permitting entry of ions when the central pore is open. Metabotropic type transmembrane receptors are coupled to *g*uanine nucleotide-binding proteins (or G proteins for short), acting via various secondary pathways that involve specific ion channels and enzymes.

Ion channels are pore-forming proteins located on plasma membranes to help facilitate or limit the diffusion of certain ions across a membrane in all living cells by allowing or restricting the flow of the ions down their electrochemical gradient. The ions of most relevance are sodium (Na^+), potassium (K^+), chloride (Cl^-), and calcium (Ca^{2+}). Also located across the membranes of certain cells (e.g., neurons, axons) are voltage-gated conductance ion channels (that to be activated by changes in electrical potential difference near the channel) and mechanosensitive ion channels which are open under the influence of stress, pressure, and the kind.

For the G protein-coupled (transmembrane) receptors, their main function is to transduce extracellular stimuli into intracellular signals. These metabotropic receptors are involved in the modulation or regulation of a wide variety of physiological systems, including the mood and behavior center, the visual and smell senses, the immunological system, and the transmission in the autonomic nervous system. They are each activated by an external stimulus in the form of binding with a ligand or another signal mediator. Upon binding, the conformational change induced in the receptor will cause activation of the G protein to either activate or inhibit a specific enzyme which then generates a second messenger. It is this second messenger that initiates the destined cellular response.

In toxicology, the importance of protein receptors may be illustrated with the activation of the *aryl hydrocarbon receptor* (AhR). This cytosolic receptor is a member of the transcription factors dictating the time at which (the expressions of) genes are to be switched on or off (i.e., to be transcribed or not). The current concept is that this Ah receptor is normally inactive until it is bound to a ligand such as TCDD (2,3,7,8-tetrachlorodibenzo-*para*-dioxin). When its activated form is complexed with the cytoplasmic chaperonins HSP90 and XAP2, AhR can be translocated into the nucleus to dimerize (combine) with an AhR nuclear translocator (ARNT) protein. This activated AhR-ARNT heterodimer complex is then capable of interacting with nuclear DNA to cause (adverse) changes in gene transcription which is to be carried out by messenger ribonucleic acid (mRNA). The affected gene expression embedded in mRNA in turn is translated into proteins of the imperfect kind (Figure 9.2). The ultimate biologic effect from this process can be carcinogenic.

140 An Introduction to Environmental Toxicology

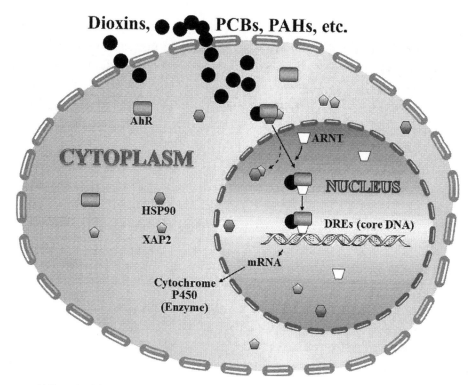

AhR ≡ Aryl hydrocarbon receptor; ARNT ≡ AhR nuclear translocator protein; DREs ≡ Dehydration-responsive elements (of the dioxin kind); HSP90 and XAP2 ≡ cytoplasmic chaperonins; PAHs ≡ polycyclic aromatic hydrocarbons; PCBs ≡ polychlorinated biphenyls; dioxins ≡ polychlorinated dibenzo-*p(ara)*-dioxins

Figure 9.2. Current Concept of Mechanism whereby Dioxins, PCBs, and PAH-type Compounds along with an Ah Receptor Can Cause Alteration of Gene Expression

9.2.4. Binding with a Cell's Constituent

Hydrogen cyanide (HCN), CO (carbon monoxide), and certain epoxides are molecules having a strong binding affinity to a cell's particular constituent and thereby capable of interfering with the normal function of that constituent. Two physiologically important cell constituents are *n*uclear deoxyribonucleic acid (*n*DNA or frequently DNA for short) and Hb (hemoglobin). Hb is the metalloprotein found in all red blood cells and contains a ferrous iron (Fe^{2+}) in its heme unit to allow the transportation of oxygen vital to many cellular functions. Working together with their mRNA, nDNA molecules will encode many more specific enzymes and other proteins compared to those DNA in the mitochondria (*see* Figure 9.1 for its cellular location).

Hydrogen cyanide is an extremely poisonous gas, which can be produced when synthetic polymers (e.g., nylon, polyacrylonitrile, polyurethane) in clothes or furnishings are burned. Once taken into the bloodstream, over 90% of the cyanide (CN^-) will occupy the oxygen-binding site in Hb, thereby making most of the Hb unable to transport oxygen to the body's various tissues and organs. Moreover, while arriving in the form of Hb-CN, the CN^- ion will preferentially bind to the heme unit of the cytochrome *c* oxidase located in the mitochondria of the host tissue to inhibit electron transport and thus will deprive the cells there of oxygen use.

The gaseous molecule CO is likewise very poisonous, given that its binding affinity to Hb (in the oxygenated Fe^{2+} form) is about 220 times stronger compared to oxygen's affinity to Hb (in the Fe^{2+} form). When existing in the Hb-CO bound form, the metalloprotein is incapable of carrying oxygen to cells in all other tissues in the body.

As stated in Chapter 8, aflatoxin B_1-8,9-epoxide and benzo[α]pyrene-7,8-dihydrodiol-9,10-epoxide are capable of binding covalently to DNA. These DNA adducts can lead to the initiation of chemical carcinogenesis.

9.3. Adverse Secondary or Indirect Actions

The presence of a relatively harmless xenobiotic in an organism's body may mechanistically or biochemically cause the production or release of certain substances that in turn can harm the cells in that body. Highlighted below are four example types included in this category: (1) allergic response; (2) side effects of medications; (3) molecular complexation; and (4) microbic invasion.

9.3.1. Allergic Response

This type of responses in or by the body is brought about when the body's immunological system responds to the presence of a normally innocuous agent (e.g., pollen, dust) that comes in contact with lymphocytes specific for that agent (technically termed *antigen*). Lymphocytes are a special group of white blood cells capable of producing antibodies (called *immunoglobulins* or Igs for short) and other substances to fight against infectious and other types of diseases. The allergic response frequently includes the release of a large amount of a biogenic amine (i.e., an organic substance with an amine group) termed *histamine*, which may lead to two major allergic symptoms: inflammation and contraction of smooth muscle (e.g., walls of blood vessels or the gastrointestinal tract). In certain allergic reactions, the release of histamine can be so much that it will cause anaphylactic (hypertensive) shock which can lead to death in a matter of minutes.

9.3.2. Side Effects of Medications

All medications come with side effects (*see also* Section 21.3.3), of which some are due to specific secondary reactions. For example, some contain dextromethorphan (DXM) as the common active ingredient for cough suppression. Yet in recent years, DXM has been notoriously known as a drug of abuse. This is because DXM can potentiate the level of the endogenous neurotransmitter called serotonin in the brain (e.g., Schwartz *et al.*, 2008), at times sufficient to induce the so-called serotonin syndrome. The syndrome starts with euphoria, hallucinations, and excitability, but at high dosage can end in life-threatening seizures. Many drugs of abuse, such as LSD (lysergic acid diethylamide), ecstasy, and cocaine, have also been linked to serotonin syndrome.

9.3.3. Molecular Complexation

This type refers to the tight-binding or, more commonly, the chelation of a ligand with a substrate. The substrate in chelation usually is a mineral or metal, whereas the ligand is typically an organic substance. The resultant complex is referred to as a chelate complex. The ligand has many names, including chelator, chelant, or chelating agent. In medicine, chelation is a therapy typically employed to remove excess toxic metals before they can cause (more) harm to the body. The removal can be done effectively because the undesired substrate (e.g., a toxic metal) can be removed along with the ligand as a single entity, with the former being held tightly by the latter. The resultant complex that contains the ligand and the substrate, though somewhat larger than the ligand itself, is still easier to be excreted from the body compared to the metal ion by itself. Otherwise, the metal ion will be freely and adversely bind to a certain cellular component or interfere with a certain biological function within the body.

Chelation can be a toxic reaction, however. In addition to causing some common side effects (e.g., skin irritation, fever, tissue damage), it can remove excess amounts of essential elements or metals (e.g., selenium, iron, zinc) from the body along the way. In particular, the application of EDTA (a.k.a. edetate disodium) has been linked to kidney damage (e.g., Cranton, 2001). EDTA is a synthetic amino acid named *e*thylene*d*iamine*t*etra*a*cetate. There have been controversies over EDTA's application as chelation therapy for reducing the risk of cardiovascular diseases (Seely *et al.*, 2005). The Asian herb cilantro is a chelator readily available in places selling fresh produce. The herb has been actively used in recent years to remove mercury (Hg) absorbed from amalgam dental fillings and other sources. As with EDTA and other chelators, cilantro comes with side effects when overused, including excess removal of essential minerals and metals.

9.3.4. Microbic Invasion

While many bacterial and viral infections are contagious (Chapter 17), the two types exert their pathogenic effects via different invasive mechanisms. For bacterial invasions, some are actually beneficial to the host organism particularly if the colonization is not aggressive. Whether a bacterial invasion can cause an infectious disease depends on the interplay between the bacterium's ability to proliferate in the host's body and the degree to which the host's body is able to defend the invasion. Most bacterial infections begin with the adherence of the pathogens (the bacteria) to specific cells on the mucous membranes of the respiratory, gastrointestinal, or genitourinary tract, followed by penetration of the epithelium to generate pathogenicity as the next stage. The third critical pathogenesis stage is for the bacteria to colonize by binding to specific tissue surface receptors and to overcome any nonspecific or immunological host defense. Some bacteria produce highly potent and lethal endotoxins or exotoxins upon invasion. Exotoxins are proteins (e.g., botulinum toxin) that may act on tissues away from the colonization site, as they are extracellular diffusible. Endotoxins are largely lipopolysaccharides localized on the outer membrane of bacteria. They are less potent compared to exotoxins and are not released until the pathogens are killed by the host's defense system.

Viruses are much smaller than bacteria and can multiply only inside a host cell. Each virus particle called virion consists of its own genetic materials (typically the RNA kind) surrounded by a protective coat of protein called capsid. As viruses are *a*cellular and do not grow via cell division or cell proliferation on their own, they produce multiple copies of themselves and certain destructive enzymes via insertion of their genetic materials into the host cell to basically hijack the latter's cell division materials and functions. When sufficient copies of a virus are so bioengineered, the new virions will burst out of the host cell, killing it and moving onward to infect other cells as well as other tissues in the host organism.

9.4. Disruption of Enzymatic Activities

The general characteristics of enzymes and their basic actions crucial to biochemical processes in a living system are highlighted in Chapter 8. Also given in that chapter is a list of substances known or suspected as capable of inhibiting or retarding the catalytic abilities of certain enzymes. Although there are several ways in which enzymatic inhibition can take place, for simplicity they can be broadly subsumed under two general modes as follows: (1) those inhibition mechanisms in which the required coenzyme or cofactor is inactivated or becomes less bioactive; and (2) those inhibitions in which the target enzyme's active site is blocked, disrupted, or otherwise becomes less bioavailable (or less bioactive).

9.4.1. Inhibition of Cofactors or Coenzymes

The function of a coenzyme can be inactivated by one or more specific toxicants. One toxicant with this ability is warfarin, an anticoagulant widely used at one time as a pesticide to kill rodents (Chapter 15). To avert life-threatening hemorrhaging, thrombin (one of the key clotting enzymes) must be sufficiently available in the animal body. Thrombin is made available from its precursor prothrombin in the liver binding with calcium ion (Ca^{2+}) being the *cofactor*. However, prothrombin is not available in the form ready for Ca^{2+} binding unless it is activated by the *coenzyme* vitamin K, which also occurs in an inactive form as vitamin K-2,3-epoxide. Warfarin, along with many other anticoagulants, is capable of antagonizing the functions of vitamin K. The inhibition is made possible likely due to warfarin's ability to bind to vitamin K-2,3-epoxide reductase (Gregus and Klaassen, 2001; Odenburg *et al.*, 2006). This reductase enzyme is responsible for catalyzing the transformation of the vitamin K epoxide to the active form of vitamin K in the liver.

For inactivation of cofactors critical to an enzyme's activation, a good example is the application of liquid citrate ($C_3H_5O[COO]_3^{3-}$) contained in a test tube for measuring *p*rothrombin *t*ime (PT). PT is a measure reflecting the clotting tendency of blood. It can be measured utilizing blood plasma drawn into a test tube in which the citrate acts as an anticoagulant by binding to the Ca^{2+} in the plasma sample. The time that the sample takes to clot is measured after an excess amount of the Ca^{2+} *cofactor* (of prothrombin leading to thrombin formation, as noted above) is added to reverse the anticoagulating effect of citrate.

As another example for inactivation of cofactors, the enzyme Mg^{2+}-ATPase needs to be activated with the cofactor Ca^{2+} or magnesium (Mg^{2+}) ion before it can catalyze the hydrolysis of ATP (adenosine-5'-triphosphate) to ADP (adenosine diphosphate) to generate energy required for many cellular reactions. This hydrolytic conversion plays a key role in supplying energy for many biochemical processes in most life forms. Mg^{2+}-ATPase is also referred to as Ca^{2+}/Mg^{2+}-ATPase or Ca^{2+}-ATPase, depending on its location in the organism's body (Ritsuko *et al.*, 1994; Zhao *et al.*, 1991). In particular, the metal cadmium (Cd^{2+}) is one that can compete with Ca^{2+} and Mg^{2+} for the binding site on Ca^{2+}/Mg^{2+}-ATPase under conducive conditions (e.g., with proper temperature,

144 An Introduction to Environmental Toxicology

proper concentration) in certain species like algae, sugar beet, mussel, and rat (e.g., Jeanne *et al.*, 1993; Lindberg and Wingstrand, 1985; Pivovarova and Lagerspetz, 1996; Zhao *et al.*, 1991).

9.4.2. Inhibition/Inactivation of Active Site

Like the active site of a protein receptor, that of an enzyme reserved for a specific substrate can be blocked or deformed. As depicted in Figure 9.3 below, the Krebs cycle (a.k.a. the citric acid cycle or the tricarboxylic acid cycle) is a complex series of enzymatic reactions in all cells that use oxygen as part of their respiration process. It is in this respiration process that the energy-rich compound ATP is mostly synthesized.

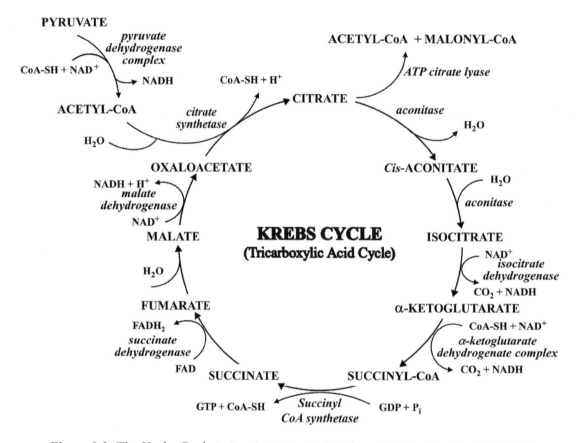

Figure 9.3. The Krebs Cycle (*a.k.a. the Citric Acid Cycle or the Tricarboxylic Acid Cycle*)

The organic compound fluorocitrate ($FC_3H_4O[COO]_3^{-3}$) is a potent Krebs cycle inhibitor by converting to 4-hydroxy-*trans*-aconitate ($C_6H_3O_7^{-3}$) which can bind tightly to the enzyme aconitase in the cycle (e.g., Lauble *et al.*, 1996). The inhibition of this enzyme shuts down the Krebs cycle crucial to many biochemical processes in aerobic organisms. Fluorocitrate can be produced as an intermediate from the rodenticide (sodium cation-based) fluoroacetate ($FCH_2CO_2^-$) under the process commonly referred to as *lethal synthesis*, in the sense that a lethal or highly toxic substance is synthesized from a relatively nontoxic precursor. The precursor fluoroacetate can also be found in certain South African plants known to cause livestock poisoning.

Organophosphates (OPs) and carbamates (CBs) are among several pesticide families (Chapter 15) known for their ability to inhibit important enzymes. The notorious effects of OP and CB pesticides come about through their ability as well as tendency of binding to the active site of the enzyme acetylcholinesterase (AChE) at the host body's brain synapses and neuromuscular junctions, where the substrate acetylcholine (ACh) acts as the neurotransmitter (i.e., substance used for stimulating the muscle to move). AChE is the enzyme that hydrolyzes (breaks down) the neurotransmitter ACh following the latter's stimulation of a nerve. More specifically, it is the enzyme that subsequently terminates the stimulation upon considerable degradation of ACh. Accordingly, inhibition or depression of AChE allows the neurotransmitter ACh to accumulate and result in initially excessive stimulation, but with death being a likely outcome when the inhibition is continuous at a sufficiently high level and long duration. Some drugs (e.g., donepezil, tacrine) developed specifically for treatment of Alzheimer's disease are known AChE inhibitors.

Metals such as lead (Pb), Hg (mercury), Cd (cadmium), and silver (Ag) are also potent enzyme inhibitors due to their high affinity for the thiol (-SH) groups present on enzymes. Many enzymes are made of peptide chains rich in cysteine ($HO_2CCH[NH_2]CH_2$-SH, or Cys-SH for short), an amino acid with a thiol (a.k.a. sulfhydryl) group on its side. When enough hydrogen (H) atoms in these -SH units are replaced by the metal (M) ions (as shown in Reactions 9.3 and 9.4 below), the tertiary structure of the enzyme's protein chain can easily be altered enough that the shape of its active site is seriously affected (distorted) as well, oftentimes to the point that the target substrate can no longer bind to this site.

$$\text{Cys-SH} + M^+ \rightarrow \text{Cys-S-M} + H^+ \tag{9.3}$$

$$2(\text{Cys-SH}) + M^{2+} \rightarrow \text{Cys-S-M-S-Cys} + 2H^+ \tag{9.4}$$

Lead is notorious for its ability to inhibit the essential enzyme *delta*-aminolevulinic acid dehydratase (δ-ALAD or ALAD) via a mechanism implicit in Reaction 9.4 (Patrick, 2006; Schafer *et al.*, 2005). The enzyme is crucial to the biosynthesis of heme, the prosthetic group of hemoglobin that carries oxygen molecules around in the blood. For most life forms, heme is also a key building block used for various biological functions in virtually every tissue in the body. Inhibition of δ-ALAD has been proposed for use as a biomarker to monitor environmental lead pollution (e.g., Kutlu and Sümer, 1998) or lead-induced effects in the heme biosynthesis pathway (e.g., Ahamed *et al.*, 2006; Alimonti and Mattei, 2008; Sakai, 2000).

9.5. Toxicodynamics of Toxicants

Toxicodynamics (TD) is technically defined (IUPAC, 1997) as *"The study of toxic actions on living systems, including the reactions with and binding to cell constituents, and the biochemical and physiological consequences of these actions."* Its focus is hence on the adverse effects and the associated toxic responses, as well as on the underlying mechanisms of action (Hodgson *et al.*, 1998). Again, inasmuch as dosage is regarded as the most crucial factor affecting toxicity, TD is interrelated closely with TK (toxicokinetics; Sections 7.5 and 9.1.2). In essence as well as in their simplest terms, TD attempts to explain how the body *reacts* to a toxicant, whereas TK is concerned with how the body *handles* the toxicant.

9.5.1. Nonspecific/Exposure-Relevant Adverse Effects

As a prelude, Table 9.1 below summarizes the various types of adverse health effects (or toxic responses) that are relevant to TD when it comes to environmental *exposure* analysis. These exposure-relevant adverse effects, along with the common underlying mechanisms of toxic action highlighted in Sections 9.2 through 9.4 above, are germane to the study of TD. Two additional relevant aspects or concepts are *dose-response relationship* and *chemical interaction*. The toxicity of a xenobiotic in a biological organism can be increased or decreased by consecutive or simultaneous exposures to one or more other toxic or harmless agents. The joint toxic effects of additivity, synergism, potentiation, and antagonism due to chemical interaction are among the numerous various affecting factors and conditions discussed in Chapter 10.

Table 9.1. Nonspecific, Exposure-Based Adverse Effects/Toxic Responses as Relevant to Toxicodynamics

Type of Effects/ Responses	General Characteristics
Local	Toxic effect/response occurring at the site of contact with the toxicant
Systemic	Toxic effect to/response by the entire body or a particular body region other than the portal of entry
Reversible	Effect that is temporary, reparable from (tissue) injury, or otherwise reversible
Irreversible	Effect that is permanent, not reparable from (tissue) injury, or otherwise irreversible
Immediate	Response or effect that develops rapidly after acute or a single exposure
Delayed	Response that develops following a short latent period from typically an acute exposure
Acute	Similar to immediate effect, but typically reserved for the kind that is usually of the severe type
Chronic	Response or effect that is developed after repeated exposures, and/or that lasts for a long time
Allergic	Effect requiring prior sensitization by an agent or by one similar in structure or in chemical/toxicological properties
Idiosyncratic	Effect or response related to abnormally high susceptibility to a specific toxicant

Amidst its analysis serving as a key component of health risk assessment (Chapter 23), dose-response relationship *per se* generally refers to a quantitative relationship between exposure to a toxicant and the severity or incidence of a toxic response. An important assertion or precaution in the analysis of dose-response relationship is that there is almost always an exposure level or dose below which no adverse effect (and thus no toxic response) occurs or can be observed. Another assertion is that once a maximum response is reached, any further increase in the exposure or dose will not result in any further increase in the effect.

In addition to carcinogenicity which generally assumes a non-threshold tumorigenic effect, allergic reaction (Table 9.1) is one adverse effect or response that does not seem to fit well into the above generalization. This type is treated as an overreaction or inappropriate response of the immunological system; it is not truly a *toxic* response. The main difference between allergy and toxic reaction is that a toxic effect is directly the result of the toxicant acting at the target site. In contrast, allergic response is typically the result of a harmless xenobiotic (termed *allergen*) stimulating a body tissue to release a protective antibody called IgE (immunoglobulin E) which will then induce an observable effect of concern. As it is frequently said, in an allergic reaction the xenobiotic at best acts as the trigger only, not the bullet. Once a person has had an allergic reaction (i.e., once sensitized to the allergen), even a very limited exposure to a very tiny dose of the allergen might trigger a life-threatening allergic reaction (e.g., anaphylaxis).

Also of special concern here is the *systemic* type of effects listed in Table 9.1, which represents a very broad category on its own (e.g., Section 9.5.2F). It includes all that can be on all of the body's internal organs, tissues, and physiological systems. Toxicants with systemic effects typically have their own target organs or tissues in which they accumulate and exert their effect(s). Many of these effects cannot be observed until a critical body burden is reached.

9.5.2. Specific/Mechanism-Based Adverse Effects

In Chapter 2, adverse health effects from environmental exposure are introduced as environmental diseases by category and in the form of concerns over their general environmental impacts. Below are those and additional adverse effects characterized in relation to, where applicable, the more specific mechanisms of (toxic) action, more unique sites of action, and/or more prominent toxicants that they are involved in or with. The adverse health effects included in this subsection are necessarily selective and brief as due to space limitation, but otherwise with the dual purpose of delineating the very broad boundary of TD while at the same time adding a place for some background materials relevant to what is known as *physiological* toxicology.

A. Irritation and Corrosive Effects

Irritation is a condition of inflammation and often painful reaction involving cell-lining damage. In most situations, it represents a localized inflammatory effect resulting from a topical exposure of an external organ (largely the eye, skin, respiratory, and genital) of the body to an agent referred to as *irritant*. Inflammation is the complex biological response of vascular tissues to the irritant, a nonspecific immunological kind involving the body's leukocytes (i.e., white blood cells) to fight off the induced effect. This type of toxic response is the body's protective attempt to remove the irritant as well as to initiate the healing process for the damaged tissue.

Irritants can be of almost any kind or form, including biological (e.g., stings, bites), chemical (e.g., phenol, metals, pesticides), mechanical (e.g., physical trauma), radioactive (e.g., ultraviolet light), and thermal (e.g., heat) stimuli. Corrosive effect refers to the production of irreversible tissue damage in the lining of the external tissue following topical exposure.

Chronic irritation is a medical term signifying the ongoing condition in which the inflammatory effect has been lingering on (and off) around the same area of the body for some time. This long-term effect as well as chronic disorder was once regarded as a very serious condition in that the irritated tissue was thought to be highly susceptible to skin lesions of the cancerous type (e.g., Dyas, 1928; Mayo, 1914). Many toxic responses can lead to chronic irritation, with the majority involving the skin and the respiratory tract.

B. Asphyxiation

Asphyxiation is a condition in which the body is deprived of oxygen, whereas asphyxia is the earlier but still serious stage characterized by an extreme decrease in oxygen supply in or to the body. Common terms for asphyxia include suffocation and inability to breathe. Several gases, including CO and HCN noted in Section 9.2.4 above, can cause asphyxia by interfering with the transport or provision of oxygen to other tissues. Symptoms of asphyxia include breathing difficulty, hypertension (high blood pressure), cyanosis, rapid pulse, convulsions, and death.

C. Narcotic and Anesthetic Effects

Narcosis, as caused by the effects of narcotics, is a condition of deep stupor or unconsciousness produced by substances (including drugs) derived from opium and those causing opiate-like addiction, such as heroin, morphine, cocaine, and barbiturates. Anesthesia, as caused by the effects of anesthetics, is a condition in which the body's sensation (including pain) in a specific anatomic region or in the entire system is blocked or temporarily taken away. Although the mechanisms of action for the two conditions are not precisely known, both mechanisms are believed to involve primarily the inhibition or activation effects of narcotic or anesthetic agents on their target receptors in the brain (e.g., Dabbagh *et al.*, 2007; Dean *et al.*, 2009; Perkins, 2005).

D. Carcinogenic/Tumorigenic Effects

These biologic effects can lead to carcinogenesis, the process by which normal cells are transformed into tumor or cancer cells. The process is caused by mutations or adverse changes of the genetic materials in normal cells, leading to the upset of the normal balance between cell proliferation (as a result of cell growth or cell division) and routine programmed cell death (termed *apoptosis*). Agents that cause carcinogenesis are called carcinogens; and those causing mutagenesis are called mutagens. Irreparable DNA molecules, as from damage by being "adducted" to an epoxide (Section 9.2.4), can disrupt the genetic programming that regulates the cell proliferation and/or apoptosis process. Further discussion on carcinogenesis and mutagenesis is given in Chapter 18.

E. Teratogenic Effects

These biologic effects can lead to teratogenesis, the process producing abnormalities or defects prior to birth. Agents that can cause birth defects or abnormalities in the embryo or fetus are specifically termed teratogens. These agents can be viruses, radiation, and chemicals (e.g., pesticides, drugs). The mechanisms of action for most teratogens are not well understood. A teratogen usually causes a specific structural or functional effect when exposure occurs within a short, definite time window after conception. Adverse effects can result when teratogens alter the normal function of DNA. Toxicants that inhibit certain enzymatic activity, that deprive the embryo or fetus of energy or oxygen supply, or that alter the placental permeability can all cause birth defects. Note that teratogenesis can also occur in plants leading to flower abnormalities (e.g., Meyer, 1966).

F. Effects on Target Body Organs or Systems

For humans (and many other mammalians), the body organs and systems of toxicological concern generally include the liver, kidneys, eyes, skin, blood, reproductive system, nervous system, immunological system, respiratory system, cardiovascular system, and the endocrine network, though not necessarily in that order. This list represents many of the basic and yet vital body organs and physiological systems in a human body. The mechanisms of action vary greatly for toxicants exerting their effects on these body parts. Collectively, these mechanisms include, but are not limited to, all those discussed earlier in Section 9.2.

Toxicants that affect the male or female reproductive system may ultimately cause adverse effects on the reproductive function of that sex, or even indirectly of the sex partner. For example, both the human papillomavirus (Walboomers *et al.*, 1999) and cigarette smoke (Pate Capps *et al.*, 2009) are risk factors, if not etiological agents, strongly linked to cervical cancer. Any practical treatment of invasive cervical cancer necessarily comes with certain risk of infertility due to some loss of the structural and functional integrity of the cervical proper. Even a small biopsy operation to remove a cone-shaped area where the cancer develops has some risk of cervical stenosis. With the stenotic cervix being very narrow and stiffened, the mucus-producing glands there become compromised and thus the survival of sperms is adversely affected (e.g., Frishman, 2002). On the males side, it has been demonstrated (e.g., Kluwe *et al.*, 1983) that the pesticide DBCP (1,2-dibromo-3-chloropropane) can reduce fertility in male rats by acting at a site in the genital tract beyond the testis.

The cardiovascular system consists of the heart and the blood vessels (e.g., arteries, arterioles, capillaries, veins, venules). Even though the heart is not a common target organ of toxic insult, its myocytes can be damaged by some pharmaceutical agents such as the cancer therapeutic drug imatinib mesylate (Kerkelä *et al.*, 2006). There are other agents that can cause cardiotoxicity: certain natural products (e.g., animal toxins); certain solvents (e.g., toluene found in paints and some household products); certain metals, such as cobalt (Co), Cd, Pb, and Hg; and certain halogenated hydrocarbons (e.g., freons). Some gaseous pollutants such as automobile exhausts, nitric oxide (NO), CO, and O_3 are found especially harmful to the vascular portion; so are some substances in the pharmaceutical and metal groups. For example, a study in Korea (Kim *et al.*, 2005) suggested that Hg could induce an increase of cholesterol in blood as a risk factor of myocardial infraction or cardiovascular diseases.

In humans and other mammalians, the nervous system consists of the central and peripheral parts, together representing a network of specialized cells termed neurons (i.e., nerve cells) that coordinate the body's biological actions and its transmission of signals across various tissues and organs. The central nervous system (CNS), which consists of the brain and the spinal cord, has a blood-brain barrier to restrict the influx of substances in the blood to the brain. However, this and the peripheral nervous system are still susceptible to damage from a variety of chemical toxicants and microbial toxins, particularly in young children whose blood-brain barrier is not yet fully developed. Neurotoxicants such as certain metals (e.g., Pb, Hg) and pesticides (e.g., organophosphates, carbamates, organochlorine insecticides) are of high health concern to environmental toxicologists. Hallucination, seizures, paralysis, coma, and death are some of the apparent as well as severe or fatal outcomes associated with poisoning of the nervous system.

Some toxic airborne residues that exist in the form of gas, vapor, liquid droplets, or solid particulate matter can induce not only localized effects on the respiratory tract, but also systemic effects after inhalation intake and distribution to other tissues. Cigarette smoke is one ill-known example of environmental toxicants that can cause cancer in general and lung cancer in particular. Respiratory diseases can be broadly classified into two types: *obstructive*, that impeding the air flow (e.g., asthma, bronchiolitis); or *restrictive*, that characterized by reduction in lung volume (e.g., lung cancer, pulmonary fibrosis). Causes of this disease group range from infectious agents and other environmental exposure to allergens and genetic origin.

The immunological system is a network of special proteins, cells, tissues, and organs working together to protect the host against foreign objects (e.g., microbes, cells, chemical substances) by using its antibodies. From this system (including bone marrow, spleen, and lymph nodes in humans), various lymphocytes and other cells with different functions are derived. Many agents are known to suppress immunological functions, leading to reduced control of abnormal tissue growth or to lowered host resistance to microbial infections. Some toxicants may provoke exaggerated responses causing systemic or localized effects, or eventually autoimmune reactions. Responses of the immunological system to toxicants are generally subsumed under the following four hypersensitivity categories: (1) *anaphylactic reactions* (Type I: acute, allergy); (2) *cytolytic reactions* (Type II: antibody-dependent); (3) *immunological complex reactions* (Type III: involving mostly IgG antibodies with soluble antigens); and (4) *delayed reactions* (Type IV: T cell-mediated, antibody-independent). Environmental allergens of concern include: certain inorganic gases (e.g., O_3); certain metals (e.g., Co, nickel, Hg); certain aromatic hydrocarbons (e.g., benzene); and certain pesticides (e.g., some organophosphates).

The liver is both the largest and a highly complex organ in the human body. As a metabolism (as well as a biotransformation) center for most nutrients, drugs, and other xenobiotics, it is the common target organ of many toxicants. These toxicants at high doses can induce a variety of harmful effects on the liver: damage to various organelles in the hepatic (liver) cells: steatosis (fatty liver); hepatic cell death; cholestasis (reduction or impaired secretion of bile or its components); liver cirrhosis (scarring); liver cancer; and hepatitis (liver inflammation). Examples of hepatotoxicants of high environmental health concern include: aflatoxins; arsenic (As); CCl_4 (carbon tetrachloride); ethanol (alcohol); and vinyl chloride.

The kidney is also a major target organ of toxic effects, insomuch as urine is the principal route by which many toxicants are (eventually) excreted from the body. Environmental toxicants of nephrotoxic concern include (certain): metals (e.g., As, Cd, Hg, Pb); halogenated hydrocarbons (e.g.,

CCl_4, chloroform); herbicides (e.g., paraquat); persistent organic pollutants (e.g., PCBs, TCDD); and mycotoxins (e.g., aflatoxins). Their mechanisms of (toxic) action include: interaction with receptors; inhibition of oxidative phosphorylation (i.e., a biochemical process producing the energy-rich compound ATP from utilizing the electron donor NADH generated in the Krebs cycle); injuries to biomembranes; and disturbance of calcium (Ca^{2+}) homeostasis (e.g., Commandeur and Vermeulen, 1990; Tarloff and Wallace, 2008; Wang et al., 2009).

In addition to skin irritation noted above, dermal contact with certain environmental toxicants can result in various types of dermal toxicity: sensitization; allergic dermatitis (including the photoallergic type); contact dermatitis (including the phototoxic type); skin lesions; skin cancer; and a variety of *systemic* effects following dermal absorption of these toxicants and their distribution to other body tissues. Environmental toxicants that can induce dermal toxicity include: ultraviolet radiation (with effects including phototoxicity and photoallergy); organochlorines such as PCBs and dioxins (with effects including notably chloracne); pesticides such as propargite and permethrin (both with effects including dermatitis); and metals such as nickel (Ni) and Hg (both with effects including allergic dermatitis), and arsenic (with effects including skin cancer).

Substances that can injure the cornea and the nearby iris include acids, alkalis, detergents, smog, and solvents. A number of toxic agents are known to compromise the transparency integrity of the lens, frequently leading to cataract formation. In addition to certain drugs (Meier-Ruge, 1972) and a number of medical conditions (e.g., arterial hypertension, diabetes, HIV-1 disease), environmental exposure to chemicals such as 4,4′-methylenedianiline aerosols (Leong et al., 1987) and carbon disulfide (Sugimoto et al., 1978) can damage the retina in humans and animals. This in turn will adversely affect visual acuity, as retina is the light sensitive tissue lining the inner surface of the eye.

In addition to HCN and CO noted above in Section 9.2.4, nitrate (NO_3^-) and hydrosulfide (HS^-) can adversely affect the hemoglobin's ability to serve as an oxygen-carrier. When the HS^- or NO_3^- ion binds to the metalloprotein to form sulf-hemoglobin (sulfHb) or met-hemoglobin (metHb), respectively, the F^{2+} ion in the Hb's heme unit is converted to F^{3+} thereby losing its ability to bind to an oxygen (O_2) molecule. A number of environmental toxicants (e.g., arsine, benzene, copper, methyl chloride, Pb) can cause (acquired) hemolytic anemia, a condition with destruction and removal of red blood cells at an abnormally high rate (prior to their normal lifespan) causing the victim to experience fatigue, dizziness, confusion, irregular heartbeat (medically termed arrhythmia), and other symptoms. In particular, exposure to benzene is strongly linked to leukemia, a cancer of the blood or bone marrow.

The endocrine network (system) controls development, metabolism, growth, and cellular regulation within the (human) body. The network consists of endocrine glands and the natural specific chemical messengers termed *hormones* that they produce and secrete. The major endocrine glands include hypothalamus, pineal gland, pituitary gland, thyroid gland, parathyroid gland, pancreas, adrenal gland, ovary, and testis (Figure 19.1). Hormones are the ones that actually regulate most major bodily functions, from hunger and reproduction to emotions and mood. Basic mechanisms of action for endocrine disruptors involving receptor binding are reflected in Section 9.2.3 above. A fuller discussion on chemical disruption of the endocrine system is given in Chapter 19.

References

Ahamed M, Verma S, Kumar A, 2006. Delta-Aminolevulinic Acid Dehydratase Inhibition and Oxidative Stress in Relation to Blood Lead among Urban Adolescents. *Human & Exper. Toxicol.* 25:547-553.

Alimonti A, Mattei D, 2008. Biomarkers for Human Biomonitoring. In *Biological Monitoring: Theory & Applications – Bioindicators and Biomarkers for Environmental Quality and Human Exposure Assessment* (Conti ME, Ed.). Billerica, Massachusetts, USA: WIT Press, Chapter 6.

Barron MG, Carls MG, Heintz R, Rice SD, 2004. Evaluation of Fish Early Life-Stage Toxicity Models of Chronic Embryonic Exposures to Complex Polycyclic Aromatic Hydrocarbon Mixtures. *Toxicol. Sci.* 78: 60-67.

Carls MG, Meador JP, 2009. A Perspective on the Toxicity of Petrogenic PAHs to Developing Fish Embryos Related to Environmental Chemistry. *Hum. Ecol. Risk Assess.* 15:1084-1098.

Commandeur JNM, Vermeulen NPE, 1990. Molecular and Biochemical Mechanisms of Chemically Induced Nephrotoxicity: A Review. *Chem. Res. Toxicol.* 3:171-194.

Cranton EM, 2001. Kidney Effects of Ethylene Diamine Tetraacetic Acid (EDTA): A Literature Review. In *A Textbook on EDTA Chelation Therapy* (Cranton EM, Ed.), 2nd Edition. Charlottesville, Virginia, USA: Hampton Roads, Chapter 26.

Crawford RL, Hess TF, Paszczynski A, 2004. Combined Biological and Abiological Degradation of Xenobiotic Compounds. In *Biodegradation and Bioremediation* (Singh A, Ward OP, Eds.). Berlin, Heidelberg, Germany: Springer-Verlag, Chapter 11.

Dabbagh A, Dahi-Taleghani M, Elyasi H, Vosoughian M, Malek B, Rajaei S, Maftuh H, 2007. Duration of Spinal Anesthesia with Bupivacaine in Chronic Opium Abusers Undergoing Lower Extremity Orthopedic Surgery. *Arch. Iranian Med.* 10:316-320.

Dean R, Bilsky EJ, Negus SS (Eds.), 2009. *Opiate Receptors and Antagonists: From Bench to Clinic*. New York, New York, USA: Humana Press.

Dyas FG, 1928. Chronic Irritation as a Cause of Cancer. *JAMA* 90:457.

Frishman GN, 2002. Treatment of Cervical Stenosis. In *Office-Based Infertility Practice* (Seifer DB, Collins RL, Eds.). New York, New York, USA: Springer-Verlag, Chapter 14.

Gregus Z, Klaassen CD, 2001. Mechanisms of Toxicity. In *Casarett and Doull's Toxicology: The Basic Science of Poisons* (Klaassen CD, Ed.), 6th Edition. New York, New York, USA: McGraw-Hill, Chapter 3.

Hodgson E, Mailman RB, Chambers JE (Eds.), 1998. *Dictionary of Toxicology*. New York, New York, USA: Grove's Dictionaries Inc.

Howell R, Wyngaarden J, 1960. On the Mechanism of Peroxidation of Uric Acids by Hemeoproteins. *J. Biol. Chem.* 235:3544-3550.

IUPAC (International Union of Pure and Applied Chemistry), 1997. Compendium of Chemical Terminology (Compiled by McNaught AD and Wilkinson A), 2nd Edition. London, Great Britain: Royal Society of Chemistry.

Jeanne N, Dazyl AC, Moreau A, 1993. Cadmium Interactions with ATPase Activity in the Euryhaline Alga *Dunaliella bioculata*. *Hydrobiologia* 252:245-256.

Kerkelä R, Grazette L, Yacobi R, Iliescu C, Patten R, Beahm C, Walters B, Shevtsov S, Pesant S, Clubb FJ, et al., 2006. Cardiotoxicity of the Cancer Therapeutic Agent Imatinib Mesylate. *Nature Med.* 12:908-916.

Kim DS, Lee EH, Yu SD, Cha JH, Ahn SC, 2005. Heavy Metal as Risk Factor of Cardiovascular Disease – An Analysis of Blood Lead and Urinary Mercury. *J. Prev. Med. Public Health* 38:401-407.

Kluwe WM, Lamb JC IV, Greenwell AE, Harrington FW, 1983. 1,2-Dibromo-3-Chloropropane (DBCP)-Induced Infertility in Male Rats Mediated by a Post-Testicular Effect. *Toxicol. App. Pharmacol.* 71:294-298.

Kutlu M, Sümer S, 1998. Effects of Lead on the Activity of δ-Aminolevulinic Acid Dehydratase in *Gammarus pulex*. *Bull. Environ. Contam. Toxicol.* 60:816-821.

Lauble H, Kennedy MC, Emptage MH, Beinert H, Stout CD, 1996. The Reaction of Fluorocitrate with Aconitase and the Crystal Structure of the Enzyme-Inhibitor Complex. *Proc. Natl. Acad. Sci. USA* 93:13699-13703.

Leong BKJ, Lund JE, Groehn JA, Coombs JK, Sabaitis CP, Weaver RJ, Griffin RL, 1987. Retinopathy from Inhaling 4,4'-Methylenedianiline Aerosols. *Fund. Appl. Toxicol.* 9:645-658.

Lindberg S, Wingstrand G, 1985. Mechanism for Cd^{2+} Inhibition of $(K^+ + Mg^{2+})$ ATPase Activity and K^+ ($^{86}Rb^+$) Uptake Join Roots of Sugar Beet (*Beta vulgaris*). *Physiologia Plantarum* 63:181-186.

Mayo WJ, 1914. Chronic Irritation A Cause of Cancer. *The New York Times*, 10 April.

Meier-Ruge W, 1972. Drug-Induced Retinopathy. *CRC Crit. Rev. Toxicol.* 1:325-360.

Meyer VG, 1996. Flower Abnormalities. *The Botanical Rev.* 32:165-218.

Oldenburg J, Bevans CG, Müller CR, Watzka M, 2006. Vitamin K Epoxide Reductase Complex Subunit 1 (VKORC1): The Key Protein of the Vitamin K Cycle. *Antioxidants & Redox Signaling* 8:347-353.

Pate Capps NJ, Stewart A, Shaw CB, 2009. The Interplay between Secondhand Cigarette Smoke, Genetics, and Cervical Cancer: A Review of the Literature. *Biol. Res. Nursing* 10:392-399.

Patrick L, 2006. Lead Toxicity Part II: The Role of Free Radical Damage and the Use of Antioxidants in the Pathology and Treatment of Lead Toxicity – Lead. *Altern. Med. Rev.* 11:114-127.

Perkins B, 2005. How Does Anesthesia Work? *Scientific America*, 7 February.

Pivovarova NB, Lagerspetz KYH, 1996. Effect of Cadmium on the ATPase Activity in Gills of *Anodonta cygnea* at Different Assay Temperatures. *J. Therm. Biol.* 21:77-84.

Ritsuko M, Mitsuoa H, Masatakaa A, Taizoua I, Hisashi T, 1994. Evidence That Both $Ca2^+$-ATP-ase and $(Ca^{2+} + Mg2^+)$-ATPase Activities in the Plasma Membrane-Rich Fraction from Bovine Parotid Gland Reside on the Same Enzyme Molecule. *Inter. J. Biochem.* 26:287-229.

Sakai T, 2000. Biomarkers of Lead Exposure. *Ind. Health* 38:127-142.

Schafer JH, Glass TA, Bressler J, Todd AC, Schwartz BS, 2005. Blood Lead Is a Predictor of Homocysteine Levels in a Population-based Study of Older Adults. *Environ. Health Perspect.* 113:31-35.

Schwartz AR, Pizon AF, Brooks DE, 2008. Dextromethorphan-Induced Serotonin Syndrome. *Clin. Toxicol.* 46:771-773.

Seely DR, Wu P, Mills EJ, 2005. EDTA Chelation Therapy for Cardiovascular Disease: A Systematic Review. *BMC Cardiovasc. Disord.* 5:32 (online journal).

Simic M, Jovanovic S, 1989. Antioxidation Mechanisms of Uric Acid. *J. Am. Chem. Soc.* 11:5778-5782.

Sugimoto K, Goto S, Kanda S, Taniguchi H, Nakamura K, Baba T, 1978. Studies on Angiopathy due to Carbon Disulfide. Retinopathy and Index of Exposure Dosages. *Scand. J. Work Environ. Health* 4:151-158.

Tarloff JB, Wallace AD, 2008. Biochemical Mechanisms of Renal Toxicity: In *Molecular and Biochemical Toxicology* (Smart RC, Hodgson E, Eds.), 4th Edition. Hoboken, New Jersey, USA: John Wiley & Sons, Chapter 29.

Wagner BA, Buettner GR, Burns CP, 1994. Free Radical-Mediated Lipid Peroxidation in Cells: Oxidizability Is a Function of Cell Lipid Bis-Allylic Hydrogen Content. *Biochemistry* 33:4449-4453.

Walboomers JM, Jacobs MV, Manos MM, Bosch FX, Kummer JA, Shah KV, Snijders PJ, Peto J, Meijer CJ, Muñoz N, 1999. Human Papillomavirus Is a Necessary Cause of Invasive Cervical Cancer Worldwide. *J. Pathol.* 189:12-19.

Wang L, Cao J, Chen D, Liu X, Lu H, Liu Z, 2009. Role of Oxidative Stress, Apoptosis, and Intracellular Homeostasis in Primary Cultures of Rat Proximal Tubular Cells Exposed to Cadmium. *Biol. Trace Element Res.* 127:53-68.

Williams AT, Burk RF, 1990. Carbon Tetrachloride Hepatotoxicity: An Example of Free Radical-Mediated Injury. *Seminars Liver Dis.* 10:279-284.

Zhao D, Elimban V, Dhalla NS, 1991. Characterization of the Purified Rat Heart Plasma Membrane Ca^{2+}/Mg^{2+}ATPase. *Mol. Cell. Biochem.* 107:151-160.

Review Questions

1. Briefly define the toxicological terms *site of (toxic) action* and *mechanism of (toxic) action*.
2. What are the six categories of common mechanisms of toxic action that are important to a general environmental toxicologist (and thereby discussed in this chapter)?
3. What is the key role of lipid peroxyl radical in lipid peroxidation?
4. Briefly characterize the two types of transmembrane receptors.
5. What are ion channels? And in these channels, what are the most relevant ions in terms of receptor modulation?
6. Briefly describe the general mechanisms in which hydrogen cyanide and carbon monoxide can adversely affect the normal functions of hemoglobin.
7. How is allergic response different from a typical toxic effect (or action)?
8. In terms of *secondary adverse actions*, what is something that can be regarded as *common* to both the application of medications and the use of chelation therapy?
9. How does bacterial invasion mechanistically differ from viral invasion?
10. What are the two basic modes in which enzymatic activities can be inhibited?
11. Name a cation that is a competitive inhibitor of Mg^{2+} for the binding site on Mg^{2+}-ATPase.
12. Briefly explain why fluorocitrate is a potent Krebs cycle killer (blocker).
13. How does lead (Pb) biochemically inhibit the enzymatic activity of δ-ALAD?
14. What is the basic difference between toxicodynamics and toxicokinetics?
15. Briefly characterize the following: a) acute effect; b) delayed effect; c) idiosyncratic effect.
16. How are cell proliferation and apoptosis mechanistically relevant to carcinogenesis?
17. Why was (is) chronic irritation treated as a serious medical condition?
18. What is the most prominent target body organ of the pesticide DBCP in male rats?
19. Name the body organ(s) and system(s) on which mercury (Hg) can exert its adverse effects (as mentioned in this chapter).
20. Name an agent that can cause: a) chloracne; b) photoallergic dermatitis; c) retinopathy.
21. Name the agent(s) that can cause both hepatotoxicity and nephrotoxicity.

CHAPTER 10

Factors and Conditions Affecting Toxicity

10.1. Introduction

Today, the term *toxicity* is coined as the state or quality of being poisonous or as the level of an agent's toxic strength or capacity, a subject matter of foremost relevance to toxicologists in all branches. Aside from its toxicological properties, a toxicant's *actual* adverse effect on or to the body of a biological organism depends on predominately three interrelated conditions: (1) the way in which the toxicant is disposed in the organism's body; (2) the toxicant's bioavailability at the site of action; and (3) the extent to which the organism's body can defend against the toxic action. These three contingencies are not mutually exclusive but somewhat convoluted. For example, the extent to which the organism responds to a toxic action depends on how and how much the toxicant is delivered to the site of action. At the same time, the toxicant's bioavailability at the site of action is contingent on the organism's ability to eliminate, detoxify, or weaken the toxicant or its toxicity during the course of the toxicant's disposition in the body.

10.1.1. Extrinsic Factors

A vast number of extrinsic factors can affect heavily one or more of the three contingencies noted above, with many involving the mechanism of (toxic) action. To facilitate the discussion in this chapter, these external factors are broadly subsumed under the following three categories based on their nature and root, or otherwise on their source: (1) environmental factors; (2) nutritional factors; and (3) physicochemical factors.

The above source categories are neither mutually exclusive, considering that as a quick example the nutritional constituents of a diet that can affect toxicity are also those coming from the environment or available to consumers as food products. Another reality is that despite the notion that a toxicant's physicochemical properties tend to be intrinsic in nature, these intrinsic properties are strongly affected by the environmental conditions in which the toxicant is present. As discussed specifically later in Section 10.4, a toxicant's chemical properties include its reactivity with other substances co-existing in the same environment. It is under this notion, or in this sense, that many physicochemical properties may be treated as involving certain extrinsic elements, if not truly as extrinsic environmental factors.

10.1.2. Intrinsic Cofactors

In contrast, biological factors such as age, gender, health status, and species differences are intrinsic in nature and are not everyday variables that fall within the realm of environmental toxicology. This is not to suggest that these intrinsic factors are not of high concern or relevance to some branches of toxicology. It only means that in practice, environmental toxicology is preoccupied as well as masterminded with finding ways to control and prevent *external* factors that affect human health and the environment. This notion is consistent with the concept as well as the paradigm of environmental health advocated by the World Health Organization (WHO) over a decade ago, a point made explicitly in Section 2.1.3.

Biological factors are included in this chapter, nevertheless, not only for a sense of completeness but also for their important role acting in many ways as *co*factors of the extrinsic variables discussed in this chapter. After all, it is not a perception, but a reality, that children being younger are generally more vulnerable to environmental exposure compared to adults. One apparent reason for such a difference is that young children's many body parts including their brain are not yet fully developed to withstand as much of the comparatively larger load of environmental exposure. Another reality is that recently there have been more clinical data available to support the emergence of gender dimorphic profiles, at least in terms of drug efficacy and adverse drug reactions (e.g., Nicolson *et al.*, 2010).

10.2. Environmental Factors

In most cases within a practical range, a positive correlation exists between the level of exposure to a toxicant and the amount or the severity of the adverse effect that the toxicant exerted on an organism, leading to the notion of dose-response relationship consistently asserted by people in the health risk assessment sector. Whether being measured directly or indirectly, environmental exposure is a function of the toxicant's concentration and the way in which the exposure is encountered. There is the consensus that for most toxic effects, their manifestation requires the dose to reach a threshold, and that beyond the maximum level no further increase in toxicity will result (Section 9.3.1). It is also intuitive that before a toxic response can be induced, there has to be exposure. Many etiological hypotheses from epidemiological studies are built on this concept. In the case of *environmental* exposure, the toxicant's concentration in a medium becomes the most influential factor affecting its toxicity. In fact, all regulatory mitigation measures developed or proposed for environmental exposure are based on this notion.

Inasmuch as environmental exposure is mostly an involuntary act, other exposure-related environmental parameters such as control measures in effect, exposure duration, and exposure frequency are all crucial and relevant. Nonexposure-related environmental factors or conditions that can affect toxicity include the environmental medium's pH, temperature, sunlight, and many (other) meteorological variables.

10.2.1. Level of Environmental Exposure

There are ample practical cases and experimental data supporting Paracelsus' notion of dose-response relationship (Chapter 1), which asserts that a contaminant's toxicity is strongly related to its environmental exposure level (though mostly within a practical range only). Four such cases are discussed in this subsection for didactic purposes, with each selected to intentionally represent a unique toxicity situation or platform.

A. London Fog of 1952

In December 1952, London and its greater metropolitan area in Britain were severely polluted with heavy smog containing high levels of sulfur dioxide (SO_2). As discussed in Chapter 11 (and elsewhere), SO_2 is not only highly toxic to plants but also a potent pulmonary irritant to humans. This air pollution episode resulted in some 4,000 *excess* (*premature*) deaths and some 100,000 *extra* cases of cardiovascular- or respiratory-related illnesses in the metropolitan area. As later reassessed by Bell and Davis (2001), the weekly mortality estimated for Greater London was highly positively correlated with the weekly air concentrations of SO_2 occurring in that area, even beyond the episode period during the first week of December 1952 (Figure 10.1). The strong positive correlation should be interpreted with caution, nonetheless, in that certain confounding effects might be inevitable as SO_2 was not (likely) the only smog pollutant present in the Greater London sky during that period.

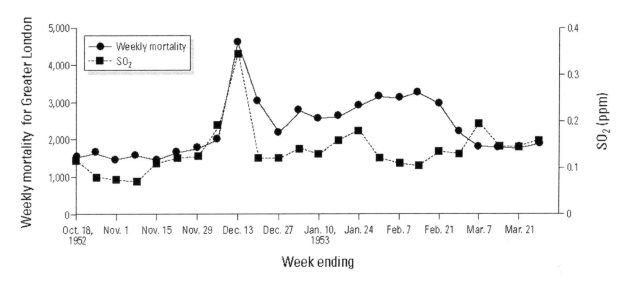

Figure 10.1. Approximate Air Concentrations of Sulfur Dioxide (SO_2) and Weekly Mortality in Greater London, 1952-1953 (*reproduced from Bell and Davis [2001] with implicit permission for public domain materials published in a U.S. government journal*)

B. Uptake of Soil Cadmium and Arsenic

Cadmium (Cd) and arsenic (As) are phytotoxic metals known to suppress plant growth (e.g., Anastasia and Kender, 1973; Farooqi *et al.*, 2009; John *et al.*, 2008; Sheppard, 1992; Woolson, 1973). There are, however, plant species that are hyperaccumulators of heavy metals without suffering (noticeable) cell damage. In a field pot-culture experiment (Sun *et al.*, 2008) on black nightshade (*Solanum nigrum* L), the field data showed that the accumulation of Cd increased with increasing soil concentration except when As was also present at a sufficiently high concentration in the same soil pot. As shown in Table 10.1, mean concentrations were increased up to *threefold* for Cd accumulation in the *S. nigrum* stems when the spike with Cd in the pot soils was increased *fivefold* (i.e., from Cd-10 to Cd-50), except when the pot soil was also spiked with As at the highest spike concentration of 250 mg/kg (i.e., except at As-250).

Table 10.1. Mean Concentrations of Cadmium (Cd) Measured in the Stems of *Solanum nigrum* Growing in Pot Soils Spiked with Various Levels of Cd and Arsenic (As)[a]

Treatment	Concentration of Cd (mg/kg)		
	Cd-10	Cd-25	Cd-50
As-0	122	208	387
As-50	170	184	385
As-250	106	124	102

[a] modified from Table 1 in Sun *et al.* (2008); spike As-50 ≡ 50 mg/kg of As added, spike Cd-25 ≡ 25 mg/kg of Cd added, and so forth.

C. LC_{50} of Polychlorinated Biphenyls for Three Fish Species

Polychlorinated biphenyls (PCBs) were sold in the United States under the eight trade names Aroclor 1221, 1232, 1242, 1248, 1254, 1260, 1262, and 1268. Their individual LC_{50} values (i.e., the lethal concentrations that killed 50% of a test population) were determined by Stalling and Mayer (1972) for three fish species using the intermittent-flow bioassay method (Adams, 1995; Chandler *et al.*, 1974; *see* also Section 22.2.2). These acute toxicity data, reproduced in Table 10.2 below, showed that while varying considerably among the eight PCB products and the three fish species tested, in all cases the LC_{50} values decreased (i.e., the potency increased) with increasing days of exposure (and thereby with increasing total exposure level).

Table 10.2. Acute Toxicity of Aroclors (PCBs) to Three Fish Species[a]

Aroclor	Species	Median Lethal Concentration (LC_{50}, in µg/L)					
		5 days	10 days	15 days	20 days	25 days	30 days
1242	Bluegills	154	72	54	–	–	–
1242	Catfish	–	174	107	–	–	–
1248	Bluegills	307	160	76	10	–	–
1248	Catfish	–	225	127	–	–	–
1248[b]	Bluegills	137	76	–	–	–	–
1248[b]	Catfish	–	94	57	–	–	–
1254	Bluegills	–	443	204	135	54	–
1254	Catfish	–	–	741	300	113	–
1254	Trout	156	8	–	–	–	–
1260	Bluegills	–	–	–	245	212	151
1260	Catfish	–	–	–	296	166	137
1260	Trout	–	240	94	21	–	–

[a] modified from Stalling and Mayer (1972); temperature at 20° C (68° F), except noted otherwise; alkalinity, 260; pH, 7.4; days are duration of exposure; Aroclor is the trade name for polychlorinated biphenyl (PCB) products sold in the United States.
[b] temperature at 27° C.

D. Cigarette Smoking and Lung Cancer Mortality

An epidemiological study (Pope *et al.*, 2011) was conducted in which adjusted relative risks (RRs) over various increments of active cigarette smoking were estimated for an analytic cohort of nearly 800,000 American adults. The analytic cohort data were a subset of the ongoing prospective cohort data collected by the American Cancer Society as part of the Cancer Prevention Study II (e.g., SBMLIC, 1992). The participants in this analytic cohort, all aged 30 years or older, were followed up for mortality for six years, including 20% of them that were active (current) smokers. Nearly 69% of the smokers had a smoking history (duration) of 30 years or longer, with the rest 31% had at least 5 years (since they must start smoking before 25 years of age to be accepted as participants). In statistical concept and in this cohort study, RR is basically the *ratio* of the lung cancer mortality (death rate) occurring in the smoker group *to* that occurring among the never-smokers. Presented in Table 10.3 are the RRs of lung cancer mortality estimated in the study for the various increments of active cigarette smoking, after adjustment for alcohol consumption, education, gender, marital status, smoking history, and several other variables. Overall, the adjusted RR estimates as shown in Table 10.3 appear to support a strong *linear* exposure-response relationship for lung cancer mortality with cigarette smoking.

Table 10.3. Adjusted Relative Risks (RRs) of Lung Cancer Mortality Estimated for Various Increments of Exposure from Cigarette Smoking[a]

Increment (Mid-Range) of Daily Exposure[b]	Estimated Daily Dose of $PM_{2.5}$ (mg)[c]	Adjusted RR (95% confidence interval)
≤3 (1.5) cigarettes	18	10.44 (7.30, 14.94)
4-7 (5.5) cigarettes	66	8.03 (5.89, 10.96)
8-13 (10) cigarettes	120	11.63 (9.51, 14.24)
13-17 (15) cigarettes	180	13.93 (11.04, 17.58)
18-22 (20) cigarettes	240	19.88 (17.14, 23.06)
23-27 (25) cigarettes	300	23.82 (18.80, 30.18)
28-32 (25) cigarettes	360	26.82 (22.54, 31.91)
33-37 (35) cigarettes	420	26.72 (18.58, 38.44)
38-42 (40) cigarettes	480	30.63 (25.79, 36.38)
≥43 (45) cigarettes	540	39.16 (31.13, 49.26)

[a] adapted and modified from Table 2 in Pole *et al.* (2011); the lung cancer risk being relative to never-smokers and adjusted for relevant variables including alcohol consumption, education, gender, marital status, and smoking history.

[b] nearly 69% of the smokers had a smoking history (duration) of 30 years or longer, with the rest 31% having at least 5 years since the participants were 30 years of age or older and started smoking before 25 years of age.

[c] based on a dose of 12 mg/cigarette, as so assumed by the authors in the study; note that inasmuch as the bulk of the carcinogens and toxic substances in $PM_{2.5}$ (*p*articular *m*atter with airborne fine particles of the diameter size 2.5 μm or smaller, *see* Chapter 12) can be found in cigarette smoke or vice versa, the inclusion of the $PM_{2.5}$ daily doses by the study authors was allegedly a design to replay the argument that high levels of air pollution is as bad as heavy cigarette smoking in terms of the risk for developing lung cancer or cardiopulmonary diseases.

10.2.2. Other Exposure-Related Factors

In addition to exposure level, other major common exposure-related factors include mode of contact with the toxicant and control measures that are in effect. There are many other factors that in some situations also have a strong influence on exposure, such as work experience and employment type. These other variables are not treated as straightly environmental in nature within the context of this book. In many cases, frequency of exposure and duration of exposure are key determinants of exposure level, as in the above two cases explicitly with PCBs (Table 10.2) and implicitly with cigarette smoking (Table 10.3). However, they should be better treated as collaborative but distinct factors for the consideration given below.

A. Frequency and Duration of Exposure

Both exposure frequency and exposure duration are collaborative with environmental exposure level, particularly for chronic effects resulting from exposure at lower levels. Here by collaborative, it presumes that the effect of (environmental) exposure level or dose obeys Haber's law (e.g., Gaylor, 2000). This law asserts the effect e equivalency of any two sets of dose concentration c_i and exposure time t_i, as long as the mathematical products of the two sets are equivalent. That is, if $c_1 \times t_1 = c_2 \times t_2$, then $e_1 = e_2$. It is apparent that such an assertion cannot hold true for all cases. For example, suppose $t_2 = t_1 + t_1$ (i.e., t_2 being twice as long as t_1). Then under Haber's law, $e_1 = e_2$ only when $c_2 = (½)c_1$ (i.e., c_1 being twice as high as c_2). However, if the toxicant from exposure at the lower level c_2 can be sufficiently eliminated from the host's body by t_1 (or now half of t_2) and the effect can be induced only from exposure at levels exceeding c_2, then no effect would likely result from the second exposure c_2 scenario. Note that in exposure assessment, duration of exposure is commonly defined as the *period* of *each* exposure event (e.g., 4 hours, 1 day) whereas frequency of exposure, as the *number* of exposure events (e.g., daily, weekly, 90 days).

In reality, the adverse effect of any given exposure is much more dynamic than what can be explained mathematically and tends to obey Haber's law within some constraints. Both the data in Table 10.2 and Table 10.3 demonstrated that exposure frequency is a crucial factor. In the case with cigarette smoking (Table 10.3), it is clear that the lung cancer deaths resulted from chronic (daily) exposure for at least 5 years. In the case with the acute toxicity of PCBs to fish (Table 10.2), the data showed that at least for the fish species and the bioassay conditions tested, *longer* exposure days were required for *lower* (lethal) exposure concentrations in order for the various PCB products each to attain the same definite (fixed) *lethality rate of 50%*.

B. Mode of Contact and Control Measure

These two factors are more subtle compared to environmental concentration or exposure time and can be highly interrelated. An example for supporting this argument is the case of young children playing on a residential lawn treated with an herbicide. At what time post-application and in what manner these children are allowed to play on a treated lawn depend on largely the health conscience of their parents concerning the herbicide's (potential) harmful effects. In general, a parent's knowledge or awareness of a pesticide's toxicity and the restrictions on reentry can come from product labeling which serves as some form of control measure.

Control measure can indeed have a substantial impact on the environmental exposure of certain (groups of) toxicants. A real case in point is the California state law for banning the use of trans fats in restaurants effective New Year's Day in 2010, as briefly discussed in Chapter 4 (Section 4.2.2C). Additional real case examples for mitigating exposure via some form of control measure can be found also in Chapter 4, such as those related to triclosan used as an antibacterial agent (Section 4.2.1A) and to lead on toy jewelry (Section 4.2.1B).

Nonetheless, in reality it is very difficult to assess the magnitude of children's exposure when it comes to something like lead on toys or toy jewelry, as it all depends on their individual habits and personality. Touching the supposedly low levels of lead coated on toys is generally not a significant exposure route. Unfortunately, toddlers up to 3 or 4 years of age often chew on their toys and put their hands in their mouths. Exposure from object-to-mouth or hand-to-mouth will increase considerably the intake of a substance compared to routine dermal contact. In most cases, the dermal absorption and acquisition of a topical dose in an incremental manner is less potent than the oral absorption and acquisition of a bolus (oral) dose (e.g., Ross *et al.*, 2000). There are ample data supporting this assertion. For instance, where available the *oral* LD_{50} (the lethal dose that killed 50% of a test population) is almost always much lower (i.e., much more potent) than the corresponding *dermal* LD_{50} specifically listed in the Material Safety Data Sheet (commonly known by its acronym MSDS) for each relevant chemical ingredient in a product.

For environmental exposure of relatively long duration and high frequency, people can be exposed to more than one contaminant with the same or a very similar adverse effect of concern. It is for this potential that the Food Quality Protection Act (FQPA) of 1996 directs U.S. EPA to consider the *cumulative* adverse effect from exposures to pesticides having a common mechanism of toxicity at issue. This type of public health concerns has strengthened and expanded U.S. EPA's practice in its pesticide risk assessment to also perform *aggregate* exposure analysis for each target population, by considering exposures to the same pesticide from work, foods, drinking water, and other sources or routes. Further discussion on this topic is given in Chapter 23. What is important to note here is that the route of exposure to (i.e., the mode of contact with) an environmental toxicant is not always well defined. This problem is not unique to the human species. Large fish can take in a persistent toxic substance not only from the contaminated water, but also from eating smaller fish that each might already have had a considerable amount of the substance concentrated in their tissues. The two familiar terms relating to this kind of environmental exposure are *bioaccumulation* and *biomagnification*, which are discussed extensively in Chapter 6.

10.2.3. Nonexposure-Related Factors

Environmental factors that are influential but not as directly related to exposure include the medium's pH, temperature, humidity, light, and other meteorological variables. Temperature variations may cause a physiological stress to the host or lead to a substantial difference in a toxicant's physicochemical properties and thus its toxicological profile as well. As shown in Table 10.2, the LC_{50} of Aroclor 1248 for both catfish and bluegills were reduced twofold when the temperature in the bioassay was increased from 20° C (68° F) to 27° C (81° F). Other studies (e.g., Barson, 1983; Bat *et al.*, 2000; Boina *et al.*, 2009; Khan *et al.*, 2007; Li *et al.*, 2006; Viswanathan and Murti,

1989) also found temperature to have a significant effect on a substance's toxicity, though mostly in insects and other invertebrates. High ambient temperature was shown to affect considerably the release and transport of those airborne substances whose presence may trigger an allergic reaction (Jacobson and Morris, 1976; Viswanathan and Murti, 1989). Furthermore, it is a familiar practice to many farmers that plants are not to be sprayed with lime sulfur at a field temperature above 29° C (85° F), as then the fungicide would become a burning agent to the foliage.

The effects of humidity and moisture on toxicity, like those of temperature, are not as well understood in humans and other mammalians as in insects. One reason is that substances like pesticides are not designed to get rid of humans or other mammalians. There tend to be greater motivations for investigating the effects of temperature and humidity on insects because a pesticide's efficacy is at stake for marketing purposes. In any case, there was one relevant study (Barson, 1983) conducted in which beetles (*Oryzaephilus surinamensis*) were exposed to each of three organophosphorus insecticides at various (30, 50, 70, 90% relative) humidity levels. The study revealed that the mortality of the test beetles increased with increasing humidity at each test temperature (5° to 30° C at 5° C intervals). It was thought that the increase in lethal effect was due to high ambient humidity's capability to cause swelling of the stratum corneum of invertebrates and thereby to allow greater penetration of a substance through their skin (Suskind, 1977).

The toxicities of many metals and other substances were reportedly affected by the pH in the aqueous test solution (e.g., Franklin *et al.*, 2000; Ho *et al.*, 1999; Kobayashi and Kishino, 1980; Michnowicz and Weaks, 1984; Sawyer *et al.*, 2007). However, this factor or condition may not be of immediate concern for terrestrial organisms.

High altitude areas are those on the Earth's surface high above sea level (above ~5,000 ft or 1,524 m), where the temperatures are cold and the atmospheric pressures are low compared to those at sea level. Altitude effects on the toxicological properties of environmental toxicants are not well understood. Nonetheless, a number of studies (e.g., Castillo and Timiras, 1964; Fischer, 1941; Singh *et al.*, 2001; Vats *et al.*, 2008) implicated that the toxicities of some toxicants could be affected considerably in humans treated and animals dosed at high altitude. It is likely that such altitude-related changes in toxicity were due to the effect on the test subject's physiological response, rather than to any modulation directly on the toxicity of the test material. In any event, it is a known fact that in humans, the risk of carbon monoxide (CO) poisoning is proportionate to high altitude (among other things). However, this is likely due to the fact that less oxygen per breath is available at high altitude.

Light is a variable that can affect a host's diurnal rhythm or the physicochemical (and thus likely the toxicological) properties of a toxicant. For instance, atmospheric SO_2 in the presence of sunlight and water vapor can readily form sulfuric acid (H_2SO_4), which is a major acidic component found in acid rain (Chapter 5). Many substances are subject to photolysis (i.e., chemical decomposition induced by light or other radiant energy; *see* Chapter 5). Both light quality and light quantity have long been shown to affect herbicide toxicity to plants (e.g., Erickson *et al.*, 1972; Pollak and Crabtree, 1976). It is apparent that temperature is closely related to (sun)light.

A number of studies have been carried out to analyze the interactions between light and the hormone melatonin (Chapter 19) in humans, animals, and plants. In humans and certain other mammalians such as nocturnal rodents, melatonin is known to regulate the circadian rhythms of several biological functions by varying its circulating levels in a daily cycle. Secretion of certain hormones including melatonin is reportedly influenced by light exposure (e.g., Bellastella *et al.*, 1998; Boyce and Kennaway, 1987; Hymer *et al.*, 2009; Kasuya *et al.*, 2008; Reiter *et al.*, 2007).

10.3. Nutritional Factors

Nutrition as a science refers to the study focusing on the physiological process by which an organism nourishes itself, or is nourished, with food for growth and health maintenance. Food toxicology, on the other hand, is the branch of toxicology or nutrition concerned with toxicants (including toxins) found in foods. In contrast, nutritional toxicology is the branch with its focus on nutritional status affected by the interactions between toxicants and nutrients in the diet (Omaye, 2004). Nourishing ingredients found in foods are known as nutrients, which in general biochemical terms include proteins, lipids, carbohydrates, vitamins, and minerals. The focus of this section is on nutrition-related factors or conditions tending to modulate the adverse effects of environmental toxicants. Such nutritional variables can be broadly divided into the two categories: (1) nutritional status of the host body; and (2) those nutrients capable of modulating a toxicant's effects.

10.3.1. Nutritional Status

Malnutrition, starvation, fasting, obesity, and nutritional disorders all reflect the nutritional status of the host in which a toxicant is present; that is, all representing a common nutritional state that the host is in. Any of these nutritional conditions can modulate significantly the adverse effect that the toxicant has on its host. For example, malnutrition can increase considerably the toxicological properties of certain metals such as cadmium (Prasad and Nath, 1995), certain pesticides such as naled (Kaloyanova and Tasheva, 1983), and certain (other) organic substances such as hexachlorocyclohexane (Agrawal *et al.*, 1992).

Starvation can be caused by famine, poverty, severe gastrointestinal disorders, coma, stroke, fasting, and the eating disorder *anorexia nervosa*, with the last two each being largely a voluntary act. In all cases, this condition can modulate the toxicity of xenobiotics what malnutrition can do and more, as it represents the worse and more dangerous form of the latter. In particular, an animal study (Dave, 1981) showed that adult fathead minnows starved for 80 days were twice more susceptible to the acute toxicity of endrin which, like hexachlorocyclohexane (HCH), is an organochlorine pesticide with high lipophilicity. During starvation, lipids stored in fatty tissues are utilized before other sources such as proteins and fats in the muscle (Czesny *et al.*, 2003). This event suggests that starvation can cause lipophilic toxicants such as endrin and HCH to become less available in the adipose tissues and likely more available at the site of toxic action instead.

10.3.2. Macro- and Micro-Nutrients

Nutrients are generally divided into macronutrients and micronutrients according to the quantity in which they are needed by the organism's body to sustain its essential biological functions. Accordingly, *micro*nutrients like potassium (K) and phosphorus (P) for mammalians (particularly humans) are *macro*nutrients for plants. Macronutrients for humans generally include the macromolecules proteins, carbohydrates, and lipids. Water is a macronutrient by definition, but frequently excluded from consideration as one of the (key) nutritional factors not only owing to its unique importance to life but also due to its abundance. Micronutrients for humans include a number of vitamins, minerals, and metals, of which some are more essential than others. Many nutrients have the ability to modulate the activities of many Phase I or Phase II enzymes (Chapter 8) and thereby also the potential to affect considerably the toxicity of xenobiotics. Below is a brief account of select studies that support this notion which is largely species-specific.

A. Macronutrients in Mammalians

Protein deficiency in quantities is a major kind of malnutrition and thus has much of the effects on toxicity as malnutrition in general has. Biochemically, these malnutrition effects are likely due to, as induced by protein deficiency, an alteration in the liver's ability to biotransform xenobiotics (e.g., Czygan *et al.*, 1974; Hayes *et al.*, 1973; Kawano and Hiraga, 1980). In addition, poor quality of dietary protein can be treated as a special form of protein deficiency. Protein quality refers to how well the essential amino acids in a protein can compensate for those required by the body. Several studies revealed that the quality of dietary protein correlated positively with cytochrome P450 activities in the rat liver (e.g., Campbell and Hayes, 1976; Kato *et al.*, 1981; Miranda and Webb, 1973), thus enhancing either the detoxification or the bioactivation of certain toxicants. In particular, a study by Schulsinger *et al.* (1989) showed that both low quantity and poor quality of protein intake were equally effective in retarding the development of hepatic preneoplastic lesions induced by aflatoxin B_1.

It was shown (Sonawane *et al.*, 1983) that high dietary carbohydrates in the male rat with low fat but normal protein content resulted in a noticeable decrease in microsomal P450 enzymes in the animal's liver. On the other hand, low levels of carbohydrate intake, whether along with alcohol (Korourian *et al.*, 1999; Tsukada *et al.*, 1998) or with high fat (Yoo *et al.*, 1991) in the diet, elevated the hepatic level of CYP2E1 in the rat. In any case, modulation of this P450 enzyme (CYP2E1) level can have a crucial effect on the toxicity of some environmental toxicants, as the enzyme plays a key role in the biotransformation of xenobiotics.

Several studies (e.g., Century, 1973; Clinton *et al.* 1984; Marshall and McLean, 1971; Wade and Norred, 1976) also demonstrated that high levels of polyunsaturated fatty acids (PUFA) in diets to rats brought about an increase in the activity of microsomal cytochrome P450 in the rat liver. In addition, one study (Saito *et al.*, 1990) found that dietary lipids containing a high concentration of linoleic acid, which is an *Omega-6* kind as well as an essential PUFA, were able to induce a higher elevation of the P450 enzyme activity in rats. These findings support the notion that lipid quality can also affect considerably the toxicity of certain xenobiotics.

B. Micronutrients in Mammalians

The effects of vitamins, minerals, and metals on the toxicity of xenobiotics can be appreciated from their role as coenzymes or cofactors of many Phase I and Phase II enzymes (Chapter 8). Among the large number of vitamins found in the human body, vitamin A (e.g., retinol), vitamin

B₁ (thiamine), vitamin B₂ (riboflavin), vitamin C (ascorbic acid), and vitamin E (e.g., tocopherol) are the more prominent ones known to affect the activities of Phase I enzymes. Some other vitamins are themselves affected by the activities of certain cytochrome P450s. In humans, vitamin D is bioactivated to its active hormonal form by certain P450s. And the cause of vitamin K deficiency can be attributed to an induction of P450s by some anticonvulsants.

Moreover, experiments with vitamin C-deficient guinea pigs consistently showed a decreased hepatic microsomal P450 content in animals fed on diets not supplemented with the vitamin (e.g., Rikans, 1982; Sato and Zannoni, 1976). On the other hand, a study in rats (Ramírez-Farías *et al.*, 2008) found that vitamin C and vitamin E were protective against alcohol-induced liver injury and capable of modulating hepatic and plasma lipid peroxidation.

In general, deficiencies in vitamin A and vitamin E reportedly can cause a decrease in cytochrome P450 activity in animal livers (Iwasaki *et al.*, 1994; Miranda *et al.*, 1979). And vitamin B_1 deficiency has been linked to an increased content of CYP2E1 in the rat liver (Yoo *et al.*, 1990). Furthermore, vitamin B_2 deficiency has been associated with an increase in the hepatic contents of cytochrome P450s and cytochrome b_5, but with a decrease in the hepatic content of NADPH-dependent cytochrome P450 reductase (Taniguchi, 1980). Other members in the vitamin B group (e.g., biotin, choline, cyanocobalamin, folic acid, niacin, pantothenic acid, pyridoxine) either do not seem to affect the activities of Phase I and Phase II enzymes, or have not been actively investigated for such effects.

Overall, a decrease in the contents or activities of P450 enzymes has been linked to a deficiency in dietary magnesium (Mg), calcium (Ca), copper (Cu), and zinc (Zn), as well as to an excess intake of iron (Fe) and iodine (I). In particular, Zn deficiency can alter the activities of some Phase II enzymes (Jagadeesan and Oesch, 1988). Even though zinc is essential for all living forms, an excess intake of this metal can be harmful to the human body (Fosmire, 1990). For instance, excessive intake of zinc can suppress copper absorption (Fosmire, 1990; Oestreicher and Cousins, 1985), thus indirectly affecting the activities of certain cytochrome P450 enzymes via the effects of copper deficiency. Studies have shown that copper has the ability to inhibit or retard the catalytic functions of CYP1A1, CYP1A2, CYP3A4, and NADPH-dependent cytochrome P450 reductase in hepatic microsomes (Kim *et al.*, 2002; Korashy and El-Kadi, 2005; Letelier *et al.* 2009). This, however, does not seem to be the case with zinc *per se* (Kim *et al.*, 2002).

As with zinc and copper, molybdenum (Mo) is an essential trace metal for virtually all life forms. In humans, this metal functions as a cofactor for sulfite oxidase, xanthine oxidase, and aldehyde oxidase. The last two oxidase enzymes reportedly play a key role in the biotransformation of certain xenobiotics (Eckhert, 2006). Significant increases were observed in brain mitochondrial and microsomal P450 contents in rats treated with magnesium (Liccione and Maines, 1989). One study (Yasukochi *et al.*, 1977) observed that the P450 contents were depressed considerably in rats injected with cobalt (Co), which is a significant component of vitamin B_{12}. Another rat study (Shivarajashankara *et al.*, 2001) found that an excess of dietary fluoride (F) caused an increase in brain and hepatic levels of glutathione S-transferase (GST), which is an important Phase II enzyme. And some effects of selenium (Se) deficiency were observed on the hepatic microsomal cytochrome P450 system in rats (Burk and Masters, 1975). At this time, it is unclear what effects, if any, that other micronutrients (e.g., boron, chloride, chromium, potassium, sodium) can have, directly or indirectly, on the biotransformation of xenobiotics.

10.4. Physicochemical Factors

Most of a toxicant's physicochemical properties are actually its nature and are what have made up its basic toxicological profile. For instance, as noted in Section 10.1, in humans most airborne particles larger than 15 μm in diameter are filtered by the nasal hairs and thereby unable to exert their toxic effects at the lower region of the lung. And sulfur spray fungicide will burn the foliage if it is applied to crops at a field temperature above 29° C (85° F), although this second case may be viewed as due to the substance's physicochemical properties coupled with an environmental condition of high temperature. Strictly speaking, a chemical property is any of a material's properties that has the potential to alter the chemical nature of matter during a chemical reaction by virtue of the material's chemical composition. A material's chemical properties therefore include its toxicity, chemical stability, flammability, and reactivity with or against other co-existing substances. Of these, the material's *reactivity* is the variable that can seriously affect its own toxicity or that of another, and thereby is the focus of this section. This reactivity, of which chemical interaction is the main part, can result in a joint toxic effect that falls into one of the four patterns: (1) additivity or additive effect; (2) synergism; (3) potentiation; and (4) antagonism.

10.4.1. Additivity of Toxic Effects

In toxicology, especially in health risk assessment, the term *additivity* (of toxic effects) refers to the joint effect that is expected from two toxicants exerting a common toxic effect at issue. More specifically, the exposure to one of the two toxicants with a toxicity level of 1 unit and concurrently (or shortly afterwards) to the other toxicant with a toxicity level of 2 units will result in a combined toxicity level of 3 units. This result implies that neither toxicant has any apparent effect on the other's toxicity. One desired outcome from such a joint effect is that in its absence, the effect of the toxicant at issue may be below the threshold of exerting harm to the host's body. It has been reported (Eaton and Klaassen, 2001) that when two organophosphate pesticides are applied together, the joint effect of acetylcholinesterase enzymatic inhibition is likely additive.

Dose-addition is currently the default approach employed to assess cumulative risks from exposures to multiple toxicants that are suspected to share a common mechanism of toxicity (e.g., Chen *et al.*, 2001). The concerns with cumulative risks by regulatory entities have come around from primarily two developments: (1) mandate of the FQPA of 1996 in the United States (e.g., Sielken, 2000); and (2) use of toxic equivalency factors advocated by WHO for estimation of health risks from dioxin-like substances (Chapter 16). The validity of such a cumulative risk approach has remained controversial until recently, when more evidence is emerging to support the dose-additive effects of the pyrethroid pesticides (Chapter 15) on motor activity in rats (Wolansky *et al.*, 2009).

10.4.2. Synergism of Toxic Effects

The term *synergism* (of toxic effects) refers to the combined effect of two toxicants that is greater than additive. Numerically, the combined toxicity level would be greater than 3 units for the example with the two hypothetical toxicants given above on additivity (Section 10.4.1). Such a joint effect outcome implies that one toxicant has an effect on the toxicity of the other, with a consequence potentially being much worse than expected. An example is the concurrent exposures to the two *hepato*toxic compounds ethanol (C_2H_5-OH) and carbon tetrachloride (CCl_4) that together produce much more *liver* injury than what would be expected from adding their individual hepatic effect (Eaton and Klaassen, 2001).

Another example of synergism is the lung cancer risk from joint exposures to asbestos and cigarette smoking. Estimates of the joint effect of the two toxicants were found to exceed the sum of their individual carcinogenic effects observed in each of the 12 epidemiological studies revisited by Erren *et al.* (1999). A field pot experiment (Agrawal *et al.*, 1981) also revealed that synergistic effect of plant injury occurred when rice plants were fumigated jointly with O_3 (ozone) and SO_2 (sulfur dioxide). In that experiment, the plant injuries were measured in terms of the reductions in chlorophylls *a* and *b* as well as in total contents of chlorophyll and carotenoid in leaves.

10.4.3. Potentiation of Toxic Effects

In keeping with the definition of the verb *potentiate* being to make (more) potent or to enhance an effect, here the term *potentiation* (of toxic effects) refers to an interaction in which one substance's presence makes the other substance toxic or more toxic to a body organ or tissue. It means that the potentiator (i.e., potentiating agent) *per se* has little or no toxic effect on the host body, but has an enhancing effect on the toxicity of the other (or another) substance. This assertion is based on the notion that if the potentiator has similar toxic effects on the same host body, then by definition the joint effect should be treated as additive or synergistic.

As case examples, isopropanol and acetone have been shown able to potentiate the hepatotoxicity of CCl_4 in rats (Plaa *et al.*, 1982), as neither potentiator is a hepatotoxicant. And the relatively nontoxic ascorbic acid (vitamin C) has been implicated for potentiating the cytotoxicity of the anticancer therapeutic drug arsenic trioxide (As_2O_3) in human leukemia cells (Yedjou *et al.*, 2009). Moreover, two cases of acute occupational poisoning have been reported (Manno *et al.*, 1996), in which severe hepatonephrotoxicity was developed from inhalation of CCl_4 present at high concentrations in the fire extinguishing liquid. The toxicity of CCl_4 was reportedly potentiated by alcohol abuse by the two patients. The study's conclusion was based on the observation that the rest of the co-workers showed no signs of the toxicity for those that were exposed to CCl_4 under the same working conditions but were verified as non-alcohol abusers. Since *nephro*toxicity was involved, alcohol and not CCl_4 was concluded as the potentiator.

10.4.4. Antagonism of Toxic Effects

Of the four types of chemical interaction discussed in this chapter, antagonism (of toxic effects) is the most desirable from a medical standpoint, given that this type is the basis of many therapeutic developments. The term refers to a chemical interaction between two substances whereby their joint effect is *less* than what one would expect from the sum of their individual effects. Antagonism itself can be subdivided into four major forms or subtypes. Chelation therapy, as discussed in

Section 9.3.3, is an example of the *chemical* form of antagonism. On the other hand, treatment of CO (carbon monoxide) poisoning with hyperbaric oxygen (O_2) is a medical therapy relying on the increased removal of CO from hemoglobin. This competition for receptor sites is an example of the *competitive* or *recept*or form of antagonism.

Functional or *physiological* antagonism is the third major form, which occurs when two agents produce opposite effects on the same physiological system or function thereby effectively counteracting each other's effect. The paper by Haag and Palmer (1928) provided a historical account of this form of antagonism between calcium (Ca) and magnesium (Mg) and between a few other ions. The paper credited the importance of this form in maintaining a physiological balance among the elements entering the animal diet. The fourth form is *dispositional* in nature, involving the alteration of chemical disposition whereby the agent at issue becomes less bioactive or bioavailable at the site of action. Dietary calcium is a dispositional antagonist known to lower the intestinal absorption of lead (Pb) in humans (Peraza *et al.*, 1998). In a way, the hyperbaric oxygen applied for treatment of CO poisoning can be classified additionally as a dispositional antagonist.

10.5. Biological Cofactors

As with the three major groups of extrinsic factors discussed above, there are numerous various biological variables acting as cofactors capable of affecting the toxicity of xenobiotics in a living system. The more crucial ones include age, gender, health status, disease condition, species, genetic makeup, strain, race, and physiological state, with some of them being highly interrelated. These biological cofactors individually or in combination play a key role in setting the effects that the extrinsic factors have on the toxicity of xenobiotics. Considering that these biological cofactors are intrinsic in nature, perhaps the most effective way to avoid or attenuate their effects on the toxicity of concern is to avoid coming in contact with the toxicant.

10.5.1. Age, Gender, and Health Status

In terms of effects on toxicity, age does matter a lot. In 2003, WHO launched a campaign on environmental health (as discussed in Chapter 2), specifically for young children with the high health concern that these future citizens possess unique biological, developmental, and behavioral vulnerabilities; and they indeed do. One argument supporting this concern is that the blood-brain barrier cellular structure in young children is not fully developed to be able to restrict the passage of harmful substances from their blood to their brain. An example for age effect in a different direction is that in the plant kingdom, young leaves of some Cucurbitaceae species (e.g., cucumber) were found more resistant to injury from acute exposure to SO_2, whereas mature leaves were more sensitive to similar exposure (Sekiya *et al.*, 1982).

Gender can affect considerably the toxicity of certain environmental toxicants as well. A study showed that the oldest females were the most difficult wild house mice to be killed by the anticoagulant warfarin compared to the males and the younger females (Rowe and Redfern, 1964, 1967). Another study (Eeva *et al.*, 2006) showed that in a population of small insectivorous passerine birds living around a copper smelter, the males had a 33% higher local survival probability. Yet the local survival rate of the females did not differ between those living in the polluted and the unpolluted environment. Still another example is the discovery, which is now a widely known fact to many toxicologists, that unleaded gasoline was capable of inducing kidney tumors only in male rats but not in females or in either sex of mice. This species- and gender-specific disorder was later confirmed as attributed to the high levels of the protein $\alpha_{2\mu}$-globulin present in male rats only, and hence is now referred to as $\alpha_{2\mu}$-globulin nephropathy. The paper by Swenberg (1993) compiled a long list of substances, including certainly unleaded gasoline, that were reported as capable of causing $\alpha_{2\mu}$-globulin nephropathy.

Health status and disease condition, both of which can lead to a certain physiological state of the host body, are simply two terms referring to the same thing but viewing it from the opposite end of the same spectrum. Either case can affect considerably the activities of certain Phase I and Phase II enzymes and thereby the toxicity of certain xenobiotics. For example, a study observed that the blood level of CYP3A4 mRNA (i.e., CYP3A4 gene expression) in a group of patients correlated positively with the progression of their viral liver disease (Horiike *et al.*, 2005). CYP3A4 is one of the most important human cytochrome P450 enzymes involved in the biotransformation of xenobiotics. There is a body of evidence supporting the positive correlation between gene expression of CYP3A4 and the enzyme's metabolic activity in the human liver (e.g., Watanabe *et al.*, 2004). Kidney is quantitatively the second major organ (after liver) that can increase the toxic potential of environmental toxicants, usually by causing slower elimination of the toxicants from the body. Renal failure can adversely affect not only the elimination, but also the metabolism and transport of xenobiotics (e.g., Sun *et al.*, 2006).

As is true of humans who are sick, unhealthy plants are more susceptible to attack by pests, pathogens, and chemical substances. Compared to the leaves of healthy plants, those of chlorotic plants (e.g., caused by iron-deficiency) generally show more signs of oxidative stress despite the argument that oxidative injury may not be as definitive or transparent (e.g., Salama *et al.*, 2009; Tewari *et al.*, 2005). In plants or animals, oxidative stress refers to the adverse condition leading to excessive production of ROS (reactive oxygen species) in their cells, likely caused by the loss of some of their physiological antioxidant mechanisms.

10.5.2. Species, Strain, Race, and Genetics

An example of species variation as a variable affecting toxicity is provided in Section 10.5.1 concerning $\alpha_{2\mu}$-globulin nephropathy on male rats but not on both sex of mice. Even within the same species, the potency of certain environmental toxicants can vary considerably among strains. For example, the LD_{50} of thiourea (CH_4N_2S) was found to differ nearly 300-fold from one strain of rats to another (e.g., tame Norway *vs.* wild Alexandrine *vs.* wild Norway) even when the animals were dosed under reportedly identical conditions (Dieke and Richter, 1945).

As noted in Section 8.6.1, around 8% of Africans/African-Americans and 7% of Caucasians are treated as "poor" metabolizers because they lack CYP2D6 or its function in their body. This cytochrome P450 is one of the most important Phase I enzymes in xenobiotic biotransformation, in that it is responsible for catalyzing the oxidative metabolism of many drugs (and other substances) in the human body. Yet there is a considerable variability of the enzyme's genetic expressions in the human liver, with some losing entirely the enzyme's ability to oxidize many xenobiotics. In essence, genetic variations in CYP2D6 activity can affect the toxicity of many xenobiotics, especially drugs. The P450 enzymes in other families and some Phase II enzymes are likewise highly polymorphic as they too are subject to considerable genetic variation.

In genetics, genotype refers to the set of genes responsible for a particular trait. In the plant kingdom, many genotypes vary in their uptake of and tolerance to toxic metals. For example, in the 99 pea genotypes tested (Belimov *et al.*, 2003; Metwally *et al.*, 2005), large variability was found in their uptake of several heavy metals and their tolerance to cadmium.

References

Adams WJ, 1995. Aquatic Toxicology Testing Methods. In *Handbook of Ecotoxicology* (Hoffman DJ, Rattner BA, Burton GA, Cairns J, Eds.). Boca Raton, Florida, USA: Lewis/CRC Publishers, pp.25-46.

Agrawal D, Sultana P, Gupta GSD, Gopal K, Khanna RN, Anand M, 1992. Effect of Hexachlorocyclohexane on Biochemical Parameters of Rats on a Protein Deficient Diet. *Toxicol. Environ. Chem.* 35:109-114.

Agrawal M, Nandi PK, Rao DN, 1981. Effect of Ozone and Sulphur Dioxide Pollutants Separately and in Mixture on Chlorophyll and Carotenoid Pigments of *Oryza sativa*. *Water, Air, Soil Pull.* 18:449-454.

Anastasia FB, Kender WJ, 1973. The Influence of Soil Arsenic on the Growth of Low-Bush Blueberry. *J. Environ. Qual.* 2:335-337.

Barson G, 1983. The Effects of Temperature and Humidity on the Toxicity of Three Organophosphorus Insecticides to Adult *Oryzaephilus surinamensis* (L.). *Pest. Magnt. Sci.* 14:145-152.

Bat L, Akbulut M, Mehmet Çulha M, Gündoğdu A, Satilmiş HH, 2000. Effect of Temperature on the Toxicity of Zinc, Copper and Lead to the Freshwater Amphipod *Gammarus pulex* (L., 1758). *Turk. J. Zool.* 24: 409-415.

Belimov AA, Safronova VI, Tsyganov VE, Borisov AY, Kozhemyakov AP, Stepanok VV, Martenson AM, Gianinazzi-Pearson V, Tikhonovich IA, 2003. Genetic Variability in Tolerance to Cadmium and Accumulation of Heavy Metals in Pea (*Pisum sativum* L.). *Euphytica* 131:25-35 (revised version published online in August 2006).

Bell ML, Davis DL, 2001. Reassessment of the Lethal London Fog of 1952: Novel Indicators of Acute and Chronic Consequences of Acute Exposure to Air Pollution. *Environ. Health Perspect.* 109(Suppl 3):389-394.

Bellastella A, Pisano G, Iorio S, Pasquali D, Orio F, Venditto T, Sinisi AA, 1998. Endocrine Secretions under Abnormal Light-Dark Cycles and in the Blind. *Hormone Res.* 49:153-157.

Boina DR, Onagbola EO, Salyani M, Stelinski LL, 2009. Influence of Posttreatment Temperature on the Toxicity of Insecticides against *Diaphorina citri* (Hemiptera: Psyllidae). *Hort. Entomol.* 102:685-691.

Boyce P, Kennaway DJ, 1987. Effects of Light on Melatonin Production. *Biol. Psych.* 22:473-478.

Burk RF, Masters BSS, 1975. Some Effects of Selenium Deficiency on the Hepatic Microsomal Cytochrome P-450 System in the Rat. *Arch. Biochem. Biophys.* 170:124-131.

Campbell TC, Hayes JR, 1976. The Effect of Quantity and Quality of Dietary Protein on Drug Metabolism. *Fed. Proc.* 35:2470-2474.

Castillo LS, Timiras PS, 1964. Electroconvulsive Responses of Rats to Convulsant and Anticonvulsant Drugs during High Altitude Acclimatization. *J. Pharmacol. Exp. Ther.* 146:160-166.

Century B, 1973. A Role of the Dietary Lipid in the Ability of Phenobarbital to Stimulate Drug Detoxification. *J. Pharmacol. Exp. Ther.* 185:185-194.

Chandler JH, Sanders HO, Walsh DF, 1974. An Improved Chemical Delivery Apparatus for Use in Intermittent-Flow Bioassays. *Bull. Environ. Contam. Toxicol.* 12:123-128.

Chen JJ, Chen Y-J, Rice G, Teuschler LK, Hamernik K, Protzel A, Kodell RL, 2001. Using Dose Addition to Estimate Cumulative Risks from Exposures to Multiple Chemicals. *Regul. Toxicol. Pharmacol.* 34:35-41.

Clinton SK, Mulloy AL, Visek WJ, 1984. Effects of Dietary Lipid Saturation on Prolactin Secretion, Carcinogen Metabolism and Mammary Carcinogenesis in Rats. *J. Nutri.* 114:1630-1639.

Czesny S, Rinchard J, Abiado MAG, Dabrowski K, 2003. The Effect of Fasting, Prolonged Swimming, and Predator Presence on Energy Utilization and Stress in Juvenile Walleye (*Stizostedion vitreum*). *Physiol. Behav.* 79:597-603.

Czygan P, Greim H, Garro A, Schaffner F, Popper H, 1974. The Effect of Dietary Protein Deficiency on the Ability of Isolated Hepatic Microsomes to Alter the Mutagenicity of a Primary and a Secondary Carcinogen. *Cancer Res.* 34:119-123.

Dave G, 1981. Influence of Diet and Starvation on Toxicity of Endrin to Fathead Minnows (*Pimephales promelas*). EPA-600/S3-81-048. U. S. Environmental Protection Agency, Environmental Research Laboratory, CERI, Duluth, Minnesota, USA.

Dieke SH, Richter CP, 1945. Acute Toxicity of Thiourea to Rats in Relation to Age, Diet, Strain and Species Variation. *J. Pharmacol. Exp. Ther.* 83:195-202.

Eaton DL, Klaassen CD, 2001. Principles of Toxicology. In *Casarett and Doull's Toxicology: The Basic Science of Poisons* (Klaassen CD, Ed.), 6th Edition. New York, New York, USA: McGraw-Hill, Chapter 2.

Eckhert C, 2006. Other Trace Elements. In *Modern Nutrition in Health and Disease* (Shils ME, Shike M, Ross AC, Caballero B, Cousins RJ, Eds.), 10th Edition. Philadelphia, Pennsylvania, USA: Lippincott, Williams & Wilkins, pp.338-350.

Eeva T, Hakkarainen H, Laaksonen T, Lehikoinen E, 2006. Environmental Pollution Has Sex-Dependent Effects on Local Survival. *Biol. Lett.* 2:298-300.

Erickson DH, Erickson LC, Seely CI, 1972. Effects of Light Quantities and Glucose on 2,4-D Toxicity to Canada Thistle. *Weed Sci.* 20:384-386.

Erren TC, Jacobsen M, Piekarski C, 1999. Synergism between Asbestos and Smoking on Lung Cancer Risks. *Epidemiology* 10:405-411.

Farooqi ZR, Iqbal MZ, Kabir M, Shafiq M, 2009. Toxic Effects of Lead and Cadmium on Germination and Seedling Growth of *Albizia Lebbeck* (L.) Benth. *Pak. J. Bot.* 41:27-33.

Fischer E, 1941. Prophylaxis against Lethal Effect of High Altitude by Means of a Digitalis Glycoside (Gitalin). *Am. Heart J.* 21:545-550.

Fosmire GJ, 1990. Zinc Toxicity. *Am. J. Clin. Nutri.* 51:225-227.

Franklin NM, Stauber JL, Markich SJ, Lim RP, 2000. pH-Dependent Toxicity of Copper and Uranium to a Tropical Freshwater Alga (*Chlorella* sp.). *Aquatic Toxicol.* 48:275-289.

Gaylor DW, 2000. The Use of Haber's Law in Standard Setting and Risk Assessment. *Toxicology* 149:17-19.

Haag JR, Palmer LS, 1928. The Effect of Variations in the Proportions of Calcium, Magnesium, and Phosphorus Contained in the Diet. *J. Biol. Chem.* 76:361-365.

Hayes JR, Mgbodile MUK, Campbell TC, 1973. Effect of Protein Deficiency on the Inducibility of the Hepatic Microsomal Drug-Metabolizing Enzyme System – I: Effect on Substrate Interaction with Cytochrome P-450. *Biochem. Pharmacol.* 22:1005-1014.

Ho K, Kuhn A, Pelletier M, Hendricks T, Helmstetter A, 1999. pH Dependent Toxicity of Five Metals to Three Marine Organisms. *Environ. Toxicol.* 14:235-240.

Horiike N, Abe M, Kumagi T, Hiasa Y, Akbar SMF, Michitaka K, Onji M, 2005. The Quantification of Cytochrome P-450 (CYP 3A4) mRNA in the Blood of Patients with Viral Liver Diseases. *Clin. Biochem.* 38: 531-534.

Hymer WC, Welsch J, Buchmann E, Risius M, Whelan HT, 2009. Modulation of Rat Pituitary Growth Hormone by 670 nm Light. *Growth Horm. IGF Res.* 19:274-279.

Iwasaki M, Iwama M, Miyata N, Iitoi Y, Kanke Y, 1994. Effects of Vitamin E Deficiency on Hepatic Microsomal Cytochrome P450 and Phase II Enzymes in Male and Female Rats. *Intern. J. Vitam. Nutri. Res.* 64: 109-112.

Jacobson AR, Morris SC, 1976. The Primary Air Pollutants: Viable Particulates, Their Occurrences, Sources and Effects. In *Air Pollution* (Stern AC, Ed.), 3rd Edition. New York, New York, USA: Academic Press, Vol.1, pp.169-196.

Jagadeesan V, Oesch F, 1988. Effects of Dietary Zinc Deficiency on the Activity of Enzymes Associated with Phase I and II of Drug Metabolism in Fischer-344 Rats: Activities of Drug Metabolising Enzymes in Zinc Deficiency. *Drug Nutri. Interact.* 5:403-413.

John R, Ahmad P, Gadgill K, Sharma S, 2008. Effect of Cadmium and Lead on Growth, Biochemical Parameters and Uptake in *Lemna polyrrhiza* L. *Plant Soil Environ.* 54:262-270.

Kaloyanova F, Tasheva M, 1983. Effect of Protein Malnutrition on Toxicity of Pesticides. In *Pesticide Chemistry, Human Welfare, and the Environment* (Miyamoto J, Kearney PC, Eds.) – Volume 3: Mode of Action, Metabolism, and Toxicology. Oxford, London, UK: Pergamon Press, pp.527-529.

Kasuya E, Kushibiki S, Yayou K, Hodate K, Sutoh M, 2008. Light Exposure during Night Suppresses Nocturnal Increase in Growth Hormone Secretion in Holstein Steers. *J. Anim. Sci.* 86:1799-1807.

Kato N, Tani T, Yoshida A, 1981. Effect of Dietary Quality of Protein on Liver Microsomal Mixed Function Oxidase System, Plasma Cholesterol and Urinary Ascorbic Acid in Rats Fed PCB. *J. Nutri.* 111:123-133.

Kawano S, Hiraga K, 1980. Effect of Dietary Protein Deficiency on Rat Hepatic Drug-Metabolizing Enzyme System. *Japan J. Pharmacol.* 30:75-83.

Khan MA, Ahmed SA, Salazar A, Gurumendi J, Khan A, Vargas M, von Catalin B, 2007. Effect of Temperature on Heavy Metal Toxicity to Earthworm *Lumbricus terrestris* (Annelida: Oligochaeta). *Environ. Toxicol.* 22:487-494.

Kim J-S, Ahn T, Yim S-K, Yun C-H, 2002. Differential Effect of Copper (II) on the Cytochrome P450 Enzymes and NADPH-Cytochrome P450 Reductase: Inhibition of Cytochrome P450-Catalyzed Reactions by Copper (II) Ion. *Biochemistry* 41:9438-9447.

Kobayashi K, Kishino T, 1980. Effect of pH on the Toxicity and Accumulation of Pentachlorophenol in Goldfish. *Bull. Japan. Soc. Sci. Fish* 46:167-170.

Korashy HM, El-Kadi AOS, 2005. Regulatory Mechanisms Modulating the Expression of Cytochrome P450 1A1 Gene by Heavy Metals. *Toxicol. Sci.* 88:39-51.

Korourian S, Hakkak R, Ronis MJ, Shelnutt SR, Waldron J, Ingelman-Sundberg M, Badger TM, 1999. Diet and Risk of Ethanol-Induced Hepatotoxicity: Carbohydrate-Fat Relationships in Rats. *Toxicol. Sci.* 47:110-117.

Letelier ME, Faúndez M, Jara-Sandoval J, Molina-Berríos A, Cortés-Troncoso J, Aracena-Parks P, Marín-Catalán R, 2009. Mechanisms Underlying the Inhibition of the Cytochrome P450 System by Copper Ions. *J. Appl. Toxicol.* 29:695-702.

Li H, Feng T, Liang P, Shia X, Gao X, Jiang H, 2006. Effect of Temperature on Toxicity of Pyrethroids and Endosulfan, Activity of Mitochondrial Na^+- K^+-ATPase and Ca^{2+}- Mg^{2+}-ATPase in *Chilo suppressalis* (Walker) (Lepidoptera: Pyralidae). *Pest. Biochem. Physiol.* 86:151-156.

Liccione JJ, Maines MD, 1989. Manganese-Mediated Increase in the Rat Brain Mitochondrial Cytochrome P-450 and Drug Metabolism Activity: Susceptibility of the Striatum. *J. Pharmacol. Exp. Ther.* 248:222-228.

Manno M, Rezzadore M, Grossi M, Sbrana C, 1996. Potentiation of Occupational Carbon Tetrachloride Toxicity by Ethanol Abuse. *Human Exp. Toxicol.* 15:294-300.

Marshall WJ, McLean AEM, 1971. A Requirement for Dietary Lipids for Induction of Cytochrome P-450 by Phenobarbitone in Rat Liver Microsomal Fraction. *Biochem. J.* 122:569-573.

Metwally A, Safronova VI, Belimov AA, Dietz K-J, 2005. Genotypic Variation of the Response to Cadmium Toxicity in *Pisum sativum* L. *J. Exp. Botany* 56:167-178.

Michnowicz CJ, Weaks TE, 1984. Effects of pH on Toxicity of As, Cr, Cu, Ni and Zn to *Selenastrum capricornutum* Printz. *Hydrobiologia* 118:299-305.

Miranda CL, Webb RE, 1973. Effects of Dietary Protein Quality on Drug Metabolism in the Rat. *J. Nutri.* 103:1425-1430.

Miranda CL, Mukhtara H, Benda JR, Chhabra RS, 1979. Effects of Vitamin A Deficiency on Hepatic and Extrahepatic Mixed-Function Oxidase and Epoxide Metabolizing Enzymes in Guinea Pig and Rabbit. *Biochem. Pharmacol.* 28:2713-2716.

Nicolson TJ, Mellor HR, Roberts RR, 2010. Gender Differences in Drug Toxicity. *Trends Pharmacol. Sci.* 31:108-114.

Oestreicher P, Cousins RJ, 1985. Copper and Zinc Absorption in the Rat: Mechanism of Mutual Antagonism. *J. Nutri.* 115:159-166.

Omaye ST, 2004. *Food and Nutritional Toxicology*, Boca Raton, Florida, USA:CRC Press, Chapter 1 (p.3).

Peraza MA, Ayala-Fierro F, Barber DS, Casarez E, Rael LT, 1998. Effects of Micronutrients on Metal Toxicity. *Environ. Health Perspect.* 106(Suppl 1):203-216.

Plaa GL, Hewitt WR, du Souich P, Caill G, Lock S, 1982. Isopropanol and Acetone Potentiation of Carbon Tetrachloride-Induced Hepatotoxicity: Single *versus* Repetitive Pretreatments in Rats. *J. Toxicol. Environ. Health* 9(Part A):235-250.

Pole CA III, Burnett RT, Turner MC, Cohen A, Krewski D, Jerrett M, Gapstur SM, Thun MJ, 2011. Lung Cancer and Cardiovascular Disease Mortality Associated with Ambient Air Pollution and Cigarette Smoke: Shape of the Exposure-Response Relationships. *Environ. Health Perspect.* 119:1616-1621.

Pollack T, Crabtree G, 1976. Effect of Light Intensity and Quality on Toxicity of Fluorodifen to Green Bean and Soybean Seedlings. *Weed Sci.* 24:571-574.

Prasad R, Nath R, 1995. Cadmium-Induced Nephrotoxicity in Rhesus Monkeys (*Macaca mulatta*) in Relation to Protein Calorie Malnutrition. *Toxicology* 100:89-100.

Ramírez-Farías C, Madrigal-Santillán E, Gutiérrez-Salinas J, Rodríguez-Sánchez N, Martínez-Cruz M, Valle-Jones I, Gramlich-Martínez I, Hernández-Ceruelos A, Morales-Gonzaléz JA, 2008. Protective Effect of Some Vitamins against the Toxic Action of Ethanol on Liver Regeneration Induced by Partial Hepatectomy in Rats. *World J. Gastroenterol.* 14:899-907.

Reiter RJ, Tan DX, Korkmaz A, Erren TC, Piekarski C, Tamura H, Manchester LC, 2007. Light at Night, Chronodisruption, Melatonin Suppression, and Cancer Risk: A Review. *Crit. Rev. Oncog.* 13:303-328.

Rikans LE, 1982. NADPH-Dependent Reduction of Cytochrome P-450 in Liver Microsomes from Vitamin C-Deficient Guinea Pigs: Effect of Benzphetamine. *J. Nutri.* 112:1796-1800.

Ross JH, Dong MH, Krieger RI, 2000. Conservatism in Pesticide Exposure Assessment. *Regul. Toxicol. Pharmaco.* 31:53-58.

Rowe FP, Redfern R, 1964. The Toxicity of 0.025% Warfarin to Wild House Mice (*Mus muscultu* L.). *J. Hyg., Camb.* 62:389-393.

Rowe FP, Redfern R, 1967. The Effect of Sex and Age on the Response to Warfarin in a Non-Inbred Strain of Mice. *J. Hyg. Camb.* 65:55-60.

Saito M, Oh-Hashi A, Kubota M, Nishide E, Yamaguchi M, 1990. Mixed Function Oxidases in Response to Different Types of Dietary Lipids in Rats. *Br. J. Nutri.* 63:249-257.

Salama Z, El-Beltagi H, El-Hariri D, 2009. Effect of Fe Deficiency on Antioxidant System in Leaves of Three Flax Cultivars. *Not. Bot. Hort. Agrobot. Cluj.* 37:122-128.

Sato PH, Zannoni VG, 1976. Ascorbic Acid and Hepatic Drug Metabolism. *J. Pharmaco. Exp. Ther.* 198: 295-307.

Sawyer TW, Vair C, Nelson P, Shei Y, Bjarnason S, Tenn C, McWilliams M, Villanueva M, Burczyk A, 2007. pH-Dependent Toxicity of Sulphur Mustard *in vitro*. *Toxicol. Appl. Pharmacol.* 221:363-371.

SBMLIC (Statistical Bulletin Metropolitan Life Insurance Company), 1992: Cancer Prevention Study II. The American Cancer Society Prospective Study. *Stat. Bull. Metrop. Insur. Co.* 73:21-29.

Schulsinger DA, Root MM, Campbell TC, 1989. Effect of Dietary Protein Quality on Development of Aflatoxin B1-Induced Hepatic Preneoplastic Lesions. *JNCI* 81:1241-1245.

Sekiya J, Wilson LG, Filner P, 1982. Resistance to Injury by Sulfur Dioxide: Correlation with Its Reduction to, and Emission of, Hydrogen Sulfide in Cucurbitaceae. *Plant Physiol.* 70:437-441.

Sheppard SC, 1992. Summary of Phytotoxic Levels of Soil Arsenic. *Water, Air, Soil Poll.* 64:539-550.

Shivarajashankara YM, Shivashankara AR, Bhat PG, Rao SH, 2001. Effect of Fluoride Intoxication on Lipid Peroxidation and Antioxidant Systems in Rats. *Fluoride* 34:108-113.

Sielken RL, 2000. Risk Metrics and Cumulative Risk Assessment Methodology for the FQPA. *Regul. Toxicol. Pharmacol.* 31:300-307.

Singh SN, Vats P, Kumria MML, Ranganathan S, Shyam R, Arora MP, Jain CL, Sridharan K, 2001. Effect of High Altitude (7,620 m) Exposure on Glutathione and Related Metabolism in Rats. *Europ. J. Appl. Physiol.* 84:233-237.

Sonawane BR, Coates PM, Yaffe SJ, Koldovsky O, 1983. Influence of Dietary Carbohydrates (Alpha-Saccharides) on Hepatic Drug Metabolism in Male Rats. *Drug Nutri. Interact.* 2:7-16.

Stalling DL, Mayer FL Jr, 1972. Toxicities of PCBs to Fish and Environmental Residues. *Environ. Health Perspect.* 1:159-164.

Sun H, Frassetto L, Benet LZ, 2006. Effects of Renal Failure on Drug Transport and Metabolism. *Pharmacol. Ther.* 109:1-11.

Sun Y, Zhou Q, Diao C, 2008. Effects of Cadmium and Arsenic on Growth and Metal Accumulation of Cd-Hyperaccumulator *Solanum nigrum* L. *Bioresource Technol.* 99:1103-1110.

Suskind RR, 1977. Environment and the Skin. *Environ. Health Perspect.* 20:27-37.

Swenberg JA, 1993. Alpha 2µ-Globulin Nephropathy: Review of the Cellular and Molecular Mechanisms Involved and Their Implications for Human Risk Assessment. *Environ. Health Perspect.* 101(Suppl 6): 39-44.

Taniguchi M, 1980. Effects of Riboflavin Deficiency on Lipid Peroxidation of Rat Liver Microsomes. *J. Nutri. Sci. Vitaminol.* 26:401-413.

Tewari RK, Kumar P, Neetu, Sharma PN, 2005. Signs of Oxidative Stress in the Chlorotic Leaves of Iron Starved Plants. *Plant Sci.* 169:1037-1045.

Tsukada H, Wang P-Y, Kaneko T, Wang Y, Nakano M, Sato A, 1998. Dietary Carbohydrate Intake Plays an Important Role in Preventing Alcoholic Fatty Liver in the Rat. *J. Hepatol.* 29:715-724.

Vats P, Singh VK, Singh SN, Singh SB, 2008. Glutathione Metabolism under High-Altitude Stress and Effect of Antioxidant Supplementation. *Aviation, Space Environ. Med.* 79:1106-1111.

Viswanathan PN, Murti CRK, 1989. Effects of Temperature and Humidity on Ecotoxicology of Chemicals. In *Ecotoxicology and Climate* (Bourdeau P, Haines JA, Klein W, Murti CRK, Eds.). New York, New York, USA: John Wiley & Sons, pp.139-154.

Wade AE, Norred WP, 1976. Effect of Dietary Lipid on Drug-Metabolizing Enzymes. *Fed. Proc.* 35:2475-2479.

Watanabe M, Kumai T, Matsumoto N, Tanaka M, Suzuki S, Satoh T, Kobayashi S, 2004. Expression of CYP3A4 mRNA Is Correlated with CYP3A4 Protein Level and Metabolic Activity in Human Liver. *J. Pharmacol. Sci.* 94:459-462.

Wolansky MJ, Gennings C, DeVito MJ, Crofton KM, 2009. Evidence for Dose-Additive Effects of Pyrethroids on Motor Activity in Rats. *Environ. Health Perspect.* 117:1563-1570.

Woolson EA, 1973. Arsenic Phytotoxicity and Uptake in Six Vegetable Crops. *Weed Sci.* 21:524-527.

Yasukochi Y, Nakamura M, Minakami S, 1977. Effect of Cobalt on the Synthesis of Liver Microsomal Cytochromes. *J. Biochem.* 81:1005-1009.

Yedjou C, Thuisseu L, Tchounwou C, Gomes M, Howard C, Tchounwou P, 2009. Ascorbic Acid Potentiation of Arsenic Trioxide Anticancer Activity against Acute Promyelocytic Leukemia. *Arch. Drug Inf.* 2:59-65.

Yoo JH, Ning SM, Pantuck CB, Pantuck EJ, Yang CS, 1991. Regulation of Hepatic Microsomal Cytochrome P450IIE1 Level by Dietary Lipids and Carbohydrates in Rats. *J. Nutri.* 121:959-965.

Yoo JS, Park HS, Ning SM, Lee MJ, Yang CS, 1990. Effects of Thiamine Deficiency on Hepatic Cytochromes P450 and Drug-Metabolizing Enzyme Activities. *Biochem. Pharmacol.* 39:519-525.

Review Questions
1. What should be considered as the most important environmental factor in terms of potential for affecting the toxicity of environmental toxicants?
2. How were the weekly air concentrations of SO_2 related to the weekly mortality in the Greater London area during October 1952 through March 1953?
3. Explain why the LC_{50} of Aroclor 1248, as shown in Table 10.2, could have such a wide range as from 10 µg/L to 307 µg/L.
4. What appears to be the shape of the exposure-response relationship for lung cancer mortality with cigarette smoking that is supported by the adjusted relative risk estimates shown in Table 10.3. (Will a person have a similar risk for lung cancer if he smokes 10 cigarettes every day *vs.* if he is exposed to $PM_{2.5}$ at a daily dose of 120 mg?)
5. Give a numerical example (along with certain assumptions) for the potential fallacy of using Haber's law to estimate (the level of) environmental exposure.

6. Why is it important to understand the mode of contact and the control measure in effect when assessing environmental exposure?
7. How can temperature, humidity, or altitude affect the toxicity of certain environmental toxicants?
8. How is light related to the diurnal rhythm in humans that can affect their exposures to certain environmental toxicants?
9. What is likely the common biochemical mode whereby many nutrients can affect the toxicity of environmental toxicants?
10. How can dietary lipids that contain linoleic acid biochemically affect the toxicity of certain environmental toxicants?
11. Briefly describe how high and low levels of dietary carbohydrates can affect the toxicity of certain environmental toxicants.
12. Give a chemical example for the potential that excessive zinc (Zn) intake can indirectly affect the toxicity of certain environmental toxicants.
13. Give a chemical example for each of the following joint toxic effect patterns: a) additivity; b) potentiation; c) synergism; d) dispositional form of antagonism; e) chemical form of antagonism.
14. Explain why unleaded gasoline can induce kidney tumor in only male but not female rats.
15. Briefly explain how kidney disease can affect the toxicity of an environmental toxicant.
16. Briefly explain why genetic polymorphism of CYP2D6 is a clinically important issue to human health.

CHAPTER 11

Air Pollutants – I: Inorganic Gases

୨•ଓ

11.1. Introduction

All air pollutants of concern are confined to the troposphere, which is the lowest layer of the Earth's atmosphere extending to about 10 miles (16 kilometers) above sea level. This air zone, in which almost all of the Earth's weather occurs, contains about 75 to 80% of the atmosphere's mass and 99% of its water (H_2O) vapor and dust particles. The cooler, second layer of Earth's atmosphere is the stratosphere, just above the troposphere and below the mesosphere. The air that humans breathe is present in the troposphere, and is a mixture of (mostly) gaseous substances containing approximately 78.1% nitrogen (N_2) and 20.9% oxygen (O_2) molecules. The substances in the remaining ~1% include roughly: 0.8% argon (Ar); 0.03% carbon dioxide (CO_2); and collectively, 0.04% of H_2O vapor, trace gases such as helium (He) and neon (Ne), as well as all air pollutants. It is with such an atmospheric composition that in most situations, any pollutant found in the air that humans breathe is not considered having concentrations sufficient to pose any *acute* or *immediate* health threat. Otherwise, inhalation is a major route of environmental exposure insomuch as an average human adult inhales over 12,000 liters of air every day.

11.1.1. Hazardous Air Pollutants

Over 200 hazardous air pollutants have been detected in the ambient air. These toxic air pollutants, also referred to as air toxics, are substances that can cause cancer or other serious health effects. Where applicable, some of these air toxics are discussed in other chapters. For instance, airborne residues such as those of the fumigant methyl bromide and the industrial chemical asbestos are discussed in Chapters 15 and 20, respectively. The list of air toxics considered by U.S. EPA, as mandated by the U.S. Clean Air Act Amendments of 1990, does not include commonly found air pollutants such as the inorganic gases discussed in this chapter or the particulate matter (PM) and the volatile organic compounds (VOCs) covered, respectively, in the next two chapters.

11.1.2. Criteria Inorganic Gaseous Pollutants

The air pollutants that U.S. EPA has found to occur commonly over the United States include sulfur dioxide (SO_2), nitrogen oxides (NO_x), ozone (O_3), carbon monoxide (CO), lead (Pb), and PM. These six air pollutants are designated as the "criteria air pollutants" due to the U.S. Clean Air Act mandate directing U.S. EPA to adopt a *National Ambient Air Quality Standard* (NAAQS) for each of these six air pollutants. According to the U.S. Clean Air Act, airborne particles of lead compounds are also treated as air toxics. The nature and effects of lead, along with those of some other toxic metals, are discussed in Chapter 14.

In this chapter, the four criteria inorganic gaseous pollutants (i.e., SO_2, NO_x, O_3, CO) are considered separately in their respective sections that follow. The discussion on each of these four inorganic gases focuses on primarily the same three fundamental aspects: (1) its sources of pollution; (2) its characteristics and physicochemical properties; and (3) its adverse effects on humans, animals, plants, and the environment, where appropriate or applicable.

Several other inorganic gases, such as ammonia (NH_3), hydrogen sulfide (H_2S), chlorine (Cl_2), hydrogen chloride (HCl), and hydrogen fluoride (HF), are also harmful or for some even more so. However, due to space limitation and their relative infrequency in occurrence, these other inorganic gases are not specifically discussed in this or other chapters.

11.2. Sulfur Dioxide

Sulfur dioxide (SO_2) is the most predominant member of a family of highly reactive gases known as sulfur oxides (SO_x). Another member that is also a significant but less common air pollutant is sulfur trioxide (SO_3). Historically, SO_2 was responsible for several acute air pollution episodes, including those occurring in Meuse Valley in October of 1930, in Donora in December of 1948, and in London in December of 1952. The London fog of 1952, as mentioned in Section 10.2.1A, resulted in around 4,000 excess deaths and 100,000 extra illness cases due to the smog's effects on their respiratory or cardiovascular system. The smog was reportedly the result of the cold, stagnant fog contaminated with chimney smoke, the particulates from vehicle exhausts, and other pollutants including especially SO_2. The death tolls from the two earlier smog disasters noted above were on a much smaller scale, with 60 to 70 deaths occurring in the populated valley near Liege, Belgium and about 20 deaths in the American mill town Donora, Pennsylvania.

11.2.1. Sources of Pollution

In the United States, around 94% of all SO_2 emissions from anthropogenic sources in 2016 were from fossil fuel combustion at electric power plants (~73%) and other industrial facilities (~21%). The remaining ~6% included emissions from industrial processes (e.g., extracting metals from ore), paper and pulp manufacturing, and the burning of high sulfur-containing fuels by trains, large ships, and diesel trucks (U.S. EPA, 2017a). The apparently good news (U.S. EPA, 2017b) is that the national annual (daily maximum 1-hour average) air levels of SO_2 declined 84% between 1980 (159.8 ppb) and 2015 (25.3 ppb).

Environmental exposure to SO_2 is usually at its highest outdoors in the summer months, when smoke pollutants will react more readily and more actively with the sun and hot temperatures to form smog. Levels of SO_2 in the air are typically higher than normal within or near facilities that release the air pollutant through heavy industrial activities (e.g., copper smelting, processing or combustion of coal and petroleum oil at electric power plants). People can also be exposed to SO_2 if they work in or are around places producing sulfuric acid (H_2SO_4), paper, pulp, fertilizers, or food preservatives.

Owing to its strong antimicrobial and antioxidant properties, SO_2 is commonly employed as food preservatives for many dried fruits, vegetables, and alcoholic drinks. It also has the following uses: as a disinfectant; as an intermediate for making other substances; for bleaching flour, textile fibers, and glue; for winemaking; and for water treatment. SO_2 is a high-volume product applied in the United States, with a market valued at 5 billion dollars in 2015 (TMR, 2016).

Natural pollution sources of SO_2 include biological or plant decays but predominately volcanoes. While emissions of SO_2 caused by human activity far exceed its natural emissions in the developed and developing countries, natural processes are responsible for roughly half of the world's atmospheric sulfur (S) which in the presence of oxygen (O_2) and high temperatures can form SO_2 (Reaction 11.1). Along with CO_2 and HF, SO_2 is the volcanic gas posing the greatest potential hazard to humankind and ecosystems. Large explosive eruptions can result in a tremendous volume of sulfur aerosols injected into the stratosphere, where the aerosols can promote depletion of the ozone layer and eventually cause lower, undesired temperatures on the Earth's surface.

11.2.2. Characteristics and Properties

Sulfur dioxide is a nonflammable, colorless, irritating, liquefied compressed gas when packaged in cylinders under its own vapor pressure (35 psig at 21.1° C or 70° F). It has an acidic, pungent, and suffocating odor, detectable at 3 to 5 ppm (parts per million); at 0.5 to 1 ppm, it leaves an acidic taste in the human mouth. This inorganic gas can cause severe chemical burns if inhaled or upon skin contact at high doses. Its general physicochemical properties are listed in Table 11.1.

Table 11.1. General Physicochemical Properties of Sulfur Dioxide $(SO_2)^a$

Molecular weight	64.1
Vapor pressure	35 psig (at 21.1° C)
Boiling point	−10° C (at 1 atm)
Vapor density (specific gravity)	2.25 (with air = 1)
Melting point	−75.5° C (at 1 atm)
Gas density	2.93 kg/m^3 (at 0° C and 1 atm)

^{a}mainly from various handbooks on physical and chemical properties of inorganic compounds.

In the laboratory, SO_2 gas can be formed by addition of hydrochloric acid (HCl-H_2O) to solid sodium sulfite ($NaSO_3$). Commercially or more commonly, the gas can be produced by burning the element S (sulfur), by combusting hydrogen sulfide (H_2S), or by roasting of sulfide ores such as pyrite (FeS_2) and chalcocite (Cu_2S), as shown below in Reactions 11.1 through 11.4 (where $s \equiv$ solid, $g \equiv$ gas):

$$S\,(s) + O_2\,(g) \rightarrow SO_2\,(g) \tag{11.1}$$

$$2\,H_2S\,(g) + 3O_2\,(g) \rightarrow 2H_2O\,(g) + 2SO_2\,(g) \tag{11.2}$$

$$4FeS_2\,(s) + 9O_2\,(g) \rightarrow 2Fe_2SO_3\,(s) + 6SO_2\,(g) \tag{11.3}$$

$$2Cu_2S\,(s) + 3O_2\,(g) \rightarrow 2Cu_2O\,(s) + 2SO_2\,(g) \tag{11.4}$$

In general, SO_2 gas is formed whenever sulfur-containing fuels (e.g., coal, petroleum oil) are burned. Pyrite (FeS_2) is the most common of the sulfide minerals. This mineral is commonly found co-existing with other sulfides or oxides, such as chalcopyrite ($CuFeS_2$). Chalcopyrite and Cu_2S (chalcocite) are the most abundant minerals found in copper (Cu) ores and hence in copper smelting plants as well.

Oxidation of SO_2 with oxygen, in the presence of a certain catalyst, can form the acid H_2SO_4. For example, when the catalyst used is vanadium pentoxide (V_2O_5), SO_3 is formed first which is then hydrated into the acid, as shown below in Reaction 11.5 (where $l \equiv$ liquid).

$$2SO_2\ (g) + O_2\ (g) \rightarrow 2SO_3\ (g), \text{ with } V_2O_5 \text{ as the catalyst} \tag{11.5a}$$

$$SO_3\ (g) + H_2O\ (l) \rightarrow H_2SO_4\ (g) \tag{11.5b}$$

In the troposphere, atmospheric SO_2 can be readily oxidized to SO_3 by hydroxyl radical (HO·) followed by O_2, as discussed in Section 5.2.3C (e.g., Reactions 5.8 through 5.10). The resultant H_2SO_4 then becomes the (principal) acidic component of acid rain. The hydroxyl radical, on the other hand, can readily become available as a by-product component of the photochemical smog reaction (Reaction 5.3) discussed in Section 5.2.3B.

11.2.3. Toxic Effects and Advisories

Sulfur dioxide (SO_2) is both a potent phytotoxicant and a strong respiratory irritant. It is largely due to such concerns that U.S. EPA (2010a) has set a maximum 1-hour average of 75 ppb (parts per billion) as the *primary* NAAQS (National Ambient Air Quality Standard) for protection of public *health* from SO_2 exposure. The guideline values set forth by the World Health Organization (WHO, 2006) are 20 and 500 µg/m^3 (i.e., ~7 ppb and ~100 ppb) for a maximum 24-hour and a 10-minute average, respectively. For *secondary* NAAQS, which is for public *welfare* (including protection against reduced visibility and damage to animals, vegetation, and buildings), U.S. EPA (2012) has set a maximum 3-hour average of 500 ppb and an annual of 20 ppb as the limits. The guideline values set forth by WHO (2000a) for vegetation protection are an average of 30 µg/m^3 for annual exposure and an average of 100 µg/m^3 for a 24-hour exposure.

As noted in Section 11.2.1, the national annual (daily maximum 1-hour average) air levels of SO_2 in the United States declined 84% between 1980 and 2015. Yet despite such a significant decline in the national levels in the country (and in many other western countries), the air pollutant still represents a threat to public health and vegetation in certain local areas. For instance, U.S. EPA recently determined (e.g., Sierra Club, 2016) that in the eastern Texas, the air levels of SO_2 around the Big Brown, Martin Lake, and Monticello coal plants violated the NAAQS.

A. Effects on Humans and Animals

In humans and many other mammalians, inhalation is the principal route of exposure to SO_2, which is readily converted to sulfite (SO_3^-) and bisulfite (HSO_3^-) in the moist mucous membrane of the upper respiratory tract. Exposure to very high concentrations ($\geq$100 ppm) of this inorganic gas can be life-threatening, especially for asthmatic children. Otherwise, common symptoms from acute exposure to SO_2 include wheezing, chest tightness, and shortness of breath. From chronic exposure at 0.5 to 3 ppm, the effects include respiratory illness, modulation of the defense mechanisms in the lungs, and aggravation of existing cardiovascular disorders.

At least two health organizations (ATSDR, 1998; WHO, 2006) had evaluated extensively the large volumes of available epidemiological and animal toxicity data concerning environmental exposure to SO_2. Their reviews came down to three points. First, it was not certain if the chronic effects observed in workers were attributed to SO_2 exposure alone since these victims might have been exposed to other pollutants as well. Second, the thresholds for the health effects of SO_2 were highly variable, depending on the nature of local sources, the prevailing meteorological conditions, and the victim's asthmatic status. And third, which is more certain, studies in a range of animal species supported strongly the human data on airway damage (e.g., epithelial hyperplasia) and pulmonary effects (e.g., bronchoconstriction) from chronic exposure to SO_2.

The available studies (ATSDR, 1998) did not seem to provide any conclusive evidence supporting the reproductive or developmental effects of SO_2 exposure in humans, in part because those human study subjects exposed to SO_2 were exposed to other air pollutants as well. Another reason is that the animal data on developmental or maternal effects of SO_2 showed either negative or inconclusive support for their extrapolation to humans.

B. Effects on Plants

Uptake of SO_2 by plants is primarily via the stomata (i.e., the microscopic pores) located between the guard cells on leaf surfaces shielded by the epidermis (Figure 7.3). The symptoms associated with acute injury appear as necrotic lesions on both (the upper and underneath) leaf surfaces that usually occur between veins, with the color of the injured areas ranging from bleached white or light tan to reddish brown depending on the prevailing environmental conditions present and the plant species affected. With chronic injury, the affected plants usually have chlorotic leaves from paling to yellow with green veins.

For some plant species, both the enlarging (young) and older leaves tend to be more resistant to acute SO_2 injury, whereas the mature as well as fully expanded ones are typically the most sensitive (e.g., Daines, 1968; Sekiya *et al.*, 1982). A number of studies showed inter- and intra-species variations in plant sensitivity to SO_2 injury. Such variations can occur in part because SO_2 usually needs to first enter the stomata before leaf injury can take place. Yet the stomatal apertures are affected considerably by the specific environmental conditions that the plant is in. It has shown (e.g., Griffiths, 2003; Schubert, 1984) that certain species of crops (e.g., alfalfa, sweet clover), flowers (e.g., cosmos, violet, zinnia), trees (e.g., apple, American elm, pear), and vegetables (e.g., radish, carrot) tend to be more susceptible to SO_2 injury.

C. Effects of Acid Rain

Rain that falls on the ground as wet deposition may contain acidic components such as H_2SO_4 (sulfuric acid), a mineral liquid readily formed by oxidation of SO_2 in the troposphere. This type of rain, more formally termed *acid rain* or *acid deposition*, can have serious detrimental effects on the environment by acidifying soils, aquatic systems, and infrastructures. Acid rain can also reduce visibility. It was largely due to this kind of environmental concerns that U.S. Congress passed the Acid Deposition Act in 1980.

When falling down on plants, acid rain can damage their leaves ending in necrotic lesions or chlorotic tissues. In most situations, acid rain can reduce or inhibit plant germination and growth. When the soil is acidified, the plant roots can be severely damaged, along with a high potential for leaching of their nutrients (e.g., calcium, potassium) present in the soil proper nearby. Moreover, many soil microbes and their enzymes can be denatured by the high acidity so generated. Otherwise, via their enzymes, these microbes can help release nutrients from decaying leaves and other debris on the soil.

Acid rain can adversely affect many aquatic organisms and land animals. Fish and other aquatic creatures are particularly vulnerable, as they all need water to breathe. When the water is acidified, an aquatic organism's life and its reproductive function can be endangered. In particular, water acidity can cause a reduction of the calcium (Ca) levels in female fish to the point that either these creatures can no longer produce eggs, or their eggs will fail to pass through from their ovaries. Even when the eggs are fertilized, the freshly hatched larvae will not develop normally when the water that they are in has an unfavorably low pH (U.S. EPA, 1980).

Acids, including particularly sulfuric acid (H_2SO_4), have a corrosive effect on limestone and marble buildings. Marble and limestone are made of calcium carbonate ($CaCO_3$) which, when reacting with H_2SO_4 long enough, will get or become dissolved. Sulfuric acid is also corrosive to copper and the metal's alloys (e.g., bronze). It is reportedly said (*Harvard Magazine*, 2000) that due to such concerns, Harvard University now hides its bronze Large Four Piece Reclining Figure (sculptured by Henry Moore) for the winter in waterproof swaddling, which otherwise has reclined on the grass in front of this American university's Lamont Library for well over 20 years.

11.3. Nitrogen Oxides: Nitrogen Dioxide

Nitrogen dioxide (NO_2) and nitric oxide (NO) are the most predominant members of another family of highly reactive gases known as nitrogen oxides (NO_x). This section has its focus on NO_2 simply because NO can be readily converted to NO_2 in the presence of O_2 (Reaction 11.6). Both NO_2 and NO, along with their related compounds ozone (O_3) and peroxyacetylnitrate (PAN), are involved heavily in the photochemical smog reaction described in Section 5.2.3B. These oxidants were responsible for several acute air pollution episodes occurring in the greater Los Angeles area in the mid-1950s. Though on smaller scales and with concerns more on O_3 being the culprit, more recent episodes of this kind can still be found in many parts of the world where traffic congestion is particularly an issue, such as Beijing (Xu *et al.*, 2011), Delhi (Sati and Mohan, 2014), Denver (Benton-Short and DeSousa, 2014), Hong Kong (Xue *et al.*, 2016), Jakarta (Suhadi *et al.*, 2005), Rome (Movassaghi *et al.*, 2012), and Santiago (Rubio *et al.*, 2005).

11.3.1. Sources of Pollution

Whether from natural or anthropogenic sources, it does not seem fair or sufficient to discuss

NO$_2$ without considering NO, as both are the predominant components of NO$_x$ present frequently together and in large quantities. The two oxides are produced from a variety of natural processes in the air, water, and soil. Atmospheric nitrogen fixation is one natural process whereby diatomic nitrogen (N$_2$) in the air is separated by lightning into monatomic N which can then react with O$_2$ in the air to form NO$_x$ (Section 5.2.3D). Biological nitrogen fixation is another natural process in which N$_2$ is converted to mostly NH$_3$ (ammonia) first and then to NO$_x$ via the actions of certain algae in water or certain bacteria in soils and plants.

The primary anthropogenic sources of NO$_x$ are exhaust fumes from automobiles and emissions from electric utilities as well as other industrial processes. Although exhaust fumes have more NO than NO$_2$, the NO released readily reacts with O$_2$ in the air to form NO$_2$ (Reaction 11.6). In 2016, 95% of the 10.5 million tons of national NO$_x$ emissions in the United States were from on-road vehicles (34%), non-road engines (23%), fuel combustion (27%), and industrial processes (11%). The remaining ~5% was from numerous minor sources including waste disposal, residential wood combustion, solvent use, wildfires, and fertilizers (U.S. EPA, 2017a).

On-road traffic is likewise the major source of NO$_x$ emissions in Europe, accounting for over half of the annual total emissions in that region (EEA, 2002). In certain European cities such as London, it accounts for over 70% of the total toll there (Font and Fuller, 2016; Holman, 1999). As with London, recently Moscow and Paris have been reportedly ranked among the most congested cities in Europe.

Unlike SO$_2$, considerable levels of NO$_2$ gas are commonly found indoors in places burning fuel. The primary indoor sources of NO$_2$ include kerosene heaters, gas heaters, gas stoves, wood-burning fireplaces, and tobacco smoke. Due to these common sources, the indoor NO$_2$ concentrations can exceed those in the outdoor ambient air in the vicinity. An Ethiopian study (Kumie et al., 2009) found that housing conditions, season of the year, fire use characteristics, frequency of cooking, and agroecological (biomass) factors were the most important determinants of indoor NO$_2$ level. That study's findings were based on over 17,000 air samples collected in 3,300 rural local residences during a two-year investigation period.

11.3.2. Characteristics and Properties

At above room temperature (>21.1° C or 70° F), NO$_2$ is present as a reddish brown gas with a pungent odor. It is nonflammable, but accelerates burning of combustible materials. This inorganic gas can be readily generated via the oxidation of NO by O$_2$ in the air (Reaction 11.6).

$$2NO + O_2 \rightarrow 2NO_2 \qquad (11.6)$$

Nitrogen dioxide is a strong oxidizing agent and readily reacts with H$_2$O vapor in the air to form nitric acid (HNO$_3$), as shown in Reaction 11.7. Nitric acid, like H$_2$SO$_4$, is a highly corrosive substance and thus is also one of the major acidic constituents of acid rain. The acid is a precursor of certain components found in PM (particulate matter). Another pathway through which NO$_2$ can form HNO$_3$ is by reacting with the hydroxyl radical (HO·) from photochemistry in the atmosphere, as shown in Reaction 11.8.

$$3NO_2 + H_2O \rightarrow 2HNO_3 + NO \tag{11.7}$$

$$NO_2 + HO\cdot \rightarrow HNO_3 \tag{11.8}$$

Nitrogen dioxide and certain other NO_x members are precursors of a number of highly toxic secondary (i.e., second-generation) air pollutants including O_3 and the organic nitrate PAN. The general physicochemical properties of NO_2 are listed in Table 11.2.

Table 11.2. General Physicochemical Properties of Nitrogen Dioxide $(NO_2)^a$

Molecular weight	46.0
Boiling point	21.1° C (at 1 atm)
Vapor density (specific gravity)	1.58 (with air = 1)
Melting point	−11.2° C (at 1 atm)
Gas density	3.4 kg/m^3 (at 22° C and 1 atm)

^{a}mainly from various handbooks on physical and chemical properties of inorganic compounds.

11.3.3. Toxic Effects and Advisories

As with SO_2, NO_2 is not only a potent phytotoxicant but also a strong respiratory irritant. The HNO_3 in acid rain formed from NO_2 (e.g., Reaction 11.7) is corrosive to building materials at high concentrations. The organic nitrate PAN generated from NO_2 can cause haze to reduce visibility. The presence of NO_2 makes smog in summer look brownish. In the United States, there was a 59% decrease (U.S. EPA, 2017b) in national average emission of NO_2 between 1980 (108.5 ppb) and 2015 (44.6 ppb). Despite such a significant decline, U.S. EPA (2010b) has set a new 1-hour, health-based NAAQS of 100 ppb for short-term exposure to NO_2 while continuing to allow an average annual of 53 ppb as the primary and secondary NAAQS. The WHO (2006) guideline values for NO_2 are 200 µg/m^3 (~100 ppb) for 1 hour and 40 µg/m^3 for an annual average.

A. Effects on Humans and Animals

Nitrogen dioxide (NO_2) can irritate and burn the skin, the eyes, the nose, the throat, and/or the lungs, depending on its air concentrations in place. Inhalation of NO_2, particularly by children, can decrease the lung's ability to defend against bacteria and viruses and thereby increase the risk of respiratory infection. Exposure to NO_2 can also aggravate asthma or worsen pulmonary function in later life. Symptoms from low levels of NO_2 exposure may include coughing, shortness of breath, tiredness, nausea, and fluid buildup in the lungs. Exposure at very high concentrations of NO_2 can result in serious effects: rapid burning and spasms of tissues in the upper respiratory tract; interference with transport of oxygen across body tissues; buildup of fluid in the lungs; collapse; and death.

Long-term exposure to sufficiently high levels of NO_2 can lead to permanent lung damage. There is some evidence linking atmospheric levels of NO_2 to increases in daily mortality (Burnett *et al.*, 2004) and daily hospital admissions for pulmonary diseases (Linn *et al.*, 2000). There are also studies showing an association of NO_2 exposure with damage in the developing fetus (Brauer *et al.*, 2008) and with decreased fertility in men (Wiwanitkit, 2007). A case-control study showed that outdoor levels of NO_2 were significantly linked to sudden infant death syndrome (Klonoff-Cohen *et al.*, 2005). Another epidemiological study found an association between daily indoor exposure to NO_2 and asthmatic symptoms in children (Smith *et al.*, 2000).

Nitrogen dioxide is not only a precursor of the corrosive nitric acid HNO_3, but can also increase atmospheric deposition of nitrogen (N_2). Nitrogen is the element most responsible for eutrophication, a term typically used for over-enrichment of nutrients in aquatic systems to the point to cause a substantial reduction in O_2 availability in the water. This environmental effect, along with the effect of acid rain, provides an aquatic ecosystem that can be highly destructive to fish and other aquatic creatures.

B. Effects on Plants

Nitrogen dioxide (NO_2) can induce a highly negative effect on photosynthesis in plants. Symptoms from this kind of plant injury include random necrotic spots between leaf veins. Brownish-yellow spots can be seen on the marginal areas of broad leaves, whereas in coniferous leaves the browning typically occurs on their tips or mid-sections.

The inorganic gas can suppress plant growth. One study (Srivastava and Ormrod, 1986) in bean plants showed that when 8-day old seedlings were exposed to NO_2 at 0.02 to 0.5 ppm for 6 hours daily for 15 days, shoot growth was inhibited. Another study (Taylor and Eaton, 1966) revealed that when Pinto bean and Pearson-improved tomato seedlings were exposed to NO_2 at levels below 1 mg/m^3 for 10 to 22 days, significant growth suppression occurred, along with an increase in total chlorophyll content and distortion of leaves. When SO_2 or O_3 was present in certain species, the adverse effects caused jointly with NO_2 on their growth were found from additive to mostly synergistic (Reinert and Gray, 1981; Tingey *et al.*, 1971; White *et al.*, 1974).

The effects of NO_2 on plants appear to be species- and dose-specific. For instance, one study (Adam *et al.*, 2008a) found that exposure of *Mulukhiya* plants to NO_2 at 0.05 ppm in a controlled chamber promoted both vegetative growth and flowering. Two other studies (Adam *et al.*, 2008b; Takahashi *et al.*, 2005) showed that at ambient levels, NO_2 stimulated the vegetative growth of sunflower, lettuce, cucumber, and pumpkin. As hypothesized by the study authors, inasmuch as flowering is controlled by developmental and environmental signals, at the appropriate levels NO_2 might act as a signaling molecule rather than as a destructive pollutant.

11.4. Tropospheric Ozone

Ozone (O_3) is a gas found at substantial levels in both the troposphere and the stratosphere. In the troposphere, O_3 is a potent air pollutant to human health and ecosystems. In the stratosphere, the O_3 layer extends upward from about 10 to 30 miles (16 to 48 kilometers) to form a shield protecting life on the Earth from the sun's harmful ultraviolet (UV) rays. Like PAN, tropospheric O_3 is (largely) a secondary air pollutant, generated predominantly from the photolysis of NO_2. As such, both of these secondary pollutants along with NO_2 are involved in most of the air pollution episodes identified as caused by photochemical oxidants.

11.4.1. Sources of Pollution

Given that NO_2 is a major precursor of most O_3 found in the troposphere, the sources of tropospheric O_3 are similar to those of NO_x discussed in Section 11.3.1. Accordingly, many urban areas tend to have high levels of O_3 in their environment as well, particularly in the summer months. Nonetheless, O_3 is subject to long-range transport carried by winds and thereby can also be found at considerable levels in some rural areas. Both VOCs (Reaction 11.9) and CO (Reason 11.10) are also precursors of O_3 produced in the tropospheric environment.

Natural sources of O_3 include the small amounts from hydrocarbons (HCs) released by plants as well as soils, and the very small quantities in the stratosphere that occasionally migrate down to the Earth's surface. In addition, O_3 can be formed by generating high-power electrical discharges in air or oxygen. Due to its strong oxidation properties, O_3 has been produced for use in medicine, as a food disinfectant or sanitizer, and for cleaning or detoxification purposes. This inorganic gas is gaining popularity as a "green" alternative to chlorine for treatment of pool water. Generators that yield a high level of O_3 are now used preferentially by restaurants and hotels for removing foul odors in the shortest time in order to satisfy their (arriving) customers.

11.4.2. Characteristics and Properties

Under normal conditions, ozone is a gas with a strong, irritating, chlorine-like odor. It is a powerful oxidant as well as a strong corrosive agent and hence overall a highly toxic air pollutant. O_3 has a bluish color in either the gas or the liquid state. The inorganic gas changes to a liquid at $-112°$ C ($-170°$ F) and to a bluish-black solid at $-193°$ C ($-315°$ F).

The formation of tropospheric O_3 from a VOC precursor may involve the two steps in Reaction 11.9, where VOC being a HC compound is commonly denoted by R-C with the symbol C representing a carbon atom to which a reactive oxygen ion (O·) may attach.

$$R\text{-}C + O\cdot + O_2 \rightarrow R\text{-}CO + O_2 \rightarrow R\text{-}CO_3\cdot \tag{11.9a}$$

$$O_2 + R\text{-}CO_3\cdot \rightarrow R\text{-}CO_2 + O_3 \tag{11.9b}$$

Note that the highly reactive O· ion in Reaction 11.9a can come from the photodissociation of NO_2 into this reactive species plus NO (Section 5.2.3B). And the peroxide radical R-CO_3· has the counter effect of enhancing the formation of NO_2 by reacting with NO. Meantime, O· can readily react with O_2 to form O_3 (Reaction 5.4).

For tropospheric CO as the precursor, the formation of O_3 begins by reacting with the radical HO· in the atmosphere. The reaction of perhydroxyl radical HO_2· with NO forms NO_2 and HO·. That is, CO can form tropospheric O_3 by enhancing the formation of O· via its formation of NO_2 (Reaction 11.10) and then via the photolysis of NO_2 (Section 5.2.3B).

$$CO + HO\cdot \rightarrow CO_2 + H^+ \tag{11.10a}$$

$$H^+ + O_2 \rightarrow HO_2\cdot \tag{11.10b}$$

$$HO_2\cdot + NO \rightarrow HO\cdot + NO_2 \qquad (11.10c)$$

For O_3 in the stratosphere, it is generated at the expense of breaking the stratospheric diatomic oxygen (O_2) apart into two monatomic oxygen ions ($O\cdot$) upon absorption of an UV photon hv (whose wavelength is shorter than 240 nm). Each of the two $O\cdot$ ions then combines with a separate O_2 molecule nearby to form an O_3 molecule.

The physical and chemical properties of O_3 are very different from those of diatomic oxygen. Its general physicochemical properties are listed in Table 11.3.

Table 11.3. General Physicochemical Properties of Tropospheric Ozone $(O_3)^a$

Molecular weight	48.0
Boiling point	$-111.3°$ C (at 1 atm)
Vapor density (specific gravity)	1.612 (with air = 1)
Melting point	$-192.5°$ C
Gas density	2.141 kg/m^3 (at $0°$ C and 1 atm)

^{a}mainly from various handbooks on physical and chemical properties of inorganic compounds.

11.4.3. Toxic Effects and Advisories

In the United States, the primary and the secondary NAAQS for ground-level (i.e., tropospheric) ozone (O_3) are both 70 ppb as the daily maximum 8-hour average (U.S. EPA, 2015). The WHO (2006) guideline value for O_3 is 100 µg/m^3 (~50 ppb) for 8 hours. A 32% decline in the national average of ground-level O_3 was observed (U.S. EPA, 2017b) in the United States between 1980 (101 ppb) and 2015 (69 ppb). In 2003, southern Europe observed almost the worst summer ozone levels, but rather unfortunately succeeded by those in 2006 (EEA, 2007). In summer 2006, a large number of southern European countries experienced 1-hour O_3 levels exceeding Europe's long-term alert threshold of 240 µg/m^3, with the highest level of 370 µg/m^3 occurring in Italy. More recently on 11 June 2014, a maximum 1-hour O_3 level of 305 µg/m^3 was reported (EEA, 2015) from Berre-I'Étang, a commune in southern France.

A. Effects on Humans and Animals

Exposure to ground-level O_3 can trigger a wide array of health problems including throat and airway irritation, chest pains, coughing, wheezing, shortness of breath, and sunburn-like inflammation of the skin. It can aggravate asthma, bronchitis, emphysema, and other respiratory disorders. Exposure to O_3 can also impair lung function and inflame the linings of the respiratory tract. Prolonged exposure to O_3 can permanently scar lung tissues.

There are many animal toxicity studies supporting the association between permanent damage to the human lungs and chronic exposure to O_3 at various levels below 0.25 ppm (for around 8 to 10 hours a day), especially those conducted in rats (Grose *et al.*, 1989; Huang *et al.*, 1988) and monkeys (Hyde *et al.*, 1989; Tyler *et al.*, 1988). There are also human data linking long-term exposure of O_3 at ambient air levels to the incidence (Beeson *et al.*, 1998) and mortality (Abbey *et al.*, 1999) of lung cancer in nonsmoker male adults. It was estimated that in 2013, around 215,000 global deaths were caused by exposure to O_3 (Brauer, 2016; Forouzanfar *et al.*, 2015). There was also implication (Caiazzo *et al.*, 2013) that O_3 exposure attributed to approximately 2,000 premature deaths occurring each year in the United States.

B. Effects on Plants

Ozone at high concentrations can cause more harm to plants and ecosystems than all other air pollutants combined can. It can injure the leaves of many plant species, suppress their growth, depress flowering, and reduce crop yields. It can interfere with the ability of sensitive plants to produce or store food and can make some of them more susceptible to certain diseases, insects, other pollutants, and harsh weather.

The symptoms from plant injuries caused by O_3 include various types of chlorotic markings and necrotic lesions such as flecking, stippling, bronzing, and reddening. There is some evidence that certain crops such as alfalfa, cotton, and soybean are more susceptible to yield loss caused by O_3 (e.g., Heagle, 1989; Rich and Tomlinson, 1974). Studies showed that SO_2 and O_3 had synergistic damage in tobacco plants (Macdowall and Cole, 1971; Menser and Heggestad, 1966). Nonetheless, the interaction observed between SO_2 and O_3 in hybrid poplar plants (*Populus deltoids* Bartr. x *P. trichocarpa* Torr. and Gray) was antagonistic instead, as SO_2 had actually reduced the toxic effect of O_3 on leaf growth in the hybrids tested (Noble and Jensen, 1980).

11.5. Carbon Monoxide

Carbon monoxide (CO) is an odorless, colorless, tasteless, and potentially lethal gas. As such, it can kill a person before the individual is aware of its presence. It is for this reason that CO is nicknamed the silent killer (gas). This inorganic gas is highly toxic to humans at high concentrations because its binding affinity to the metalloprotein hemoglobin (Hb) is about 220 times greater than that of oxygen to Hb (Section 9.2.4). When existing in the Hb-CO bound form, the metalloprotein is incapable of carrying oxygen to cells in other body tissues. As its sources of emission being so numerous indoors as well as outdoors, CO is both an indoor poisonous gas and a notorious outdoor air pollutant. In the United States, historically one major acute outdoor episode was documented (Hexter and Goldsmith, 1971) linking CO air pollution to daily mortalities observed in Los Angeles County during the years 1962 to 1965. In two other acute outdoor episodes occurring around that period (December 1962 and October 1963), CO along with SO_2 and total HCs was also implicated for the cause of family illness in New York City (Ingram *et al.*, 1965). In more recent reports on O_3 air pollution, such as the one occurring in southern Europe in 2006 (Section 11.4.3), CO could actually be blamed as the culprit instead inasmuch as it is one of the key precursors for the formation of tropospheric O_3 (Section 11.4.2).

11.5.1. Sources of Pollution

Carbon monoxide (CO) is formed wherever incomplete combustion of a carbonaceous fuel occurs. This means that in a situation where oxygen supply is not proportionally in its fullness, burning a fossil fuel or the kind can lead to a substantial amount of CO in the area. Fossil fuels include coal, petroleum, and natural gas, which all are rich in carbon. Even wood, tobacco, and kerosene are HC (hydrocarbon) materials thus highly rich in carbon. In unvented areas where oxygen supply is limited, worn or poorly maintained combustion devices can be significant sources of CO. Burning devices that are commonly found to use carbonaceous fuel indoors include wood stoves, fireplaces, kerosene heaters, gas furnaces, and any gasoline-powered equipment.

Automobile exhausts around the garages, parking areas, and nearby roadways are major outdoor sources of CO. This is particularly true of exhausts from diesel engines which are powered directly by controlling the fuel rather than air supply. Even for vehicles using non-diesel fuel, the air-to-fuel ratios can be too low in the engine during starting or when the automobile is not maintained properly. These concerns are the main reasons why many countries require on-road motor vehicles each to be equipped with a catalytic converter to help cut down the emission of CO and other by-product toxic substances coming off their engine.

In the United States, even with the catalytic converter requirement in effect for well over 20 years, on-road motor vehicle exhausts continue to contribute about 60% of all CO mobile emissions nationwide (U.S. EPA, 2014). A much higher percentage (85 to 95%) from this source can be seen in cities with heavy traffic congestion. One explanation for such high percentages still being seen is that both the number of vehicles on the road and the distances that they have driven have more than doubled in the past 20 some years. Other sources of CO emission include industrial processes, non-road engines, wildfires, and residential wood burning.

11.5.2. Characteristics and Properties

In addition to its special characteristics being odorless, colorless, and tasteless, CO is a flammable, non-irritating gas soluble in ethanol (C_2H_6O) and benzene (C_6H_6) but sparingly in water. This inorganic gas has considerable industrial importance due to its widespread application as a fuel or as a reducing agent. Among other applications, CO can be utilized to make aldehydes (R-CHO, where R ≡ any organyl group) which can be used to make detergents or to be mixed with methanol (CH_3OH) to form acetic acid (CH_3COOH). Acetic acid in turn can be used to make certain polymers to be applied in paints and adhesives.

The flammable range of CO is 13 to 74%, with the characteristic that it will quickly ignite in the presence of air and a spark. Its general physicochemical properties are listed in Table 11.4.

Table 11.4. General Physicochemical Properties of Carbon Monoxide (CO)[a]

Molecular weight	28.0
Boiling point	$-191.5°$ C (at 1 atm)
Vapor density (specific gravity)	0.97 (with air = 1)
Melting point	$-205°$ C
Gas density	1.25 kg/m^3 (at 0° C and 1 atm)

[a]mainly from various handbooks on physical and chemical properties of inorganic compounds.

Several methods can be employed to produce CO in the laboratory, including dehydration of formic acid (HCO_2H) with H_2SO_4 (Reaction 11.11) and heating calcium carbonate ($CaCO_3$) with zinc (Zn) metal (Reaction 11.12). The dehydration method (Reaction 11.11) is, however, regarded as the standard procedure for experimental or laboratory production of CO.

$$HCO_2H + H_2SO_4 \rightarrow CO + H_2O + H_2SO_4 \tag{11.11}$$

$$CaCO_3 + Zn \rightarrow ZnO + CaO + CO \tag{11.12}$$

The most common method for industrial production of CO is by combustion of carbon (C) either in air at high temperatures with an excess supply of C over O_2 (Reaction 11.13a), or by utilizing CO_2 in place of O_2 also at high temperatures (Reaction 11.13b).

$$O_2 + 2C \rightarrow 2CO \ (>800° \text{ C or } >1,470° \text{ F}) \tag{11.13a}$$

$$2CO \leftrightarrows C + CO_2 \ (\leftarrow \text{ when at temperatures } >800° \text{ C}) \tag{11.13b}$$

11.5.3. Toxic Effects and Advisories

In the United States, no federal standards have been reached for CO either in indoor air or for public welfare protection. The primary (i.e., public health-based) NAAQS for CO in outdoor air has been set at 9 ppm (40 mg/m^3) for 8 hours, and 35 ppm for 1 hour (U.S. EPA, 2011). The WHO (2000b) guideline values for CO are 10 ppm for 8 hours and 90 ppm for 15 minutes. Average CO levels in residential areas without gas stoves reportedly ranged from around 0.5 to 5 ppm. Yet levels measured near properly-adjusted and poorly-adjusted gas stoves were up to 15 ppm and above 30 ppm, respectively. The outdoor levels of CO generally peak during the colder months when inversion conditions are more frequent. During those months, the air pollutant will likely get trapped near the ground beneath a layer of warm air.

A. Effects on Humans and Animals

Carbon monoxide (CO) is known as the most potent and common asphyxiant, as it can deprive Hb (hemoglobin) of the ability to carry oxygen to cells in various body tissues. The adverse effects of CO exposure can vary considerably from person to person, particularly at low concentrations. At low levels of exposure, CO likely causes mild effects that are frequently mistaken for the common flu without fever. Symptoms from mild effects include headaches, disorientation, dizziness, nausea, and tiredness, frequently with no motivation to work. The health threat from CO at low levels is most serious for people suffering from cardiovascular diseases (e.g., angina pectoris or congestive heart failure).

At moderate levels of exposure, angina, vision impairment, and reduced brain function may result, whereas at sufficiently high levels even healthy people will be seriously affected. The symptoms from high levels include vision impairment, disorientation, headaches, dizziness, nausea, confusion, and death. Acute fatal effects are mainly due to asphyxiation.

Carbon monoxide at ambient air levels may trigger serious respiratory problems largely due to its contribution to the formation of (ground-level) ozone smog. In a person with a cardiovascular disease, even a short-term exposure to CO at ambient air levels may cause chest pains in the affected person and suppress his or her ability to work. Prolonged exposure at low levels may induce other cardiovascular effects, sleepiness, light-headedness, memory problems, and changes in mood in the affected person.

B. Effects on Plants

Under most conditions, CO is not harmful to plants in that it can be rapidly oxidized to form CO_2 which is quickly utilized for photosynthesis. The increase in atmospheric CO_2 actually would have a substantial positive environmental effect, as atmospheric CO_2 can help fertilize plants thus enabling them to grow faster as well as larger and to withstand drier climates. Several studies revealed that CO induced not only the initiation or stimulation of root formation in certain plant species (Cao *et al.*, 2007; Zimmerman *et al.*, 1993), but also a change in the sex expression pattern in certain (other) plant species (Heslop-Harrison and Heslop-Harrison, 1957; Minina and Tylkina, 1947). Some other studies (e.g., Webster, 1954) nonetheless showed that CO had the potential to inhibit the enzymatic activity of cytochrome oxidase in plant tissues and thereby the capability of damaging the cellular respiratory functions there (an effect briefly described in Section 9.2.4).

References

Abbey DE, Nishino N, McDonnell WF, Burchette RJ, Knutsen SF, Beeson WL, Yang JX, 1999. Long-Term Inhalable Particles and Other Air Pollutants Related to Mortality in Nonsmokers. *Am. J. Respir. Crit. Care Med.* 159:73-382.

Adam SEH, Abdel-Banat BMA, Sakamoto A, Takahashi M, Morikawa H, 2008a. Effect of Atmospheric Nitrogen Dioxide on Mulukhiya (*Corchorus olitorius*) Growth and Flowering. *Am. J. Plant Physiol.* 3:180-184.

Adam SEH, Shigeto J, Sakamoto A, Takahashi M, Morikawa H, 2008b. Atmospheric Nitrogen Dioxide at Ambient Levels Stimulates Growth and Development of Horticultural Plants. *Botany* 86:213-217.

ATSDR (U.S. Agency for Toxic Substances and Disease Registry), 1998. Toxicological Profile for Sulfur Dioxide. U.S. Department of Health and Human Services, Atlanta, Georgia, USA.

Beeson WL, Abbey DE, Knutsen SF, 1998. Long-term Concentrations of Ambient Air Pollutants and Incident Lung Cancer in California Adults: Results from the ASHMOG Study. *Environ. Health Perspect.* 106: 813-823.

Benton-Short L, DeSousa C, 2014. Cities and Pollution. In *Cities of North America: Contemporary Challenges in U.S. and Canadian Cities* (Benton-Short L, Ed.). Lanham, Maryland, USA: Rowman & Littlefield, Chapter 12.

Brauer M, 2016. The Global Burden of Disease from Air Pollution. AAAS (American Association for the Advancement of Science) 2016 Annual Meeting – Global Science Engagement (Presented 13 February 2016, Washington DC, USA).

Brauer M, Lencar C, Tamburic L, Koehoorn M, Demers P, Karr C, 2008. A Cohort Study of Traffic-Related Air Pollution Impacts on Birth Outcomes. *Environ. Health Perspect.* 116:680-686.

Burnett RT, Stieb D, Brook JR, Cakmak S, Dales R, Raizenne M, Vincent R, Dann T, 2004. Associations between Short-Term Changes in Nitrogen Dioxide and Mortality in Canadian Cities. *Arch. Environ. Health* 59:228-236.

Caiazzo F, Ashok A, Waitz IA, Yim SHL, Barrett SRH, 2013. Air Pollution and Early Deaths in the United States. Part I: Quantifying the Impact of Major Sectors in 2005. *Atmos. Environ.* 79:198-208.

Cao Z-Y, Xuan W, Liu Z-Y, Li X-N, Zhao N, Xu P, Wang Z, Guan RZ, Shen W-B, 2007. Carbon Monoxide Promotes Lateral Root Formation in Rapeseed. *J. Intl. Plant Biol.* 49:1070-1079.

Daines RH, 1968. Sulfur Dioxide and Plant Response. *J. Occup. Environ. Med.* 10:516-524.

EEA (European Environment Agency), 2002. Annual European Community CLR-TAP Emission Inventory 1990-2000 (Technical Report No. 91). Copenhagen, Denmark.

EEA (European Environment Agency), 2007. Air Pollution by Ozone in Europe in Summer 2006 (Technical Report No. 5). Copenhagen, Denmark.

EEA (European Environment Agency), 2015. Summer 2014 Ozone Assessment – Overview of Exceedances of EC Ozone Thresholds Values for April-September 2014 (Technical Report No. 10). Copenhagen, Denmark.

Font A, Fuller GW, 2016. Did Policies to Abate Atmospheric Emissions from Traffic Have a Positive Effect in London? *Environ. Poll.* 218:463-474.

Forouzanfar MH, Alexander L, Anderson HR, Bachman VF, Biryukov S, Brauer M, Burnett R, Casey D, Coates MM, Cohen A, *et al.*, 2015. Global, Regional, and National Comparative Risk Assessment of 79 Behavioral, Environmental and Occupational, and Metabolic Risks or Clusters of Risks in 188 Countries, 1990-2013: A Systematic Analysis for the Global Burden of Disease Study 2013. *Lancet* 386:2287-2323.

Griffiths H, 2003. Air Pollution on Agricultural Crops. Ministry of Agriculture, Food & Rural Affairs, Ontario, Canada.

Grose EC, Stevens MA, Hatch GE, Jaskot RH, Selgrade MJK, Stead AG, Costa DL, Graham JA, 1989. The Impact of a 12-Month Exposure to a Diurnal Pattern of Ozone on Pulmonary Function, Antioxidant Biochemistry and Immunology. In *Atmospheric Ozone Research and Its Policy Implications* (Schneider T, Lee TS, Wolters GJR, Grant LD, Eds.). Nijmegen, The Netherlands: Elsevier, pp.535-544.

Harvard Magazine, 2000. Art under Wrap. Vol.102, March-April.

Heagle AS, 1989. Ozone and Crop Yield. *Ann. Rev. Phytopathol.* 27:397-423.

Heslop-Harrison J, Heslop-Harrison Y, 1957. The Effect of Carbon Monoxide on Sexuality in *Mercurialis ambigua* L. fils. *New Phytol.* 56:352-355.

Hexter AC, Goldsmith JR, 1971. Carbon Monoxide: Association of Community Air Pollution with Mortality. *Science* 172:265-267.

Holman C, 1999. Sources of Air Pollution. In *Air Pollution and Health* (Holgate ST, Samet JM, Koren HS, Maynard RL, Eds.). London, UK: Academic Press, pp.115-148.

Huang Y, Chang LY, Miller FJ, Graham JA, Ospital JJ, Crapo JD, 1988. Lung Injury Caused by Ambient Levels of Oxidant Air Pollutants: Extrapolation from Animal to Man. *Am. J. Aerosol. Med.* 1:180-183.

Hyde DM, Plopper CG, Harkema JR, St. George JA, Tyler WS, Dungworth DL, 1989. Ozone-Induced Structural Changes in Monkey Respiratory System. In *Atmospheric Ozone Research and Its Policy Implications*, (Schneider T, Lee TS, Wolters GJR, Grant LD, Eds.). Nijmegen, The Netherlands: Elsevier, pp. 523-534.

Ingram W, McCarroll JR, Cassell EJ, Wolter D, 1965. Health and the Urban Environment: Air Pollution and Family Illness. II. Two Acute Air Pollution Episodes in New York City. *Arch. Environ. Health* 10:364-366.

Klonoff-Cohen H, Lam P, Lewis A, 2005. Outdoor Carbon Monoxide, Nitrogen Dioxide, and Sudden Infant Death Syndrome. *Arch. Dis. Child.* 90:750-753.

Kumie A, Emmelin A, Wahlberg S, Berhane Y, Ali A, Mekonen E, Worku A, Brandstrom D, 2009. Sources of Variation for Indoor Nitrogen Dioxide in Rural Residences of Ethiopia. *Environ. Health* 8:51 (online journal).

Linn WS, Szlachcic Y, Gong H Jr, Kinney PL, Berhane KT, 2000. Air Pollution and Daily Hospital Admissions in Metropolitan Los Angeles. *Environ. Health Perspect.* 108:427-434.

Macdowall FDH, Cole AFW, 1971. Threshold and Synergistic Damage to Tobacco by Ozone and Sulfur Dioxide. *Atmos. Environ.* 5:553-554.

Menser HA, Heggestad HE, 1966. Ozone and Sulfur Dioxide Synergism: Injury to Tobacco Plants. *Science* 153:424-425.

Minina EG, Tylkina LG, 1947. Physiological Study of the Effect of Gases upon Sex Differentiation in Plants. *Compt. Rend. Acad. Sci. URSS* 55:169-172.

Movassaghi K, Russo MV, Avino P, 2012. The Determination and Role of Peroxyacetil Nitrate in Photochemical Processes in Atmosphere. *Chem. Cent. J.* 6(Suppl 2):S8 (online journal).

Noble RD, Jensen KF, 1980. Effects of Sulfur Dioxide and Ozone on the Growth of Hybrid Poplar Leaves. *Am. J. Bot.* 67:1005-1009.

Reinert RA, Gray TN, 1981. The Response of Radish to Nitrogen Dioxide, Sulfur Dioxide, and Ozone, Alone and in Combination. *J. Environ. Qual.* 10:240-243.

Rich S, Tomlinson H, 1974. Mechanisms of Ozone Injury to Plants. In *Air Pollution Effects on Plant Growth* (Dugger M, Ed.). Washington DC, USA: American Chemical Society, Chapter 6.

Rubio MA, Lissi E, Villena G, Caroca V, Gramsch E, Ruiz A, 2005. Estimation of Hydroxyl and Hydroperoxyl Radicals Concentrations in the Urban Atmosphere of Santiago. *J. Chil. Chem. Soc.* 50:471-476.

Sati AP, Mohan M, 2014. Analysis of Air Pollution during a Severe Smog Episode of November 2012 and the Diwali Festival over Delhi, India. *Intl. J. Remote Sens.* 35:6940-6954.

Schubert TS, 1984. Sulfur Dioxide Injury to Plants. Plant Pathology Circular No. 257. Division of Plant Industry, Florida Department of Agriculture and Consumer Services, The Capitol, Tallahassee, Florida, USA.

Sekiya J, Wilson LG, Filner P, 1982. Resistance to Injury by Sulfur Dioxide: Correlation with Its Reduction to, and Emission of, Hydrogen Sulfide in Cucurbitaceae. *Plant Physiol.* 70:437-441.

Sierra Club, 2016. New EPA Safeguards Address Unsafe Texas Coal Plant Pollution (press release dated 30 November). http://content.sierraclub.org/press-releases/2016/11/new-epa-safeguards-address-unsafe-texas-coal-plant-pollution (retrieved 6 June 2017).

Smith BJ, Nitschke M, Pilotto LS, Ruffin RE, Pisaniello DL, Willson KJ, 2000. Health Effects of Daily Indoor Nitrogen Dioxide Exposure in People with Asthma. *Eur. Respir. J.* 16:879-885.

Srivastava HS, Ormrod DP, 1986. Effects of Nitrogen Dioxide and Nitrate Nutrition on Nodulation, Nitrogenase Activity, Growth, and Nitrogen Content of Bean. *Plant Physiol.* 81:737-741.

Suhadi DR, Awang M, Hassan MN, Abdullah R, Muda AH, 2005. Review of Photochemical Smog Pollution in Jakarta Metropolitan, Indonesia. *Am. J. Environ. Sci.* 1:110-118.

Takahashi M, Nakagawa M, Sakamoto A, Ohsumi C, Matsubara T, Morikawa H, 2005. Atmospheric Nitrogen Dioxide Gas Is a Plant Vitalization Signal to Increase Plant Size and the Contents of Cell Constituents. *New Phytol.* 168:149-154.

Taylor OC, Eaton FM, 1966. Suppression of Plant Growth by Nitrogen Dioxide. *Plant Physiol.* 41:132-135.

Tingey DT, Reinert RA, Dunning JA, Heck WW, 1971. Vegetation Injury from the Interaction of Nitrogen Dioxide and Sulfur Dioxide. *Phytopathol.* 61:1506-1511.

TMR (Transparency Market Research), 2016. Sulfur Dioxide Market by Application (Sulfuric Acid, Bleaching Agent, Refrigerating Agent, Food Preservative and Others), by End Use (Chemical, Textiles, Food & Beverages and Others) – North America Industry Analysis, Size, Share, Growth, Trends, and Forecast – 2016-2024. TMR, State Tower, 90 State Street, Suite 700, Albany, NY, 12207, USA.

Tyler WS, Tyler NK, Last JA, Gillespie MJ, Barstow TJ, 1988. Comparison of Daily and Seasonal Exposures of Young Monkeys to Ozone. *Toxicology* 50:131-144.

U.S. EPA (U. S. Environmental Protection Agency), 1980. Acid Rain. EPA-600/9-79-036. Office of Research and Development, Washington DC, USA.

U.S. EPA (U.S. Environmental Protection Agency), 2010a. Primary National Ambient Air Quality Standard for Sulfur Dioxide. *Federal Register* 75:35520-35603.

U.S. EPA (U.S. Environmental Protection Agency), 2010b. Primary National Ambient Air Quality Standard for Nitrogen Dioxide. *Federal Register* 75:6474-6537.

U.S. EPA (U.S. Environmental Protection Agency), 2011. Review of National Ambient Air Quality Standards for Carbon Monoxide. *Federal Register* 76:54294-54343.

U.S. EPA (U.S. Environmental Protection Agency), 2012. Secondary National Ambient Air Quality Standards for Oxides of Nitrogen and Sulfur. *Federal Register* 77:20218-20272.

U.S. EPA (U.S. Environmental Protection Agency), 2014. 2014 National Emissions Inventory (NEI) Data. https://www.epa.gov/air-emissions-inventories/2014-national-emsissions-inventory-nei-data/ (retrieved 11 August 2017).

U.S. EPA (U.S. Environmental Protection Agency), 2015. National Ambient Air Quality Standards for Ozone. *Federal Register* 80:65292-65468.

U.S. EPA (U. S. Environmental Protection Agency), 2017a. All Criteria Pollutants National Tier 1 for 1970 –2016. http://www.epa.gov/sites/production/files/2016-12/national_tier1_caps.xlsx (retrieved 7 June 2017).

U.S. EPA (U. S. Environmental Protection Agency), 2017b. National Air Quality: Status and Trends of Key Air Pollutants (webpage updated 26 July 2017). https://www.epa.gov/air-trends (retrieved 30 July 2017).

Webster GC, 1954. The Effect of Carbon Monoxide on Respiration in Higher Plants. *Plant Physiol.* 29:399-400.

White KL, Hill AC, Bennett JH, 1974. Synergistic Inhibition of Apparent Photosynthesis Rate of Alfalfa by Combination of Sulfur Dioxide and Nitrogen Dioxide. *Environ. Sci. Technol.* 8:574-576.

WHO (World Health Organization), 2000a. WHO Air Quality Guidelines for Europe, Second Edition: Effects of Sulfur Dioxide on Vegetation – Critical Levels (Chapter 10). WHO European Centre for Environment and Health, Bonn, Germany.

WHO (World Health Organization), 2000b. WHO Air Quality Guidelines for Europe, Second Edition: Carbon Monoxide (Chapter 5.5). WHO European Centre for Environment and Health, Bonn, Germany.

WHO (World Health Organization), 2006. WHO Air Quality Guidelines for Particular Matter, Ozone, Nitrogen Dioxide and Sulfur Dioxide: Global Update 2005, Summary of Risk Assessment. Geneva, Switzerland.

Wiwanitkit V, 2007. Sexual Fertility and Its Relationship to Occupational Hazards. *Sexual. & Disab.* 25:45-47.

Xu Z, Zhang J, Yang G, Hu M, 2011. Acyl Peroxy Nitrate Measurements during the Photochemical Smog Season in Beijing, China. *Atmos. Chem. Phys. Discuss.* 11:10265-10303.

Xue L, Gu R, Wang T, Wang X, Saunders S, Blake D, Louie PKK, Luk CWY, Simpson I, Xu Z, et al., 2016. Oxidative Capacity and Radical Chemistry in the Polluted Atmosphere of Hong Kong and Pearl River Delta Region: Analysis of a Severe Photochemical Smog Episode. *Atmos. Chem. Phys.* 16:9891-9903.

Zimmerman PW, Crocker W, Hitchcock AE, 1933. Initiation and Stimulation of Roots from Exposure of Plants to Carbon Monoxide Gas. *Contrib. Boyce Thompson Inst.* 5:1-17.

Review Questions
1. Name the six criteria air pollutants designated by U.S. EPA.
2. When and where did the acute air pollution take place that resulted in 4,000 excess deaths and 100,000 extra people getting sick largely due to the effects of SO_2-related smog on their cardiopulmonary system?
3. In addition to SO_2, which two volcanic gases pose the greatest potential hazard to humans and ecosystems?
4. What are the major anthropogenic sources of SO_2 emissions in the United States?
5. Briefly explain how H_2SO_4 can be formed from SO_2 in the troposphere.
6. What can H_2SO_4 in acid deposition do chemically to limestone and marble buildings?
7. What is the primary anthropogenic source of NO_2, given that automobile exhaust fumes typically contain more NO than NO_2 by volume?
8. Which of the inorganic gases discussed in this chapter is (are) also considered as a common indoor air pollutant? And what is (are) its (their) primary indoor sources?
9. Briefly describe the adverse health effects of NO_2 on humans.
10. Briefly describe the symptoms from plant injuries induced by exposure to NO_2, particularly when either SO_2 or O_3 is also present.
11. How are tropospheric and stratospheric O_3 generally formed?
12. Briefly describe the major characteristics of O_3.
13. What are the three common precursors of O_3? And in each case, with which chemical component in the air does the diatomic oxygen (O_2) molecule eventually react to form O_3?
14. With respect to joint effect on leaf growth, what is likely to happen to *hybrid poplar* plants that have been exposed to SO_2 and O_3 simultaneously?
15. Why is carbon monoxide nicknamed the silent killer? And how is it generally produced?
16. Briefly explain why on-road motor vehicle exhausts continue to contribute over 50% of all CO emissions nationwide in the United States, even after the nationwide catalytic converter requirement has been in effect for well over 20 years.
17. Briefly describe the symptoms from acute CO poisoning in humans.
18. Briefly describe the effects of CO on plants.
19. Briefly describe separately the beneficial effects of O_3 and of CO on or to the environment.

CHAPTER 12

Air Pollutants – II: Particulate Matter

12.1. Introduction

To many people, the word *aerosol* refers to an aerosol spray or a canister containing the spray material. In atmospheric chemistry, aerosol actually refers to a suspension of fine solid particles, tiny liquid droplets, or a mixture of both in a gas medium; and by default, air is the gas medium of common interest. Particulate matter (PM), the subject matter of this chapter, is atmospheric aerosol without specifically referring to or considering the gas medium portion. Otherwise, for all practical purposes and within the context of this chapter as well as this book, the terms *PM* and (atmospheric) *aerosol* are synonymous with each other.

With respect to air pollution, the various forms of aerosols under consideration include dust, smoke, smog, fume, haze, fog, and mist. Dust aerosol typically refers to tiny solid particles produced by disintegration or decomposition, whereas the relatively tinier smoke particles are generated from fire or spark of light. Fume particles are similar to smoke particles in size, but can be generated by any material coming in contact with air. Haze is an atmospheric phenomenon where dust, smoke, or other airborne matters are in amounts sufficient to obscure visibility. Mist and fog are composed of liquid droplets and differ from each other only in density and visibility. Smog is fog that has been polluted mostly with smoke. In all cases, the solid particles and liquid droplets, namely the PM, that are of health concern include primarily those that as a group are directly or indirectly harmful to human health or the environment. By convention, they are collectively treated as a single air pollutant entity. Due to its common occurrence across the United States, PM has been designated by U.S. EPA as one of the six criteria air pollutants.

12.1.1. Composition of Airborne Particulates

The composition of primary airborne particulates can vary substantially depending on their sources. In areas such as the tropical and desert regions, wind-blown solid dust aerosols are the principal source of particulate loading. This type is composed of primarily mineral oxides and other materials blown from the Earth's crust. Another common source is sea spray (away from the desert regions), with the particulates consisting of largely the sodium chloride (NaCl) salt along with small quantities of organic substances and other mineral constituents of sea salt.

By definition, PM includes biological particles, such as viruses, bacteria, molds, and any tiny metallic, radioactive, or carcinogenic molecules carried by these microbes (or vice versa, depending on their size and other factors such as physicochemical properties). Secondary particulates are formed from the oxidation of primary gases, such as from oxidation of sulfur oxides (SO_x) into sulfuric acid (H_2SO_4) and of nitrogen oxides (NO_x) into nitric acid (HNO_3). In the presence of ammonia (NH_3), secondary particulates can take the form of ammonium salts (e.g., ammonium sulfate NH_2SO_4, ammonium nitrate NH_4NO_3). Organic matter (OM) is a collection of primary and secondary particulates, with the former being biogenic or anthropogenic in origin. Secondary OM particulates generally derive from the oxidation of volatile organic compounds (VOCs). Another significant particulate type consists of predominately black (i.e., elemental) carbon and is commonly called soot. Soot and OM together constitute the carbonaceous portion of particulates.

12.1.2. Basic Characteristics of Airborne Particulates

Most PM under investigation has particulates ranging from 0.01 μm (micrometer or micron) to less than 100 μm in diameter. As a point of reference, tobacco smoke particles are at about the middle of this size range. Like biological particulates, particles in tobacco smoke are capable of picking up many tiny substances such as indoor radon and its progenies (Chapter 14). Most airborne particles will eventually fall onto the ground or get washed down by precipitation. Yet some are able to rise to almost the highest levels of the atmosphere, stay for a long time, or travel for long distances. Except for those of ultra-tiny size (*see* Section 12.2.5 and Table 12.1), the lighter and smaller (<1 μm) a particle is, the longer (in weeks) it tends to stay in the air. In contrast, the heavier and larger ones will settle onto the ground by gravity in hours. Particulates like the diesel aerosol kind are usually found at their peak levels near the emission source.

Not all airborne particulates are harmful. Because most aerosols reflect sunlight back into space, they have a positive global cooling effect by lowering the amount of solar radiation that is to reach the Earth's surface. Particulates containing large amounts of sulfate and nitrate molecules are strong light-scatters (due to the larger sizes of these components) that help make the particulate proper more effective as a deflector. OM (organic matter) can affect the atmospheric radiation field by light absorption or scattering. Soot, on the other hand, includes strong light-absorbing materials capable of yielding a large positive radiative forcing (i.e., a large positive balance between radiations traveling into and out of the atmosphere). Atmospheric deposition of particulates is also a significant source of nutrients (e.g., minerals, trace metals) to oceans where carbon sequestration and aquatic productivity can then be enhanced.

12.2. Sizes of Particulate Matter

As alluded to earlier, PM includes many kinds and forms of substances that together thus can cause a wide spectrum of toxic effects to human health and the ecosystem. Yet in spite of such a concern, these substances are almost always treated as a single complex mixture. This is because to many health regulatory entities, it is not the types of particulates involved that matters the most. Rather, it is their size that is deemed most relevant to health threats. This notion is based on the large body of evidence (e.g., Section 12.4) supporting the strong link between the sizes of airborne particles and their potential for causing numerous various health problems.

Amidst the fact that airborne particles have irregular shapes with geometric diameters difficult to be measured, for simplicity but more by convention, their dynamic behavior and impacts in the immediate space are generally expressed in terms of the aerodynamic diameter of an idealized spherical particle. Airborne particles are thus typically collected and characterized in terms of their aerodynamic equivalent diameter which is utilized to represent their size. The aerodynamic diameter of a perfect spherical object is roughly equivalent to the product of its diameter multiplied by the square root of its density. This approach means that airborne particles designated or measured with the same (*aerodynamic*) diameter will may not have a similar shape or dimension.

12.2.1. Sizes of Regulatory Importance

There are broadly four particulate size categories employed by the health regulatory sector to characterize PM in relation to its impacts on environmental health. These four categories are: (1) non-inhalable coarse particles; (2) inhalable coarse particles; (3) fine particles; and (4) nano- or ultrafine particles. In practice, however, not all agencies opt to use these four sizes to the fullness. For example, U.S. EPA earlier was most concerned with particles that were only 10 μm in (henceforth aerodynamic) diameter or smaller because the agency then concluded that these were the ones capable of passing through at least the human's upper respiratory tract. That is, U.S. EPA's position then was that those airborne particles larger than 10 μm were non-inhalable and therefore would have no apparent health threats as an air pollutant entity. The agency now has a focus more on particulates in both the inhalable coarse and the fine particle groups, which by sampling limitations automatically include those in the nano or ultrafine group.

By convention, inhalable coarse particles in the atmosphere are those each have a diameter between 2.5 and 10 μm and are put in the category denoted by $PM_{2.5-10}$. Fine particles are those that are also inhalable (as due to their size) but each have a diameter of 2.5 μm or smaller and accordingly are denoted by $PM_{2.5}$. For very fine particles each with a diameter of 0.1 μm or less and now known to have more serious health implications, they are specifically termed *ultrafine* particles (UFPs) and denoted by $PM_{0.1}$. Nano-particles, denoted by PM_{nano}, are considered having a similar particle size range as the UFPs have, except to a small group of scholars (e.g., Chang *et al.*, 2008) who specifically refer to particles with a diameter of 0.056 μm (i.e., 56 nm) or smaller as nano-particles. As explained later in Section 12.2.5, the sources of UFPs and of PM_{nano} may be treated as different, at least to some scholars. In any event, it is more certain that PM_{10} used to be the size group having the most regulatory attention. This group refers to all inhalable particles with a diameter of 10 μm or *smaller* and may include the fine, ultrafine, and nano-particles, depending on the context. Lastly, non-inhalable coarse particles as a group are denoted by PM_{10+}, which is not a notation used often enough by the health and aerosol science sectors as the health concern with particles in this size group is minimal.

Particle size is of regulatory importance because it is the principal parameter governing the motions and depositions of aerosols by affecting the inertial, gravitational, or Brownian diffusional force that applies. For airborne particles on the micron (μm) scale, inertial and gravitational forces dominate. Inertia is the tendency of a moving object to resist acceleration without settling down until it runs into another object (e.g., the walls of an airway conduit) resulting in an impaction or interception. Gravitational force occurs when the object's motion is governed or affected by gravity leading to sedimentation. As the particle size is down to the nano scale, diffusional force dominates, with the particles acting much like gas or vapor molecules. Diffusion occurs when smaller particles are in Brownian (i.e., jiggling-like) motion to hit another object's surface. The general composition and basic properties of particulates in $PM_{2.5-10}$, $PM_{0.1-2.5}$, and $PM_{0.1}$ are summarized in Table 12.1. More specific characteristics of airborne particulates in the various size groups, starting with those of PM_{10+}, are discussed separately in the subsections that follow.

12.2.2. Non-Inhalable Coarse Particles (PM_{10+})

The terms *non-inhalable* and *inhalable* are somewhat subjective particularly in relation to size cutoff (e.g., Kumar, 2008; Raabe, 1982). About 50% of the particles with a diameter of around 10 μm (i.e., irrespective of their shape) were historically found capable of penetrating down below the pharynx region and thereby are now treated as inhalable for size cutoff and monitoring purposes. Yet some literature also has treated particles of 15 to 30 μm (e.g., cotton fiber) as inhalable in the sense that they can penetrate through the nose or the mouth. Another inconsistency in PM jargon is that, according to the U.S. Occupational Safety and Health Administration and the U.S. Mine Safety and Health Administration, respirable dust particles are those small enough to penetrate deep into the lung. And, as defined by the two agencies, they all supposedly have a diameter just less than 10 μm. In contrast, U.S. EPA includes the 10 μm particles in its inhalable group. Such a size cutoff preference suggests that the terms *respirable* and *inhalable* have (or should have) different connotations. Adding to the confusion, in some places such as Europe, *fine* particles are denoted by PM_{10-}, not $PM_{2.5-}$ (e.g., van Zelma *et al.*, 2008).

Historically, for air monitoring purposes as well as by sampling limitation, only those airborne particles with a diameter of about 100 μm or less were collected as total suspended particles or particulates (TSP) which as a group is a collective and an inclusive term for a mixture of solid particles and liquid droplets measured in the air. Yet in reality, particles in PM_{10+} frequently have an upper-bound diameter of about 40 or 50 μm instead. This is because particles larger than 50 μm tend to settle quickly (in minutes to hours) and thus likely near their sources of emission not readily collectible in the air zone often far away from the emission source.

The group called TSP is actually an archaic regulatory measure of the *mass* concentration of all particles collected in an area's ambient air. As the monitoring interest then was mostly in the total *weight* of all airborne particles collected in a sample, the air samplers available then were typically designed without preference in particle size other than the filter's capacity to capture and retain particles in a certain size (diameter) range. Many high-volume air samplers have the ability to retain particles up to about 100 μm (e.g., U.S. EPA, 1999). Unfortunately, the actual size cutoff varies with wind speed and wind direction in the field, thereby frequently ending with an actual capture of lighter particles of 50 μm or smaller.

With a size-select *inlet* to the filter collecting the airborne particles, even a high-volume air sampler (U.S. EPA, 1999) can be utilized to collect particles of 10 μm or smaller in diameter. The concentration and the mass of PM_{10+} therefore can be analyzed by subtraction of the PM_{10} level from the TSP level measured. Consequently, PM_{10+} generally contains particles collectible as TSP with a diameter >10 but practically <50 μm. The depositions of most PM_{10+} particles are by gravitational sedimentation, with a residence time in minutes to hours and a travel distance not far from their emission source.

Table 12.1. Comparison of Fine and Coarse Inhalable Airborne Particulates[a]

	PM$_{2.5}$ (Fine)		PM$_{2.5-10}$ (Coarse)
	PM$_{0.1}$ (Ultrafine)	PM$_{0.1-2.5}$ (Accumulation)[b]	
Formation processes	Combustion, high-temperature processes, atmospheric reactions		Break-up of large solids and large droplets
Formation	Nucleation Condensation Coagulation	Condensation Coagulation Reaction of gases in or on particles Evaporation of cloud/fog droplets in which gases have dissolved and reacted	Mechanical disruption (crushing, grinding, abrasion of surfaces) Evaporation of sprays Suspension of dust reactions of gases in or on particles
Composition	Sulfate Elemental (black) carbon Metal compounds Organics with very low saturation vapor pressure at ambient temperature	Sulfate, nitrate, ammonium, and hydrogen ions Elemental (black) carbon Large variety of organic compounds Metals: compounds of lead, of cadmium, of nickel, of vanadium, of manganese, of copper, of iron, of zinc, etc. Particle-bound water	Suspended soil or street dust Fly ash from uncontrolled combustion of coal, oil, or wood Nitrates/chlorides from hydrochloric acid/nitric acid Oxides of crustal elements (iron titanium, aluminum, silicon) Calcium carbonate, sea salt, sodium chloride Pollen, molds, fungal spores Plant/animal fragments Tire, brake pad, or road wear debris
Solubility	Probably less than those of PM$_{0.1-1}$	Often soluble, hygroscopic and deliquescent	Largely insoluble and non-hygroscopic
Sources	Combustion Atmospheric transformation of sulfur dioxide or some organic compounds High-temperature processes	Combustion of coal, of oil, of gasoline, of diesel fuel, of wood Atmospheric transformation products of sulfur dioxide, nitrogen oxides, or organic carbon (e.g., terpenes) High-temperature processes, smelters, steel mills, etc.	Resuspension of industrial dust or of soil tracked onto roads and streets Suspension from disturbed soil (e.g. farming, unpaved roads, mining) Uncontrolled coal or oil combustion Biological sources Ocean spray Construction or demolition
Half-life (in air)	Minutes to hours[c]	Days to weeks	Minutes to days
Removal processes	By growing in accumulation mode Diffusion to raindrops	Formation of cloud droplets and then deposition in rain Dry deposition	Dry deposition by fallout Scavenging by falling rain drops
Travel distance	<1 to 10s of km	100s to 1,000s of km	<1 to 100s of km

[a] adapted and modified from Table 2.1 in WHO (2006b), which was based on the analysis report by U.S. EPA (2004).

[b] diameter size cutoff used by WHO (2006b) for accumulation of fine particles was 0.1 μm to 1.0 μm while acknowledging that the upper size limit extending to 2.5 μm is sometimes fixed by convention for measurement purposes.

[c] these ultrafine particles tend to have a very short residence time likely due to their transient nature being removed by diffusion at high rates.

12.2.3. Inhalable Coarse Particles ($PM_{2.5-10}$)

Airborne particles in this coarse group are supposedly the largest among all the inhalables; they are mostly produced by decomposition or disintegration of larger solid particles or liquid droplets, such as by crushing, grinding, spray evaporation, or suspensions of dusts from construction and agricultural operations. These particulates are inhalable but also the coarse fraction of the entire PM_{10} group. Note that by definition PM_{10} includes the fine and smaller particle fractions unless the notation is specifically intended for particles of exactly 10 μm, in which case it can be denoted by $PM_{[10]}$ for clarity purposes. $PM_{2.5-10}$, or $PM_{[10]}$, is known as the inhalable group as well as the thoracic fraction. This is because the particles in this group are considered having the ability to penetrate into at least the larynx region. The cutoff for the low end for coarse particles is 2.5 μm because energy considerations typically limit coarse particle size to >2 μm.

Examples of $PM_{2.5-10}$ particles include dust particles, bacteria, molds, pollen, spores, fly ashes, and insect parts. The residence time of these inhalable coarse particles in the atmosphere, at least in certain regions such as Europe, is about 1 to 6 days (van Zelma *et al.*, 2008), with a travel distance less than 10 km (6.2 miles). In the United States, the primary (i.e., public health-based) and the secondary (i.e., public welfare-based) NAAQS (National Ambient Air Quality Standard) for PM_{10} are both set at 150 μg/m^3 averaged over a 24-hour period (U.S. EPA, 2013). The World Health Organization (WHO, 2006b) guideline values for this size group are 50 and 20 μg/m^3 averaged over a 24-hour and a one-year period, respectively.

12.2.4. Fine Particles ($PM_{0.1-2.5}$)

Airborne particles in this size group are different from those in $PM_{2.5-10}$ both in origin and in physicochemical properties. Once inhaled, these *fine* particles can reach into the gas-exchange (alveolar) region of the lung and hence are often referred to as the *respirable* fraction. In addition to evaporation of fog or cloud droplets being a major source, these particles can originate from a gas nucleated into particles of ultrafine size. The gas may come from either a natural or an anthropogenic source. The UFPs (ultrafine particles) so generated can then become fine particles by growing up to a size of about 1 μm or a bit larger via one of the two accumulation processes termed condensation and coagulation. In condensation, additional gas molecules are required to condensate on the UFPs generated from nucleation. In contrast, coagulation is the process whereby multiple UFPs *gather* to form larger ones.

$PM_{0.1-2.5}$ particles are composed of various combinations of nitrate (NO_3^-) compounds, sulfate (SO_4^{2-}) compounds, ammonium (NH_4^+) ions, hydrogen (H^+) ions, metals (e.g., Pb, Cd), polycyclic aromatic hydrocarbons (PAHs), and particle-bound water. The major sources of $PM_{0.1-2.5}$ are fossil fuel combustion, burning of vegetation, and smelting as well as processing of metals. Unlike the inhalable coarse $PM_{2.5-10}$, they tend to be soluble in water.

The residence time of $PM_{0.1-2.5}$ in terms of half-life in air is from days to weeks (Table 12.1), with a travel distance ranging from hundreds to thousands of kilometers (1 kilometer = 0.62 mile). In the United States (U.S. EPA, 2013), the *primary* NAAQS for $PM_{2.5}$ are 35 μg/m^3 averaged over a 24-hour period and 12 μg/m^3 averaged over a one-year period, whereas the *secondary* NAAQS are 35 μg/m^3 averaged over a 24-hour period and 15 μg/m^3 averaged over a one-year period. The

WHO (2006b) guideline values for $PM_{2.5}$ are 25 and 10 $\mu g/m^3$ averaged over a 24-hour and a one-year period, respectively.

12.2.5. Nano- and Ultrafine Particles ($PM_{0.1}$)

Airborne particles in this group have the size of a molecule or virus, which are each less than 100 nm (0.1 μm) or about one-thousandth the width of a human hair. For consistency with other PM size groups, the diameters of UFPs (ultrafine particles) usually are still expressed in units of micrometers (microns). These UFPs can be either carbon-based or metallic. Within each subclass, they can be further divided according to their magnetic properties. Their concentrations can be measured using a condensation nucleus counter (e.g., McMurry, 2000) which can detect particles as tiny as 2 nm in diameter. The morphology of these nano-particles can be observed using transmission electron microscopy under certain physical laboratory conditions.

Ultrafine particles are mostly found in the atmospheric environment where most of them originate from combustion sources (e.g., vehicle exhaust fumes, forest fires) and volcanic ashes. These ultra-tiny particles are frequently the end products of a wide variety of physical, chemical, and biological processes, of which some are commonplace and traditional whereas some others are novel and radically different (Aitken *et al.*, 2004). UFPs can originate from nucleation, an initial physical reaction stage whereby a gas from anthropogenic or natural source becomes a particle of nano size. These ultra-tiny particles are the major constituents of airborne particulates, though with a rather short residence time (likely due to their transient nature being removed by diffusion at high rates, *see* Table 12.1). Owing to their vast quantities found in the atmosphere and their strong ability to penetrate deep into the lungs, they are a major health concern.

In some literature, there seems to be a technical distinction between nano- and ultrafine particles, although the two groups are practically in the same size range. To some scholars, the term *nano-particles* refers to solely those particles manufactured intentionally for their specific material properties. These are typically some forms of polymers or metals acting as a thermal spray or coating for another material. In contrast, UFPs are referred to by these scholars as particles found in the natural environment (e.g., volcanic ashes) or produced unintentionally such as during thermal processes (e.g., candlelight burning, welding) and machining of materials.

12.3. Issues on Urban Airborne Particulate Pollution

In the United States (U.S. EPA, 2017a), the national annual average level of PM_{10} declined 31% from 84.9 $\mu g/m^3$ in 1990 (the first year this index was used to replace TSP) to 51.9 $\mu g/m^3$ in 2015. For the $PM_{2.5}$, the annual average declined 31% from 13.5 $\mu g/m^3$ in 2000 (the first year this index was used) to 8.5 $\mu g/m^3$ in 2015. Despite these impressive downward trends, the health issues on urban (airborne) particulate pollution remain a high concern in major cities. For one thing, the national annual average of PM_{10} that the American people experienced in 2015 still exceeded the guideline value (20 $\mu g/m^3$) set forth by WHO (2006b).

Worldwide, the health problems with urban particulate pollution are due to the very fact that well over half of the global population now lives in urban areas, a trend that is now accelerating rapidly particularly in the developing countries. Urban cities tend to use large quantities of energy and synthetic materials, resulting in inevitably the generation of large volumes of waste materials and pollutants. Noteworthy is the reality that for large urban cities around the world (e.g., Beijing, London, Los Angeles, Mumbai, New York, Tokyo), they are merging into even huger megalopolitan areas especially along highways with heavy traffic.

Air pollution in urban areas comes from a vast variety of sources. In general, fossil fuel combustion is the single most abundant source for PM, as well as for many other classic air pollutants such as sulfur dioxide (SO_2), nitrogen oxides (NO_x), and carbon monoxide (CO) discussed in Chapter 11. Of particular importance is the burning of fuels for road transport and electricity generation. In addition to direct emissions, PM particles can be generated from SO_2, VOCs, and vehicle exhausts released into the atmosphere. The particles that are emitted directly are called primary particulates, whereas those generated from gases and other substances are referred to as secondary particulates. Anthropogenic sources of primary PM include transportation, industrial processes, smelting, heating, burning of vegetation, and dust particles from disturbed land or soil surfaces. Natural sources include wind-blown dusts from deserts, natural vegetation, volcanoes, wildfires, and sea spray salt. Directly or indirectly, industrial developments and human-related events can have a significant impact on these natural and anthropogenic emissions.

In general, or in more simplified terms, there are three main source categories of airborne particulate pollution in urban areas. These are mobile sources, stationary sources, and open-burning sources, which collectively can be further categorized into several more specific source types such as motor traffic, industrial processes, power plants, and domestic fuel. The investigation published by Mage *et al.* (1996) found that motor traffic was one of the major sources, if not the major source, of air pollution in megacities. In addition, a recent literature review by Gulia *et al.* (2015) concluded that over 70 to 80% of air pollution in megacities in developing countries was attributed to vehicular emissions.

12.3.1. Episodes of Particulate Pollution

Urban (airborne) particulate pollution is inevitably an ongoing major environmental health issue, inasmuch as motor traffic remains a principal anthropogenic source of airborne particulates. As a case in point, despite the extensive emission control efforts made to improve the air quality in greater Los Angeles for the past 30 years, thick hazes can still be seen obscuring the metropolitan's skylines. In fact, the South Coast Air Basin, which includes all of Los Angeles and its nearby counties Riverside, Orange, and San Bernardino, currently is still designated as one of the worst regions in the United States for nonattainment of PM_{10} (U.S. EPA, 2017b).

In Europe, the year 2003 experienced several serious wintertime pollution episodes due to PM on France's Paris Basin (Bessagnet *et al.*, 2005). Moreover, according to a World Bank study in 1999 (Pandey *et al.*, 2006), approximately 85% of the 3,226 residential areas under investigation had an estimated annual average level of PM_{10} exceeding the WHO (2006b) guideline limit of 20 $\mu g/m^3$, with 46% of these areas having levels exceeding by twofold or more. The worldwide residential areas included in that study were those in cities each reported having a population larger than 100,000 residents.

The somewhat outdated findings from the World Bank study also implicated PM_{10} as a major problem in all Asian countries except Japan. The study further found that many cities worldwide, such as Tegucigalpa and Montevideo in Latin America, experienced an annual average PM_{10} level well over 300 µg/m³. Overall, the findings from the World Bank study were consistent with those observed by Baldasano *et al.* (2003), who assessed similarly the air quality for a number of major cities in the developed and developing countries. More recently, it has estimated (Brauer, 2016; Brauer *et al.*, 2016; WHO, 2016) that nearly 90% of the world's population currently lives in areas where the particulate pollution exceeds WHO's air quality guideline, with people in China, India, and the southeast Asian countries taking a heavier toll.

Motor traffic is not the only major source of PM pollution in urban areas. For instance, one large Asian city with the most serious urban particulate pollution problem is Beijing, the national capital of China. In addition to both the high volume of daily motor traffic in the megacity and the persistent industrial pollution from many large facilities located there (Dillner *et al.*, 2006), each spring Beijing experiences dust storms that cause high levels of PM. Two of the recent serious episodes reported in the news worldwide occurred on 28 February 2013 and 15 April 2015, when Beijing residents reportedly woke up to only find the capital blanketed in yellow dusts, amidst a sandstorm sweeping relentlessly into the megacity. The sweeps were in a manner similar to the ones experienced by residents living in Sydney, Australia on 23 September 2009 and 11 January 2013. The two huge outback dust storms swept across much of Australia and blanketed Sydney aggressively on those two days, seriously disrupting flights and ground transportation as well as forcing residents to stay indoors from the gale-force winds.

Still another major source of PM polluting urban areas is industrial processing. This was (and likely still is) the case with Greece in its northwestern region where lignite mining operations and lignite-fired power stations are located. According to the study by Triantafyllou *et al.* (2006) not too long ago, the particulate pollution problems in that region with flying dusts and ashes were not only serious but also more complicated as the region is located near the mining activities. Their analysis concluded that a complex system of sources (e.g., as due to additional contribution from urban pollution) coupled with poor meteorological conditions had simply worsened the particulate pollution in that region.

12.3.2. Monitoring of Particulate Matter

The term *urban air pollution episode* generally implies a short-term increase in ambient pollution that is greater than what would be expected as part of a day-to-day variation. In their most extreme form, urban air pollution episodes are accompanied by physical discomfort, disruption of daily living, public fear, illness, and in some instances even death. In any event, it is important to have the airborne particulate levels monitored periodically for all urban areas.

As summarized in Table 12.1, different size particulates (e.g., $PM_{2.5-10}$, $PM_{0.1-2.5}$) have different properties especially with respect to their deposition patterns and penetration in the human respiratory tract. In addition to size and physical properties, the chemical and biological composition of PM can have a strong influence on its adverse health effects. For example, metals such as cobalt (Co), copper (Cu), iron (Fe), and vanadium (V) are reportedly the major contributors of cellular response induced by ambient PM (Chen *et al.*, 1999). Therefore, monitoring of PM even at ambient levels is important and relevant.

Mass measurements of PM were first performed in the late 1800s by drawing ambient air through filter paper that was weighed before and after sampling. In the United States, measurements of TSP (total suspended particulates) for radioactivity analyses were first carried out during the 1950s to evaluate the effects of tests for above-ground nuclear weapons. The technology was soon utilized for measuring mass concentrations of particulates in major urban areas. The availability of these data was the basis for designating TSP (i.e., all those particles with a practical aerodynamic diameter of <50 μm or so) as the first indicator of PM for the NAAQS adopted in the United States in 1970.

Measurement of PM concentrations, identification of their sources, and evaluation of the effects of emission-reduction measures are difficult tasks under any circumstance, particularly in developing (as well as underdeveloped) countries where many small industries lack the appropriate pollution-control devices to provide an emission inventory. Many urban areas in those countries currently still use some unquantifiable combination of fuel sources (e.g., bottled gas, natural gas) for cooking and heating. Burning of vegetation and waste incineration are also common events even in places where such activities are prohibited. For these and other reasons, monitoring of TSP remains to be the only practical, yet less accurate or precise, particulate measurement method available in many developing countries (Krzyzanowski and Schwela 1999).

12.3.3. Airborne Microbes

As noted repeatedly earlier, airborne particulates are not confined to chemical matters. They may include biological materials (e.g., bacteria, molds, viruses, along with indoor radon and the kind that these microbes can carry or be adsorbed to). Although under normal conditions air does not contain the nutrients and moisture required for airborne microbes to colonize and growth, it can still abound in their numbers in that these tiny organisms can be evaporated or blown off from soils or other dry decomposed materials on the ground (e.g., excrete).

Microbes in decomposed materials or in soils can become an important source of particulates contaminating food products and places such as schools and hospitals. Contaminations of this type can cause food spoilage and diseases when the spoiled food products are ingested. People can also be exposed to airborne microbes directly via inhalation.

A more active exposure pathway for airborne microbes is actually their transmission from person to person through coughs and sneezes. During a sneeze, millions of tiny droplets of water and mucus containing the microbes can be sprayed into the air. Even though the droplets initially are each about 10 to 100 μm, they can rapidly dry to the more floatable, inhalable droplet nuclei of less than 5 μm. These tiny nuclei can still contain the microbial particles. Environmental diseases transmitted in this manner include Legionnaires' disease, the 2009 H1N1 flu, and SARS (severe acute respiratory syndrome).

The ultimate fate of airborne microbes is governed by a complex set of conditions involving many variables such as sunlight, temperature, wind speed, size and nature of the particulate carriers, ability of microbes to form resistant spores, and adaptability of a microbe species to the new physical environment. Even the slightest air current can extend the residence time of airborne microbes to a sufficiently long one.

Both the quantity and quality of airborne microbes vary considerably with location as well as with time of the day, the month, and the year. For one thing, the microbial flux and hence the microbial quantity in the air are likely conditioned on a solar environment that affects the release of microbes into the air (Karra and Katsivela, 2007; Lighthart, 2000). Phylogenetic analyses showed that the atmospheric microbial community structure was linked to particle size (Polymenakou *et al.*, 2008).

Only limited data are available concerning the relationship of urban areas to the particulates in their ambient air or to the natural microbial communities in their soils. It was speculated that the ambient air in a congested urban area would harbor a greater number of microbes. Indeed, a study (Brodie *et al.*, 2007) was available to support this speculation to some extent after monitoring ambient air for about four months in 2003 in two U.S. cities (Austin and San Antonio) in the state of Texas. Its data revealed that the airborne particulates from the two cities contained over 1,800 diverse bacterial species, a richness approaching that of the bacterial communities found in many soils. The study found that meteorological and temporal factors, rather than location, tended to be key determinants in shaping the composition of airborne biological materials.

In terms of absolute quantity and composition, it has estimated that as many as a quarter of the total particulates present above ground are made up of biological materials ranging from 0.02 to 100 μm in (diameter) size (Jones and Harrison, 2004). In general, viruses are each smaller than 0.1 μm and bacteria are each mostly between 0.3 and 8 μm. Pollen particles and fungal spores tend to be larger, each up to 60 μm (Stanley and Linskins, 1974).

At the moment, studies with a special focus on bioaerosols in urban ambient air are even more limited. Of the couple dozens published, one was a cross-sectional study (Mopuang *et al.*, 2005) conducted to assess the microbial counts (expressed as cfu ≡ colony forming units) and the PM_{10} levels in air samples collected from roadsides of the Bangkok Fashion City Area in Thailand. This Thai study showed that ~5% of the bacterial counts and ~26% of the PM_{10} levels exceeded the recommended targets of 1,000 cfu/m^3 and 120 μg/m^3, respectively.

Another study (Zheng *et al.*, 2009) related to microbial counts was performed to analyze the average contents of airborne microbes in half of the 16 Chinese cities located in the region known as Pearl River Delta Urban Agglomeration. The region covering 47,525 km^2 has become one of the most flourishing places in economic development in China. In this Chinese study, the average contents of airborne microbes (mainly bacteria and fungi) measured were found statistically correlated with each of the environmental factors investigated. The factors under analysis included wind speed, humidity, temperature, TSP, rate of pedestrian trafficking, rate of vehicle trafficking, and population density. These factors were found having, as where expected, either a significantly negative effect or a significantly positive effect on the microbial content.

In terms of particle size distribution, a study (Polymenakou *et al.*, 2008) was carried out to determine the quality of airborne microbes over a coastal city along the eastern Mediterranean Sea during an intensive north African dust storm. This Mediterranean study demonstrated that airborne microbes of particle size >3.3 μm were predominantly spore-forming bacteria (e.g., Firmicutes), whereas those respirable and smaller were bacteria commonly found in soils or widely distributed in the environment.

More recently, a study (Kobayashi *et al.*, 2015) was conducted to investigate the bioprocess of airborne bacteria brought around by the Asian dust nicknamed Kosa, a well-known meteorological phenomenon whereby aerosols are carried by the westerly winds from inland China to East Asia. This Kosa study found that compared with the soil bacteria and their spores, the dust bioaerosol bacteria and their spores were more tolerant to ultraviolet (UV) radiation, suggesting that the bio-aerosols were transported across the atmosphere as living spores.

12.4. Toxic Effects of Airborne Particulates

The strong link between airborne particulate pollution and mortality goes back to at least the year 1930, when the then heavily industrialized areas in Belgium's Meuse Valley were blanketed by thick fog during the first week of December. That air pollution episode reportedly caused more than 60 deaths in the valley, an area located east of the city of Liege. Although SO_2 and H_2SO_4 were the respiratory irritants blamed for causing those deaths, fine soot particles such as those found in diesel exhaust fumes were also considered a likely contribution (Nemery *et al.*, 2001). Those fine diesel-like particles were thought to have been coated with much of the ultrafine particulate sulfates formed from oxidation of SO_2 in the atmosphere.

Other historical links included acute air pollution episodes occurring in the mill town Donora, Pennsylvania in 1948, in London in 1952, in New York in 1953, and in London again in 1962. Among these episodes, the London fog of 1952 has since become a notorious landmark in air pollution epidemiology as it reportedly led to the most excess deaths (~4,000) and most excess morbidity (~100,000) of this kind in the world's history. Several studies also revealed a specific link between increase in daily mortality and exposure to certain levels of PM_{10} and $PM_{2.5}$. Those studies included a time series analysis by Daniel *et al.* (2000), which supported the findings by others showing a positive link between daily mortality and particulate pollution even at levels below regulatory limits. In addition, recent epidemiological studies on urban particulate pollution have all pointed to the direction that inhalation of particulates, especially those of the $PM_{2.5}$ portion, has serious chronic health effects in humans and reportedly (WHO, 2016) causes worldwide approximately 3 million premature deaths each year.

The Global Burden of Disease (GBD) data compiled by the Institute for Health Metrics and Evaluation (Brauer, 2016; Brauer *et al.*, 2016; Forouzanfar *et al.*, 2015) showed that in 2013, there were 2.9 million global deaths (5.3% of all deaths) caused by outdoor fine particulate air pollution. These data further showed that in the United States, ambient air pollution was ranked the 13th highest risk factor for deaths with 79,000 estimated for 2013.

At any rate, available data all suggest that the mortality and the morbidity events that were linked to particulate air pollution may fall under three adverse effects categories: those related or due to (1) effects on the respiratory tract; (2) effects on the cardiovascular system; and (3) other serious adverse health effects such as cancer and sudden infant death syndrome (SIDS). Particulate air pollution can also have serious adverse effects on the natural environment, such as prevention of photosynthesis in plants, impairment of visibility, and soiling of surface materials (e.g., paints) on building structures.

12.4.1. Mechanisms and General Trends

As reflected in the analysis and status report by Lippmann *et al.* (2003), a vast number of epidemiological and toxicological studies were carried out about two decades ago, largely in a collaborative manner, to investigate the mechanisms of toxic action underlying the PM-associated health effects. This collaborative activity led to the development of certain common mechanism hypotheses (e.g., Section 12.4.3) and certain common toxic endpoints for testing (e.g., lung function, heart rate, arterial oxygen saturation, cardiac dysrhythmias, respiratory symptoms, tissue biomarkers of effects). On the other hand, results from such collaborative efforts repeatedly offered strong links between $PM_{2.5}$ exposure and a variety of acute responses, with implications that $PM_{2.5}$ might be biologically active at current peak exposure levels.

Several studies also demonstrated higher PM-associated health risks for certain susceptible subpopulations such as the elderly and individuals with pre-existing cardiopulmonary diseases. Results from some (e.g., Zanobetti and Schwartz, 2000) of those studies showed specifically that while socioeconomic factors and race did not affect susceptibility to PM-associated mortality, females were found at a higher risk. Children were also found more susceptible to PM exposure, particularly for those with asthma. There were data (Yu *et al.*, 2000) showing that an increment of 10 $\mu g/m^3$ in PM_{10} and in $PM_{1.0}$ increased the children's risk of having asthma symptoms by 11% and 18%, respectively.

Diabetics too were identified as a major susceptible subpopulation. In two single-city studies (Zanobetti and Schwartz, 2001, 2002), the risk of PM-associated hospitalization for cardiovascular diseases for diabetics was found two times higher compared to the general population. Individuals having other types of diseases were also found at higher risks of the specific cardiopulmonary diseases at issue. For example (Zanobetti *et al.*, 2000), heart failure and respiratory disorders elevated the PM-associated risks of hospital admission for chronic obstructive pulmonary disease (COPD) and for cardiovascular diseases, respectively.

12.4.2. Effects on the Respiratory Tract

According to the GBD (Global Burden of Disease) database (Forouzanfar *et al.*, 2015), in 2013 there were worldwide 1.27 million deaths from pulmonary-related (COPD and lower respiratory infections combined) diseases caused by (exposure to) ambient air pollution. Airborne particulates of special concern to the protection and maintenance of pulmonary health are those known as fine particles ($PM_{2.5}$), which each by strict notation have a diameter of 2.5 μm or smaller (i.e., including UFPs and nano-particles). Fine particles are easily inhaled deep into the gas-exchange (alveolar) region of the lung, where they can enter the bloodstream or remain embedded in the recessed areas for a long time. The particle's size is a key determinant governing the location at which the particle would come to rest in the respiratory tract once inhaled. Larger particles (>15 μm) are generally filtered in the nose or the throat and therefore generally do not cause much health concern other than potential nuisance. In contrast, particulates smaller than about 10 μm (i.e., PM_{10-}

can settle in the bronchi as well as the lungs and can therefore cause a variety of health problems. As mentioned earlier, the 10 μm size does not represent a strict cutoff between those that are inhalable and non-inhalable, but has been followed by many regulatory agencies primarily for monitoring convenience (see Section 12.2.2). Regardless, ultra-tiny particles on the nano scale are the ones most capable of passing through and beyond the human lung to adversely affect other organs and tissues including the brain. In fact, a newly emerging technique for transporting drug molecules across the blood brain barrier is with the aid of nano-particles

According to a time series analysis (Anderson et al., 2004) performed for WHO, an increase of 10 $\mu g/m^3$ in PM_{10} level would cause a 1.3% increase in mortality from respiratory diseases. It is important to note that even levels of particulates that otherwise may not affect healthy people can cause breathing difficulties for people with asthma or pulmonary disease (e.g., COPD), especially for children. Particulate pollution can trigger asthma attack and cause wheezing, coughing, as well as respiratory irritation. It can also aggravate respiratory conditions in persons with sensitive airways. In fact, some individuals with chronic bronchitis can experience a worsening of their pulmonary conditions upon exposure to dust or smoke.

More recent studies have repeatedly linked increase of premature death with exposure to relatively low levels of PM. As noted earlier, individuals at a higher risk are the elderly and those with pre-existing cardiopulmonary disorders. The elderly are typically more susceptible in part because they are those likely to have pre-existing lung or heart disease. Cigarette smokers, especially those smoking for years, generally have reduced lung function and thus can be affected more seriously by particulate pollution.

Children tend to be more susceptible to particulate pollution because their lungs and immunological system are still being developed. These youngsters are the ones found frequently engaging in vigorous outdoor activities, thus making them more vulnerable to particulate air pollution compared to healthy adults. In the recent past, a number of studies (e.g., Avol et al., 2001; DeFranco et al., 2016; Gauderman et al., 2000, 2002, 2004; Kaiser et al., 2004; UNICEF, 2016; Woodruff et al., 1997, 2006; Yu et al., 2000) were published linking airborne particulate pollution with a wide variety of adverse health effects specifically on children. These various adverse effects included reduced lung function, asthma exacerbation, impairment of lung function growth, increased episodes of coughing and breathing difficulty, premature death, and preterm birth risk.

12.4.3. Effects on the Cardiovascular System

The GBD database (Forouzanfar et al., 2015) revealed slightly worse adverse effects of ambient air pollution on the cardiovascular system compared to the respiratory tract. In 2013, there were 1.5 million global deaths from cardiovascular-related diseases (ischemic heart disease and stroke combined) caused by ambient air pollution, out-numbering those from pulmonary-related diseases (caused by ambient air pollution) by 230,000.

In the United States, a nationwide study (Dominici et al., 2006) on 204 urban counties showed that people with short-term exposure to $PM_{2.5}$ had an increased risk of hospital admission not only for respiratory but also for cardiovascular diseases. The highest admission increase observed was for heart failure, with a 1.3% increase in risk of hospitalization per 10 $\mu g/m^3$ increase in same-day

PM$_{2.5}$ concentration. The study found that the risk of cardiovascular diseases tended to be higher in counties located in the Northeast, the Southeast, the Midwest, and the South of the United States.

According to a literature review by Brook *et al.* (2004), several epidemiological studies revealed a consistent elevated risk of cardiovascular events in relation to short-term and long-term exposures to PM at ambient levels. The review ended with a discussion of several plausible pathophysiological mechanisms (e.g., acute arterial vasoconstriction, enhanced thrombosis, propensity for arrhythmia) for the increased risk.

On the other hand, an animal study (Sun *et al.*, 2005) demonstrated that compared to the controls breathing filtered air, mice inhaling air polluted with PM$_{2.5}$ had more plaque (i.e., fatty deposits) in their arteries. The health effects of PM$_{2.5}$ exposure in this mouse study were found more dramatic when the test animals were put on a high-fat diet.

12.4.4. Other Serious Health Effects

Some UFPs (ultrafine particles) can be found in diesel exhaust fumes and fireplace soot. These ultra-tiny particles may be more damaging to the cardiopulmonary system than previously speculated by some scientists. There is now strong evidence that particles <100 nm (i.e., <0.1 μm) can pass through biomembranes to migrate into other body tissues. Studies showed that airborne particulates in this size range were able to cause brain damage similar to those found in patients with Alzheimer's disease. In addition to their ability to disrupt cellular processes, these ultra-tiny particles can bypass the respiratory tract's natural defense mechanisms to become embedded in the deepest recesses of the lung. It is important to note that in terms of *number* of particles, many more UFPs than PM$_{2.5-10}$ are inhaled into the lungs (e.g., Oberdorster *et al.*, 1995). This is because it is supposed to take about 1 million particles of 0.1 μm to fill up the same *volume* (3-D space) as to be occupied by a single particle of 10 μm.

Particles found in diesel exhausts, more commonly known as diesel particulate matter, are typically in the size range of 100 nm. This type is made up of inorganics, hydrocarbons, but predominately carbon particles; it thus has the nickname *soot* or *black carbon* particulate matter. Soot is a principal component of diesel exhausts emitted by on-road (e.g., trucks, buses) and off-road (e.g., ships, trains, construction equipment) diesel engines. U.S. EPA (2005) has estimated that each year soot pollution causes approximately 4,700 premature deaths in nine major cities in the nation (Boston, Detroit, Los Angeles, Philadelphia, Phoenix, Pittsburgh, San Jose, Seattle, St. Louis). As with biological agents, soot particles can serve as carriers for whichever tinier carcinogenic matter (e.g., benzopyrenes from tobacco smoke) adsorbed onto their surfaces.

Several studies showed that long-term exposure to airborne particulates significantly (Avol *et al.*, 2001; Gauderman *et al.*, 2000, 2002) and permanently (Gauderman *et al.*, 2004) impaired lung function growth in children. Some other studies (Kaiser *et al.*, 2004; Woodruff *et al.*, 1997, 2006) linked PM to SIDS (sudden infant death syndrome) and to postneonatal infant mortality. SIDS is defined as the sudden death of a one-year old infant or younger, for which the cause remains unexplainable after both a thorough case analysis and a complete autopsy investigation (Willinger *et al.*, 1991).

A study by Woodruff *et al.* (1997) estimated that American infants had a 12% higher risk of SIDS for each 10 µg/m^3 increase in PM$_{10}$. That study analyzed the relationship between the levels of PM$_{10}$ and the SIDS observed within a population of 4 million infants born in 86 metropolitan areas in the United States between 1989 and 1991. Based on the risk factors derived in that study, the Environmental Working Group (EWG, 1997) jointly with Physicians for Social Responsibility re-determined that about 500 SIDS cases occurring each year were related to airborne particulate pollution. Their re-analysis also revealed that PM$_{10}$ pollution was associated with nearly one out of every five SIDS cases in the top 12 metropolitan areas (leading by the greater Los Angeles) where SIDS and particulate pollution were both more severe. Nevertheless, several subsequent studies (e.g., Dales *et al.*, 2004; Tong and Colditz, 2004; Woodruff *et al.*, 2006) were unable to find any significant link between particulate pollution and SIDS. A more recent cohort study by DeFranco *et al.* (2016), on the other hand, found that exposure to high levels of PM$_{2.5}$ during pregnancy was associated with a 19% increased risk of preterm birth, with the highest risk being from high levels of exposure during the third trimester.

12.4.5. Effects/Impacts on the Environment

Plants exposed to wet and dry deposition of airborne particulates can be injured depending on what air pollution constituents are contained. The leaves of a plant can be coated with PM that falls onto their surfaces to block their gas-exchange function, and hence to reduce their exposure to sunlight for photosynthesis which is a life-sustaining process for plants. This type of coating can also cause abrasion as well as radiative heating and can reduce the active photon flux reaching the photosynthetic sites. In addition, strong acidic or alkaline materials contained in the PM can cause direct damage to the leaf's surface as well as its cellular components.

Some investigators have considered the rhizosphere (i.e., the soil zone surrounding the plant roots) to be a more probable route as well as source for uptake of nutrients by plants and thereby to have a greater impact on vegetation and ecosystems. For instance, those toxic metals present in the particulates, when deposited onto this soil zone, can inhibit the process in the soil there that makes nutrients available to plants. Moreover, the availability of alkaline cations and aluminum is affected by soil pH which can be altered considerably by the various types of particulates in the PM deposited onto the rhizosphere. For terrestrial ecosystems, in most cases particulate pollution has its strongest impact in the vicinity of its emission source.

It is a known fact that particulates in acid precipitation can contribute to the soiling and erosion of property and other structural materials including notably surface paints. These environmental effects can lead to a considerable increase in cleaning and maintenance costs, as well as a substantial loss of (physical) properties and their values. When acidic particulates eventually settle onto (and then into) lakes, rivers, or oceans, they can acidify the water there to a pH level less suitable for aquatic life. These acidic particulates can also have similar adverse effects on forests and crops that are sensitive to an acidic climate.

Furthermore, fine particles have the ability to scatter light, thereby having the strongest impact on visibility impairment which has negative effects on property values and traffic safety. When light is scattered away or absorbed, such as by certain fine particulates, both the clarity and the

212 An Introduction to Environmental Toxicology

color of what can be visioned are reduced. In the United States, fine particulates are blamed for causing the infamous Brown Cloud that has remained a complex urban pollution problem for the metropolitan area in Denver, Colorado for well over three decades. The thick, smoggy brownish cloud that hovers above that area typically occurs in the winter days as part of a seasonal air inversion. In the meantime, on the other side of the globe in the megacity Delhi in India, visibility impairment reportedly has been caused more by carbonaceous particulates (elemental and organic carbon) followed by sulfate (e.g., Singh *et al.*, 2008). In many cities across the world, including Delhi, the main sources of carbonaceous aerosols are emissions from traffics and residential combustion of coal as well as other solid fuels.

References

Aitken RJ, Creely KS, Tran CL, 2004. Nanoparticles: An Occupational Hygiene Review. Health and Safety Executive Research Report 274. Prepared by the Institute of Occupational Medicine, Research Park North, Riccarton, Edinburgh, UK.

Anderson HR, Atkinson RW, Peacock JL, Marston L, Konstantinou K, 2004. Meta-Analysis of Time Series Studies and Panel Studies of Particulate Matter (PM) and Ozone (O_3). Report of a WHO Task Group. WHO Regional Office for Europe, Copenhagen, Denmark.

Avol EL, Gauderman WJ, Tan SM, London SJ, Peters JM, 2001. Respiratory Effects of Relocating to Areas of Differing Air Pollution Levels. *Am. J. Respir. Crit. Care Med.* 164:2067-2072.

Baldasano JM, Valera E, Jiménez P, 2003. Air Quality Data from Large Cities. *Sci. Total Environ.* 307: 141-165.

Bessagnet B, Hodzic A, Blanchard O, Lattuati M, Le Bihan O, Marfaing H, Rouil L, 2005. Origin of Particulate Matter Pollution Episodes in Wintertime over the Paris Basin. *Atmos. Environ.* 39:6159-6175.

Brauer M, 2016. The Global Burden of Disease from Air Pollution. AAAS (American Association for the Advancement of Science) 2016 Annual Meeting – Global Science Engagement (Presented 13 February 2016, Washington DC, USA).

Brauer M, Freedman G, Frostad J, van Donkelaar A, Martin RV, Dentener F, van Dingenen R, Estep K, Amini H, Apte JS, Balakrishnan K, *et al.*, 2016. Ambient Air Pollution Exposure Estimation for the Global Burden of Disease 2013. *Environ. Sci. Technol.* 50:79-88.

Brodie EL, DeSantis TZ, Parker JPM, Zubietta IX, Piceno YM, Andersen GL, 2007. Urban Aerosols Harbor Diverse and Dynamic Bacterial Populations. *Proc. Natl. Acad. Sci. USA* 104:299-304.

Brook RD, Franklin B, Cascio W, Hong Y, Howard G, Lipsett M, Luepker R, Mittleman M, Samet J, Smith SC Jr, Tager I, 2004. Air Pollution and Cardiovascular Disease. *Circulation* 109:2655-2671.

Chang L-P, Tsai J-H, Chang K-L, Lin JJ, 2008. Water-Soluble Inorganic Ions in Airborne Particulates from the Nano to Coarse Mode: A Case Study of Aerosol Episodes in Southern Region of Taiwan. *Environ. Geochem. Health* 30:291-303.

Chen LC, Su WC, Qu Q, Cheng TJ, Chan CC, Hwang JS, 1999. Composition of Particulate Matter as the Determinant of Cellular Response. In *Proceedings of the Third Colloquium on Particulate Air Pollution and Human Health*. Prepared for/sponsored by the California Air Resources Board, California Environmental Protection Agency, Sacramento, California, USA.

Dales R, Burnett RT, Smith-Doiron M, Stieb DM, Brook JR, 2004. Air Pollution and Sudden Infant Death Syndrome. *Pediatrics* 113:628-631.

Daniels MJ, Dominici F, Samet JM, Zeger SL, 2000. Estimating Particulate Matter – Mortality Dose-Response Curves and Threshold Levels: An Analysis of Daily Time-Series for the 20 Largest US Cities. *Am. J. Epidemiol.* 152:397-406.

DeFranco E, Moravec W, Xu F, Hall E, Hossain M, Haynes EN, Muglia L, Chen A, 2016. Exposure to Airborne Particulate Matter during Pregnancy Is Associated with Preterm Birth: A Population-Based Cohort Study. *Environ. Health* 15:6 (online journal).

Dillner AM, Schauer JJ, Zhang Y, Zeng L, Cass GR, 2006: Size-Resolved Particulate Matter Composition in Beijing during Pollution and Dust Events. *J. Geophys. Res.* 111:D05203 (online journal).

Dominici F, Peng RD, Bell ML, Pham L, McDermott A, Zeger SL, Samet JM, 2006. Fine Particulate Air Pollution and Hospital Admission for Cardiovascular and Respiratory Diseases. *JAMA* 295:1127-1134.

EWG (Environmental Working Group), 1997. Particulate Pollution and Sudden Infant Death Syndrome in the United States. Policy memorandum prepared on 10 July by M. Evans of EWG jointly with Physicians for Social Responsibility. EWG, 1436 U Street NW, Suite 100, Washington DC, USA.

Forouzanfar MH, Alexander L, Anderson HR, Bachman VF, Biryukov S, Brauer M, Burnett R, Casey D, Coates MM, Cohen A, *et al.*, 2015. Global, Regional, and National Comparative Risk Assessment of 79 Behavioral, Environmental and Occupational, and Metabolic Risks or Clusters of Risks in 188 Countries, 1990-2013: A Systematic Analysis for the Global Burden of Disease Study 2013. *Lancet* 386:2287-2323.

Gauderman WJ, McConnell R, Gilliland F, London S, Thomas D, Avol E, Vora H, Berhane K, Rappaport EB, Lurmann F, *et al.*, 2000. Association between Air Pollution and Lung Function Growth in Southern California Children. *Am. J. Respir. Crit. Care Med.* 162:1383-1390.

Gauderman WJ, Gilliland GF, Vora H, Avol E, Stram D, McConnell R, Thomas D, Lurmann F, Margolis HG, Rappaport EB, *et al.*, 2002. Association between Air Pollution and Lung Function Growth in Southern California Children: Results from a Second Cohort. *Am. J. Respir. Crit. Care Med.* 166:76-84.

Gauderman WJ, Avol E, Gilliland F, Vora H, Thomas D, Berhane K, McConnell R, Kuenzli N, Lurmann F, Rappaport E, *et al.*, 2004. The Effect of Air Pollution on Lung Development from 10 to 18 Years of Age. *NEJM* 351:1057-1067.

Gulia S, Shiva Negendra SM, Khare M, Khanna I, 2015. Urban Air Quality Management – A Review. *Atmos. Pollut. Res.* 6:286-304.

Jones AM, Harrison RM, 2004. The Effects of Meteorological Factors on Atmospheric Bioaerosol Concentrations – A Review. *Sci. Total Environ.* 326:151-180.

Kaiser R, Romieu I, Medina S, Schwartz J, Krzyzanowski M, Künzli N, 2004. Air Pollution Attributable Postneonatal Infant Mortality in U.S. Metropolitan Areas: A Risk Assessment Study. *Environ. Health* 3:4 (online journal).

Karra S, Katsivela E, 2007. Microorganisms in Bioaerosol Emissions from Wastewater Treatment Plants during Summer at a Mediterranean Site. *Water Res.* 41:1355-1365.

Kobayashi F, Maki T, Kakikawa M, Yamada M, Puspitasari F, Iwasaka Y, 2015. Bioprocess of Kosa Bioaerosols: Effect of Ultraviolet Radiation on Airborne Bacteria within Kosa (Asian Dust). *J. Biosci. Bioeng.* 119:570-579.

Krzyzanowski M, Schwela D, 1999. Patterns of Air Pollution in Developing Countries. In *Air Pollution and Health* (Holgate ST, Samet JM, Koren HS, Maynard RL, Eds.). London, UK: Academic Press, pp. 105-113.

Kumar RS, 2008. Cotton Dust – Impact on Human Health and Environment in the Textile Industry. *Textile Magazine* 49:55-60.

Lighthart B, 2000. Mini-Review of the Concentration Variation Found in the Alfresco Atmospheric Bacterial Populations. *Aerobiologia* 16:7-16.

Lippmann M, Frampton M, Schwartz J, Dockery D, Schlesinger R, Koutrakis P, Froines J, Nel A, Finkelstein J, Godleski J, *et al.*, 2003. The U.S. Environmental Protection Agency Particulate Matter Health Effects Research Centers Program: A Midcourse Report of Status, Progress, and Plans. *Environ. Health Perspect.* 111:1074-1092.

Mage D, Ozolins G, Peterson P, Webster A, Orthofer R, Vandeveerd V, Gwynne M, 1996. Urban Air Pollution in Megacities of the World. *Atmos. Environ.* 30:681-686.

McMurry PH, 2000. The History of Condensation Nucleus Counters. *Aerosol Sci. Technol.* 33:297-322.

Mopuang M, Kongtip P, Sujirarat D, Luksamijarulkul P, 2005. Microbial Count and Particulate Matter Level in Roadside Air of Bangkok Fashion City. *Thai Environ. Engr. J.* 20:31-34.

Nemery B, Hoet PH, Nemmar A, 2001. The Meuse Valley Fog of 1930: An Air Pollution Disaster. *Lancet* 357:704-708.

Oberdorster G, Gelein RM, Ferin J, Weiss B, 1995. Association of Particulate Air Pollution and Acute Mortality: Involvement of Ultrafine Particles? *Inhal. Toxicol.* 7:111-124

Pandey KD, Wheeler D, Ostro B, Deichmann U, Hamilton K, Bolt K, 2006. Ambient Particulate Matter Concentrations in Residential and Pollution Hotspot Areas of World Cities: New Estimates Based on the Global Model of Ambient Particulates (GMAPS). The World Bank Development Economics Research Group and the Environment Department Working Paper, The World Bank, Washington DC, USA.

Polymenakou PN, Mandalakis M, Stephanou EG, Tselepides A, 2008. Particle Size Distribution of Airborne Microorganisms and Pathogens during an Intense African Dust Event in the Eastern Mediterranean. *Environ. Health Perspect.* 116:292-296.

Raabe OG, 1982. Comparison of the Criteria for Sampling 'Inhalable' and 'Respirable' Aerosols. *Ann. Occup. Hyg.* 26:33-44.

Singh T, Khillare PS, Shridhar V, Agarwal T, 2008. Visibility Impairing Aerosols in the Urban Atmosphere of Delhi. *Environ. Monit. Assess.* 141:67-77.

Stanley RG, Linskins HF, 1974. *Pollen: Biology, Chemistry and Management*. Berlin, Germany: Springer Verlag.

Sun Q, Wang A, Jin X, Natanzon A, Duquaine D, Brook RD, Aguinaldo J-G, Fayad ZA, Fuster V, Lippmann M, *et al.*, 2005. Long-Term Air Pollution Exposure and Acceleration of Atherosclerosis and Vascular Inflammation in an Animal Model. *JAMA* 294:3003-3010.

Tong S, Colditz P, 2004. Air Pollution and Sudden Infant Death Syndrome: A Literature Review. *Paediatr. Perinat. Epidemiol.* 18:327-335.

Triantafyllou AG, Zoras S, Evagelopoulos V, 2006. Particulate Matter over a Seven Year Period in Urban and Rural Areas within, proximal and far from Mining and Power Station Operations in Greece. *Environ. Monit. Assess.* 122:41-60.

UNICEF (United Nations International Children's Fund), 2016. Clear the Air for Children – The Impact of Air Pollution on Children. UNICEF Division of Data, Research and Policy, 3 United Nations Plaza, New York, New York, 10017, USA.

U.S. EPA (U.S. Environmental Protection Agency), 1999. Sampling of Ambient Air for Total Suspended Particulate Matter (SPM) and PM_{10} Using High Volume (HV) Sampler. Compendium Method IO-2.1, EPA/625/R-96/010a. Office of Research and Development, Cincinnati, Ohio, USA.

U.S. EPA (U.S. Environmental Protection Agency), 2004. Air Quality Criteria for Particulate Matter, Volume I. EPA/600/P-99/002aF. Office of Research and Development, Research Triangle Park, North Carolina, USA.

U.S. EPA (U.S. Environmental Protection Agency), 2005. Particulate Matter Health Risk Assessment for Selected Urban Areas. EPA 452/R-05-007A. Office of Air Quality Planning and Standards, Research Triangle Park, North Carolina, USA.

U.S. EPA (U.S. Environmental Protection Agency), 2013. National Ambient Air Quality Standards for Particulate Matter. *Federal Register* 78:3086-3287.

U.S. EPA (U. S. Environmental Protection Agency), 2017a. National Air Quality: Status and Trends of Key Air Pollutants (webpage updated 26 July 2017). https://www.epa.gov/air-trends (retrieved 30 July 2017).

U.S. EPA (U.S. Environmental Protection Agency), 2017b. Green Book: PM-10 (1987) Designated Area by State/Area/County/Area (data current as of 20 June 2017). https://www3.epa.gov/airquality/greenbook/pbcty.html (retrieved 4 August 2017).

van Zelma R, Huijbregtsa MAJ, den Hollanderc HA, van Jaarsveldd HA, Sautere FJ, Struijsb J, van Wijnenc HJ, van de Meent D, 2008. European Characterization Factors for Human Health Damage of PM_{10} and Ozone in Life Cycle Impact Assessment. *Atmos. Environ.* 42:441-453.

WHO (World Health Organization), 2006a. Health Risks of Particulate Matter from Long-Range Transboundary Air Pollution. WHO Regional Office for Europe, Copenhagen, Denmark.

WHO (World Health Organization), 2006b. WHO Air Quality Guidelines for Particular Matter, Ozone, Nitrogen Dioxide and Sulfur Dioxide: Global Update 2005, Summary of Risk Assessment. Geneva, Switzerland, Chapter 2.

WHO (World Health Organization), 2016. Ambient Air Pollution: A Global Assessment of Exposure and Burden of Disease. Geneva, Switzerland.

Willinger M, James LS, Catz C, 1991. Defining the Sudden Infant Death Syndrome (SIDS): Deliberations of an Expert Panel Convened by the National Institute of Child Health and Human Development. *Pediatr. Pathol.* 11:677-684.

Woodruff TJ, Grillo J, Schoendorf KC, 1997. The Relationship between Selected Causes of Postneonatal Infant Mortality and Particulate Air Pollution in the United States. *Environ. Health Perspect.* 105:608-612.

Woodruff TJ, Parker JD, Schoendorf KC, 2006. Fine Particulate Matter ($PM_{2.5}$) Air Pollution and Selected Causes of Postneonatal Infant Mortality in California. *Environ. Health Perspect.* 114:786-790.

Yu O, Sheppard L, Lumley T, Koenig JQ, Shapiro GG, 2000. Effects of Ambient Air Pollution on Symptoms of Asthma in Seattle-Area Children Enrolled in the CAMP Study. *Environ. Health Perspect.* 108:1209-1214.

Zanobetti A, Schwartz J, 2000. Race, Gender, and Social Status as Modifiers of the Effects of PM_{10} on Mortality. *J. Occup. Environ. Med.* 42:469-474.

Zanobetti A, Schwartz J, 2001. Are Diabetics More Susceptible to the Health Effects of Airborne Particles? *Am. J. Respir. Crit. Care Med.* 164:831-833.

Zanobetti A, Schwartz J, 2002. Cardiovascular Damage by Airborne Particles: Are Diabetics More Susceptible? *Epidemiology* 13:588-592.

Zanobetti A, Schwartz J, Gold D, 2000. Are There Sensitive Subgroups for the Health Effects of Airborne Particles? *Environ. Health Perspect.* 108:841-845.

Zheng Z, Xie X, Ouyang Y, Wang C, Zeng H, Chen Y, Chen T, 2009. Study on the Relativity between Airborne Microbes and Environmental Factors in Pearl River Delta' Urban Agglomeration, Guangdong. *J. Sustain. Develop.* 2:106-113.

Review Questions

1. What do the terms *dust, smoke, smog, fume, haze, fog,* and *mist* refer to in relation to atmospheric aerosol pollution?
2. What are the main differences between airborne particulates formed from wind-blown dust particles in tropical regions and those from sea spray, in terms of their composition?
3. What are the main differences between primary and secondary particulate matter?
4. Briefly characterize the various sizes of airborne particulate matter that are of regulatory importance.
5. Which of the following is nonhygroscopic and likely has an atmospheric half-life of minutes to days? a) $PM_{0.1}$; b) $PM_{0.1-1}$; c) $PM_{2.5}$; d) $PM_{2.5-10}$; e) $PM_{[2.5]}$.
6. Give at least three examples for the sources of $PM_{2.5-10}$.
7. Briefly describe the two accumulation processes *condensation* and *coagulation* for formation of $PM_{0.1}$.
8. What might be the technical differences between ultrafine and nano-particles?
9. What is generally the single most abundant source of PM in urban areas? And what is the more specific, major source of PM in megacities?
10. Name a region in the United States that currently is designated as (one of) the worst for nonattainment of PM_{10}.
11. Name three episodes of urban airborne particulate pollution that were caused by dust storms or industrial processing, as covered in this chapter.
12. Briefly discuss some of the major concerns, issues, or problems with monitoring PM concentrations, particularly in the developing countries, as discussed in this chapter.
13. Briefly explain why airborne microbes should be treated as a major and significant constituent of urban airborne particulate pollution.
14. What type(s) of particles was (were) considered responsible for causing the deaths in the acute air pollution episode that occurred in Belgium's Meuse Valley in 1930?
15. List the human subpopulations that tend to be more susceptible to PM-associated health problems.
16. It has estimated that approximately _____ of the world population currently breathes air that does not comply with the WHO air quality guidelines: a) 60%; b) 70%; c) 80%; d) 90%.
17. Briefly explain why children are especially susceptible to adverse health effects of PM on their respiratory system.
18. What may be a plausible mechanism that promotes atherosclerosis leading to cardiovascular diseases when humans or mice are subjected to chronic exposure to air polluted by $PM_{2.5}$, especially when the exposure is coupled with a high-fat diet?
19. What is the key determinant that will direct or cause an airborne particle to rest in the respiratory tract once inhaled?
20. Briefly explain what diesel particulate matter is, and briefly describe its impacts on human health.
21. List the major types or forms of adverse effects on the environment that can be caused by airborne particulate pollution.

CHAPTER 13

Volatile Organic Compounds

ა·ა

13.1. Introduction

In general terms, volatile organic compounds (VOCs) refer to a huge group of diverse hydrocarbon (and hence *organic*) solid or liquid substances that readily evaporate and remain in the air as gases at ambient temperature. These hydrocarbons (HCs), including those fully halogenated, generally have a sufficiently high vapor pressure with a boiling point between $50°$ to $250°$ C ($122°$ to $482°$ F). Organic compounds in this group include a vast variety of biological substances from plants, synthetic chemicals from industrial processes, ingredients from household products, and components from protective coatings as well as paints in building or other structural materials. More bluntly, VOCs of environmental health concern can be found virtually everywhere indoors and outdoors, such as in the air, the water, soils, waste dumps, industrial products, and household as well as consumer goods. Yet in practice, as due to limited resources but largely to the complexities involved in tracking the emission quantity of each VOC, many regulatory agencies (e.g., U.S. EPA) focus on only a handful that have been determined to pose serious health threats while at the same time their occurrence is with alarmingly high frequency around residential areas.

13.1.1. As Precursors of Ozone and Particulate Matter

As noted in Chapters 11 and 12, some VOCs are precursors of ozone (O_3) and secondary particulate matter (PM). The formation of O_3 with VOCs as precursors can occur via the reaction between oxygen (O_2) and peroxyacyl radicals R-CO_3·, where R stands for any organic substituent group (Reaction 11.9). Many atmospheric VOCs can also react directly with sunlight and nitrogen oxides (NO_x) to form O_3.

In the urban atmospheric environment, the most abundant secondary species of PM include sulfate (SO_4^{2-}), nitrate (NO_3^-), and ammonium (NH_4^+) compounds, as well as secondary organic matter (SOM). The formation of SOM from oxidation of atmospheric VOCs can contribute significantly to the airborne particulate load. Although the formation of SOM is not well understood in part due to the perturbation with the wide array of VOC species available, one accepted mechanism is the oxidation of HC compounds with six or more carbon (C) atoms to form products with lower vapor pressure. When such an atmospheric VOC is oxidized (e.g., by hydroxyl radical HO·), the resultant oxidation product has relatively higher polarity and lower volatility due to the addition of oxygen or nitrogen to the parent compound regardless of the species involved. Because of their lower volatility, these "semi-volatile" oxidation products will eventually condense on preexisting PM. Some of these oxidation products can "nucleate" directly and homogeneously to form new ultra-tiny particles (Seinfeld and Pankow, 2003).

13.1.2. Sources of Environmental Pollution

As VOCs are available in a wide array of products, nearly every person is inevitably exposed to some of these substances to some level. Smokers and individuals working at dry cleaners, photograph laboratories, industrial facilities, or similar settings tend to face the highest risk. In addition to consumer products such as automotive cleaners, spot removers, and degreasing fluids, many VOCs can be found in groundwater.

Contamination of groundwater with certain VOCs can be traced to sources such as industrial facilities, home septic tanks, municipal landfills, and (hazardous) waste dumps. Some VOCs can also be found in groundwater when fuel such as gasoline is spilled on the ground or leaks from an underground storage tank. These substances can readily evaporate into indoor air when contaminated water is used for drinking or during cooking, showering, and washing dishes, particularly when the water is heated. Accordingly, the levels of VOCs can be higher indoors than in outdoor ambient air, sometimes by as much as tenfold or more under certain circumstances such as in a confined, closed-door area.

There are two prominent groups of VOCs when all common anthropogenic sources are considered: (1) chlorinated solvents; and (2) fuel components. Chlorinated solvents are widely used in industry and as components of common consumer products, such as carbon tetrachloride (CCl_4), methylene chloride (CH_2Cl_2), tetrachloroethylene ($Cl_2C=CCl_2$), trichloroethylene ($HC=CCl_3$), and vinyl chloride ($CH_2=CHCl$). Fuel components, those found largely in petroleum, include benzene (C_6H_6), toluene ($C_6H_5CH_3$), the isomers of xylene ($C_6H_4C_2H_6$), and methyl *tert(iary)*-butyl ether ($C_5H_{12}O$). Many VOCs, including notably formaldehyde (CH_2O), can also be by-products from indoor combustion or certain natural processes. Other by-products of less concern to environmental health include those formed by chlorination in water treatment, such as chloroform ($CHCl_3$).

13.2. Use Standards and Environmental Health Concerns

There are global concerns with VOCs not only because of their high emission volumes found compromising the ambient as well as the indoor air quality everywhere, but also for the fact that many of these substances are fairly or highly toxic to humans. No country or region has yet established standards for use of VOCs in non-commercial or non-industrial settings. However, a number of countries including the United States have set a maximum contaminant level (MCL) or the kind for a handful of VOCs in groundwater. In addition, U.S. Occupational Safety and Health Administration (OSHA) has regulated formaldehyde (CH_2O) as a carcinogen, by adopting a permissible exposure limit (PEL) of 0.75 ppm (parts per million) for exposure in workplaces (Table 20.1). Switzerland and Australia are among the other two dozen nations also setting a standard for worker exposure to formaldehyde.

13.2.1. Standards for Consumer/Commercial Products

In April 2004, the European Union (EU) finalized the EU-wide VOC content limits on solvent paints, varnishes, and vehicle refinishing products. The EU legislation (under The Paints Directive 2004/42/EC) sets limits for the maximum contents of VOCs in 12 categories of decorative paints and varnishes, as well as in 5 categories of products used in vehicle refinishing (e.g., the coating of road vehicles used as part of vehicle repair).

For certain consumer and commercial products available in the United States, federal *emission* standards for their VOC content limits were issued by U.S. EPA (1988) three decades ago. These certain products included vehicle refinish coatings, air fresheners, fabric protectants, flea and tick insecticides, oven cleaners, hair styling gels, shaving creams, and more. California was the first state passing its own law in 2000 to limit the VOC contents in paints and coatings. Arizona, New Jersey, New York, and Texas were the other few states that shortly followed suit to adopt their own content limits for VOCs in similar products.

Effective 1 January 2009, the states of California, Maine, Maryland, Michigan, New Jersey, and Pennsylvania all impose more stringent content limits for product categories already covered in their existing VOC regulations, while in some cases also expanding their list of product categories per their existing regulation (Balek, 2009). The VOC limits in California (actually effective 31 December 2008) are 1% of the product content by weight for non-aerosol sanitizers, disinfectants, as well as bathroom and tile cleaners. There does not seem to be any content limits set for VOCs in consumer products outside of the United States, except those proposed by the Canadian government (Environment Canada, 2013).

13.2.2. Select Compounds of Environmental Health Concern

Aside from being the precursors of O_3 and secondary PM to either of which exposure can pose public health threats, VOCs as a group have their own wide range of health effects on humans ranging from being carcinogenic to relatively harmless. For a considerable number of these HC compounds, long-term exposure can damage the liver, the kidneys, and the nervous system. Due to their use mostly being the components of consumer and commercial products, their toxic effects on plants, vegetation, and wildlife generally receive less public health attention. It is on this notion that the characteristics, pollution sources, and health effects of the six select VOCs are so (not) discussed in this chapter. The select six VOCs are formaldehyde (CH_2O), benzene (C_6H_6), methyl *tert(iary)*-butyl ether ($C_5H_{12}O$), methylene chloride (CH_2Cl_2), tetrachloroethylene (C_2Cl_4), and trichloroethylene (C_2HCl_3). They have been selected due to their certain unique applications, large production, relatively high toxicity to humans, and in some case didactic merit.

More specifically, this chapter has a special concern with formaldehyde because the solvent is commonly utilized (as a component) to manufacture a variety of consumer (e.g., upholstery cleaners, nail polish removers) and textile products (e.g., those fabrics treated with its resins to become crease-resistant) found in homes. For benzene, the high health concern is with its use in the United States being in the top 20 in terms of production volume for synthesis of other chemicals, along with the fact that it is a ubiquitous natural component of crude oil, gasoline, and cigarette smoke. Methyl *tert(iary)*-butyl ether is still being produced in huge quantities outside of the United States for use predominantly as a fuel additive (i.e., as an oxygenate) in motor gasoline. The other three VOCs (methylene chloride, tetrachloroethylene, trichloroethylene) selected for discussion in this chapter are among the handful toxic *chlorinated* solvents still being applied widely in the industry today, at least in some parts of the world.

The chemical structures of the six select VOCs are given in Figure 13.1 below. Their physicochemical and toxicological characteristics are discussed systematically in their own sections that follow. For their physicochemical and toxicological properties, much of the specific information presented in this chapter is from the individual documents prepared for their toxicological profiles by the U.S. Agency for Toxic Substances and Disease Registry (ATSDR). Major sources for supplementary information are U.S. EPA and the World Health Organization (WHO).

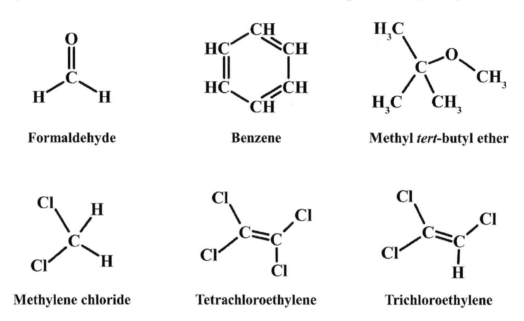

Figure 13.1. Chemical Structures of Six Select Volatile Organic Compounds

13.3. Formaldehyde

At ambient temperature (21.1° C or 70° F), formaldehyde (CH_2O) is a flammable, nearly colorless gas with a suffocating, pungent smell. It is the simplest aldehyde (R-CHO, where R is an organyl group and for formaldehyde an hydrogen atom instead), and is known by several other names including formic aldehyde, methanal, and methyl aldehyde. This VOC is soluble in water but does not stay in a water solution for long. In sunlight, most of its molecules in the air will decompose into formic acid (CH_2O_2). While formaldehyde does not accumulate in animals or plants, it is produced in small quantities in the human body. In liquid (≥37% solution), it has a boiling point of 96° C (205° F) and a vapor pressure of ~25 mm Hg at 25° C (77° F).

13.3.1. Sources and Uses

Formaldehyde (CH_2O) is used in many industrial processes. It is a component of many consumer products (e.g., automobile body polishes, synthetic resins, carpets, disinfectants, personal care products, cosmetics). The VOC is also a common building block for the synthesis of many other more complex materials, particularly for the production of polymers. It has projected (MRC, 2014) that the global CH_2O production in 2017 would exceed 52 million tons.

Formaldehyde (CH_2O) gas at room temperature readily converts to a variety of derivatives, of which many are applied extensively in the industry. One important or popular derivative is the stable cyclic 1,3,5-trioxane ($C_3H_6O_3$). This cyclic trimer is commonly used as a stable source of anhydrous CH_2O and for polymerization of certain thermoplastics (e.g., polyacetal). A polymer formed from formaldehyde is termed *paraformaldehyde* ($OH[CH_2O]_nH$; typically, n = 9 to 100). When reacting with certain substances (e.g., melamine, phenol, urea), this simple aldehyde produces resins that have wide applications as adhesives and binders in the wood product, pulp and paper, and fiberglass industries. The textile industry frequently uses CH_2O-based resins as finishers to make fabrics crease-resistant.

Formaldehyde can be formed naturally with atmospheric carbon (C), hydrogen (H), and oxygen (O_2). This natural source may account for as much as 90% of its total volume in a certain environment. The VOC is a major intermediate in the combustion of methane (CH_4) and many other HC substances (e.g., those in wildfires, automobile exhausts, tobacco smoke). Formaldehyde can be a major component of photochemical smog when accumulated in the air following the oxidation of atmospheric CH_4 (Reactions 13.1) and other HC substances, provided that O_3 (ozone), nitric oxide (NO), sunlight (hv), and water (H_2O) vapor are all sufficiently available.

$$O_3 + hv \rightarrow O_2 + O\cdot \quad (13.1a)$$

$$O\cdot + H_2O \rightarrow 2HO\cdot \quad (13.1b)$$

$$CH_4 + HO\cdot \rightarrow CH_3\cdot + H_2O \quad (13.1c)$$

$$CH_3\cdot + O_2 \rightarrow CH_3O_2\cdot \quad (13.1d)$$

$$CH_3O_2\cdot + NO \rightarrow CH_3O\cdot + NO_2 \quad (13.1e)$$

$$CH_3O\cdot + O_2 \rightarrow CH_2O + HO_2\cdot \quad (13.1f)$$

Subreactions 13.1a and 13.1b above are part of those given in Section 5.2.3B for photochemical reaction. The three methane-based radicals involved in the above subreactions are methyloxy radical ($CH_3O\cdot$), methyl peroxy radical ($CH_3O_2\cdot$), and methyl radical ($CH_3\cdot$). As cyclic and complex as the process seems to be, following CH_2O (formaldehyde) formation (Subreaction 13.1f) the resultant perhydroxyl (a.k.a. hyperoxy) radical $HO_2\cdot$ can combine with NO to form nitrogen dioxide (NO_2) and hydroxyl radical $HO\cdot$.

Formaldehyde is used widely as a disinfectant owing to its capability of eliminating many fungi, many bacteria, and some viruses. Topical solutions containing CH_2O derivatives as active ingredients are applied as medicines for treatment of warts and some other skin conditions. Some topical creams, cosmetics, and personal hygiene products specifically contain CH_2O derivatives for prevention of bacterial infection. For example, methenamine ($N_4[CH_2]_6$) is a cyclic HC (hydrocarbon) compound that in acid medium can be hydrolyzed into ammonia (NH_3) and CH_2O.

This cyclic HC is commonly used to prevent and treat urinary tract infections. On the other hand, it is not an unknown fact that formaldehyde has been widely applied as an embalming agent for the temporary preservation of human and animal remains from decay.

13.3.2. Exposures and Toxic Effects

As far back as in the 1980s, animal studies revealed that long-term exposure to CH_2O (formaldehyde) caused nasal cancer in rats (ATSDR, 1999, 2010a; NCI, 2009). Some 25 years later, after many more carcinogenicity data have been reassessed thoroughly by its 26 scientists from 10 countries, WHO's International Agency for Research on Cancer (IARC, 2006, 2012, 2017) has classified CH_2O as a human (Group 1) carcinogen. The IARC experts have concluded that there is now sufficient evidence linking CH_2O exposure to the development of nasopharyngeal cancer in humans, which is a rare kind occurring predominantly in the developing countries. The experts have also found limited evidence linking CH_2O exposure to leukemia as well as to cancers at other sites including oral cavity, lung, and brain.

The main concern with CH_2O exposure is for workers in the facilities that manufacture or process the VOC, in the healthcare industry, and in the embalming business. A considerable number of workers are exposed to CH_2O every day in the developed and developing countries. It has estimated that around 152,000 Canadians (CAREX Canada, 2012) and 235,000 Australians (Driscoll, 2014) may be exposed to CH_2O at work. It has also projected that over 1 million workers may be exposed to some level of CH_2O across the European Union (IARC, 2006). In the meantime, China is reportedly the largest producer as well as consumer of this VOC in the world (e.g., Tang *et al.*, 2009).

Occupational exposure to CH_2O (formaldehyde) is from three major sources: during (1) decomposition of CH_2O-based resins; (2) emission of CH_2O from embalming fluids or other aqueous solutions; and (3) production of CH_2O via the combustion of a variety of organic substances (e.g., as included in automobile exhaust fumes). In addition to carcinogenic harm, CH_2O can cause allergy and other short-term adverse health effects. Inasmuch as its resins are used in many textile and construction materials, formaldehyde is one of the common indoor air pollutants. When present in the air at levels exceeding 0.1 ppm, it can irritate the human eyes and mucous membranes. As a result, some people may experience watery eyes, burning sensations (in the eyes, nose, or throat), coughing, wheezing, nausea, and skin irritation. Severe exposure can cause death from burns to the lungs, as proven in test animals (ATSDR, 1999, 2010a). Some people are particularly sensitive to CH_2O. For them, exposure to even very small amounts of the VOC can trigger asthma symptoms or cause breathing difficulties. It is for these health concerns that EU has banned the commercial use of formaldehyde since September 2007.

In the United States, at least three incidents were reported to have been caused by exposure to CH_2O-based resins used to build trailers (and mobile homes). The occupants were victims of the Iowa floods in 2008, Hurricane Katrina in 2005, and Hurricane Rita in 2005. The trailers that the victims moved into were provided by the U.S. Federal Emergency Management Agency (FEMA) in response to the evacuation crises. Some of the trailer occupants complained of violent coughing, nosebleeds, breathing difficulties, and persistent headaches. Analytical tests reportedly (e.g., CDC,

2010; Hsu, 2008) revealed that the formaldehyde levels in some of these trailers exceeded the maximum limit of 16 ppb (parts per billion) adopted by FEMA (e.g., DHS, 2009).

13.4. Benzene

Benzene (C_6H_6) is a colorless, flammable liquid with an aromatic (i.e., sweet) smell. This VOC is a *mono*aromatic (i.e., that with *one* benzene ring) HC (hydrocarbon) substance available as a natural constituent of crude oil and can be synthesized from other chemical components present in petroleum. It is structurally famous for its highly poly*un*saturated *benzene* ring which is constructed with one hydrogen (H) atom for each of the six carbon (C) atoms forming the ring (Figure 13.1). Benzene is insoluble in water (0.19% at 25° C), but miscible with many (other) organic solvents (e.g., alcohol, carbon disulfide, chloroform, oils). It has a boiling point of 80.1° C (176° F) and a vapor pressure of 75 mm Hg at 20° C (68° F).

13.4.1. Sources and Uses

Benzene is commonly found in automobile exhaust fumes, industrial emissions, fumes from automobile service stations, tobacco smoke, and household products such as glues, paint strippers, and detergents. Because the VOC has been more recently and actively treated as a human carcinogen, its application as an additive in gasoline is now limited in many countries. However, it is still widely utilized as an industrial solvent and a precursor in the production of drugs, dyes, plastics, rubbers, and pesticides.

Many important chemicals are derived from benzene by replacing one or more of its H atoms with functional groups (e.g., $-NH_2$, $-OH$, $-CH_3$). Examples of simple benzene derivatives include toluene ($C_6H_5CH_3$), the isomers of xylenes ($C_6H_4C[CH_3]_2$), and phenol (C_6H_5OH). On the other hand, linking two benzene rings gives the biphenyl (C_6H_5-C_6H_5) molecule, which is the core structural unit present in PCBs (polychlorinated biphenyls). Further loss of the two H and C atoms at this linkage gives the "fused" two-ring aromatic HC substance named naphthalene ($C_{10}H_8$). Anthracene ($C_{14}H_{10}$) is a fused three-ring aromatic HC substance (with one of its three rings being fused to the other two at its opposite sides). All HC substances with two or more benzene rings are termed *polynuclear* or *polycyclic* aromatic hydrocarbons (PAHs). For those substances referred to as *hetero*cyclic hydrocarbons (i.e., *hetero*cycles), at least one C atom in the benzene ring is replaced with a different chemical element (e.g., nitrogen).

In the United States, gasoline used to contain a small percent of benzene as an antiknock additive until it was replaced by tetraethyl lead ($[CH_3CH_2]_4Pb$) in the 1950s. However, these days with the worldwide phase-out of leaded gasoline, benzene has been used once again as a gasoline additive in some countries. Recent concerns with benzene's adverse health effects and the potential for its entering groundwater have led to more stringent regulations of its content in all forms of gasoline in Europe (Ubrich and Jeuland, 2007) and the United States (U.S. EPA, 2006), with national limits being set at respectively 1% and 0.62% by content.

Benzene is now used primarily as an intermediate to synthesize other chemicals, with styrene ($C_6H_5CH=CH_2$) being one of the most widely produced derivatives. Styrene, also known as vinyl benzene, is commonly utilized to make polystyrene (a thermoplastic substance) and copolymers (those made from two or more monomeric species). Other benzene derivatives include phenol and the fully saturated cyclohexane (C_6H_{12}). Phenol is widely used for resins and adhesives, and is an important precursor for large groups of herbicides and pharmaceuticals. Cyclohexane is applied mostly as raw material for the production of nylon.

In laboratory research, toluene is now commonly used in place of benzene. Even though the chemical properties of the two monoaromatics are similar, toluene has a wider liquid range and, due to its methyl unit (-CH_3), is relatively less toxic. The methyl group in toluene is subject to rapid oxidation, thereby causing the aromatic to undergo a relatively more rapid enzymatic degradation to result in a lower observed toxicity.

13.4.2. Exposures and Toxic Effects

Exposure to benzene may come from several sources. Outdoor air may contain low levels of benzene from tobacco smoke, wildfires, automobile exhausts, fumes from automobile service stations, and industrial emissions. Air with higher levels of benzene can be found around toxic waste dumps or near older, not well-constructed gasoline stations. Naturally, the indoor sources include indoor tobacco smoking and vapors from household products that contain the VOC as one of their components (more commonly referred to as ingredients).

Workers in various industries processing or producing benzene are at a higher risk of exposure to this carcinogenic aromatic. Industries engaging in the use of benzene include shoe making, rubber production, paint production, leather manufacturing, oil refinery, and adhesive production. In the United States, OSHA has set a PEL of 1 ppm for an 8-hour workday, 40-hour workweek exposure (i.e., on a time-weighted average basis), and a short-term exposure limit of 5 ppm for 15 minutes. Discussion on OSHA's PELs, including sources of their values set for benzene and other toxic substances, is given in Chapter 20 on occupational toxicology.

At times, water and soil contaminations are also major sources of exposure to benzene. For example, it was reported (GWPC, 2007) that over 100,000 underground storage tank sites across the United States involved groundwater or soil contamination by some form of benzene as a result of industrial seepage. In the United States, federal regulations require that reports be submitted to U.S. EPA for spills or accidental releases of benzene into the environment if they each amount to 10 pounds (4.5 kg) or more. U.S. EPA (2012) has set the nation's MCL of benzene in drinking water at 5 µg/L. As a more specific case, the water supply to the greater city of Harbin in China (the tenth largest in the nation with a population of nearly 10 million people) was shut down for five days in November 2005 (UNEP, 2005). The shutdown was due to a chemical explosion occurring 10 days earlier in a petrochemical plant located nearby. The explosion led to a chemical spill of roughly 100 tons of toxic mixture of benzene, nitrobenzene ($C_6H_5NO_2$), and aniline (C_6H_5-NH_2) into the nearby Songhua River supplying the city's drinking water.

Human exposure to benzene is a global health concern. This monoaromatic targets several vital body organs including the liver, kidneys, lungs, blood cells, heart, and brain. In addition, it can cause breakage of DNA strand as well as damage to chromosomes. The major health concern with benzene exposure, however, is its effects on the blood. Benzene is known to cause leukemia, a cancer involving the blood-forming organs. Chronic exposure to benzene can cause bone marrow damage, lower white blood cell count, and a decrease in red blood cells that can lead to anemia. Benzene can cause excessive bleeding and increase the chance of infection by depressing the immunological system. The organic solvent is also linked to other hematological malignancies (i.e., those cancers that affect the blood, bone marrow, and lymph nodes). Overall, there does not appear to be any controversy or dispute over the body of evidence linking benzene to acute myeloid leukemia or to acute nonlymphocytic leukemia. According to the toxicological profile prepared by ATSDR (2007, 2015), several studies collectively showed that benzene caused cancer in both sexes of multiple species of animals exposed via various routes. IARC (1987, 2012, 2017) has long listed benzene as a human (Group 1) carcinogen.

In humans, benzene is biotransformed into several metabolites including *trans, trans*-muconic acid ($C_6H_6O_4$) which can be accurately measured in the urine if the test is performed shortly following exposure. Despite the fact that this urine test may not be sufficiently specific for benzene exposure, as the metabolite can come from other sources, it is a practical and relatively inexpensive biomonitoring tool. Pure benzene in the human body can also be oxidized to produce the metabolite benzene epoxide. This epoxide is not readily excreted out of the body, but can readily interact with a guanine base on the DNA to form a DNA adduct which has the potential to cause cancer.

Acute exposure to benzene at high concentrations can lead to unconsciousness (as it can cause narcosis) and hence even death, whereas at low concentrations it can cause drowsiness, dizziness, rapid heart rate, tremors, and confusion. If the exposure is via drinking water or eating foods with high levels of benzene, the symptoms can include vomiting, nausea, and irritation of the gastrointestinal tract.

13.5. Methyl *tert(iary)*-Butyl Ether

Methyl *tert(iary)*-butyl ether ($C_5H_{12}O$), known to the public more commonly by its acronym MTBE, is a volatile, flammable, and colorless liquid. MTBE has a minty odor somewhat reminiscent of diethyl ether ($[CH_3\text{-}CH_2]_2O$), leading to unpleasant taste and odor in water. The VOC is only moderately soluble in water (4.8% at 20° C), but miscible with gasoline and certain (other) organic solvents (e.g., alcohol, other ethers). It has a boiling point of 55.2° C (131° F) and a vapor pressure of 245 mm Hg at 25° C.

13.5.1. Sources and Uses

MTBE is currently being investigated for its potential use as an inexpensive solvent for dissolving gallstones by utilizing a special surgical tube to deliver the solvent directly to the patient's gall bladder. This minty ether can be produced via the chemical reaction of methanol (CH_3OH) with isobutylene (C_4H_8). Methanol is derived from the methane-rich natural gas whereas isobutylene can be made available from butane (C_4H_{10}) in crude oil or natural gas, thereby qualifying MTBE as a (product or component of) fossil fuel. MTBE is commonly used as an oxygenate in gasoline to raise the octane rating. However, the gasoline additive recently has been increasingly noticed to quickly and easily pollute large quantities of groundwater when gasoline oxygenated with MTBE is spilled or leaked around gasoline stations. Due to such rising environmental health concerns, its production in the United States has declined substantially in recent years.

MTBE was produced in the United States in huge quantities during its high use as a fuel additive, with over 200,000 barrels per day in 1999. However, due to the numerous state bans of its application as a gasoline oxygenate, MTBE's daily production in the nation has since reduced substantially, with about 41,000 barrels in 2015 (USEIA, 2017). The state bans were enacted in response to high concerns over the widespread contamination by MTBE-containing gasoline detected in many drinking water aquifers within the affected states. The widespread releases of MTBE-containing gasoline reportedly came from underground storage tanks, with the most infamous cases being in Santa Monica and South Lake Tahoe (both places located in California).

To a certain extent, the decline of MTBE production in the United States is also due to the alternative ethanol-derived ethyl *tert(iary)*-butyl ether ($C_6H_{14}O$) being given a more favorable tax break in many states. The use and production of MTBE are declining in western Europe at a similar rate. However, MTBE's market is expected to continue to grow in other parts of the world. In 2011, Asia alone reportedly accounted for approximately 35% (5.25 tons) of the global MTBE supply in volume terms (PRWeb, 2014).

As an organic solvent, MTBE possesses a distinct advantage over most other ethers by having a higher boiling point coupled with a much lower tendency to form explosive organic peroxides. This minty ether is biodegradable to carbon dioxide (CO_2) and water (H_2O) molecules under aerobic conditions with bacteria that usually are of the slow-growing type. In any event, MTBE can be removed rapidly and affordably from water to undetectable levels by means of a fluidized bed reactor designed specifically to carry out multiphase chemical reactions.

13.5.2. Exposures and Toxic Effects

Given that MTBE offers water an unpleasant taste even at very low levels (~10 µg/L), it can render large quantities of groundwater non-potable. MTBE is frequently introduced into water-supply aquifers either by leakage from underground storage tanks around gasoline stations, or by MTBE-treated gasoline spilling onto the ground nearby. Despite the fact that nowadays the storage tanks are much better designed and better constructed than in the 1980s, a substantial number of accidental releases still occur since many of the older tanks are still being used. Owing to its high solubility and persistence, MTBE travels faster and farther than many other gasoline components released into the same aquifer. Another reality is that MTBE's high water solubility will cause it to seep through soils with ease, thereby polluting large quantities of ground and surface waters rather quickly.

The views amongst scientists concerning the adverse health effects of MTBE are inconsistent at the moment, in part because of the limited toxicity data available. The animal data reviewed by ATSDR (1996) supported the link between inhalation exposure to MTBE and certain adverse respiratory effects. Acute health effects such as coughing, nose or throat burning, headaches, and nausea were reported by people exposed to the fuel vapors while pumping MTBE-treated gasoline into automobile tanks or while driving on the road (ATSDR, 1996; NRC, 1996). At any rate, there was (and still is) the contention that symptoms of this type as observed in the human studies could come from concurrent exposure to other gasoline components.

IARC (1999, 2017) has listed MTBE as a Group 3 carcinogen (i.e., an agent not classifiable as to its carcinogenicity to humans; *see* Box 18.1 for the classification scheme used by IARC). U.S. EPA (1997), on the other hand, has reached a different decision on the VOC's carcinogenicity to humans. The federal agency has classified MTBE as a potential human carcinogen at high doses, after receiving the support of an interagency assessment (Melnick *et al.*, 1997). The data available to U.S. EPA showed that when test animals inhaled high doses of MTBE, some developed cancers or experienced other health effects, including depression of the central nervous system (CNS), decreased muscle tone, impaired treadmill performance, labored respiration, ataxia, and decreased hind-limb grip. As of today, U.S. EPA has not set a national health advisory limit for MTBE in drinking water, based on the argument that the limited animal data on hand were insufficient to quantify the VOC's health risks from the low exposure levels anticipated in drinking water.

13.6. Methylene Chloride (Dichloromethane)

The molecular formula of methylene chloride (MC) is CH_2Cl_2, which thus gives the VOC the other equally popular chemical name *dichloro*methane (DCM). MC is a colorless, nonflammable liquid widely used as an industrial solvent. The chlorinated solvent is slightly soluble in water (20 g/L at 20° C), but fairly miscible with many (other) organic solvents (e.g., acetone, alcohol, carbon tetrachloride, chloroform). MC has a sweet aroma, a boiling point of 40° C (104° F), and a vapor pressure of 349 mm Hg at 20° C.

13.6.1. Sources and Uses

Methylene chloride (a.k.a. dichloromethane) is a useful organic solvent for many industrial processes owing to its low boiling point and high solvency power to dissolve a wide array of other organic substances. The chlorinated solvent is used principally as a paint remover, as an aerosol spray propellant, as a degreasing agent, and in the manufacture of pharmaceuticals (e.g., vitamins, antibiotics, steroids, tablet coating). In the food industry, it is used as an extraction solvent for coffee decaffeination, hops, and spices. Some consumer products in aerosol form may contain the VOC as an ingredient, such as in room deodorants and household cleaners. MC (a.k.a. DCM) is used in the garment screen printer industry for removal of heat-seal transfers on garments. The solvent is also used for cleaning metal surfaces. Due to its chemical ability to weld plastic parts, MC is commonly applied to seal the casing of electric meters.

Nearly two decades ago, the annual global production of MC was estimated (WHO, 2000a) at over 500,000 tons, of which over 50% was used in the western Europe. While more recent estimates of global MC production are not (readily) available, it has estimated (U.S. EPA, 2017a) that the annual usage of MC in the United States is (still) over 130,000 tons. In the meantime, rising concerns over MC's adverse health effects have led various sectors in many countries to search for alternatives to many of its industrial applications. For example, measures were approved by the EU in 2009 to ban MC in most paint strippers used by consumers and professionals outside of the industrial premises. The EU ban (European Parliament, 2009), which took full effect on 6 June 2012, applies to MC-based mixtures used for stripping paint, varnish, or lacquer. As of 2017, pure MC or mixtures containing the solvent for other types of use applications (e.g., aerosol spray propellant, degreasing) can continue to be sold and used in Europe.

13.6.2. Exposures and Toxic Effects

Methylene chloride (MC) can be an air pollutant of major global health concern, considering the assessment by WHO (2000a) that up to 80% of the solvent's global production is released into the atmosphere. A similar annual percentage release of the MC production is also experienced in the United States (ATSDR, 2000, 2010b). Although MC may be formed from natural sources, such sources do not make a significant contribution compared to the global release. In the atmosphere, MC generally has a residence life of about six months prior to complete degradation with photochemically-produced hydroxyl radical (WHO, 2000a). Accordingly, the main environmental exposure concern for the general population is inhalation of ambient air. For workers (and consumers), indoor exposure to the chlorinated solvent is expected to be much higher, particularly during the formulation of paint strippers and other spray aerosols. In the United States, it has estimated (U.S. EPA, 2017b) that 32,600 workers may be exposed to MC vapors annually during paint and coating removal activities, with about 46% of them being exposed during furniture refinishing. In addition, it has projected (U.S. EPA, 2017b) that each year about 1.3 million American consumers use paint removal products containing MC.

Methylene chloride (MC) is among the many chlorinated solvents known to impair the CNS if inhaled at high doses. The solvent used to be a general anesthetic until fatalities were reported (IPCS, 1997). Like those of other VOCs, MC vapors are more harmful to humans when present in poorly ventilated areas. Despite the fact that the solvent is the least toxic of the chloromethane group (IPCS, 1997), it still has a potential for acute inhalation hazard owing to its high volatility. In fact, inhalation of MC vapors at high levels can potentially lead to CO (carbon monoxide) poisoning since the solvent will be biotransformed to chloride (Cl^-) ion and CO in the body. Acute inhalation exposure to MC can also lead to severe optic neuropathy (Kobayashi *et al.*, 2008) and hepatitis (Cordes *et al.*, 1988), whereas dermal contact with the solvent in sufficient amount and duration can cause chemical burns on the skin (Wells and Waldron, 1984).

Laboratory studies revealed that MC (methylene chloride) induced liver and lung cancers in several animal species. Based on this body of evidence, IARC (2016, 2017) and U.S. EPA (2011) have classified MC, respectively, as a probable human (Group 2A) carcinogen and as an agent "likely to be carcinogenic in humans".

There is a general consensus that even when the primary adverse health effect from short-term exposure to MC is impairment of CNS functions, such impairment does not normally cause permanent disability. The acute toxicity of MC by inhalation or other routes is therefore not expected to be substantial. Chronic exposure to MC was found to associate with induction of fatty liver in guinea pigs (Morris *et al.*, 1979) and with increased incidences of hepatic hemosiderosis, necrosis, granulomatous inflammation, as well as bile duct fibrosis in rats (NTP, 1986). Several other animal studies (Narotsky *et al.*, 1992; Nishio *et al.*, 1984; WHO, 2000a) implicated MC's potential harm for its ability to cross the placental barrier, amidst the fact that the VOC had not been found teratogenic in rats and mice at even high doses.

13.7. Tetrachloroethylene

Tetrachloroethylene ($Cl_2C=CCl_2$) is also known by its IUPAC (International Union of Pure and Applied Chemistry) name *tetrachloroethene*, but is preferentially referred to as *per*chloroethylene (with *per*-chloro ≡ *all*-chlorinated) largely due to its acronym PCE or PERC being distinguishable from TCE which is customarily reserved for its structurally as well as chemically related cousin trichloroethylene (as discussed in Section 13.8 below). PCE (PERC) is a colorless, nonflammable liquid widely used for dry cleaning of fabrics, and is thus nicknamed *the* dry-cleaning fluid. The VOC is slightly soluble in water (0.15 g/L at $25°$ C), but miscible with many (other) organic solvents (e.g., alcohol, benzene, ether). It has a low vapor pressure of 18.5 mm Hg at $25°$ C but a high boiling point of $121°$ C ($250°$ F), as well as a sweet odor detectable by most people at ≥1 ppm.

13.7.1. Sources and Uses

Tetrachloroethylene (PCE or PERC) is used in the dry cleaning industry as a degreaser and as an ingredient in other industrial and consumer products. PCE is widely employed in dry cleaning, particularly in the small-business sector, owing to its excellent solvency for organic materials. The chlorinated solvent has a long history of use in spot removers and paint strippers. When included in a mixture with other chlorohydrocarbons, its application is mainly to degrease metal parts in the automotive and other metalworking shops.

Although PCE has been the dry cleaning fluid of choice for many decades, it has suffered a dramatic reduction in global production in recent years (Lacson and Toki, 2006), by 70 to 80% from 1990 to 2005. In the United States, the decline in PCE use for dry cleaning from 1990 (103,000 tons) to 2005 (17,000 tons) was 83%. The reductions over the same period in Japan and the western Europe were around 75% and 70%, respectively. The reduction in global production of PCE has been reportedly due to more efficacious work practices coupled with the utilization of more efficient equipment designed to minimize loss of the solvent.

It has estimated (ATSDR, 2014a) that about 85% of PCE produced is released into the environment, primarily into the atmosphere. PCE in the air is degraded by hydroxyl radical (HO·), yielding phosgene ($COCl_2$), trichloroacetyl chloride (C_2Cl_4O), hydrogen chloride (HCl), and other by-products. The half-life of PCE in the air varies with latitude, season, and level of atmospheric HO·, but typically between 1 and 8 months (ATSDR, 2014a; WHO, 2000b). In water, PCE is degraded very slowly by hydrolysis, and is persistent under aerobic conditions. PCE can be degraded via reductive dechlorination under anaerobic conditions, yielding vinyl chloride ($CH_2=CHCl$), dichloroethylene ($C_2H_2Cl_2$), trichloroethylene (C_2HCl_3; *see* Section 13.8 below), and a few other by-products. Release of PCE into the environment is largely via industrial emissions, but may also be from building materials and consumer products. When released onto surface water and land in sewage sludge, PCE readily evaporates to the atmosphere owing to its relatively low solubility in water and moderately high mobility in soils.

13.7.2. Exposures and Toxic Effects

Due to tetrachloroethylene's (PCE's) pervasiveness and ability to persist under certain conditions, the potential for human exposure to the chlorinated solvent can be substantial. The major routes of exposure for the general population are inhalation of ambient air and consumption of contaminated drinking water. Available data suggest that dermal uptake is not a principal route for most people. Exposure to PCE (PERC) from inhalation of ambient air can vary considerably depending on location. In general, levels of PCE in the air are higher in urban areas and places near point sources than in rural areas and away from the sources. As expected, PCE poses the highest risk to workers in dry cleaning facilities. PCE is also one of the common soil contaminants due to the high volume of its discharges from industrial processing.

According to the toxicity data reviewed by ATSDR (2014a), the adverse health effects from (chronic) exposure to PCE include mainly neurological problems, development of cancer, and damage to the liver as well as kidneys. At high concentrations, PCE is both a potent anesthetic agent and a cardiac epinephrine sensitizer. Teratogenicity studies in rats, rabbits, and mice collectively showed that PCE caused fetotoxicity and embryotoxicity at high doses. On the other hand, inconclusive adverse reproductive effects from occupational exposure were reported. Coupled with the mechanistic support by a number of animal studies, a handful of epidemiological studies on dry cleaning workers implicated an increased risk for several types of cancer including liver, kidney, and leukemia. Based on this body of evidence, IARC (1995, 2012, 2014, 2017) has listed PCE as a probable human (Group 2A) carcinogen.

As with many other chlorinated hydrocarbons, PCE can dissolve fat from the human skin with the potential for skin irritation. Intense irritation of the upper respiratory tract was observed in human volunteers exposed to high concentrations (>1,000 ppm) of PCE (Carpenter 1937; Rowe *et al.*, 1952). In addition, a population-based study (Goldman, 2010) of 198 twin pairs, along with available relevant animal data, provided substantial circumstantial evidence linking PCE and TCE (trichloroethylene) to Parkinson's disease.

13.8. Trichloroethylene

Trichloroethylene (ClCH=CCl$_2$) is also known as trichloroethene (TCE) under its systematic (i.e., IUPAC) name. This volatile chlorinated solvent is a clear liquid with a sweet smell. It is not soluble in water, but miscible with a number of (other) organic solvents (e.g., alcohol, chloroform, ether). TCE is nonflammable under normal conditions. It has a boiling point of 86.7° C (188° F) and a vapor pressure of 74 mm Hg at 25° C.

13.8.1. Sources and Uses

Trichloroethylene (TCE) is an effective solvent for a variety of organic materials, having many of the chemical functions and industrial applications offered by PERC (a.k.a. PCE ≡ tetrachloroethylene) and DCM (a.k.a. MC ≡ methylene chloride). As such, TCE is an excellent extraction solvent for greases, oils, fats, tars, waxes, and the kind. Up to 90% of its use is reportedly for degreasing and cold cleaning of metal parts (WHO, 2000c). The remaining 10% or so is largely for printing ink production, paint production, textile printing, and large-scale industrial dry-cleaning (*vs.* small business type with PERC). The textile industry has used this VOC to scour fabrics (e.g., cotton, wool) and as a solvent in waterless dyeing and finishing operations. As a solvent or a component of some solvent blends, TCE is used in pesticides, adhesives, lubricants, paint strippers, and cold metal cleaners (ATSDR, 2014b).

Virtually all (99%) TCE from industrial and consumer uses is released into the environment, primarily into the atmosphere with only a negligible percentage entering the water (WHO, 2000c). Owing to its relatively high vapor pressure, the chlorinated solvent can readily evaporate from surface waters when contaminated from direct industrial discharges. TCE in soils has the potential to seep into groundwater due to its moderate water solubility. Some low levels of TCE are hence commonly found in drinking water supplied by groundwater aquifers. TCE can be released into indoor air during the use of consumer products containing the solvent as an ingredient, or due to vapor migration (i.e., vapor intrusion) from subsurfaces such as underground walls or water supply lines. In the United States, much of the TCE is released into the atmosphere from vapor degreasing operations. Even more so than for PCE and DCM in the air, the predominate degradation process for atmospheric TCE is via reaction with hydroxyl radical (HO·), accordingly having a much shorter atmospheric residence half-life of about one week (ATSDR, 2014b).

13.8.2. Exposures and Toxic Effects

According to ATSDR (2014b), the atmospheric levels of TCE, like those of PERC (PCE), are much higher in industrial and populated places than in rural or remote areas. The general population is exposed to TCE through consumption or use of water contaminated by the chlorinated solvent, largely due to evaporation and leaching from waste disposal sites. In addition to consuming contaminated water, showering and bathing can be significant sources of indoor exposure to TCE. This is because TCE can readily volatilize into the air from hot water. Another major source of indoor exposure to TCE is through use of consumer products containing the chlorinated solvent as an ingredient.

Inhalation is the major route through which workers are exposed to the highest levels of TCE, particularly those working in the degreasing industry. Workers can be exposed to TCE in facilities where this VOC is manufactured or processed. Bystanders too can be exposed to TCE from inhaling air around these facilities.

In humans, short-term and long-term inhalation exposures to TCE can affect the CNS, with the common signs and symptoms being dizziness, headaches, fatigue, facial numbness, and euphoria. Other adverse health effects, particularly from chronic exposure, may include damage to the liver and kidneys as well as impairment to the developmental, immunological, and endocrine systems (ATSDR, 2014b).

When inhaled, TCE can induce CNS depression resulting in general anesthesia, but at a slow rate due to its high lipid solubility and consequently with less desirable effect as an anesthetic agent. The symptoms of acute non-medical exposure are similar to those of alcohol intoxication, starting with headaches, dizziness, and likely confusion. With increasing exposure, the effect can progress to unconsciousness. The associated respiratory and circulatory depression can result in death. TCE at low levels is relatively non-irritating to the respiratory tract. However, at high levels of exposure it can cause rapid breathing and lower the threshold for epinephrine-induced cardiac arrhythmias (WHO, 2000c).

Several epidemiological studies (e.g., Watson et al., 2006; Yauck et al., 2004) suggested an association between congenital heart defects and maternal exposure to TCE. Increase in incidence of congenital cardiac defects was claimed in those studies with communities exposed to TCE contamination in groundwater, amidst the fact that the exact exposure levels involved could not be determined. Nevertheless, such findings reportedly were by and large consistent with the adverse health effects observed in laboratory animals.

Several other epidemiological studies associated TCE exposure with several types of tumors in humans (e.g., cervical, kidney, lymphatic). Some animal studies also linked TCE exposure to lung, kidney, and liver cancers in mice and rats (e.g., Fukuda et al., 1983; Maltoni et al., 1986, 1988; NTP, 1988, 1990). Based on these and more recent data, IARC (1995, 2012, 2014, 2017) has relisted TCE from a probable human (Group 2A) to a human (Group 1) carcinogen.

Recent public health concerns with exposures to TCE and PERC (PCE) have extended to the appreciation and prediction of their toxicokinetics (TK) via the application of physiologically-based toxicokinetics (PB-TK) modeling. TCE and PERC are among the few environmental toxicants whose TK parameters have been studied extensively and successfully using PB-TK modeling. One reason for such a high modeling potential or success is that TCE and PERC are two of the few lipophilic solvents rapidly absorbed and metabolized to a variety of metabolites, including those that are toxic to the liver and kidneys. As alluded to in Chapter 7, PB-TK (a.k.a. PB-PK) modeling may be utilized to help discern the quantitative distribution of both the parent compound and its metabolites within a living organism's body. Accordingly, many human and animal PB-TK models have been developed and updated for TCE to further appreciate its quantitative disposition and that of some of its prominent metabolites in the human and animal bodies (e.g., Evans et al., 2009; Isaacs et al., 2004; Simmons et al., 2002; WHO, 2000c).

As for any other toxicant, a well-designed PB-TK model can be utilized to help unfold the relationship between the internal dose of TCE measured and its toxic effects observed. Available PB-TK human models for TCE have been applied specifically for cancer risk assessment by utilizing results observed in animal studies (WHO, 2000c). Animal results utilized in such human models included tumor incidence in mouse liver (Bogen, 1988; Fisher and Allen, 1993), tumor incidence in rat kidneys (Bogen, 1988), and kinetics data in rats (Koizumi, 1989). Some of the human and animal PB-TK models developed for PCE (tetrachloroethylene) can be found in the guidance document published by WHO (2000b). Apparently, the PB-TK models discussed in that WHO document can easily be extended for use on TCE (trichloroethylene), a chemical cousin of PCE.

References

ATSDR (U.S. Agency for Toxic Substances and Disease Registry), 1996. Toxicological Profile for Methyl *tert*-Butyl Ether. U.S. Department of Health and Human Services, Atlanta, Georgia, USA.

ATSDR (U.S. Agency for Toxic Substances and Disease Registry), 1999. Toxicological Profile for Formaldehyde. U.S. Department of Health and Human Services, Atlanta, Georgia, USA.

ATSDR (U.S. Agency for Toxic Substances and Disease Registry), 2000. Toxicological Profile for Methylene Chloride. U.S. Department of Health and Human Services, Atlanta, Georgia, USA.

ATSDR (U.S. Agency for Toxic Substances and Disease Registry), 2007. Toxicological Profile for Benzene. U.S. Department of Health and Human Services, Atlanta, Georgia, USA.

ATSDR (U.S. Agency for Toxic Substances and Disease Registry), 2010a. Addendum to the Toxicological Profile for Formaldehyde. U.S. Department of Health and Human Services, Atlanta, Georgia, USA.

ATSDR (U.S. Agency for Toxic Substances and Disease Registry), 2010b. Addendum to the Toxicological Profile for Methylene Chloride. U.S. Department of Health and Human Services, Atlanta, Georgia, USA.

ATSDR (U.S. Agency for Toxic Substances and Disease Registry), 2014a. (Draft) Toxicological Profile for Tetrachloroethylene (PERC). U.S. Department of Health and Human Services, Atlanta, Georgia, USA.

ATSDR (U.S. Agency for Toxic Substances and Disease Registry), 2014b. (Draft) Toxicological Profile for Trichloroethylene (TCE). U.S. Department of Health and Human Services, Atlanta, Georgia, USA.

ATSDR (U.S. Agency for Toxic Substances and Disease Registry), 2015. Addendum to the Toxicological Profile for Benzene. U.S. Department of Health and Human Services, Atlanta, Georgia, USA.

Balek B, 2009. New VOC Limits for Cleaning Products Effective Beginning of 2009. ISSA (International Sanitary Supply Association – The Worldwide Cleaning Industry Association): News Release (21 January). ISSA Headquarters, 7373 N. Lincoln Avenue, Lincolnwood, Illinois, USA.

Bogen KT, 1988. Pharmacokinetics for Regulatory Risk Analysis: The Case of Trichloroethylene. *Regul. Toxicol. Pharmacol.* 8:447-466.

CAREX Canada, 2012. Formaldehyde – Occupational Estimate (published November 2012). http://www.carecanada.ca/en/formaldehyde/occupational_estimate/ (retrieved 3 April 2017).

Carpenter CP, 1937. The Chronic Toxicity of Tetrachloroethylene. *J. Ind. Hyg. Toxicol.* 19:323-336.

CDC (U.S. Centers for Disease Control and Prevention), 2010. Final Report on Formaldehyde Levels in FEMA-Supplied Travel Trailers, Park Models, and Mobile Homes (released 2 July 2008, amended 15 December, 2010). U.S. Department of Health and Human Services, Atlanta, Georgia, USA.

Cordes DH, Brown WD, Quinn KM, 1988. Chemically Induced Hepatitis after Inhaling Organic Solvents. *West J. Med.* 148:458-460.

DHS (U.S. Department of Homeland Security), 2009. FEMA Response to Formaldehyde in Trailers (Redacted). OIG-09-83 (June 2009). DHS Office of Inspector General, Washington DC, USA.

Driscoll TR, 2014. The Australian Work Exposures Study (AWES): Formaldehyde. Canberra: Safe Work Australia, GPO Box 641 Canberra ACT 2601, Australia.

Environment Canada, 2013. *Consultation Document*: Revisions to the Proposed Volatile Organic Compound (VOC) Concentration Limits for Certain Products Regulations. Environment Canada Products Division, Place Vincent Massey, 9th Floor, 351 St-Joseph Blvd, Gatineau, Quebec, KIA 0H3, Canada.

European Parliament, 2009. Decision No 455/2009/EC of the European Parliament and the Council of 6 May 2009 – Amending Council Directive 76/769/EEC as Regards Restrictions on the Marketing and Use of Dichloromethane. *Off. J. Eur. Un.* L137(3 June):3-6.

Evans MV, Chiu WA, Okino MS, Caldwell JC, 2009. Development of an Updated PBPK Model for Trichloroethylene and Metabolites in Mice, and Its Application to Discern the Role of Oxidative Metabolism in TCE-Induced Hepatomegaly. *Toxicol. Appl. Pharmacol.* 236:329-340.

Fisher JW, Allen BC, 1993. Evaluating the Risk of Liver Cancer in Humans Exposed to Trichloroethylene Using Physiological Models. *Risk Anal.* 13:87-95.

Fukuda K, Takemoto K, Tsuruta H, 1983. Inhalation Carcinogenicity of Trichloroethylene in Mice and Rats. *Ind. Health* 21:243-254.

Goldman S, 2010. Parkinson's Disease Risk Is Increased in Discordant Twins Exposed to Specific Solvents. Presented at the American Academy of Neurology's 62nd Annual Meeting in Toronto, Canada, 10-17 April.

GWPC (Groundwater Protection Council), 2007. Groundwater Report to the Nation: A Call to Action – Groundwater and Underground Storage Tanks. GWPC, 13308 N. MacArthur Boulevard, Oklahoma City, Oklahoma, USA.

Hsu, SS, 2008. Toxicity in FEMA Trailers Blamed on Cheap Materials, Low Construction Standards. Reported in *Washington Post*, 3 July.

IARC (International Agency for Research on Cancer), 1987. IARC Monographs on the Evaluation of Carcinogenic Risks to Humans, Supplement 7: Overall Evaluations of Carcinogenicity – An Updating of IARC Monographs Volumes 1 to 42. Lyon, France: WHO Press.

IARC (International Agency for Research on Cancer), 1995. IARC Monographs on the Evaluation of Carcinogenic Risks to Humans, Volume 63: Dry-Cleaning, Some Chlorinated Solvents and Other Industrial Chemicals. Lyon, France: WHO Press.

IARC (International Agency for Research on Cancer), 1999. IARC Monographs on the Evaluation of Carcinogenic Risks to Humans, Volume 73: Some Chemicals That Cause Tumours of the Kidney or Urinary Bladder in Rodents and Some Other Substances. Lyon, France: WHO Press.

IARC (International Agency for Research on Cancer), 2006. IARC Monographs on the Evaluation of Carcinogenic Risks to Humans, Volume 88: Formaldehyde, 2-Butoxy-Ethanol and 1-tert-Butoxy-2-Propanol. Lyon, France: WHO Press.

IARC (International Agency for Research on Cancer), 2012. IARC Monographs on the Evaluation of Carcinogenic Risks to Humans, Volume 104F: Chemical Agents and Related Occupations. Lyon, France: WHO Press.

IARC (International Agency for Research on Cancer), 2014. IARC Monographs on the Evaluation of Carcinogenic Risks to Humans, Volume 106: Trichloroethylene, Tetrachloroethylene, and Some Other Chlorinated Agents. Lyon, France: WHO Press.

IARC (International Agency for Research on Cancer), 2016. IARC Monographs on the Evaluation of Carcinogenic Risks to Humans, Volume 110: Some Chemicals Used As Solvents and in Polymer Manufacture. Lyon, France: WHO Press.

IARC (International Agency for Research on Cancer), 2017. IARC Monographs on the Evaluation of Carcinogenic Risks to Humans, Volume 1-119: List of Carcinogens. Lyon, France: WHO Press.

IPCS (International Programme on Chemical Safety), 1997. INCHEM Poisons Information Monographs (PIM) 343 – Methylene Chloride. IPCS World Health Organization, Geneva, Switzerland.

Isaacs KK, Evans MV, Harris TR, 2004. Visualization-Based Analysis for a Mixed-Inhibition Binary PBPK Model: Determination of Inhibition Mechanism. *J. Pharmacokin. Pharmacodyn.* 31:215-242.

Kobayashi A, Ando A, Tagami N, Kitagawa M, Kawai E, Akioka M, Arai E, Nakatani T, Nakano S, Matsui Y, Matsumura M, 2008. Severe Optic Neuropathy Caused by Dichloromethane Inhalation. *J. Ocular. Pharmacol. Therap.* 24:607-612.

Koizumi A, 1989. Potential of Physiologically Based Pharmacokinetics to Amalgamate Kinetic Data of Trichloroethylene and Tetrachloroethylene Obtained in Rats and Man. *Br. J. Ind. Med.* 46:239-249.

Lacson J, Toki G, 2006. C2 Chlorinated Solvents (CEH Marketing Research Report Abstract). *Chemical Industrial Newsletter* by SRI Consulting (February Issue). http://chemical.ihs.com/nl/Public/2006Feb.pdf (retrieved 3 April 2013).

Maltoni C, Lefemine G, Cotti G, 1986. Experimental Research on Trichloroethylene Carcinogenesis. In *Archives of Research on Industrial Carcinogenesis* (Maltoni C, Mehlman MA, Eds.), Volume 5. Princeton, New Jersey, USA: Princeton Scientific Publishing, p.393.

Maltoni C, Lefemine G, Cotti G, Perino G, 1988. Long-Term Carcinogenicity Bioassays on Trichloroethylene Administered by Inhalation to Sprague-Dawley Rats and Swiss and B6C3F1 Mice. *Ann. NY Acad. Sci.* 534:316-342.

Melnick RL, White MC, Davis JM, Hartle RW, Ghanayem B, Ashley DL, Harry GJ, Zeiger E, Shelby M, Ris CH, 1997. Potential Health Effects of Oxygenated Gasoline. In *Interagency Assessment of Oxygenated Fuels*, National Science and Technology Council, Washington DC, USA.

Morris JB, Smith FA, Garman RH, 1979. Studies on Methylene Chloride-Induced Fatty Liver. *Exp. Mol. Path.* 30:386-393.

MRC (Merchant Research & Consulting Ltd), 2014. World Formaldehyde Production to Exceed 52 Mln Tonnes in 2017 (news release 27 June). http://mcgroup.co.uk/news/20140627/formaldehyde-production-exceed-52-mln-tonnes.html (retrieved 13 March 2017).

Narotsky MG, Hamby BT, Mitchell DS, Kavlock RJ, 1992. Full-Litter Resorptions Caused by Low-Molecular Weight Halocarbons in F-344 Rats (Abstract 67). *Teratology* 45:472-473.

NCI (U.S. National Cancer Institute), 2009. Formaldehyde and Cancer Risk. NCI FactSheet (issued 20 November). U.S. National Institutes of Health (NCI Public Inquiries Office, 6116 Executive Boulevard, Rm 3036A), Bethesda, Maryland, USA.

Nishio A, Yajema S, Yahogi M, Sasaki Y, Sawano Y, Miyao N, 1984. Studies on the Teratogenicity of Dichloromethane in Rats. *Gakujutsu Hikoku-Kagoshima Daigaku Nogakubu* 34:95-103 (in Japanese).

NRC (U.S. National Research Council), 1996, *Toxicological and Performance Aspects of Oxygenated Motor Vehicle Fuels*. Washington DC, USA: National Academy Press.

NTP (U.S. National Toxicology Program), 1986. Toxicology and Carcinogenesis Studies of Dichloromethane (Methylene Chloride) (CAS No. 75-09-2) in F344/N Rats and B6C3F1 Mice (Inhalation Studies). TR-306. U.S. Department of Health and Human Services, Research Triangle Park, North Carolina, USA.

NTP (U.S. National Toxicology Program), 1988. Toxicology and Carcinogenesis Studies of Trichloroethylene (CAS No. 79-01-6) in Four Strains of Rats (ACI, August, Marshall, Osborne-Mendel) (Gavage Studies). TR-273. U.S. Department of Health and Human Services, Research Triangle Park, North Carolina, USA.

NTP (U.S. National Toxicology Program), 1990. Carcinogenesis Studies of Trichloroethylene (without Epichlorohydrin) (CAS No. 79-01-6) in F344/N Rats and B6C3F1 Mice (Gavage Studies). TR-243. U.S. Department of Health and Human Services, Research Triangle Park, North Carolina, USA.

PRWeb, 2014. Global MTBE Production to Decline by 0.2% Annually through 2017, According to Indemand Report by Merchant Research & Consulting (news release 26 February). http:/www.prweb.com/releases/2014/03/prweb11675466.htm (retrieved 13 March 2017).

Rowe VK, McCollister DD, Spencer HC, Adams EM, Irish DD, 1952. Vapor Toxicity of Tetrachloroethylene for Laboratory Animals and Human Subjects. *AMA Arch. Ind. Hyg. Occup. Med.* 5:566-579.

Seinfeld JH, Pankow JF, 2003. Organic Atmospheric Particulate Material. *Ann. Rev. Phys. Chem.* 54:121-140.

Simmons JE, Boyes WK, Bushnell PJ, Raymer JH, Limsakun T, McDonald A, Sey YM, Evans MV, 2002. A Physiologically Based Pharmacokinetic Model for Trichloroethylene in the Male Long-Evans Rat. *Toxicol. Sci.* 69:3-15.

Tang X, Bai Y, Duong A, Smith MT, Li L, Zhang L, 2009. Formaldehyde in China: Production, Consumption, Exposure Levels, and Health Effects. *Environ. Intl.* 35:1210-1224.

Ubrich E, Jeuland N, 2007. Panorama 2008: Perspectives for Post-Euro 4 Standards for Passenger and Light Commercial Vehicles (Euro 5, Euro 5+, Euro 6). IFP Headquarters, 1 & 4, Avenue de Bois-Préau, 92852 Rueil-Malmaison, Cedex, France.

UNEP (United Nations Environment Programme), 2005. The Songhua River Spill, China, December 2005: Field Mission Report. United Nations Avenue, Gigiri, PO Box 30552, 00100, Nairobi, Kenya.

USEIA (U.S. Energy Information Administration), 2017. Methyl Tertiary Butyl Ether (MTBE) Oxygenate Production. Pet_pnp_oxy_a_epooxt_yop_mbbl_m.xls (webpage 31 January 2017). http://www.eia.gov/dnav/pet/pet_ pnp_ oxy_ a_ epooxt_yop_mbbl_m.htm (retrieved 13 March 2017).

U.S. EPA (U.S. Environmental Protection Agency), 1988. National Volatile Organic Compound Emission Standards for Consumer Products. *Federal Register* 63:48819-48847.

U.S. EPA (U.S. Environmental Protection Agency), 1997. Drinking Water Advisory: Consumer Acceptability Advice and Health Effects Analysis on Methyl Tertiary-Butyl Ether (MtBE). EPA-822-F-97-009. Office of Water, Washington DC, USA.

U.S. EPA (U.S. Environmental Protection Agency), 2006. Control of Hazardous Air Pollutants from Mobile Sources. *Federal Register* 71:15804-15963.

U.S. EPA (U.S. Environmental Protection Agency), 2011. Toxicological Review of Dichloromethane (Methylene Chloride) – In Support of Summary Information on the Integrated Risk Information System (IRIS). EPA/635/R-10/003F. Office of Research and Development, Washington DC, USA.

U.S. EPA (U.S. Environmental Protection Agency), 2012. 2012 Edition of the Drinking Water Standards and Health Advisories. EPA 822-S-12-001. Office of Water, Washington DC, USA.

U.S. EPA (U.S. Environmental Protection Agency), 2017a. Fact Sheet: Methylene Chloride or Dichloromethane (DCM) (webpage last updated 6 February 2017). http://www.epa.gov/assessing-and-manging-chemicalsunder-tsca/fact-sheet-methylene-chloride-or-dichloromethane-dcm (retrieved 4 March 2017).

U.S. EPA (U.S. Environmental Protection Agency), 2017b. Methylene Chloride and N-Methylpyrrolidone; Regulation of Certain Uses under TSCA Section 6(a). *Federal Register* 82:7464-7533.

Watson RE, Jacobson CF, Williams AL, Howard WB, DeSesso JM, 2006. Trichloroethylene-Contaminated Drinking Water and Congenital Heart Defects: A Critical Analysis of the Literature. *Reprod. Toxicol.* 21: 117-147.

Wells GG, Waldron HA, 1984. Methylene Chloride Burns. *Br. J. Ind. Med.* 41:420.

WHO (World Health Organization), 2000a. *Air Quality Guidelines for Europe*, Second Edition, Chapter 5.7: Dichloromethane. WHO Regional Publication, European Series, No. 91, Copenhagen, Denmark.

WHO (World Health Organization), 2000b. *Air Quality Guidelines for Europe*, Second Edition, Chapter 5.13: Tetrachloroethylene. WHO Regional Publication, European Series, No. 91, Copenhagen, Denmark.

WHO (World Health Organization), 2000c. *Air Quality Guidelines for Europe*, Second Edition, Chapter 5.15: Trichloroethylene. WHO Regional Publication, European Series, No. 91, Copenhagen, Denmark.

Yauck JS, Malloy ME, Blair K, Simpson PM, McCarver DG, 2004. Proximity of Residence to Trichloroethylene-Emitting Sites and Increased Risk of Offspring Congenital Heart Defects among Older Women. *Birth Defects Res.* 70(A):808-814.

Review Questions

1. Briefly distinguish the definition for VOCs in general terms from that for VOCs of regulatory concern.
2. List the two series of chemical reactions through each of which VOCs can serve as precursors for the formation of ozone.
3. What is the general mechanism whereby VOCs can serve as precursors for the formation of secondary organic aerosols?
4. What are the three main sources of occupational exposure to formaldehyde?
5. How may formaldehyde chemically become a major component of photochemical smog?
6. What happened to the health of those victims of Hurricane Katrina and Hurricane Rita that moved to live in trailers provided by the U.S. federal government?
7. Name three substances that are simple derivatives of benzene, and the one regarded as being among the most widely produced (using benzene as the intermediate).
8. What happened to the greater city of Harbin in China following the Songhua River pollution in 2005?
9. What are the major sources for environmental release of benzene into the atmosphere?
10. Explain why toluene is less toxic than benzene under normal circumstances.
11. What may be the one main health concern regarding benzene exposure?
12. What may be the metabolic fate of benzene in the human body?
13. What is the major industrial use of MTBE? And why is this VOC treated more as a water contaminant than as an air pollutant?
14. What are the major uses and health effects of MTBE?
15. What are the major uses and health effects of methylene chloride?
16. What are the major health effects of PERC vapors when inhaled at high concentrations?
17. Which of the following VOCs is best known as *the* dry-cleaning fluid?

    a) benzene; b) formaldehyde; c) MTBE; d) dichloromethane; e) PERC; f) TCE.

18. Give a chemical example for vapor intrusion as a potential source of indoor air exposure to VOCs.
19. What are the major uses and health effects of TCE?
20. Which of the following VOCs is (are) classified by IARC, if any, as a: (I) Group 1 human carcinogen; (II) Group 2A probable human carcinogen; (III) Group 2B possible human carcinogen?

    a) formaldehyde; b) benzene; c) MTBE; d) methylene chloride; e) PERC; f) TCE.

21. Which of the following VOCs whose degradation in the atmosphere is *the most* via reaction with hydroxyl radical?

    a) methylene chloride; b) MTBE; c) TCE; d) PCE; e) formaldehyde; f) benzene.

CHAPTER 14

Toxic and Radioactive Metals

14.1. Introduction

The history of metals dates back to 6000 BC or earlier, reportedly beginning with gold ($_{79}$Au). Metals may be chemically defined as all the elements in the periodic table (Figure 14.1) with an atomic number above 86, plus all the *non*-hydrogen ($_{1}$H) elements appearing on the left of the stairstep line bordered by boron ($_{5}$B), silicon ($_{14}$Si), germanium ($_{32}$Ge), antimony ($_{51}$Sb), and polonium ($_{84}$Po). That is, as many as 93 (79%) of the 118 elements (as of 2017) can be treated as metals. Even the five elements forming the stairstep line, along with arsenic ($_{33}$As) and tellurium ($_{52}$Te), may be chemically treated as metals as they are metalloids having some of the chemical properties of a metal. Those metals in the cation state (i.e., ion with positive charge) can form salts with acids, basic oxides with oxygen, and alloys with one another. Nevertheless, to a large number of people, metals are more commonly known as (electropositive) elements that generally have a shiny surface, tend to be competent thermal and electrical conductors, and can be hammered, melted, or otherwise processed into thin sheets or wires.

1 H																		2 *He*
3 Li	4 Be												5 B	6 C	7 N	8 O	9 F	10 *Ne*
11 Na	12 Mg												13 Al	14 Si	15 P	16 S	17 Cl	18 *Ar*
19 K	20 Ca		21 Sc	22 Ti	23 V	24 Cr	25 Mn	26 Fe	27 Co	28 Ni	29 Cu	30 Zn	31 Ga	32 Ge	33 As	34 Se	35 Br	36 *Kr*
37 Rb	38 Sr		39 Y	40 Zr	41 Nb	42 Mo	43 Tc	44 Ru	45 Rh	46 Pd	47 Ag	48 Cd	49 In	50 Sn	51 Sb	52 Te	53 I	54 *Xe*
55 Cs	56 Ba	57-70	71 Lu	72 Hf	73 Ta	74 W	75 Re	76 Os	77 Ir	78 Pt	79 Au	80 Hg	81 Tl	82 Pb	83 Bi	84 Po	85 At	86 *Rn*
87 Fr	88 Ra	89-102	103 Lr	104 Rf	105 Db	106 Sg	107 Bh	108 Hs	109 Mt	110 Ds	111 Rg	112 Cu	113 Nh	114 Fl	115 Mc	116 Lv	117 Ts	118 Og

57 La	58 Ce	59 Pr	60 Nd	61 Pm	62 Sm	63 Eu	64 Gd	65 Tb	66 Dy	67 Ho	68 Er	69 Tm	70 Yb
89 Ac	90 Th	91 Pa	92 U	93 Np	94 Pu	95 Am	96 Cm	97 Bk	98 Cf	99 Es	100 Fm	101 Md	102 No

Figure 14.1. A Simplified Version of the Periodic Table (*primarily for illustration of metals vs. nonmetals: solid gray background ≡ metal; two-tone ≡ metalloid; light background ≡ nonmetal; italicized ≡ noble gas*)

14.1.1. Concepts of Minerals and Heavy Metals

In the literature, the terms *mineral* and *heavy metal* are generally ill defined when referred to in discussing metal chemistry or metal toxicology. The term *mineral* is commonly used to refer to chemical elements including metals. Yet in many references, a mineral is specifically defined as a *naturally* occurring *solid* formed from geological processes ending with a characteristic chemical composition as well as a highly ordered molecular structure. Accordingly, at least some 25 chemical elements (primarily elements 93 through 118) in the periodic table may not be treated as minerals since they are *synthetic* in origin. The statement that metals are minerals neither *created* nor *destroyed* by humans is thus misleading. Moreover, at ambient temperature a few elements (e.g., mercury, gallium) occur in *liquid* form. Perhaps a close analogy for the taxonomic relationship between minerals and metals or elements is that between animals and humans.

Likewise, the so-termed *heavy* metals are at best members of an ill-defined subset of chemical elements that exhibit certain *user-defined* metallic or toxicological properties. It seems that the elements in such a subset can be defined by any of the various combinations of their atomic number, their toxicity, their density, and their chemical properties that a scientific sector prefers.

14.1.2. Metals of Environmental Health Concern

Not all metals are toxic to humans, wildlife, or the ecosystem. Calcium ($_{20}$Ca), copper ($_{29}$Cu), chromium III ($_{24}$Cr^{3+}), iron ($_{26}$Fe), magnesium ($_{12}$Mg), and zinc ($_{30}$Zn) are examples that are essential to human health as long as they are not excessively accumulated in the body. Regardless of how they are defined, in environmental toxicology the main concerns with metals are their health threats, sources of pollution, and frequency of occurrence in the environment. In this chapter, the 11 metals selected from four categories are thus discussed along this line of concerns. The selection made here does not suggest in any way that those metals not discussed are harmless. At most, it means that their toxicities receive relatively less public health attention. It is also important to know that many metals discussed here (as well as many not discussed here) are also toxic to plants or lower-order animals at high levels of exposure. For example, as noted in Chapter 10, cadmium ($_{48}$Cd) and arsenic are phytotoxic metals known to retard plant growth. Additional references for their effects on species of this kind can be found in Chapter 10 and some other chapters.

14.2. The Three Heavy Metals

Whether defined by density, atomic number, toxicity, or some other criteria, the elements lead ($_{82}$Pb), mercury ($_{80}$Hg), and Cd (cadmium) are in the group so-called the three most toxic heavy metals. These three musketeers are treated as the metal pollutants of most concern to environmental health, both in terms of their toxicity and ubiquity. There is no known biological need in humans for any of the three metals. In fact, these three and many of the other so-called heavy metals all have a strong affinity for sulfhydryl (-SH) functional groups which many proteins as well as enzymes are structurally rich in. In most cases, the binding of foreign molecules to these sulfhydryl (a.k.a. thiol) units can interfere with the normal functions of enzymes in the body to ultimately result in serious or even fatal health consequences (Section 9.4.2).

14.2.1. Lead

Lead (Pb) is a soft, malleable metal with a bluish-gray color when freshly cut. It will tarnish to a dull grayish color on exposure to air, and to a shiny silver luster when melted into a liquid. Since its discovery some 9,000 years ago, lead has been used in artwork, plumbing, gasoline, batteries, paints, and manufacturing of metal products. Today, the metal can be found everywhere in the environment, owing to the vast variety of human activities involving its processing and use, such as mining, burning fossil fuel, and manufacturing. Due to its ubiquity in the air as well as the high concerns over its health effects and persistence in the environment, lead is designated as one of the six criteria air pollutants in the United States (along with the four inorganic gases discussed in Chapter 11 and particular matter discussed in Chapter 12). In recent years, lead exposures from paints and ceramic products, caulking, and pipe solder have been dramatically reduced. In 1996, the United States banned the use of lead as an additive to gasoline.

Like many other metals, lead as a free element (Pb^0) does not break down; only its compounds will be changed primarily by sunlight, air, and water. Therefore, when lead is released into the atmosphere, the metal in its free element form can travel long distances prior to settling onto the ground or water. Once it falls onto soils, lead generally sticks to the particles there. Food plants thereby can be contaminated with lead through uptake from soils.

Transport of lead from soils into groundwater depends on the type of Pb compounds and the characteristics of the soil particles involved. Water pipes in some older homes may contain lead solder from which lead can leach out into the drinking water. Some people may inhale Pb dust particles from deteriorating Pb-based paint. Some others may be exposed to lead when working in a job where the metal is used, or when engaging in hobbies that involve its use, such as in making stained glass. Still some other people may be exposed to lead from using healthcare products or folk remedies that contain lead.

Of all the metals available, lead is specifically referred to as a *systemic* poison, as it can affect virtually every organ and system in the human body. The adverse health effects of lead are the same whether it enters the body via inhalation, ingestion, or dermal contact. The main target organ for lead toxicity is the nervous system in both adults and children, despite the fact that well over 90% of its content in the body eventually ends up in the bones. Recent cases continue to show that acute Pb poisoning (a.k.a. plumbism) in children, such as from lead coated on children's jewelry and toys, can get misdiagnosed initially as viral gastroenteritis (Berg *et al.*, 2006; VanArsdale *et al.*, 2004; *see also* Section 21.4.2).

Lead exposure at low to moderate levels can cause anemia, weakness in ankles, fingers, or wrists, as well as a small increase in blood pressure, particularly in middle-aged and older people. Exposure to high levels of lead can cause severe damage to the kidneys and brain in humans and ultimately death. In pregnant women, high levels of exposure to lead can cause miscarriage. In men, exposure to high levels of lead can cause damage in body tissues and organs that are responsible for sperm production (ATSDR, 2007a; U.S. EPA, 2004). Long-term exposure to lead can decrease a person's ability to perform certain nervous system functions.

Due to its strong affinity for the thiol (-SH) group, lead can inhibit or retard the enzymatic activity of δ-aminolevulinic acid dehydratase (δ-ALAD) at low blood levels (<10 μg/dL) in adults and children. Accordingly, the activity of δ-ALAD has been treated as a sensitive indicator of Pb poisoning (e.g., Berny *et al.*, 1992; Gurer-Orhan *et al.*, 2004; Pattee and Pain, 2003). As part of the second step in the porphyrin and heme biosynthetic pathway, the δ-ALAD enzyme is responsible for catalyzing the conversion of δ-aminolevulinic acid (δ-ALA) to porphobilinogen, a precursor of heme. Heme is not only a component of the oxygen-carrying hemoglobin, but also the building block of many other hemoproteins that are likewise critical to a number of biological functions. When the enzymatic activity of δ-ALAD is sufficiently inhibited, as by lead, it will cause anemia since heme synthesis will be inhibited as well. On the other hand, δ-ALA will be accumulated in the body and thus can be monitored in the urine for Pb poisoning or porphyria, the latter referring to a condition where heme is not made properly.

There is no conclusive evidence that elemental (metallic) lead (Pb^0) can cause cancer in humans. However, laboratory studies evaluated by U.S. EPA (2004) showed a significant increase in the incidences of renal carcinoma and some other tumors in rats and mice when given large doses of lead acetate ($Pb[C_2H_3O_2]_2$) or lead phosphate ($Pb_3[PO_4]_2$). U.S. EPA (2004) hence has assigned both lead and its inorganic compounds a weight-of-evidence carcinogen classification of B2 ($\approx$ probable human) carcinogen. The World Health Organization's International Agency for Research on Cancer (IARC, 1987, 2006, 2017), on the other hand, has listed lead as possible (Group 2B) and its inorganic compounds as probable (Group 2A) human carcinogens. (IARC's classification for carcinogenicity potential is summarized in Box 18.1 in Chapter 18.)

14.2.2. Mercury

Mercury (Hg) occurs naturally in several forms. The metallic (elemental) form at ambient temperature is a shiny, whitish-silver, odorless liquid. If this elemental liquid or its compound is heated, it will give off a colorless, odorless vapor. When this heavy metal combines with chlorine ($_{17}Cl$), sulfur ($_{16}S$), or other elements to form salts, the resultant inorganic compounds usually appear as white powder or crystals. Mercury can also combine with carbon ($_6C$) to form organic compounds, of which some like methylmercuric (CH_3Hg^+) cation are colorless. Methylmercury, which is produced in large amounts by bacteria in the soil and water, is the most toxic form of Hg compounds. It is also the form most easily bioaccumulated in many living organisms.

Elemental Hg^0 is used in electrolytic process to synthesize chlorine gas (Cl_2), with caustic soda (NaOH) being formed as a co-product. In some countries, mercury is widely used in amalgams (e.g., for dental fillings), barometers, batteries, and thermometers. The heavy metal and its compounds have been utilized in medicine as a preservative in vaccine, in topical antiseptic, and for treatment of syphilis.

Mercury and its inorganic compounds can enter the atmosphere from mining of ores, manufacturing plants, and waste incineration. From natural deposits, waste disposal, and volcanic activity, these Hg compounds can contaminate the nearby waters and soils.

One major source of human exposure to mercury and its compounds is via consumption of seafood contaminated with organic Hg compounds, particularly at levels when bioaccumulation can become a phenomenon of concern. Other major sources include inhalation of and dermal contact with Hg vapors in various occupational or environmental settings, such as the air from chemical spills, incinerators, and industries burning fuel that contains Hg compounds. Mercury can also be released from dental work and medical treatments (e.g., from treatment with certain Chinese herbal medicines).

The various forms of mercury collectively can cause a wide array of adverse health effects in humans (ATSDR, 1999, 2013; U.S. EPA, 1997), including neurotoxicity (e.g., CH_3Hg^+, Hg^0), teratogenicity (e.g., CH_3Hg^+), nephrotoxicity (e.g., Hg^0, $HgCl_2$), and death (e.g., Hg^0, CH_3Hg^+). To this date, the most widespread Hg poisoning (a.k.a. mercurialism) has been the epidemic occurring in the rural region of Iraq in the winter of 1971, when farmers there used a seed grain mistreated with a CH_3Hg^+-based fungicide to make bread. In that epidemic, more than 6,000 cases of food poisoning and at least 459 deaths were reportedly caused by consumption of bread made from the contaminated grain (Bakir *et al.*, 1973).

Short-term exposure to high levels of metallic Hg^0 vapors can cause lung damage, vomiting, diarrhea, nausea, high blood pressure, and rapid heart rate, in addition to irritation to the skin, eyes, and respiratory tract. The nervous system is especially sensitive to metallic (Hg^0) and organic (e.g., CH_3Hg^+) mercury, as in these forms more Hg molecules can enter the brain. In any case, exposure to high levels of mercury in any form can be very harmful, such as causing permanent damage to the brain, the kidneys, and the fetus. Effects on brain functioning may result in tremors, irritability, shyness, poor vision, poor hearing, and memory difficulties, which represent most of the signs and symptoms first becoming evident from the Hg poisoning disaster occurring in the 1950s in a Japanese village named Minamata (e.g., Hachiya, 2006; Ishimure, 1990).

The Minamata incident was caused by the discharge of methylmercury in industrial wastewater beginning in the 1930s from a chemical factory located in Kumamoto, Japan. Over some 20 years, this highly toxic metal had bioaccumulated heavily in fish and shellfish in the nearby Minamata Bay, which is part of the Shiranui Sea. After consuming the contaminated seafood for many years through the mid-1950s, more than 2,000 villagers in the Minamata area reportedly had suffered from a degeneration of their nervous system, with symptoms being largely those described in the preceding paragraph. The second major outbreak of Minamata disease occurred again in Japan. It took place in Niigata in 1965, involving nearly 700 victims residing along the basin of the Agano River (Hachiya, 2006).

The available data on human and animal cancers are deemed insufficient for most forms of mercury. However, there were studies (ATSDR, 1999, 2013) able to link a significant increase in kidney tumors in male mice to methylmercuric chloride (CH_3HgCl) and an alarming increase in several types of tumors in rats and mice to mercuric chloride ($HgCl_2$). In line with these findings, IARC (1993, 2017) has classified CH_3Hg^+ compounds as possible human (Group 2B) carcinogens while having metallic Hg^0 and its other compounds listed as Group 3 carcinogens (i.e., agents not classifiable as to their carcinogenicity to humans).

14.2.3. Cadmium

Cadmium (Cd) is a soft, whitish-silver metal with high resistance to corrosion. As such, the metal has many commercial and industrial applications including electroplating and manufacture of metal coatings. It is widely used in batteries, pigments, plastics, solders, jewelry, and nuclear reactors. Cadmium is commonly found as a mineral containing other elements such as oxygen (as in CdO), chlorine (as in $CdCl_2$), and sulfur (as in CdS, $CdSO_4$). It can be extracted during the production of zinc (Zn) and some other metals from ores.

As with mercury, cadmium enters the atmosphere, water, and soil mostly from mining of ores, industrial facilities, and waste incineration. Its airborne residues can travel long distances prior to settling onto the ground or water surface. Although Cd residues in some forms may dissolve in water, in most cases they bind strongly to soil particles. Cadmium in the environment can build up in plants, fish, and other animal tissues.

Low levels of cadmium are found in most foods, with the liver, shellfish, and kidney meats having the highest. There is usually less cadmium found in tobacco smoke than in foods. Nonetheless, because the human lungs absorb cadmium more efficiently than the stomach does, tobacco smoke is frequently regarded as the single most significant source of Cd exposure to humans. Despite the common observation that food plants in non-industrial areas contain only small amounts of cadmium, high levels of this heavy metal can still be found in the liver and kidneys of adult herbivorous animals including humans. This is possible owing to cadmium's high propensity for long-term buildup in the animal's tissues.

Other sources of human exposure to cadmium include inhalation of air and consumption of water contaminated with the metal. Buildup of Cd levels in the air, water, and soil is not uncommon in industrial areas. People are therefore at a higher risk if they live near or work in facilities that discharge cadmium into the environment.

Exposure to cadmium can result in various serious health effects, including emphysema, renal failure, cardiovascular diseases, and cancer. Eating food or drinking water with high levels of cadmium can severely irritate the stomach, leading to vomiting, diarrhea, and other symptoms. Of all the human organs, the kidney is regarded as the most vulnerable to cadmium.

Chronic exposure to low levels of cadmium in the air, water, or foods can lead to a buildup of cadmium in the kidneys at concentrations that can cause severe renal diseases, such as proteinuria and increased formation of kidney stone (ATSDR, 2012a). Other long-term effects include bone fracture and lung damage. Data from human and animal studies suggest that exposure to high, or sometimes even moderate or low, levels of cadmium can cause osteopenia and osteoporosis (e.g., Bhattacharyya, 2009; Brzóska and Moniuszko-Jakoniuk, 2004; Gallagher *et al.*, 2008; Satarug *et al.*, 2010). Osteoporosis is the major cause of bone fractures in elderly women (and men as well), a common occurrence worldwide.

Historically, the largest outbreak involving Cd-induced osteoporosis and renal failure occurred also in Japan and likewise around the 1950s. The syndrome experienced from that incident led to a chemically-induced disorder referred to as *itai-itai byo* in Japanese (meaning *ouch-ouch pain* or *sickness* in English). The term *itai-itai* (*byo*) was coined by Japanese local residents living in the Jinzū River basin region, where most of the consumed rice was grown in fields irrigated with river water. Unfortunately, beginning in 1910 and continuing through 1945 or so, the rivers in the basin were constantly polluted with cadmium discharged in significant quantities by mining companies operating up in the mountains. The river water was also used for drinking, washing, and fishing by the downstream residents. Many of those residents, particularly the postmenopausal older women, reportedly suffered from pains induced in their joints and spine. Their pains and sufferings were not linked to Cd exposure until the mid-1950s (Kobayashi, 1978; Nogawa, 1981).

As seen in victims in the *itai-itai* incident, one of the major adverse health effects of long-term Cd poisoning is a painful skeletal condition resulting from weak, brittle, or deformed bones. Leg and spinal pains are generally the first complaints, eventually accompanied by a waddling gait due to bone deformities. These symptoms typically progress for several years until the patient is eventually unable to walk. The pains then become debilitating, with fractures becoming more common as the bone weakens. Other complications include (but are not limited to) coughing, anemia, renal failure, and death.

The adverse health effects of cadmium in humans are somewhat unique even among the toxic heavy metals. Owing to its long half-life (>30 years) within the human body, chronic exposure to even very low levels of cadmium can result in the buildup to concentrations that can result in severe health problems. The human body can store cadmium in the liver, kidneys, and other tissues by first binding the metal to a low-molecular-weight, cysteine-rich protein named metallothionein (MT) which is present in virtually all forms of life and normally binds to certain essential metals such as zinc. Due to its higher affinity for thiol groups, cadmium can competitively displace these essential metals and bind to MT more tightly. Therefore, to some extent, the Cd-MT binding may be treated as a way of reducing the bioavailability and hence the toxicity of cadmium in the body. Yet certain other (essential) metals such as copper have an even higher affinity for thiol groups and hence can replace cadmium on these binding sites. A serious concern with the Cd-MT binding is that when transported to and retained in the kidney, the protein portion of the Cd-MT complex is rapidly degraded. This then leaves the free cadmium to accumulate in the kidney, which is the metal's notorious site of toxic action.

Laboratory studies showed low fetal weight, impaired neurological development, skeletal malformations, and other developmental effects linking to Cd exposure in animals, amidst inconclusive evidence from human studies (ATSDR, 2012a). In addition, several animal and occupational studies (ATSDR, 2012a; U.S. EPA, 1999a) asserted an increase in lung cancer from chronic inhalation exposure to cadmium, although the evidence from the occupational data was not deemed sufficiently convincing as due to several confounding factors inherent in the study designs (U.S. EPA, 1999a). Nevertheless, IARC (2012a, 2017) has listed cadmium and its compounds as human (Group 1) carcinogens, whereas U.S. EPA (1999a) has classified the heavy metal as a probable human carcinogen.

14.3. Select Secondary/Pseudo Heavy Metals

The term *secondary* or *pseudo heavy metal* used here is even more ill defined than the term *heavy metal*. Regardless, in environmental toxicology this term (or another one with a similar notion) is often necessarily reserved for separating metals in this group from the three heavy metals discussed above in Section 14.2. The reality is that many of these other so-called "heavy" metals are also ubiquitous in the environment and abundant in the Earth's crust, despite the fact that their health impacts are not as devastating. Yet as with the toxic trace and radioactive metals discussed later in Sections 14.4 and 14.5, some of the so-called pseudo or secondary heavy metals are still important and relevant to environmental toxicology.

Aluminum is considered in this section largely due to the controversies over its toxicity, particularly in relation to Alzheimer's disease. Arsenic is included because it has an ancient and villainous history for being "heavy", with its name coined to king of poisons. And beryllium, as with aluminum, is one of the least dense elements and therefore may not be qualified as a heavy metal by *density* criterion. This second lightest element is included in this section because it is one of the few highly toxic *industrial* metals around.

14.3.1. Aluminum

Aluminum ($_{13}$Al) is the most abundant metal in the Earth's crust, followed by silicon (Si). Pure aluminum is highly malleable and ductile, with a silvery-white appearance. It is commonly found as a trivalent cation (Al^{3+}) in natural waters and in the tissues of most biological organisms. The metal is most available initially in the form of a mineral or an alloy that contains also oxygen, silicon, fluorine, and some other elements, as from such it can be extracted. In the air, aluminum can stay attached as a component of small particulate matter for days. Under most conditions, only a small fraction of aluminum in water will get dissolved. Some plants can take up much of the metal from contaminated soils.

Compounds of aluminum have many different uses and applications, such as aluminum sulfate ($Al_2[SO_4]_3$) in treatment of drinking water and aluminum oxide (Al_2O_3) in extraction of the metal as well as in polishing applications. Al compounds are also used for beverage cans, cooking utensils, aircrafts, siding for buildings, roofing, foil, and in many consumer products such as antacids, buffered aspirin, food additives, cosmetics, and antiperspirants. Although aluminum is ubiquitous in the diet, it does not accumulate in persons with normal physiological functions. In the United States, the average dietary intake of aluminum for adults is less than 10 mg per day. Urban water supplies may contain a higher level of aluminum since water of this kind is usually treated with aluminum sulfate or other Al compounds.

People at the highest risk of Al exposure are those staying in or near areas where the air is dusty, where ore deposits are mined or processed into the metal, or where certain toxic waste sites are located. Children and adults can be exposed to small amounts of aluminum from vaccinations or from consumption of substances containing high levels of aluminum (e.g., antacids). However, under normal physiological conditions, only a small fraction of the absorbed doses will enter the bloodstream.

To date, much of the toxicity of aluminum to humans has been controversial. Exposure to aluminum generally is not harmful, although at high levels it may cause neuromuscular and skeletal problems, digestive disorders, coughing, and minor pulmonary effects. As with Pb (lead) exposure, in some instances inhalation of Al dusts or fumes by workers can cause a decrease in their ability to perform certain nervous system functions (ATSDR, 2008).

People with renal failure are likely to retain excess amounts of aluminum in their body, a condition alleged to have caused certain bone and brain diseases in some cases. Studies showed that the nervous system was a sensitive target of Al toxicity in certain test animals. Yet obvious signs and symptoms of neurological damage were not observed in test animals treated even at high oral doses. After finding traces of aluminum in the brains of patients with Alzheimer's disease, a few studies in the mid-1970s (e.g., Crapper *et al.*, 1973, 1976) implicated that Al exposure at high levels would cause the disease. Several studies conducted shortly afterwards had either failed to confirm a similar correlation (e.g., Markesbury *et al.*, 1981; McDermott *et al.*, 1979; Trapp *et al.*, 1978) or offered minimal supportive results (e.g., Peri, 1985). On the other hand, a recent study (Mirza *et al.*, 2017) seemed to have confirmed the metal's important role in cognitive decline. Meanwhile, IARC (2012b) has decided that occupational exposures during Al production are carcinogenic to humans (i.e., with the metal Al being listed as a Group 1 carcinogen).

14.3.2. Arsenic

Arsenic (As) is found primarily in three crystalline forms. Its most predominant form is a brittle, metallic gray solid. The other two forms are a black solid structurally similar to red phosphorus and a yellow solid produced from abrupt cooling of As vapors. As compounds, which collectively are often referred to as *arsenicals*, are each present in one of several oxidation states with strikingly different toxicological profiles. Most arsenicals occur in the +3, +5, or −3 oxidation state, chemically known as arsenites (e.g., $NaAsO_2$), arsenates (e.g., KH_2AsO_4), and arsenides (e.g., Na_3As), respectively.

The metalloid is widely distributed in the Earth's crust. In the environment, arsenic is commonly combined with oxygen, chlorine, sulfur, or some other elements to form inorganic compounds. Some inorganic As compounds such as chromated copper arsenate (CCA) are used as heavy duty wood preservatives. In the United States, CCA is no longer used for residential outdoor wood structures. However, this inorganic compound is still being used in industrial applications. And the outdoor structures treated with CCA can still be found in older homes. In the tissues of living organisms, arsenic can combine with hydrogen and carbon to form organic compounds. Both As organics and inorganics have been utilized as pesticides, such as lead arsenate ($PbHAsO_4$), arsenic pentoxide (As_2O_5), and monosodium methyl arsenate (CH_4AsNaO_3). Arsenic was once used as an antiseptic to treat syphilis (Lockhart and Atkinson, 1919).

Arsenic present in minerals may enter the air, water, and soil from wind-blown dusts and may enter groundwater from runoff and leaching. In the air, As dust particles get dropped onto lands or into waters via wet depositions by rain and snow. In the water, many common arsenicals get dissolved and then ultimately end up in sediments. Fish and shellfish can accumulate arsenic which occurs mostly in a less harmful, organic form named arsenobetaine ($C_5H_{11}AsO_2$). Certain bacterial species can use their own enzymes known as glutaredoxin (a.k.a. arsenate reductase) to derive energy for growth by catalyzing the reduction of arsenates to form arsenites.

Although arsenate may be the more common form found in humans, it can be readily reduced to the more toxic arsenite (Kingston *et al.*, 1993). Arsenite is more toxic owing to its stronger affinity for the thiol group. More specifically, it can inhibit an essential metabolic enzyme named pyruvate dehydrogenase, which is responsible for the conversion of pyruvate to acetyl CoA. With the enzyme's catalytic activity being inhibited, acetyl CoA can no longer be available for use in the Krebs cycle (Figure 9.3) to carry out the critical function of cellular respiration.

People are at the highest risk when working in or living near places where there are high levels of As (arsenic) minerals found in rocks, or where large As production or use is involved (e.g., pesticide application, copper smelting, wood treatment). Small quantities of arsenic are almost always present in the diet and drinking water.

Arsenic has had its nefarious name as king of poisons since the Renaissance days, when the Spanish-Italian noble family Borgias frequently employed the metalloid as poison of choice for political assassinations. Acute exposure of inorganic arsenicals at high levels can cause irritation in the throat and lungs, and even death. Chronic or subchronic exposure (to low levels) of arsenic can cause various systemic effects including nausea, vomiting, decrease in red and white blood cell counts, irregular heartbeats, damage to blood vessels, and a tingling sensation in hands and feet. Long-term exposure can also cause a darkening of the skin and the development of small warts on the palms, soles, and/or torso. Skin contact with inorganic arsenicals can cause redness and swelling (ATSDR, 2007b, 2016).

Arsine (AsH_3) is a flammable, highly toxic gaseous compound. Acute inhalation exposure to the gas by people, even at 25 to 50 ppm (parts per million) for half an hour, can result in death (U.S. EPA, 1999b). A chelating agent known as British anti-Lewisite (BAL) was developed by a group of British biochemists during World War II as the antidote to an arsine-based chemical warfare agent named Lewisite.

Little information is available regarding the adverse health effects of arsenic's organic compounds in humans. However, methyl and dimethyl As compounds through ingestion were found to cause diarrhea and damage to the hepatic and renal systems in animals (ATSDR, 2007b, 2016). Animal studies also showed that several simple organic As compounds were less toxic than most inorganic arsenicals known.

According to IARC (2012a), a number of epidemiological studies implicated that exposure to inorganic arsenicals had a significant risk of cancer in the human skin, lungs, bladder, and likely liver as well. Based on this body of evidence, IARC (2012a, 2017) has listed both arsenic and inorganic arsenicals as human (Group 1) carcinogens, whereas U.S. EPA (1999b) has classified only inorganic arsenicals as human (Group A) carcinogens.

14.3.3. Beryllium

Beryllium ($_4Be$) is a brittle, steel-grayish metal commonly found in volcanic ashes, petroleum, soils, coal, and certain rock minerals. While beryllium is the second lightest chemical element, it has one of the highest melting points (>1,200° C or 2,190° F) and as such offers an ideal material in the aerospace and manufacturing industries. Owing to its high transparency to X-rays, the metal has made good applications in the fields of nuclear medicine and radiation physics.

Alloys and ores of beryllium are commonly employed in microcircuits, dental plates, golf club, thermal castings, and more. The metal itself, which can be extracted from the Be minerals mined, owns many desirable properties. In particular, beryllium is more elastic than steel and is nonmagnetic along with an excellent thermal conductivity.

Beryllium dust particles are released into the atmosphere from burning coal and petroleum oil, and eventually will settle onto the land and water. It can get into natural waters from erosion of rocks and soils as well as from industrial wastes. Although some Be compounds will get dissolved in the water, most will adsorb to the sediment. Like lead, beryllium tends to stick to soil particles and thus, under normal conditions, is not taken up by plants in any large amount. Beryllium rarely accumulates in a food chain.

Individuals at the highest risk to Be (beryllium) exposure are those working in industries where Be ores are mined, processed, extracted into the metal, or converted into its alloys. Residents living near these places or around uncontrolled hazardous waste dumps may also inhale higher than normal levels of beryllium.

Depending on their atmospheric levels, Be dusts and fumes may be harmful to people inhaling them. At sufficiently high concentrations (>1 mg/m^3) for even a short interval, a condition resembling acute chemical pneumonitis can result. Acute chemical pneumonitis is an inflammation of the lungs confined to the walls in the air sac (i.e., the alveolar) region. This acute condition caused by Be exposure is specifically termed *acute beryllium disease*. The condition varies in severity, but including death. The less severe form of this disease can result from skin contact with Be dusts or fumes, ending with signs and symptoms similar to those of contact dermatitis.

For some (<15%) people sensitive to beryllium, they may later develop an inflammatory reaction in the respiratory system long (10-15 years) after termination of their months- or even years-long exposure to the metal at levels above 0.5 μg/m^3. This chronic lung disorder, characterized by noncancerous nodular lesions, is called chronic beryllium disease or *berylliosis* in medical terms. Such a chronic exposure may also affect other organs as beryllium can be transported to other body parts via the bloodstream. In fact, the advanced berylliosis cases may involve formation of kidney stones as well as enlargement of the liver, spleen, and right heart. In any case, the common symptoms of berylliosis generally involve irritation of the mucous membranes, reduced lung capacity, breathing difficulties, coughing, chest pains, and fatigue (ATSDR, 2002, 2015; U.S. EPA, 1998, 1999c).

Both berylliosis and the acute condition are often treated as *industrial* diseases. This is because the ambient air levels of beryllium are typically very low, usually at the nanogram (<0.2 ng/m^3) levels (ATSDR, 2002, 2015). Several epidemiological and animal studies implicated chronic exposure to beryllium as a cause for higher risk of lung cancer (ATSDR, 2002, 2015; U.S. EPA, 1998, 1999c). Whereas U.S. EPA (1999c) has classified beryllium alone (i.e., not including its compounds) as a probable human (Group B1) carcinogen, IARC (2012a, 2017) has listed both the metal and its compounds as human (Group 1) carcinogens.

14.4. Select Toxic Trace Metals

In addition to the six metals discussed thus far, there are still many that may be regarded as "heavy metals" by different criteria. Nonetheless, a large number of these and other metals are essential to human health and thus are expected to be available in the human body at least in trace amount. As with all other substances, regardless of their importance, these *trace* metals are harmful to humans if they are too much in excess in the body. Some sources (e.g., Goyer and Clarkson, 2001; Reilly, 2004) have suggested that the list of metallic elements essential to human health, in one form or another (e.g., in certain oxidation state), should include but might not be limited to: calcium (Ca); cobalt ($_{27}$Co); copper (Cu); chromium (Cr); iron (Fe); magnesium (Mg); manganese ($_{25}$Mn); molybdenum ($_{42}$Mo); nickel ($_{28}$Ni); potassium ($_{19}$K); sodium ($_{11}$Na); and zinc (Zn). Among these dozen elements deemed essential to biological functions, calcium, magnesium, potassium, and sodium are generally available to the human body in large quantities (e.g., from foods) and thus not regarded as truly essential metals or in the sense of being in trace amounts.

Among the remaining seven elements on the above list, chromium, copper, and nickel appear to be of higher concern to environmental health and are thus discussed the three subsections that follow. Note that although iron overdose has been a leading cause of death among children, such as from accidentally swallowing large amounts of iron-supplemented vitamin pills, a common human health problem with this metal is its deficiency frequently seen in women and children. Iron deficiency can cause notably anemia and hence fatigue as well as other related symptoms (e.g., weight loss). Selenium ($_{34}$Se) is an essential trace element with no metallic property.

14.4.1. Chromium

Chromium (Cr) is a steely-grayish, lustrous, hard metal naturally occurring in most rocks. It can be found in animals, plants, and soils. Although the metal exists in several oxidation states, its commonly encountered forms are elemental or metallic Cr(0), trivalent Cr(III), and hexavalent Cr(VI). Elemental Cr is used largely for steel production whereas Cr(III) and Cr(VI) are used mostly for chrome (electro)plating, dyes, pigments, leather tanning, and wood preserving. All Cr compounds known are odorless and tasteless.

Chromium enters the atmosphere, water, and soil predominantly in its trivalent Cr(III) or hexavalent Cr(VI) form. In the air, Cr compounds are present mostly as fine dust particles which eventually settle onto the land or water. Chromium can attach firmly to soil particles. Only a small fraction of soil chromium can dissolve in water to seep into the underground water layer. No significant amount of chromium from waters has been found to accumulate in fish.

Trivalent chromium, denoted by Cr(III) or Cr^{3+}, in trace amounts is an essential nutrient required for metabolism of sugar, fat, and protein molecules in humans and animals. Actually, insufficient dietary intake of Cr(III) can lead to increase in certain hematological disorders and hyperinsulinemia (Anderson, 1994; Pechova and Pavlata, 2007).

In contrast, acute inhalation of Cr(VI), also denoted by Cr^{6+}, at high levels can cause irritation to the respiratory tract including predominately the nose. The symptoms typically involve coughing, shortness of breath, and wheezing. Perforations and ulcerations of the septum, asthma, bronchitis, decreased lung function, and pneumonia are commonly seen as associated with chronic inhalation of Cr(VI). Exposure to large amounts of Cr(VI) from ingestion can lead to gastrointestinal (GI) disorders, neurological effects, convulsions, damage to liver and kidneys, or death (ATSDR, 2012b). Dermal contact with certain Cr(VI) compounds can cause skin ulcers and contact dermatitis. The human body can detoxify some fraction of Cr(VI) to form Cr(III). Some people are extremely sensitive to Cr(VI) or even Cr(III), frequently with allergic reactions resulting in severe redness and swelling of the skin. Damage to sperms and the male reproductive system have been observed (ATSDR, 2012b) in laboratory animals exposed to Cr(VI).

The more important industrial sources of airborne chromium are those related to the production of ferrochrome (FeCr) alloy. Other industrial sources include: ore mining and refining; refractory and chemical processing; brake lining and catalytic converters for automobiles; leather tanneries; and chrome pigments (ATSDR, 2012b). Individuals may be exposed to chromium via dermal contact during the application or processing of the metal in the workplace. People in the general population are usually exposed to chromium by ingestion of foods and drinking water containing the metal or its compounds. Other potential sources of exposure for the general population are residing around uncontrolled hazardous waste sites or near industries that apply or process chromium or its compounds.

Several occupational and laboratory studies implicated Cr(VI) as a carcinogen of the human lung (ATSDR, 2012b; U.S. EPA, 1999d). An increase in stomach tumor was observed in humans and animals exposed to Cr(VI) in drinking water. The mechanism of Cr(VI) carcinogenicity in the lung is thought to be via its reduction to Cr(III) leading to the generation of a number of reactive intermediates. Based on these and other related findings, IARC (2012a, 2017) and U.S. EPA (1999d) both have classified Cr(VI) as a human (Group 1 and Group A, respectively) carcinogen. The human carcinogenicity of Cr(VI) in drinking water was publicized in 2000 in the American movie *Erin Brockovich*.

14.4.2. Copper

Copper (Cu) is a highly malleable and ductile metal with a very high electrical and thermal conductivity. Pure copper has a freshly exposed surface in pinkish or peachy color. The metal occurs naturally in the environment and is one of the few metals occurring naturally as (part of) an uncompounded mineral. Copper is one of the oldest civilizations in humankind history, with a use history dating back to some 7,000 years ago in the cultural period commonly known as the Copper Age.

Copper is an essential nutrient in humans, animals, and higher-order plants. In humans and many other mammals, copper deficiency can cause neurodegeneration and a form of anemia specifically related to pancytopenia (i.e., low in red and white blood cells). The neurological disease can be seen most commonly in human infants with Menkes (kinky hair) syndrome, which is a genetic recessive disorder affecting Cu levels in the body to eventually cause its deficiency. Copper is involved in the incorporation of iron into the heme center in hemoglobin.

Owing to largely its high thermal and electrical conductivity, copper is used extensively as a thermal or an electrical conductor to make various kinds of wiring products. Other products made with copper include plumbing fittings, sheet metal, roofing, rainspouts, cookware, doorknobs, and other fixtures in the house. Copper is also combined with zinc and tin to make brass and bronze products, respectively. Some Cu compounds have been applied as fungicides to treat plant diseases, for water treatment, and as preservatives for leather and wood.

As with many other metals, copper is released into the environment largely from mining and manufacturing operations or through wastewater discharging into rivers and lakes. Copper is also released from natural sources such as volcanoes, wind-blown dusts, decaying vegetation, farming, and forest fires. Copper released into the environment generally attaches to the clay, soil, sand, or organic matter particles. As with lead, copper itself does not break down in the environment. However, its compounds can break down easily to release free (elemental) copper (Cu^0) into the air, soil, or water.

People can be exposed to copper from various common sources, such as by inhaling contaminated air, drinking contaminated water, and ingesting foods with high Cu content. In addition, they can be exposed to copper via skin contact with the metal as well as with particulates or compounds containing the metal. High levels of copper can be found in drinking water when the house has copper pipes filled with acidic water, or in lakes and rivers that have been treated with Cu compounds to control algae. Soils located near Cu smelting plants may also contain high levels of the metal. Furthermore, people can be exposed to copper by ingesting vegetation treated with Cu-containing fungicides, or if they reside close to or work in Cu mines or facilities where the metal is processed into alloys or other products.

Ingestion of large amounts of copper sulfate ($CuSO_4$) can cause hepatic necrosis and death. Even at moderate levels, inhalation of copper can induce irritation of the nose and throat. Experimental studies on humans showed that ingestion of drinking water containing copper at 3 mg or higher per liter produced GI symptoms including nausea, vomiting, and diarrhea (Pizaro *et al.*, 1999). Studies also implicated that people with deficiency in the enzyme glucose-6-phosphate dehydrogenase would have a higher risk for the hematological effects of copper, although the magnitude of the risk remained largely unknown (Goldstein *et al.*, 1985).

Available epidemiological studies have not indicated any link between Cu exposure and cancer risk (IPCS, 1998). To this date, neither IARC (2017) nor U.S. EPA has (yet) classified copper or its compounds as potential human or animal carcinogens.

By most standards, the health effects of copper are not severe compared to those of nickel or chromium VI. Copper is included in this chapter mainly because of the emerging concerns over the dramatic increase of environmental exposure to the metal. There is a rising health concern that the widely applied oral contraceptives by women can promote copper absorption leading to an increase in the level of copper in their blood (e.g., Akinloye *et al.*, 2011; Berg *at al.*, 1998; Liukko *et al.*, 1988). Studies also revealed that copper released from the equally widely applied copper IUDs (intrauterine devices) would increase menstrual blood loss and pains in women (e.g., Cox and Blacksell, 2000; Hubacher *et al.*, 2006, 2009). Another rising health concern is that copper, along with iron and zinc, can act as a pro-oxidant to promote the generation of free radicals such as ROS (reactive oxygen species) that have been implicated in the pathogenesis of several degenerative disorders including Alzheimer's disease (e.g., Brewer, 2007; Christen, 2000; Jellinger, 2013) and the cardiovascular disease atherosclerosis (e.g., Brewer, 2007).

Furthermore, there is the prevailing concern that copper is among the few best (or worst) examples showing how an essential nutrient can become very harmful to people with certain hereditary disorders. For instance, Wilson's disease (medically referred to as hepatolenticular degeneration) is an autosomal recessive genetic disorder that can result in a buildup of excess copper in tissues to cause damage in the eyes, kidneys, brain, and notably liver. Individuals with this genetic disorder therefore can suffer from severe neurological or psychiatric symptoms as well as liver disease (e.g., Bandmann *et al.*, 2015). Severe cases need to be treated with chelation therapy and/or other medications to remove the excess copper from the body and/or reduce its absorption into the body. In all cases, where the liver becomes severely damaged, a liver transplant may be the only treatment option (Kaler, 2007).

14.4.3. Nickel

Nickel (Ni) is a silvery-white, lustrous metal with a slight tinge of gold color. It is an abundant element occurring predominantly in the form of nickel sulfide (NiS), nickel oxide (NiO), and nickel silicate (a.k.a. garnicrite, [Ni, Mg]$_3$Si$_2$O$_5$[OH]) minerals in the Earth's crust. The use of nickel dates back to around 3500 BC. Small quantities of this metal are commonly found in the air, soil, water, and foods because of its widespread applications. Nickel can be combined with other metals, such as iron, copper, chromium, and zinc, to form alloys. These alloys in turn are utilized to make coins, jewelry, and other items such as valves, spark plugs, catalysts, batteries, and heat exchangers. Most elemental nickel (Ni^o) is used to make stainless steel, particularly in the early days. Nickel and its compounds have no characteristic odor or taste.

Small amounts of nickel are found in the ambient air as a result of releases from oil-burning power plants, sewage sludge incineration, and metal refining, as well as from other manufacturing facilities involving the application of nickel (ATSDR, 2005; IPCS, 1991). In the atmosphere, nickel frequently attaches to small dust particles which will settle onto the ground or get removed out of the air through precipitation. From industrial wastewater, nickel usually ends up in soils or sediments where the metal will attach strongly to particles that contain iron or manganese. Nickel does not appear to accumulate in food chains in any considerable amount.

Individuals can be exposed to the metal from tobacco smoke and via contact with jewelry containing nickel or with stainless steel utensils made of nickel. Inhalation is the major route of occupational exposure to nickel and its compounds. Foods and drinking water are the main sources of Ni exposure for the general population, with an average daily intake of 100 to 300 µg estimated for adults (ATSDR, 2005).

In humans, the most common health effect from chronic dermal exposure to nickel is allergic dermatitis, with skin eczema (e.g., rash and itching of the hands and forearms) being the most characteristic symptom. Despite nickel's potential essentiality to human health, it has estimated that approximately 15% of American people are sensitive (allergic) to the metal. People can become sensitive to nickel when their skin comes in contact for a sufficiently long time with jewelry or other items containing the metal. Once a person is sensitized to nickel, further contact with the metal may cause the allergic reaction to flare up. Some people sensitive to nickel can also have the allergic reaction when they consume foods and water containing the metal or inhale contaminated dusts. Less frequently, certain sensitized individuals can have attacks following Ni exposure by whatever route feasible (ATSDR, 2005).

As implicated by a number of animal studies, chronic exposure to nickel or its compounds can cause GI distress (e.g., vomiting, nausea, diarrhea) as well as adverse effects on the blood, liver, kidneys, central nervous system, and immunological system. Long-term exposure to nickel via inhalation can result in certain adverse respiratory effects such as bronchitis, decrease in lung function, and a type of asthma specific to Ni exposure. Laboratory studies showed that Ni compounds that are soluble tended to be more toxic (though not necessarily more carcinogenic) than those less soluble, particularly from inhalation exposure (ATSDR, 2005).

In particular, nickel carbonyl (Ni[CO]$_4$) is a highly toxic soluble compound. Headaches, chest pains, and GI distress are commonly observed in patients of nickel carbonyl poisoning, followed by coughing, cyanosis, hyperpnoea (i.e., increase in the depth or rate of breathing), and weakness. These symptoms may be accompanied by fever and leukocytosis, with the more severe cases progressing to pneumonia, respiratory failure, cerebral edema, and death (IPCS, 1991). Lung tumors were observed in rats exposed to nickel carbonyl via inhalation (U.S. EPA, 1999e).

Along with a handful of animal experiments, several epidemiological studies implicated an increase in the risks of lung and nasal cancers from chronic exposure to nickel subsulfide (Ni$_3$S$_2$) and nickel refinery dust (ATSDR, 2005). And risks of lung and nasal cancers were found highest among workers exposed either to metallic nickel (Ni^o) over a long period or to high levels of the more soluble nickel oxide (NiO) and nickel sulfide (NiS). Accordingly, IARC (1990, 2012a, 2017) has listed all Ni compounds as human (Group 1) carcinogens and nickel as a possible human (Group 2B) carcinogen. U.S. EPA (1999e, 1999f, 1999g), on the other hand, has classified nickel subsulfide and nickel refinery dust as human (Group A) carcinogens and nickel carbonyl as a probable human (Group B2) carcinogen.

14.5. Select Radioactive Metals

Radioactive metals are metallic elements each with an unstable nucleus that can spontaneously emit its protons, neutrons, or photons to generate the so-termed *alpha* (α), *beta* (β), or *gamma* (γ) ray (or radiation). When two protons and two neutrons in the unstable nucleus are bound together as a particle, their emission is referred to as an α-radiation, α-ray, or the radiation of an α particle. A β-radiation, on the other hand, involves the emission of *either* one electron that has been converted from an excess neutron *or* one positron that has been converted from an excess proton, all in a nucleus containing an unbalanced number of protons or neutrons. When a nucleus emits an α or a β particle, the nucleus is sometimes left in a highly excited state. Gamma decay or radiation occurs whenever an excited nucleus, as a result of falling down to a lower energy state, emits an electromagnetic type of high energy photon (hv) known as γ particle.

Although these three types of radiation are capable of penetrating to some degree matters impervious to ordinary light, rays of α and β particles are relatively non-penetrating. In fact, a thin sheet of aluminum is sufficient to halt their penetration. Yet sufficient external exposure to these particles can still cause localized damage (e.g., radiation burns to the exposed skin). In contrast, γ rays are more penetrating to the skin as they have the shortest wavelengths and hence the most energy in the electromagnetic spectrum. As such, γ rays can cause *diffuse* damage throughout the human or animal body, and hence have been used clinically to destroy cancer cells.

As of 2017, a total of 38 radioactive elements have been officially identified, including technetium ($_{43}$Tc), promethium ($_{61}$Pm), and all those elements with atomic number above bismuth ($_{83}$Bi) in the periodic table (Figure 14.1). Actually, the most recent nine elements from 110 through 118 (i.e., those from Darmstadtium [$_{110}$Ds] through Oganesson [$_{118}$Og]) may be more correctly referred to as *suspected* radioactive elements for now, in the sense that their chemical and radioactive properties have yet to be fully unfolded and/or confirmed. In any event, radium ($_{88}$Ra) and radon ($_{86}$Rn) are specifically highlighted below not only because they are ubiquitous in the environment, but also because they are highly carcinogenic.

14.5.1. Radium

Radium (Ra), with a silvery-white appearance, is both the *most* heaviest alkaline earth element (i.e., the heaviest in the heaviest series) and an extremely radioactive metal. It can exist in more than 20 atomic forms, each with a nucleus containing the same number of protons (thus the same atomic number 88) but a variable number of neutrons (thus resulting in a different atomic mass number). Each of these atomic forms is chemically referred to as an isotope, or loosely as a progeny especially when it has a relatively short half-life. Radium is formed as a decay product of uranium ($_{92}$U) or thorium ($_{90}$Th) in the environment. Uranium and thorium are found in trace amounts in most rocks and soils. ^{226}Ra (a.k.a. 226-Ra or Ra-226, that with 88 protons and 138 neutrons and hence the atomic mass of 226 = 88 + 138) and ^{228}Ra (i.e., that still with 88 protons) are two principal radium isotopes found in the environment.

As with any other radioactive metal, when radium undergoes radioactive decay, it divides into two parts. One part is the radiation and the other, a daughter nucleus. The daughter nucleus *per se*, like that of radium, may be highly radioactive and thus may continue to undergo radioactive decay until a relatively stable, nonradioactive (grand)daughter is born. The most stable isotope of radium is ^{226}Ra (formed from the decay of ^{238}U), with a half-life of about 1,600 years. ^{226}Ra's daughter is 222-radon (^{222}Rn, with 86 protons).

Radium was formerly utilized as a component of self-luminous paint for compasses, for instrument panels, and for watch as well as clock dials. It was added to some household products (e.g., toothpastes) or foods for taste or as a preservative until the late 1950s. Radium, mostly in the form of radium chloride (RaCl$_2$), has been used in medicine as a radiation source for treatment of cancer and certain non-neoplastic diseases, such as the chronic inflammatory rheumatic disease termed *ankylosing spondylitis* involving primarily arthritis of the spine (Alberding *et al.*, 2006; Lassmann *et al.*, 2002). Radium has been used in radiography of other metals and as a neutron source for laboratory research.

Aside from being present in trace amounts in most rocks and soils, radium may be found in the air and water in certain areas, such as near uranium and thorium mines. The radioactive metal hence may be found in plants through uptake from contaminated soils or in fish and other aquatic creatures through intake from contaminated water. Consequently, humans can be exposed to at least a trace amount of the metal in the air, water, or foods. Uranium and thorium miners and those engaging in grinding of the two radioactive metals are expected to have the highest risk of occupational as well as environmental exposure to radium.

Little information on health effects is available for short-term exposure to radium, especially at low levels. However, as pointed out by ATSDR (1990), chronic or subchronic exposure to high levels of radium can cause anemia, teeth fracture, cataracts, necrosis of the jaw, abscess in the brain, and terminal bronchopneumonia. German patients who were injected with radium between

1946 and 1950 for treatment of certain diseases (e.g., tuberculosis) were found significantly shorter as adults compared to those not treated with the radioactive metal.

Long-term exposure to high levels of radium by the oral route is known to cause cancer in the lung, bone, head, and nasal passage (ATSDR, 1990). Accordingly, IARC (2012c, 2017) has listed ^{224}Ra, ^{226}Ra, ^{228}Ra, and their progenies as human (Group 1) carcinogens.

14.5.2. Radon

Radon (Rn) is a colorless, odorless, and tasteless radioactive noble gas. It occurs naturally as the decay product of radium and, as such, is thought to form somewhat midway via the radioactive decay chain beginning with uranium or thorium. Therefore, inasmuch as uranium has been around likely since the Earth was formed and its most common (primordial) isotope (^{238}U) has a half-life of some 4.5 billion years (or reportedly about the Earth's age), both radium and radon likewise continue to be around for billions of years. Radon is one of the densest elements remaining a gas under normal conditions. Its most stable isotope is ^{222}Rn, with a half-life of about 4 days. Strictly speaking, radon is not a metallic element under normal conditions or definition. However, its parent ^{226}Ra is certainly a true metal; radon is therefore treated in this subsection as if it were a radioactive metal (rather than as a radioactive *gas*), for the sake of simplicity.

Radon accounts for the majority of exposure to ionizing radiation by the general population. It is typically the single largest source of a person's background radiation dose. This noble gas from natural sources can accumulate in buildings, predominantly in confined areas such as cracks in a basement. As a *noble* gas with *low* chemical reactivity, radon can release itself easily from almost any type or form of chemical binding. And as a gas, it can travel freely and far enough to reach the air, water, and soil. Like radium, radon at high levels is typically found near uranium or thorium mines where milling operations of these grandparent radioactive metals occur.

When radon or its isotope undergoes radioactive decay, some of the decays involved will expel α particles which will become the major cause of human health concerns. Many epidemiological studies implicated that this type of radiation from long-term residential exposure could or would increase the risk of developing lung cancer (Darby *et al.*, 2005; Krewski *et al.*, 2005). Accordingly, radon is now regarded as a significant indoor pollutant worldwide. In the United States, radon is treated as the second most frequent cause of lung cancer, only after cigarette smoking. It accounts for some 21,000 lung cancer deaths among non-smokers each year (U.S. EPA, 2003). IARC (2012c, 2017) has listed radon as a human (Group 1) carcinogen. Other significant or major health effects caused by acute (or even chronic) exposure to radon, if any, are not well known or documented at the present time.

References

Akinloye O, Adebayo TO, Oguntibeju OO, Oparinde DP, Ogunyemi EO, 2011. Effects of Contraceptives on Serum Trace Elements, Calcium and Phosphorus Levels. *West Indian Med. J.* 60:308-315.

Alberding A, Stierle H, Brandt J, Braun J, 2006. Effectiveness and Safety of Radium Chloride in the Treatment of Ankylosing Spondylitis. Results of an Observational Study. *Z. Rheumatol.* 65:245-251 (in German).

Andersen RA, 1994. Stress Effects on Chromium Nutrition of Humans and Farm Animals. In *Proceedings of Alltech's 10th Annual Symposium, Biotechnology in Feed Industry* (Lyons TP, Jacques KA, Eds.). Loughborough, Leics, UK: Nottingham University Press, pp.267-274.

ATSDR (U.S. Agency for Toxic Substances and Disease Registry), 1990. Toxicological Profile for Radium. U.S. Department of Health and Human Services Atlanta, Georgia, USA.

ATSDR (U.S. Agency for Toxic Substances and Disease Registry), 1999. Toxicological Profile for Mercury. U.S. Department of Health and Human Services, Atlanta, Georgia, USA.

ATSDR (U.S. Agency for Toxic Substances and Disease Registry), 2002. Toxicological Profile for Beryllium. U.S. Department of Health and Human Services, Atlanta, Georgia, USA.

ATSDR (U.S. Agency for Toxic Substances and Disease Registry), 2005. Toxicological Profile for Nickel. U.S. Department of Health and Human Services, Atlanta, Georgia, USA.

ATSDR (U.S. Agency for Toxic Substances and Disease Registry), 2007a. Toxicological Profile for Lead. U.S. Department of Health and Human Services, Atlanta, Georgia, USA.

ATSDR (U.S. Agency for Toxic Substances and Disease Registry), 2007b. Toxicological Profile for Arsenic. U.S. Department of Health and Human Services, Atlanta, Georgia, USA.

ATSDR (U.S. Agency for Toxic Substances and Disease Registry), 2008. Toxicological Profile for Aluminum. U.S. Department of Health and Human Services, Atlanta, Georgia, USA.

ATSDR (U.S. Agency for Toxic Substances and Disease Registry), 2012a. Toxicological Profile for Cadmium. U.S. Department of Health and Human Services, Atlanta, Georgia, USA.

ATSDR (U.S. Agency for Toxic Substances and Disease Registry), 2012b. Toxicological Profile for Chromium. U.S. Department of Health and Human Services, Atlanta, Georgia, USA.

ATSDR (U.S. Agency for Toxic Substances and Disease Registry), 2013. Addendum to the Toxicological Profile for Mercury. U.S. Department of Health and Human Services, Atlanta, Georgia, USA.

ATSDR (U.S. Agency for Toxic Substances and Disease Registry), 2015. Addendum to the Toxicological Profile for Beryllium. U.S. Department of Health and Human Services, Atlanta, Georgia, USA.

ATSDR (U.S. Agency for Toxic Substances and Disease Registry), 2016. Addendum to the Toxicological Profile for Arsenic. U.S. Department of Health and Human Services, Atlanta, Georgia, USA.

Bakir F, Damluji SF, Amin-Zaki L, Murtadha M, Khalidi A, Al-Rawi NY, Tikriti S, Dahahir HI, Clarkson TW, Smith JC, Doherty RA, 1973. MethylHg Poisoning in Iraq. *Science* 181:230-241.

Bandmann O, Weiss KH, Kaler SG, 2015. Wilson's Disease and Other Neurological Copper Disorders. *Lancet Neurol.* 14:103-113.

Berg G, Kohlmeier L, Brenner H, 1998. Effect of Oral Contraceptive Progestins on Serum Copper Concentration. *Eur. J. Clin. Nutri.* 52:711-715.

Berg KK, Hull HF, Zabel EW, Staley PK, Brown MJ, Homa DM, 2006. Death of a Child after Ingestion of a Metallic Charm – Minnesota, 2006. *MMWR* (U.S. Centers for Disease Control and Prevention Morbidity and Mortality Weekly Report) 55:1-2.

Berny PJ, Côté LM, Buck WB, 1992. Erythrocyte δ-Aminolevulinic Acid Dehydratase (ALAD) Activity as an Indicator of Lead Exposure in Dogs and Cats: Optimal Test Conditions. *Toxicol. Mech. Mthds.* 2:57-68.

Bhattacharyya MH, 2009. Cd Osteotoxicity in Experimental Animals: Mechanisms and Relationship to Human Exposures. *Toxicol. Appl. Pharmacol.* 238:258-265.

Brewer GJ, 2007. Iron and Copper Toxicity in Diseases of Aging, Particularly Atherosclerosis and Alzheimer's Disease. *Exp. Biol. Med.* 232:323-335.

Brzóska MM, Moniuszko-Jakoniuk J, 2004. Low-Level Lifetime Exposure to Cadmium Decreases Skeletal Mineralization and Enhances Bone Loss in Aged Rats. *Bone* 35:1180-1191.

Christen Y, 2000. Oxidative Stress and Alzheimer Disease. *Am. J. Clin. Nutri.* 71(suppl):621-629.

Cox M, Blacksell SE, 2000. Clinical Performance of the Nova-T380 IUD in Routine Use by the UK Family Planning and Reproductive Health Research Network: 2-Month Report. *Br. J. Fam. Plann.* 26:148-151.

Crapper DR, Krishnan SS, Dalton AJ, 1973. Brain Aluminum Distribution in Alzheimer's Disease and Experimental Neurofibrillary Degeneration. *Science* 180:511-513.

Crapper DR, Krishnan SS, Quittkat S, 1976. Aluminum, Neurofibrillary Degeneration and Alzheimer's Disease. *Brain* 99:67-80.

Darby S, Hill D, Auvinen A, Barros-Dios JM, Baysson H, Bochicchio F, Deo H, Falk R, Forastiere F, Hakama M, *et al.*, 2005. Radon in Homes and Risk of Lung Cancer: Collaborative Analysis of Individual Data from 13 European Case-Control Studies. *Brit. Med. J.* 330:223-227.

Gallagher CM, Kovach JS, Meliker JR, 2008. Urinary Cd and Osteoporosis in U.S. Women ≥50 Years of Age: NHANES 1988-1994 and 1999-2004. *Environ. Health Perspect.* 116:1338-1343.

Goldstein BD, Amoruso MA, Witz G, 1985. Erythrocyte Glucose-6-Phosphate Dehydrogenase Deficiency Does Not Pose an Increased Risk for Black Americans Exposed to Oxidant Gases in the Workplace or General Environment. *Toxicol. Ind. Health* 1:7-80.

Goyer RA, Clarkson TW, 2001. Toxic Effects of Metals. In *Casarett and Doull's Toxicology: The Basic Science of Poisons* (Klaassen CD, Ed.), 6th Edition. New York, New York, USA: McGraw-Hill, Chapter 23.

Gurer-Orhan H, Sabırb HU, Özgüne H, 2004. Correlation between Clinical Indicators of Lead Poisoning and Oxidative Stress Parameters in Controls and Lead-Exposed Workers. *Toxicology* 195:147-154.

Hachiya N, 2006. The History and the Present of Minamata Disease – Entering the Second Half a Century. *JMAJ (Japan Med. Assoc. J.)* 49:112-118.

Hubacher D, Reyes V, Lillo S, Pierre-Louis B, Zepeda A, Chen P-L, Croxatto H, 2006. Preventing Copper Intrauterine Device Removals due to Side Effects among First-Time Users: Randomized Trial to Study the Effect of Prophylactic Ibuprofen. *Hum. Reprod.* 21:1467-1472.

Hubacher D, Chen PL, Park S, 2009. Side Effects from the Copper IUD: Do They Decrease Over Time? *Contraception* 79:356-362.

IARC (International Agency for Research on Cancer), 1987. IARC Monographs on the Evaluation of Carcinogenic Risks to Humans, Supplement 7: Overall Evaluations of Carcinogenicity – An Updating of IARC Monographs Volumes 1 to 42. Lyon, France: WHO Press.

IARC (International Agency for Research on Cancer), 1990. IARC Monographs on the Evaluation of Carcinogenic Risks to Humans, Volume 49: Chromium, Nickel and Welding. Lyon, France: WHO Press.

IARC (International Agency for Research on Cancer), 1993. IARC Monographs on the Evaluation of Carcinogenic Risks to Humans, Volume 58: Beryllium, Cd, Hg, and Exposures in the Glass Manufacturing Industry. Lyon, France: WHO Press.

IARC (International Agency for Research on Cancer), 2006. IARC Monographs on the Evaluation of Carcinogenic Risks to Humans, Volume 87: Inorganic and Organic Lead Compounds. Lyon, France: WHO Press.

IARC (International Agency for Research on Cancer), 2012a. IARC Monographs on the Evaluation of Carcinogenic Risks to Humans, Volume 100C: Arsenic, Metals, Fibres and Dusts. Lyon, France: WHO Press.

IARC (International Agency for Research on Cancer), 2012b. IARC Monographs on the Evaluation of Carcinogenic Risks to Humans, Volume 100F: Chemical Agents and Related Occupations. Lyon, France: WHO Press.

IARC (International Agency for Research on Cancer), 2012c. IARC Monographs on the Evaluation of Carcinogenic Risks to Humans, Volume 100D: Radiation. Lyon, France: WHO Press.

IARC (International Agency for Research on Cancer), 2017. IARC Monographs on the Evaluation of Carcinogenic Risks to Humans, Volumes 1-119: List of Carcinogens. Lyon, France: WHO Press.

IPCS (International Programme on Chemical Safety), 1991. Environmental Health Criteria 108 – Nickel. World Health Organization, Geneva, Switzerland.

IPCS (International Programme on Chemical Safety), 1998. Environmental Health Criteria 200 – Copper. World Health Organization, Geneva, Switzerland.

Ishimure M, 1990. *Paradise in the Sea of Sorrow: Our Minamata Disease*. Kyoto, Honshū, Japan: Yagamuchi Publishing House (translated by L. Monnet).

Jellinger KA, 2013. The Relevance of Metals in the Pathophysiology of Neurodegeneration, Pathological Considerations. *Intl. Rev. Neurobiol.* 110:1-47.

Kaler SG, 2007. Wilson's Disease. In *Cecil (Textbook of) Medicine*. (Goldman L, Asiello D, Eds.), 23rd Edition. Philadelphia, Pennsylvania, USA: Saunders Elsevier, Chapter 230.

Kingston RL, Hall S, Sioris L, 1993. Clinical Observations and Medical Outcome in 149 Cases of Arsenate Ant Killer Ingestion. *J. Toxicol. Clin. Toxicol.* 31:581-591.

Kobayashi J, 1978. Pollution by Cadmium and the Itai-Itai Disease in Japan. In *Toxicity of Heavy Metals in the Environment* (Oeheme FW, Ed.). New York, New York, USA: Marcel Dekker. pp.199-260.

Krewski D, Lubin JH, Zielinski JM, Alavanja M, Catalan VS, William FR, Klotz JB, Létourneau EG, Lynch CF, Lyon JI, *et al.*, 2005. Residential Radon and Risk of Lung Cancer: A Combined Analysis of 7 North American Case-Control Studies. *Epidemiology* 16:137-145.

Lassmann M, Nosske D, Reiners C, 2002. Therapy of Ankylosing Spondylitis with 224Ra-Radium Chloride: Dosimetry and Risk Considerations. *Rad. Environ. Biophys.* 41:173-178.

Liukko P, Erkkola R, Pakarinen P, Järnström S, Näntö V, Grönroos M, 1988. Trace Elements during 2 Years' Oral Contraception with Low-Estrogen Preparations. *Gynecol. Obstet. Invest.* 25:113-117.

Lockhart WT, Atkinson JR, 1919. Administration of Arsenic in Syphilis. *Can. Med. Assoc. J.* 9:129-135.

Markesbury WR, Ehmann WD, Hossain TI, Allauddin M, Goodin DT, 1981. Instrumental Neutron Activation Analysis of Brain Aluminum in Alzheimer Disease and Aging. *Ann. Neurol.* 10:511-516.

McDermott JR, Smith AI, Iqbal K, Wisniewski HM, 1979. Brain Aluminum in Aging and Alzheimer Disease. *Neurology* 29:809-814.

Mirza A, King A, Troakes C, Exley C, 2017. Aluminium in Brain Tissue in Familial Alzheimer's Disease. *J. Trace Elem. Med. Biol.* 40:30-36.

Nogawa K, 1981. Itai-Itai Disease and Follow-up Studies. In *Cadmium in the Environment. II: Health Effects* (Mariagu JO, Ed.). New York, New York, USA: John Wiley, pp.1-37.

Pattee OH, Pain DJ, 2003. Lead in the Environment. In *Handbook of Ecotoxicology* (Hoffman DJ, Rattner BA, Burton GA Jr, Cairns J Jr, Eds.). Boca Raton, Florida USA: Lewis Publishers, Chapter 15.

Pechova A, Pavlata L, 2007. Chromium as an Essential Nutrient: A Review. *Veterinarni Medicina* 52:1-18.

Peri DP, 1985. Relationship of Aluminum to Alzheimer's Disease. *Environ. Health Perspect.* 63:149-153.

Pizarro F, Olivares M, Uauy R, Contreras P, Rebelo A, Gidi V, 1999. Acute Gastrointestinal Effects of Graded Levels of Copper in Drinking Water. *Environ. Health Perspect.* 107:117-121.

Reilly C, 2004. *The Nutritional Trace Metals.* Oxford, UK: Blackwell Publishing, Chapter 1.

Satarug S, Garrett SH, Sens MA, Sens DA, 2010. Cd, Environmental Exposure, and Health Outcomes. *Environ. Health Perspect.* 118:182-190.

Smith WE, Smith AM, 1975. *Minamata.* New York, New York, USA: Holt, Rinehart & Winston.

Trapp GA, Miner GD, Zimmerman RL, Mastri AR, Heston LL, 1978. Aluminum Levels in Brain in Alzheimer's Disease. *Biol. Psychiatry* 13:709-718.

U.S. EPA (U.S. Environmental Protection Agency), 1997. Hg Study Report to Congress – Volume V: Health Effects of Hg and Hg Compounds. EPA-452/R-97-007. Office of Air Quality Planning & Standards and Office of Research and Development, Washington DC, USA.

U.S. EPA (U.S. Environmental Protection Agency), 1998. Toxicological Review of Beryllium and Compounds (in Support of Summary Information on IRIS). National Center for Environmental Assessment, Washington DC, USA.

U.S. EPA (U.S. Environmental Protection Agency), 1999a. Integrated Risk Information System (IRIS) on Cd. National Center for Environmental Assessment, Washington DC, USA.

U.S. EPA (U.S. Environmental Protection Agency), 1999b. Integrated Risk Information System (IRIS) on Arsine. National Center for Environmental Assessment, Washington DC, USA.

U.S. EPA (U.S. Environmental Protection Agency), 1999c. Integrated Risk Information System (IRIS) on Beryllium. National Center for Environmental Assessment, Washington, DC, USA.

U.S. EPA (U.S. Environmental Protection Agency), 1999d. Integrated Risk Information System (IRIS) on Chromium VI. National Center for Environmental Assessment, Washington DC, USA.

U.S. EPA (U.S. Environmental Protection Agency), 1999e. Integrated Risk Information System (IRIS) on Nickel Carbonyl. National Center for Environmental Assessment, Washington DC, USA.

U.S. EPA (U.S. Environmental Protection Agency), 1999f. Integrated Risk Information System (IRIS) on Nickel Refinery Dust. National Center for Environmental Assessment, Washington DC, USA.

U.S. EPA (U.S. Environmental Protection Agency), 1999g. Integrated Risk Information System (IRIS) on Nickel Subsulfide. National Center for Environmental Assessment, Washington DC, USA.

U.S. EPA (U.S. Environmental Protection Agency), 2003. EPA Assessment of Risks of Radon in Homes. EPA-402-R-2003. Office of Radiation and Indoor Air, Washington DC, USA.

U.S. EPA (U.S. Environmental Protection Agency), 2004. Integrated Risk Information System (IRIS) on Lead and Compounds (Inorganic). National Center for Environmental Assessment, Washington DC, USA.

VanArsdale JL, Leiker D, Kohn M, Merritt TA, Horowitz BZ, 2004. Lead Poisoning from a Toy Necklace. *Pediatrics* 114:1096-1099.

Review Questions

1. Approximately how many chemical elements in the periodic table can be classified as having metallic properties?
2. What are metalloids? List the elements in the periodic table that may be considered as metalloids.
3. What are the three most toxic heavy metals? And what do they have in common in terms of their interference with the normal functions of enzymes in the human body?

4. Briefly describe the relationship between blood lead levels and the enzymatic activity of δ-ALAD in the human body.
5. What is a systemic poison? And which metal is most commonly referred to as such?
6. What is the most toxic form of mercury? And what are the likely adverse human health effects caused by this form, as evident from the Minamata disaster?
7. What are the adverse human health effects commonly caused by the metal responsible for the *itai-itai* disease?
8. What appears to be the main controversy over the toxicity of aluminum in humans?
9. Which metal has its nefarious name as king of poisons? And in what oxidation state is this metal most toxic to humans?
10. Name a metal that, like lead, tends to stick to soil particles and at high levels can cause acute chemical pneumonitis.
11. Name the chemical elements that are commonly regarded as essential trace metals.
12. Briefly describe the adverse human health effects caused by hexavalent chromium.
13. What is likely to happen to individuals who, sensitized to nickel, now have come in contact with foods or jewelry containing the metal?
14. What can happen to people exposed to high levels of copper, especially if they have Wilson's disease?
15. What can be a potential major health problem for women who use oral contraceptives and engage in copper smelting operations?
16. What are radioactive metals? And how do they emit alpha, beta, or gamma radiation?
17. Which of the following types of radiation is most penetrating to the human skin? a) alpha; b) beta; c) gamma; d) non-ionizing.
18. What is a radon progeny? And what human health effects can be caused from long-term exposure to radon or some of its progenies?
19. List all the metals (whether or not due to their compounds only) discussed in this chapter that have been classified by IARC as a human (Group 1) carcinogen.
20. What human health effects can be caused from long-term exposure to radium?
21. Which of the metals in the periodic table are radioactive? And which are synthetic in origin?

CHAPTER 15

Pesticides and Pesticide Residues

15.1. Introduction

Pests of public health and agricultural concerns are nuisances specifically defined as organisms other than humans that are destructive, troublesome, or residing where they are unwelcome. They hence represent a wide variety of species including insects, weeds, fungi, bacteria, viruses, fleas, ticks, and rodents (as well as other unwanted small animals). Pesticides are active ingredients of products employed to prevent, destroy, repel, mitigate, or otherwise control these pests. Most of these active ingredients are synthetic substances while many are highly toxic, carcinogenic, and capable of disrupting the endocrine system (Chapter 19) in humans and (other) animals. The term *pesticide residues* refers to those *applied* pesticide particles remaining in the environment, especially in foods or food crops and on or around the workers. In practice, it is the pesticide residues left behind, not the pesticides to be applied, that are most relevant to environmental toxicology.

15.1.1. Health Impacts and Concerns

As of today, there have been little or no reliable statistics on global annual incidences of pesticide-related poisoning, largely due to a lack of standardized case definition and reporting scheme for incidences of this kind. Nonetheless, three decades ago, the World Health Organization (WHO, 1990) did make an estimation that roughly 3 million cases of acute severe pesticide poisoning occurred worldwide each year, of which about one-third were non-suicidal. That estimation did not include the many cases of chronic effects, those not reported, or those occurring in a non-agricultural setting. In fact, it estimated (Murray *et al.*, 2002) that the under-reporting rate of pesticide poisoning in Central America was up to 98% in those years, largely due to poor access to hospitals and other healthcare facilities. The excessive use of many pesticides, along with their acute toxicity to humans, was emphasized by Rachel Carson (1962) in her classic *Silent Spring*. It was for these and similar concerns that the U.S. Federal Insecticide, Fungicide, and Rodenticide Act (FIFRA) was rewritten in 1972 to regulate not only the efficacy of pesticides but also their sale and use, in an effort to protect the nation's human health and preserve its natural environment. This federal statute has since been amended several times, including some significant changes in the form of the Food Quality Protection Act (FQPA) of 1996.

The FIFRA provides U.S. EPA with the specific authority to: (1) strengthen the pesticide registration process by shifting the burden of proof to the pesticide registrants; (2) enforce regulatory compliance against unregistered pesticide products; and (3) promulgate the regulatory framework missing from the original version of the law. The FQPA of 1996 amended both the FIFRA and the U.S. (Federal) Food, Drug, and Cosmetic Act of 1938 (Chapter 21) by changing the way in which

U.S. EPA assesses and regulates pesticide safety. The FQPA specifically mandates U.S. EPA to consider cumulative exposures (Chapter 23) to all pesticides that share a common mechanism of toxicity at issue, particularly for young children who tend to be more sensitive and vulnerable to chemical exposure compared to adults.

15.1.2. Pesticide Residues as Pollutants

Many pesticides used today can be treated not only as soil-borne but also as water-borne pollutants. As hinted in Chapter 5 (and a couple other chapters), many pollutants from a variety of natural and anthropogenic sources are subject to mobilization and distribution across environmental compartments via various biological and chemical processes. The pesticides as well as their residues discussed in this chapter for the most part are no exceptions. Many pesticides are used on or for agricultural commodities in the form of pellet, powder, dust, and predominantly spray solution. By convention, the residues of these pesticides are perceived more as soil- or land-borne than as water-borne pollutants due to their major uses or disposal sites being on land or soil properties (e.g., farmlands, landfills). Yet in reality, the residues of the more persistent members of pesticides can be found eventually at substantial levels in ground waters, estuaries, rivers, and other water bodies, as through leaching and runoff. In fact, one of the most alarming effects of pesticide contamination of drinking water came to light around 2002, when the residues of many organochlorine (OC) and organophosphate (OP) pesticides were detected in bottled water sold in the Delhi region in India (Mathur *et al.*, 2003).

The residues of some pesticides, particularly those of the soil fumigant type, can be detected in the air as well if they are persistent and volatile enough to evaporate off the soil, land properties, or water. Methyl bromide (CH_3Br), for example, was once widely applied as a soil and structural fumigant in many countries. A global full phase-out of this fumigant was scheduled for 2005 under the global treaty *Montreal Protocol on Substances That Deplete the Ozone Layer*. The main global concern with methyl bromide is that the fumigant is readily photolyzed in the air to release elemental bromine (Br) which is highly destructive to stratospheric ozone (O_3). Ozone in the stratosphere has the function to protect life on the Earth by absorbing over 95% of the sun's harmful ultraviolet light (Chapter 11).

15.2. Usage and Classification of Pesticides

Literally well over 800 different pesticide active ingredients are currently available in the market worldwide (e.g., Tomlin, 2015). Most of these active ingredients used are synthetic organic substances, while comparatively a very small number are inorganics or from natural sources such as sulfur (S), chlorine (Cl), mercury (Hg), copper (Cu), rotenone, and neem.

15.2.1. Statistics on Pesticide Usage

As summarized in Table 15.1 below, the pesticide active ingredients employed in the United States between 1993 and 2012 were consistently around 1.2 billion pounds per year. The use estimates for the more recent years after 2012 are not yet publicly available. There is, nonetheless, the

Table 15.1. Estimates of Annual Amounts of Pesticide Active Ingredients Employed in the World, the United States, and the State of California (USA), in Million Pounds from 1993 through 2015, in All Market Sectors[a]

Year	World[b]					United States[c]					California[d]
	Herbicide	Insecticide	Fungicide	Others[e]	Total	Herbicide	Insecticide	Fungicide	Others[e]	Total	Total
1993						527	115	80	440	1,162	200
1994						583	124	79	443	1,229	191
1995	2,210	1,500	550	1,450	5,710	556	125	77	452	1,210	205
1996						578	116	79	456	1,229	198
1997	2,254	1,470	539	1,421	5,684	568	112	81	467	1,228	208
1998	2,148	1,427	553	1,522	5,650	555	103	86	462	1,206	217
1999	2,040	1,417	556	1,666	5,679	534	126	79	505	1,244	203
2000	1,944	1,355	516	1,536	5,351	542	122	74	486	1,234	188
2001	1,870	1,232	475	1,469	5,046	553	105	73	472	1,203	151
2002						527	130	71	478	1,206	168
2003						527	115	76	485	1,203	175
2004						521	114	75	500	1,210	180
2005						513	104	78	457	1,152	195
2006	2,018	955	519	1,705	5,197	498	99	73	457	1,127	188
2007	2,096	892	518	1,705	5,211	531	93	70	439	1,133	172
2008	2,083	972	737	1,058	4,850	540	63	80	452	1,135	164
2009	2,189	1,016	784	1,019	5,008	560	70	72	448	1,151	158
2010	2,120	996	811	1,249	5,177	570	63	90	526	1,249	175
2011	2,508	1,070	735	1,100	5,414	609	62	98	513	1,282	192
2012	2,847	1,065	799	1,110	5,821	678	64	105	435	1,182	187
2013											195
2014											190
2015											213

[a] for years 2008 on, estimates were provided "at the producer level" by U.S. EPA, which are treated in this table as equivalent to "in all market sectors"; [b] U.S. EPA (1997a, 1999, 2002, 2004a, 2011, 2017); [c] U.S. EPA (2011, 2017); [d] California Department of Pesticide Regulation (CDPR, 2017), which did not (and still does not) provide the public with direct use statistics by target pest type or pesticide category; [e] from years 2008 on as based on a different source (i.e., U.S. EPA, 2017), the above pesticide type *Others* included fumigants only (i.e., not including the other "minor use" pesticides such as wood preservatives, specialty biocides, vertebrate pesticides, etc.) and hence the annual *total* amounts estimated for these later years should be slightly higher than those shown above under the *Others* category.

consensus that the annual pesticide usage in the United States has remained roughly 1 billion pounds in the recent years. Underlying this consensus is the fact that the annual amounts of pesticides used in the state of California have not reduced since 2012. California is regarded as having one of the most extensive databases on pesticide usage in the world; and hence its recent trend in pesticide usage (Table 15.1) should be able to reflect closely the nation's.

Another supporting fact is that California usage contributes nearly 20% of the total pesticide usage in the United States (Table 15.1.). This is actually a startling statistic as the state's cropland represents less than 4% of the total planted acreage in the nation. The estimates provided by U.S. EPA revealed that the pesticide active ingredients employed annually in the United States represented about a quarter of the world's annual usage of ~5 billion pounds. U.S. EPA's data by pesticide type further showed that the large uses of herbicides, insecticides, and fungicides, in that order, collectively accounted for 60% or more of pesticide active ingredients used in the United States and worldwide. And the agricultural market sector alone was responsible for about 75% of the annual usage in the United States and worldwide. The home/garden, commercial, industrial, and government represented the various major non-agricultural market sectors.

15.2.2. Classification of Pesticides

A common scheme in which pesticides are classified or grouped together is according to the specific type(s) of pests that they each destroy or control. Pesticides thereby are commonly referred to as insecticides, herbicides, fungicides, rodenticides (a.k.a. predatorcides), bactericides, algaecides, piscicides, nematocides, miticides, tickicides, avicides, molluscicides, and so forth. There are, however, pesticides either belonging to a common product group or having unique biological functions that can be classified more effectively as such on their own. These pesticides include, but are not limited to, antibiotics, anticoagulants, botanicals, fumigants, petroleum oils, pheromones, and plant growth regulators (e.g., Ware and Whitacre, 2004). In Table 15.1, the plant growth regulators are subsumed under the *Herbicides* group.

Nonetheless, in environmental toxicology, pesticides may be better classified or characterized according to the chemical class or family that they belong to. This is because pesticides in the same chemical group tend to have more pesticidal and toxicological properties in common. Of the numerous chemical groups involved, a handful are most frequently implicated in symptomatic illnesses (e.g., NEETF, 2002; Reigart and Roberts, 1999) and hence are considered to have greater public health concerns. The more prominent pesticides in these various special chemical families are therefore discussed systematically in the sections that follow, with a focus specifically on their applications, pesticidal actions, and adverse health effects.

15.3. Organochlorine (OC) Pesticides

Until the beginning of World War II, when organochlorines (OCs) and organophosphates (OPs) started being used as insecticides, substances used to control insects were limited to a few from the so-called multipurpose group consisting of primarily arsenicals, sulfur, nicotine, rotenone, and hydrogen cyanide gas. The OC pesticides are chlorinated *hydrocarbon* (hence *organic*) substances.

Because of their strong covalent chlorine-carbon (Cl-C) bonds and high lipophilicity, these OC substances break down very slowly in the environment and tend to accumulate in the fatty tissues of humans and (other) animals. Consequently, they tend to remain in the environment or the food web long after they have been applied. Most OCs were (and some still are) utilized as insecticides, with all being applied extensively from the 1940s through the 1960s in agriculture or for mosquito type control. DDT was the first OC insecticide used on a large scale in the United States, until it was banned in 1973 after reconsideration of its harm to the health of wildlife and humankind. Some OC insecticides have been determined or suspected as capable of disrupting the endocrine system in the mammalian body (Chapter 19). Although most of these substances are no longer used in the United States as many are treated as potent neurotoxicants, some are still being produced by U.S. companies for use elsewhere, mostly in the developing countries.

As with many pesticides in other chemical classes, the OCs collectively are used on a wide variety of crops in various formulations. Whether in the form of spray, dust, powder, or pellet, some OCs are applied to foliar surfaces to get rid of insects settling there. Some others are utilized to preserve wood from insect damage; and still some others are employed to control insects found in grain storage facilities. Structurally and broadly, the OC pesticides can fall into the following three subclasses: (1) the diphenylethane-related OCs; (2) the cyclodiene-related OCs; and (3) the cyclohexane-related OCs.

15.3.1. Diphenylethane-Related OCs

The most prominent member in this diphenylethane subclass is *d*ichloro*d*iphenyl*t*richloroethane ($C_{14}H_9Cl_5$), known to most people by its acronym DDT. Some other members are methoxychlor, methlochlor, ethylan, chlorobenzilate, and dicofol. The last two are examples of OC pesticides applied more specifically as acaricides or miticides than as general (conventional) insecticides. Some of the OC substances noted above, such as dicofol and ethylan, do not contain exactly the bare bone structure *dichlorodiphenylethane* found in DDT (Figure 15.1), but only with the bulk of their core structure looking similar to this nucleus. They are put in this subclass largely for their sharing similar toxicological properties with DDT.

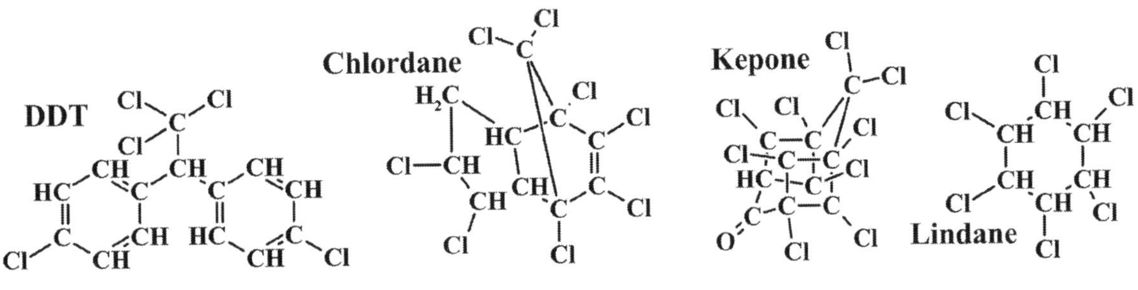

Figure 15.1. Chemical Structures of Four Select Organochlorine Pesticides

Of all the OC members in this subclass, DDT is the most widely known and the most notorious chemical substance in modern pesticide history. Approximately 1.4 billion pounds of DDT were applied in the United States for insect control between 1940 and 1970, with the peak annual usage reaching nearly 80 million pounds in 1959 (U.S. EPA, 1975). DDT proved to be extremely effective against flies and mosquitoes. The insecticide works by binding to the voltage-gated sodium (Na) channel in the insect's nerve cell, thereby locking the channel there in the open state to allow prolonged influx of Na^+ ions (Section 9.2.3). Such an "ion leakage" in turn will cause the nerve to fire repeatedly the electrical impulses expressed as muscle tremors, with the ultimate consequence being the insect's death. DDT is considered a practical and powerful insecticide all owing to its high specificity of binding to the Na^+-channel proteins in *insects*, but not so in higher-order animals (including humans).

This species-specific binding property that DDT possesses may explain in part why this and some other chlorodiphenyl OCs are found to be less toxic to mammalians from acute exposure when compared to OPs or pesticides in many other chemical groups. Nonetheless, due to their greater chemical stability and tendency to accumulate in animals, these chlorodiphenyls tend to cause more severe *chronic* effects compared to pesticides in many other chemical groups. In general, exposure to the chlorodiphenyl OCs at high doses can affect the nervous system in humans, with acute signs of excitability, tremors, and seizures. Even at low doses, chronic exposure to OCs in this subclass, especially to DDT, can affect the liver (ATSDR, 2002a; 2008).

DDT is remarkably stable in the environment except when in the air under sunlight, where it will break down quickly (with a half-life of 2 or 3 days) to TDE ≡ DDD (dichlorodiphenyldichloro*ethane*, $C_{14}H_{10}Cl_4$) and DDE (dichlorodiphenyldichloro*ethylene*, $C_{14}H_8Cl_4$). Both metabolites are equally persistent in the environment with physicochemical and toxicological properties very similar to those of DDT. A study with limited data indicated a possible link between DDE exposure and Parkinson's disease (Koldkjaer et al., 2004). Due to the way in which the two chloride atoms on their two benzene rings can be positioned, DDT, DDD, and DDE each have isomers in the *o,p'*- and *p,p'*-forms. The term *total DDTs* (or *total DDT products*) generally refers to all the isomers of DDT, DDD, and DDE in a mixture. WHO's International Agency for Research on Cancer (IARC (2016, 2017a) has listed DDT as a probable human (Group 2A) carcinogen.

15.3.2. Cyclodiene-Related OCs

This subclass (commonly referred to as *cyclodienes* for short) includes aldrin, chlordane, chlordecone (historically more commonly known by its trade name Kepone), dieldrin, endosulfan, endrin, heptachlor, mirex, and toxaphene. The structural nucleus of this subclass is a chlorinated methylene group forming a bridge across a six-member carbon ring, as in chlordane (Figure 15.1). Cyclodienes are fairly stable in soils and moderately stable to sunlight. As such, they have been widely applied for control of termites and soil-borne insect larvae that feed on plant roots. Due to their persistence often resulting in a large amount of residues present beyond the time for harvest, many cyclodienes were restricted from application on most crops.

Cyclodienes are prominent blockers of *gamma*-aminobutyric acid (GABA)-activated chloride (Cl) channels present in insects, in that these OCs have the ability to antagonize the neurotransmitter GABA's inhibitory (i.e., dampening) action. Otherwise, GABA would facilitate the intake of Cl^- ions by having its molecules bind to their specific receptors. GABA receptors are present in the brains of invertebrates and vertebrates, as well as in insect muscles. These receptors possess

Cl-channels which, if not open as in the absence of GABA, would reduce the intake of Cl^- ions leading to hyperexcitation, convulsions, and ultimately death. This is because the influx of Cl^- ions has the effect of significantly lowering the transmembrane potential and thereby the effect of dampening the firing of nerve impulses.

The cyclodienes produced in the highest quantity were aldrin ($C_{12}H_8Cl_6$), its metabolite dieldrin ($C_{12}H_8Cl_6O$), and chlordane ($C_{10}H_6Cl_8$). Chlordane (Figure 15.1) is a broad-spectrum contact insecticide once widely applied for non-agricultural purposes and on select field crops (e.g., maize, potatoes) as well as on livestock. In the mid-1970s, roughly a third of this OC's use in the United States was on agricultural crops, with the rest being used in or around homes and by structural pest control operators (ATSDR, 1994, 2013). In 1974, over 20 million pounds of chlordane were produced in the United States (IARC, 1979). In 1986, two years prior to the cancellation of almost all of its applications, only about 4 million pounds of chlordane were distributed in the United States (ATSDR, 1994, 2013). Today, the use of chlordane in the United States is limited to the control of fire ants. Chlordane affects the nervous system, the digestive system, and the liver in humans and laboratory animals. People exposed to high doses of chlordane reportedly experienced headaches, irritability, confusion, gastrointestinal (GI) disorders, weakness, vision problems, and even convulsions or death. Some metabolites or by-products of chlordane, such as oxychlordane, heptachlor, and heptachlor epoxide, are known as more toxic than this parent compound (ATSDR, 1994, 2013). Chlordane and heptachlor are also regarded as among the most potent cyclodiene carcinogens tested in animal models. IARC (2001, 2017a) has listed both of these cyclodienes as possible human (Group 2B) carcinogens.

In the United States, aldrin usage reached a peak in 1966, close to 20 million pounds (ATSDR, 2002b). Environmental exposure to aldrin is mostly from consumption of contaminated root crops or seafood. This is equally true for dieldrin, as aldrin can rapidly break down to dieldrin within the animal body or in the environment. Convulsions and deaths were seen in people ingesting large quantities of either cyclodiene. The health effects caused by the two cyclodienes, including on the nervous system, can occur from exposure to even very small amounts if for a long period, since their residues will build up in the host's body for years. Some workers exposed to moderate levels of aldrin or dieldrin for a long period experienced headaches, irritability, and uncontrolled muscle movements (ATSDR, 2002b). As both cyclodienes were shown to cause liver cancer in mice, U.S. EPA (1987) and IARC (2017a, 2017b) have classified the two cyclodienes as probable human (Group B2 and Group 2A, respectively) carcinogens.

Historically, the cyclodiene member most notorious for causing environmental pollution was chlordecone ($C_{10}Cl_{10}O$), more commonly known by its trade name Kepone (Figure 15.1). Kepone, a structural cousin of aldrin, chlordane, and dieldrin, is chemically similar to mirex. It is a carcinogen and can cause damage to the liver, kidneys, and reproductive system in humans and animals if exposed at high doses, in addition to the acute signs of irritability, tremors, and headaches. From 1966 to 1973, each year around 400,000 pounds of Kepone were produced by a U.S. manufacturing facility located in the state of Virginia for application primarily as ant and roach baits. In late 1975, it was discovered that the manufacturer not only had its workers exposed to substantial amounts of the cyclodiene, but also had the wastes illegally dumped into the nearby James River (which flows into the Chesapeake Bay). Due to the high pollution concern, the river from around the state capital Richmond to the Chesapeake Bay was then shut down for commercial fishing. Many businesses and restaurants along the river thus suffered considerably. Four decades later in 2016, Kepone (chlordecone) was still measurable in the majority (65%) of the 85 white perch and striped bass samples taken (periodically) from the James River (Unger and Vadas, 2017).

15.3.3. Cyclohexane-Related OCs

This cyclohexane subclass includes primarily the single hexachlorobenzene (HCB), also known as benzene hexachloride (BHC), and eight (theoretically possible) isomers of hexachlorocyclohexane (HCH). As their names imply, the main structural difference between HCB (C_6Cl_6) and HCH ($C_6H_6Cl_6$) is that the former has all its six Cl atoms on a benzene ring and hence without any hydrogen possible, whereas the latter contains a non-double bond cyclohexane ring instead (*see*, e.g., the lindane structure in Figure 15.1).

Hexachlorobenzene is a substance once widely employed to manufacture fireworks, ammunitions, and rubbers. It had been applied also extensively as a fungicide to protect sorghum seeds, onion seeds, wheat, and other grains until 1965. In the United States, no HCB has been produced for commercial use since the late 1970s. HCB is reportedly highly toxic to aquatic organisms. In humans, chronic oral exposure to the OC substance was linked to skin lesions with discoloration, ulceration, thyroid effects, photosensitivity, bone effects, loss of hair, and a liver disease termed *porphyria cutanea tarda* (PCT). PCT is a subtype of porphyria caused by a deficiency of the cytosolic enzyme uroporphyrinogen decarboxylase, whose action is required for completion of the synthesis of heme. The symptoms of PCT are confined to mostly the skin, along with liver function abnormalities which can lead to cirrhosis and even liver cancer. Studies showed that HCB was capable of crossing the human placenta to accumulate in fetal tissues and transferring itself in human breast milk, in addition to causing teratogenic effects, neurological changes, as well as embryolethality in animals (ATSDR, 2015). Laboratory data revealed an increase in the incidences of liver, kidney, and thyroid cancers in test animals (ATSDR, 2015). IARC (2001, 2017a) has listed HCB (hexachlorobenzene) as a possible human (Group 2B) carcinogen.

The predominant form of the cyclohexane HCH is its γ-isomer commercially known as lindane (Figure 15.1). In the United States, lindane has been applied in various ways from protecting crop seeds against insects to controlling household pests. It is also the active ingredient in many soaps and shampoos medicated for control of head lice and scabies. Over 200,000 pounds of lindane were used annually in the United States, mostly on corn and wheat seeds (ATSDR, 2005). The γ-isomer is now banned or severely restricted in over 50 countries. In the United States, it is now restricted to seed treatment for a few grain crops, but still widely employed for control of head lice and scabies except in the state of California.

Lindane is a neurotoxicant that, like (most of) the cyclodienes, interferes with the action of GABA neurotransmitter by blocking the GABA receptor-chloride channel complex at the binding site specific to picrotoxin (a phytochemical known for its ability to block GABA receptors). All HCH isomers, including specifically lindane, can affect the nervous system, liver, and kidneys. Prenatal exposure to *beta* (β)-HCH, another isomer frequently available as a by-product of lindane production, can affect brain development and has been linked to altered thyroid hormone levels (ATSDR, 2005). IARC (1987, 2016, 2017a) has classified lindane as a human (Group 1) carcinogen and all other HCH isomers as possible human (Group 2B) carcinogens.

Lindane and HCB (hexachlorobenzene) have a common biologic metabolite named pentachlorobenzene (PeCB; C_6Cl_5H), which is also a main product of HCB chemical dechlorination. The synthetic form of PeCB is registered in the United States as a fungicide, and was utilized predominantly as an intermediate for the production of the fungicide pentachloronitrobenzene (a.k.a. quintozene; $C_6Cl_5NO_2$). While having one Cl atom fewer than HCB (or lindane) has, PeCB shares some toxicological properties with HCB (or lindane), including certain adverse effects on the central nervous system (CNS), liver, and reproductive system (in the animal body).

15.4. Organophosphate (OP) Pesticides

As a chemical family of now ending with about 40 active members, organophosphorus compounds (organophosphates or OPs for short) are still among the most widely applied insecticides in the world. Each OP member contains the structural nucleus *phosphate* or a core component resembling a phosphoric salt or acid (e.g., parathion in Figure 15.2). More specifically, each OP is an ester of phosphoric acid (H_3O_4P), phosphonic acid ($H_2O_3P^+$), or a related acid. (*see*, e.g., Corbett *et al.*, 1984 for further examples). Many important macromolecules are structurally of the OP kind, including DNA (Chapter 18). OPs are also the basis of many herbicides and nerve (gas) agents. In addition, they are widely utilized as solvents, plasticizers, and extreme pressure additives for lubricants.

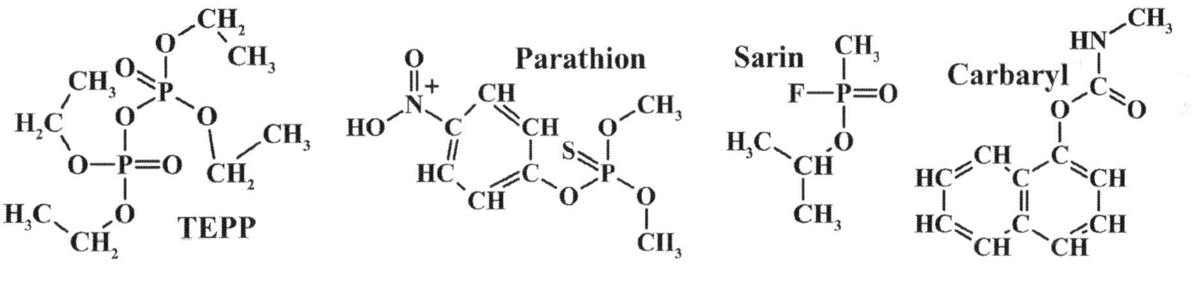

Figure 15.2. Chemical Structures of Three Select Organophosphates and One Select Carbamate

To many entomologists and environmental toxicologists, the term *OPs* refers to the group of insecticides or nerve agents that can affect the nerve function in humans, other mammalians, but primarily insects. As mentioned in Section 9.2.4, the notorious health effects of these insecticides come about through their ability of binding to the active site of the enzyme acetylcholinesterase (AChE) at the brain synapses and neuromuscular junctions, where the enzyme's substrate acetylcholine (ACh) acts as a neurotransmitter. Mechanistically, the inhibition of AChE by an OP molecule is via an attack by the OP's relatively positive phosphorus (P) atom onto the hydroxyl group (OH) of the enzyme's amino acid serine ($C_3H_7NO_3$) residue. When an OP molecule binds to the OH active site, this affected site on the enzyme can be reactivated by a strong nucleophile such as pralidoxime (2-PAM) which, together with atropine (otherwise a poisonous alkaloid), is the mainstay of treatment for OP poisoning. Another possible fate is that the OP molecule will undergo endogenous hydrolysis by the enzyme paraoxonase or esterase. Yet in most cases, the affected AChE will "age or wear out" to become functionless as the binding tends to be *irreversible*.

15.4.1. Delayed Neurotoxic OP Agents

Historically, the first OP (organophosphate) applied as an insecticide was the extremely potent AChE inhibitor tetraethyl pyrophosphate (TEPP, $C_8H_{20}O_7P_2$; Figure 15.2) developed in Germany in 1942. Other some 200 OPs available at one time included the now commonly used insecticides malathion ($C_{10}H_{19}O_6PS_2$) and diazinon ($C_{12}H_{21}N_2O_3PS$), as well as the once widely applied liquid plasticizer tri-*ortho*-cresyl phosphate (TOCP, $C_{21}H_{21}O_4P$). TOCP has never been knowingly utilized as a pesticide. It is discussed here mainly to illustrate the significance of its delayed neuropathy effect shared by a number of OP insecticides such as chlorpyrifos ($C_9H_{11}Cl_3NO_3PS$) and dichlorvos ($C_4H_7Cl_2O_4P$) when ingested at near lethal doses. TOCP was reportedly responsible for the infamous ginger Jake paralysis episode occurring in the United States in 1930. This paralysis, nicknamed Jake leg, is characterized by unsteady gait, ataxia, muscular weakness, and flaccid paralysis of the limbs. Through its metabolic products formed one to four weeks later thereby resulting in a *delayed* onset, TOCP will become capable of inhibiting AChE. The delayed paralysis is typically manifested by wrist and foot drops. Tri-*ortho*-tolyl phosphate was one of TOCP's neurotoxic metabolites observed as conclusively linked to the ginger Jake syndrome.

Before the year 1930, TOCP was widely utilized in the United States as an adulterant to boost the potability of Jamaica ginger extract (the so-called "Jake", containing ~75% alcohol by weight) that was made available to circumvent the Prohibition laws. In the early part of 1930, thousands of American consumers began to lose the use of their hands and feet. The toxicity of TOCP was studied extensively soon after its use was linked to the episode. TOCP, along with some OP insecticides, can induce a delayed neuropathy after a single high dose. This is particularly the case in chickens of about 60 days old, which are the species and the age that are now employed by default as the standard animal model for assuring the negative *o*rgano*p*hosphate-*i*nduced *d*elayed *n*europathy (OPIDN) potential of OPs intended (to be registered) for use as insecticides. The initial effects of OPIDN do not seem to involve the inhibition of AChE, but that of the neurotoxic esterase (NTE) enzyme (Johnson, 1975, 1976). The exact role of NTE inhibition in the initiation of OPIDN remains unclear (Jamal, 1997), although its enzymatic activity is known to be highest in nervous tissue (Hodgson *et al.*, 1998).

15.4.2. Acetylcholinesterase OP Inhibitors

Many OPs not involved in delayed neuropathy induction are still regarded as the most *acutely* toxic pesticides today owing to their ability to inhibit the enzyme AChE directly, rapidly, and effectively, though not all to the same extent. For example, parathion ($C_{10}H_{14}NO_5PS$; Figure 15.2) is one of the first OPs commercialized and is many times more potent than malathion, the latter being applied frequently in combating Mediterranean fruit flies and mosquitoes that transmit West Nile virus. Signs and symptoms of OP poisoning generally include tremors, muscle twitching, myosis, and those subsumed in the mnemonic acronym SLUDGE: *s*alivation, *l*acrimation, *u*rinary incontinence, *d*efecation, *G*I upset/diarrhea, and *e*mesis.

The popularity of OP insecticides increased after many OC insecticides were banned worldwide in the 1970s. In the recent decade, chlorpyrifos has been one of the few largest selling OP insecticides worldwide. In the United States, although this insecticide was banned from residential use in 2001, it is still used intensively on some field crops such as corn and soy. It has estimated (U.S. EPA, 2017) that in the United States, the nation's annual usage of chlorpyrifos in 2012 was 5 to 8 million pounds and ranked the highest among all the OP insecticides used.

Studies have associated chlorpyrifos with delays in learning, reduced physical coordination, and behavioral problems in children, including particularly *a*ttention *d*eficit *h*yperactivity *d*isorder (ADHD) and pervasive developmental disorder (e.g., Rauh *et al.*, 2006). More recent studies (Hayden *et al.*, 2010; Yadav *et al.*, 2016; Yan *et al.*, 2016; Yu *et al.*, 2015) have linked exposures of many pesticides, particularly those of OPs, to an increased risk of Alzheimer's disease. On the other hand, partly because by chemical nature OPs tend to degrade rapidly in both the environment and the animal body, not many of them have been found to profoundly cause cancer or other severe chronic health effects.

Some other commonly used OP pesticides (primarily as insecticides) are acephate, azinphos-methyl, diazinon, dichlorvos, ethion, fenthion, fonofos, malathion, and terbufos. OP-based nerve (gas) agents include sarin ($C_4H_{10}FO_2P$; Figure 15.2), soman, tabun, and VX. Some of these nerve agents were not simply mass destruction weapons of the long past. In 1995, the Japanese domestic perpetrators known as the Aum Shinrikyo cult terrorized their local communities by releasing sarin gas on several train lines of the Tokyo Metro subway, killing 13 people and injuring some 6,000 others. Moreover, as also reported all over the news, in April 2017 the Syrian government was blamed by many (western) nations to have applied sarin-like gas in a chemical weapons attack that killed some 80 people and hurt hundreds in one of its villages held by the rebels.

15.5. Major Carbamate (CB) Pesticides

In general terms, an ester is derived from an organic acid reacting with an alcohol. Carbamates (CBs) are esters of one of the simplest amino acids named (N-methyl) carbamic acid (NH_2COOH; *see*, e.g., that in carbaryl in Figure 15.2). Over 50 CBs have been synthesized for use mainly as insecticides. There is now an increasing use of these esters in medicinal chemistry (e.g., as anticonvulsants). As insecticides, CBs generally interact with AChE in the same manner as OPs do, with their carbamic moiety attacking the same -OH group in the serine residue at the enzyme's active site. Yet unlike the binding of OPs to AChE's active site, that of CBs is generally *reversible*.

15.5.1. Carbaryl

Carbaryl (1-naphthyl methylcarbamate, $C_{12}H_{11}NO_2$; Figure 15.2), the first successful insecticide in the CB family, was introduced in 1956. Worldwide, it has been used more than all the other CBs combined. In the United States, about 4 million pounds of carbaryl are employed annually, with about half for agricultural use (U.S. EPA, 2004b, 2017). Carbaryl, also known by its trade name Sevin, is registered for use on over 400 different sites including vegetables, nurseries, fruit trees, nut trees, grain crops, landscapes, lawns, home gardens, and pet collars. Although carbaryl is readily absorbed via the human skin, it has low to moderate toxicity in humans other than its moderate ability to inhibit AChE. U.S. EPA (2007a) has classified carbaryl as a possible human (Group C) carcinogen based on vascular cancer observed in mice. IARC (1987, 2017a), however, has not listed the carbamate as a potential human or animal carcinogen.

15.5.2. Propoxur and Some Other CBs

Examples of CB insecticides that are used less frequently but commonly referenced in the pesticide literature include aldicarb, carbofuran, carbosulfan, ethiofencarb, methomyl, propoxur, pirimicarb, alanycarb, and indoxacarb. Of these, the last three are newer CBs, with the very last one being designated by U.S. EPA (2000) as a "reduced-risk" pesticide. Propoxur, on the other hand, is perhaps the most toxic insecticide in the CB family (especially via the oral route), as well as one of the most widely applied home and garden pesticides in the United States (Grossman, 1995). Propoxur is a non-systemic insecticide used to control a broad-spectrum of pests including fleas, ticks, mosquitoes, ants, crickets, flies, cockroaches, and insects on lawns and turfs. While U.S. EPA (1997b) has long listed propoxur as a probable human (Group B2) carcinogen, IARC (2017a) has not yet considered the CB's carcinogenicity to humans or animals.

15.6. Pyrethrin and Pyrethroid Pesticides

Much like the above three chemical families, most pyrethroids have been used as insecticides only. This newer insecticide subfamily accounts for a large percentage of today's pesticide market. Pesticides in this subfamily are *synthetic* compounds with structural and chemical as well as toxicological properties very similar to pyrethrins. Pyrethrins are naturally occurring substances found in some species of the plant *chrysanthemum*. The word *pyrethrum* generally refers to any of these plant species but is often used synonymously with *pyrethrin*. Both the pyrethrins and the pyrethroids act by altering an insect's nerve function to ultimately cause its death.

When rats were exposed to pyrethroids at high doses, one of two symptom patterns was generally observed, depending on the chemical configuration of these modified pyrethrins. The Type I pyrethroids, which each *lack* a cyano (CN) group, were found to induce the so-called T syndrome including primarily *t*remors, aggressive sparring, and enhanced startle response. In contrast, the Type II variants, which each *contain* a cyano group, were found to produce the so-called CS syndrome including primarily *c*horeoathetosis, *s*alivation, and seizures. As with DDT, both types of pyrethroids interact with the sodium channel on neuronal biomembranes, delaying closure of this channel. Moreover, like the cyclodiene OCs, Type II pyrethroids are specifically capable of blocking the neurotransmitter GABA's dampening action on the chloride channel.

15.6.1. Pyrethrins

The natural pyrethrum extract that possesses insecticidal function is actually a mixture of six esters (WHO, 2009): three closely related esters of chrysanthemic acid named chrysanthemates or

Pyrethrins I; and three corresponding esters of pyrethrin acid named pyrethrates or Pyrethrins II. The three Pyrethrins I (esters) are specifically named pyrethrin I ($C_{21}H_{28}O_3$), cinerin I ($C_{20}H_{28}O_3$), and jasmolin I ($C_{21}H_{30}O_3$), whereas the three Pyrethrins II (esters) are specifically named pyrethrin II ($C_{22}H_{28}O_5$), cinerin II ($C_{21}H_{28}O_5$), and jasmolin II ($C_{22}H_{30}O_5$).

All six botanical active ingredient esters degrade rapidly in sunlight, typically within 24 hours, and accordingly are not economical to be used extensively for control of agricultural pests due to the high cost of reapplying them. When made available as insecticides, pyrethrin products are hence likely formulated with synergists, such as piperonyl butoxide or MGK-264, to enhance their insecticidal properties. Piperonyl butoxide is a known inhibitor of several key microsomal oxidase enzymes. As such, it is often added to the pyrethrin products to prevent these enzymes from clearing the pyrethrin off the insect's body, thereby prolonging the botanical substance's activity for acting as an insect neurotoxicant. MGK-264 (*N*-octyl bicycloheptene dicarboximide), which is an esterase inhibitor used as a mosquito repellent, also has been found as a very successful synergist (or more correctly, potentiator) of pyrethrins.

15.6.2. Pyrethroids

Pyrethroids have been synthesized to be very similar in structure to, but more stable in the environment than, pyrethrins. These synthetic substances, especially when formulated with synergists (or potentiators), such as again piperonyl butoxide or MGK-264, are comparatively more toxic to insects and inadvertently to mammals as well. Even though more than 1,000 pyrethroids have been synthesized, only some two dozens of them are actively employed in the United States and worldwide. The following are the more popular ones among the actively used: the allethrin stereoisomers, bifenthrin, *beta*-cyfluthrin, *cis*-permethrin, cyfluthrin, cypermethrin, cyphenothrin, *delta*-methrin, esfenvalerate, fenpropathrin, *gamma*-cyhalothrin, imiprothrin, *lambda*-cyhalothrin, permethrin, prallethrin, resmethrin, sumithrin, *tau*-fluvalinate, tefluthrin, tetramethrin, tralomethrin, and *zeta*-cypermethrin.

The history of pyrethroids involves three or four periods over the past 60 some years. Yet often for simplicity, they are categorized into just two generations according to their pesticidal efficacy. The first generation began with allethrin in 1949, the first pyrethroid available at that time, to several more effective ones used in agriculture in the early 1970s. The newer ones of this group included *beta*-cyfluthrin, fenvalerate, and permethrin, with effective insecticidal activity of roughly 0.1 down to 0.02 lb of active ingredient per acre treated (not for all applications). They were relatively unaffected by sunlight, lasting about 1 week as efficacious foliar residues.

The second, more recent generation appears to be even more promising to the agricultural sector for two reasons. First, the photostability of the pyrethroids in this second group is up to 10 days. Second and the more important, their insecticidal efficacy is roughly in the range of 0.02 down to 0.005 lb of active ingredient per acre treated (not for all applications); that is, up to 20 times more effective than those in the first group. Some of the pyrethroids in this second generation include cypermethrin, *delta*-methrin, *lambda*-cyhalothrin, and esfenvalerate.

Among all the pyrethroids available, permethrin ($C_{21}H_{20}Cl_2O_3$; Figure 15.3) is by far the most widely applied. In agriculture, permethrin is mostly applied to maize, cotton, wheat, and alfalfa crops, and to kill parasites on chicken and other poultry. This pyrethroid is employed extensively in Europe as a timber treatment against wood-boring beetles. In many parts of the world, it is used in healthcare products to eradicate head lice and mites responsible for scabies, as well as in homes and industrial settings to control ants and termites. Permethrin is highly toxic to fish and particularly to cats, as many cats died either after being given flea treatments with the pyrethroid intended for dogs or by coming in contact with dogs recently treated with it (Dymond and Swift, 2008; Linnett, 2008; Sutton *et al.*, 2007). U.S. EPA (2007b) has classified permethrin as a possible human carcinogen on the basis of two reproducible benign tumors (liver and lung) observed in mice along with equivocal evidence of carcinogenicity observed in rats. This classification is different from the decision made by IARC (1991, 2017a), which has not considered the pyrethroid as a potential human or animal carcinogen for lack of sufficient evidence.

Contrary to the common health effects seen from the naturally occurring pyrethrins, very few cases of allergic contact dermatitis have been reported for exposure to pyrethroids. The most documented adverse health effect from pyrethroids to humans appeared to be paresthesia (ATSDR, 2003; O'Malley, 2007). Unlike allergic contact dermatitis (which is evidenced by skin rash, itching, and sometimes blisters), paresthesia is an abnormal cutaneous sensation involving feelings of pins and needles on the exposed skin.

Among all insecticides used, pyrethroids are considered the least acutely toxic to mammals, in that they are applied at very low rates and are quickly detoxified by metabolic processes. Nonetheless, they are an excitatory nerve poison that still can cause convulsions and even death to animals when exposed to at sufficiently high doses for a long period. While the general scientific consensus is that most pyrethroids (and pyrethrins) are unlikely to be carcinogenic (e.g., ATSDR, 2003; IARC, 2017a), some are shown able to cause liver damage (e.g., Abdul-Hamid *et al.*, 2017) or capable of inducing unfavorable effects on the endocrine or the immunological system (ATSDR, 2003). Many pyrethroids are also found toxic to fish, other aquatic organisms, and birds.

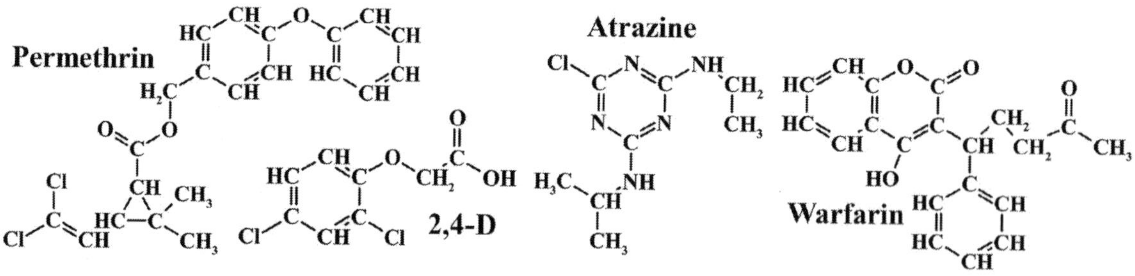

Figure 15.3. Chemical Structures of Four Select Pesticides, with One from Each of the Pyrethroid, Phenoxy, Triazine, and Coumarin Families

15.7. Major Phenoxy Pesticides

The number of chemical classes available in eliminating weeds or undesired plants is greater than those involved in controlling any other type of pests. Of all the herbicides available today, the *phenoxy* ($C_6H_5O^-$) compounds are among the most studied largely due to the environmental health concerns with their two prominent members, which are more commonly known by their acronyms 2,4-D (2,4-dichlorophenoxyacetic acid; $C_8H_6Cl_2O_3$) and 2,4,5-T (2,4,5-trichlorophenoxyacetic acid; $C_8H_5Cl_3O_3$). The structural difference between 2,4-D (Figure 15.3) and 2,4,5-T is only that the latter has an additional chlorine (and thereby 1 hydrogen fewer) attaching to its benzene ring in the number 5 position and accordingly is named 2,4,5-*trichloro*phenoxyacetic acid. Most phenoxy herbicides have some phytohormone or plant growth regulator properties as they all have some resemblance to the natural growth hormone indoleacetic acid ($C_{10}H_9NO_2$). All members in the indoleacetic acid class act by inducing rapid, uncontrolled growth of treated broadleaf weeds, ultimately killing them. Some less familiar representatives of phenoxy herbicides include MCPA (2-methyl-4-chlorophenoxyacetic acid), 2,4-DB (4-[2,4-dichlorophenoxy]-butyric acid), and Silvex (2-[2,4,5-trichlorophenoxy]-propionic acid).

15.7.1. Dichlorophenoxyacetic Acid (2,4-D)

2,4-D (dichlorophenoxyacetic acid) is one of the most widely used herbicides in the world, with approximately 40 million pounds being applied annually in the United States alone (U.S. EPA, 2005a, 2017). In non-agricultural settings, it is widely used on lawns, rangelands, and rights-of-way for control of unwanted broadleaf plants. In agriculture, it is used mainly in fields where cereal, grain, sugarcane, and other row crops are planted or to be planted. No alarming acute adverse effects to human or animal health have been associated with the use of 2,4-D (or most other phenoxy herbicides including 2,4,5-T). However, increased risks of amyotrophic lateral sclerosis and non-Hodgkin lymphoma have been linked to long-term exposure to 2,4-D. Accordingly, several phenoxy members including 2,4-D and 2,4,5-T have been listed as possible human (Group 2B) carcinogens (IARC, 1987, 2016, 2017a). Recently, 2,4-D (and 2,4,5-T to some extent) has become the subject of extended investigation for at least two subtle reasons.

One subtle reason is that both 2,4-D and 2,4,5-T were widely used as a mixture defoliant coded Agent Orange between 1962 and 1971 during the Vietnam War. During that war period, the U.S. military there sprayed millions of gallons of herbicides including mostly the defoliant mixture to remove leaves from trees that would otherwise provide camouflage cover for enemy forces. Following exposure to these herbicides, a number of U.S. Vietnam veterans subsequently reported to have suffered a number of diseases including chloracne, acute and subacute peripheral neuropathy, chronic lymphocytic leukemia, non-Hodgkin lymphoma, and prostate cancer (e.g., IOM, 2010). A government report estimated that for some 5 million Vietnamese exposed to Agent Orange, as many as 400,000 were later found to have disabilities or early death, along with some 500,000 babies born with certain birth defects (York and Mick, 2008). Some samples from Agent Orange production were later detected to contain measurable amounts of some forms of a highly toxic impurity known as 2,3,7,8-TCDD (2,3,7,8-tetrachlorodibenzo-*para*-dioxin, or dioxin for short). The environmental health impacts of 2,3,7,8-TCDD and the other dioxin congeners, along with other persistent organic pollutants, are discussed in the next chapter.

Another subtle reason for the extended investigation of 2,4-D is due to its widespread use on home lawns and golf courses. Owing to the increasing concern with children health, especially in the United States as evident from the passage of the FQPA in 1996, more attention is now given to assess the health risk for children playing on lawns treated with herbicides. Increased efforts also have been made to ensure that golfers are free from significant exposure to harmful pesticides since these clients are often charged a high fee for playing on a golf course which is repeatedly used by many players and is frequently treated with herbicides at high rates. Yet more importantly, herbicide contamination on golf courses can easily extend to the nearby groundwater through run-off and leaching.

15.7.2. Trichlorophenoxyacetic Acid (2,4,5-T)

The reality that 2,4,5-T was phased out completely in the United States by 1985 might serve as evidence that this herbicide was treated as more toxic and problematic than 2,4-D. In fact, it was 2,4,5-T and its salts or esters, not 2,4-D, that were among the substances restricted for international trade by the global treaty *Rotterdam Convention (on the Prior Informed Consent Procedure for Certain Hazardous Chemicals and Pesticides in International Trade)*, which entered into force in 2004. These cancellation and trade restriction actions likewise had the implication that the contamination of the Agent Orange defoliant by 2,3,7,8-TCDD was more likely from the production of 2,4,5-T than from that of 2,4-D.

The global use of 2,4,5-T was phased out or restricted not only due to its production tending to be contaminated with 2,3,7,8-TCDD, but also due to its potent teratogenicity found in mice at the time (Courtney *et al.*, 1970). Otherwise, much like its structural cousin 2,4-D, 2,4,5-T may not be considered to have high acute toxicity in mammals at low doses, despite the fact that IARC (1987, 2016, 2017a) has listed both herbicides as possible human (Group 2B) carcinogens.

15.8. Major Triazine Pesticides

Like the phenoxies, the triazine compounds are a widely known class of herbicides though with fewer members. Herbicides in this group recently have received increasing attention largely due to the heavy use and notoriety of its member atrazine ($C_8H_{14}ClN_5$; Figure 15.3). All triazines contain a "pseudo-benzene" ring nucleus, with three of the carbons in the benzene ring replaced with nitrogen (N) atoms (and hence with the prefix "tri" added to the part "azine" which refers to the nitrogen-containing ring). All triazines are strong inhibitors of photosynthesis at photosystem II site A, where they block the transport of electrons and light energy. Some less notorious triazine members are simazine, propazine, prometon, prometryn, ametryn, and terbutryne, with the first two being closer to atrazine in terms of chemical and toxicological properties. In fact, just a little over a decade ago, U.S. EPA (2006a) performed a cumulative risk assessment for atrazine, simazine, and propazine after reaching the decision that the three chlorinated triazines share a common mechanism of toxicity at issue.

15.8.1. Atrazine

Even though the use of atrazine is now prohibited in the European Union (EU) states (nations), it is one of the most heavily used herbicides in some 80 other nations including the United States. Between 70 and 80 million pounds of atrazine were applied in the United States in 2003 (U.S.

EPA, 2011), predominantly in cornfields. Recently, it has been the second most widely applied herbicide in the United States, only after glyphosate (Section 15.10.2), at around 70 million pounds per year (U.S. EPA, 2017). Its use remains controversial due to its adverse effects on non-target species, such as amphibians, and to its widespread contamination of waterways and drinking water supplies. Nonetheless, as noted in a U.S. EPA (2003) document, the total national economic impact in the United States would exceed $2 billion a year if atrazine were banned from use as a weed killer in corn and other row crop fields.

Atrazine was banned in the EU in 2004 not so much for the public's high concerns over its persistent groundwater contamination, but more so due to a number of significant findings on its adverse health effects. The herbicide has been alleged as a strong endocrine disruptor. While IARC (1999, 2017a) has not classified it as a potential human or animal carcinogen, studies (e.g., Fan *et al.*, 2007) showed that atrazine increased the risk of testicular cancer and the aromatase levels in animal cells. Aromatase is an enzyme that converts the male sex hormone testosterone to an estrogen; its excessive elevation thus can increase the risk of feminization in animals (e.g., fish, amphibians). As evidenced in a study conducted by Hayes *et al.* (2010), 4 of the 40 male tadpoles grown in test water tainted with atrazine at 2.5 ppb (parts per billion) became functionally female. Atrazine was also linked to low sperm counts in men. Findings of several epidemiological studies (e.g., Munger *et al.*, 1997; Ochoa-Acuña *et al.*, 2009) implicated that even when atrazine's water levels came to near the U.S. federal MCL (maximum contaminant level) of 3 ppb, they would still be harmful, with implications for birth defects or low birth weights in humans.

U.S. EPA (2003, 2006a) initially maintained that atrazine would pose no harm to the public including children, and would not adversely affect amphibian gonadal development. Yet a decade later, the agency drafted a reassessment for atrazine's environmental impacts, and now has largely concurred that the herbicide poses a potentially serious reproductive risk to mammals, frogs, birds, fishes, and many nontarget plants. The draft reassessment report (U.S. EPA, 2016) was released for public comments in 2016, and supposed to be followed shortly by a similar report specifically on atrazine's human health effects. In July 2016, California added atrazine, propazine, simazine, and their breakdown triazine products to the state's Proposition 65 list of chemicals known to cause reproductive toxicity.

15.8.2. Simazine and Propazine

Simazine ($C_7H_{12}ClN_5$) is predominately a pre-emergence herbicide applied to get rid of or otherwise control annual grasses and broadleaf weeds in soils where almonds, apples, avocados, corn, established Christmas trees, grapes, and other crops will be planted, and in non-cropped areas such as around buildings, lawns, and rights-of-way. One of simazine's major uses is in cornfields where it is frequently applied as a mixture with atrazine. Simazine is highly toxic if inhaled and slightly toxic via dermal contact. Some people who drank water that contained the herbicide exceeding the MCL of 4 ppb were found having problems with their blood (*U.S. CFR*, 2010). Skin rashes and dermatitis were observed in workers exposed to simazine (Stevens and Summer, 1991). Like its chemical cousin atrazine, simazine has not been classified as a potential human or animal carcinogen (IARC, 1999, 2017a).

Propazine ($C_9H_{16}ClN_5$), another chemical cousin of atrazine, is applied as a post-emergence selective systemic herbicide in fields where carrots, celery, and fennel are planted. It is also applied as a pre-emergence herbicide for control of broadleaf weeds and annual grasses but mostly in sweet sorghum fields. Propazine is less toxic to mammals compared to atrazine and simazine. There is evidence, though, linking the three triazines to neuroendocrine disruption (U.S. EPA, 2006b). U.S. EPA (1998) has classified propazine as a possible human (Group C) carcinogen on the basis of significant increases in mammary gland adenomas and carcinomas observed in female Sprague-Dawley rats. IARC (2017a), on the other hand, has not yet evaluated propazine's carcinogenicity to humans or animals.

15.9. Coumarin and Indandione Pesticides

Pesticides in these two classes are anticoagulants used to control rodent pests by inhibiting prothrombin formation, the process in blood responsible for clotting (Section 9.4.1). Vitamin K is commonly used as the choice of antidote for accidental poisoning caused by most anticoagulants belonging to these two classes. Anticoagulant poisoning is a major safety and health problem for young children in the United States. In 2014, around 8,500 nonpharmaceuticals-exposure cases were reported to various poison control centers across the nation. Of these cases, over 80% occurred in children younger than 6 years old (Mowry *et al.*, 2015). To protect American children from accidental ingestion of these anticoagulants, registered labels thus require that the treated baits be inaccessible to children or placed in a tamper-proof box. There are rodenticides (predatorcides) available without anticoagulant properties, such as bromethalin, thallium sulfate, DDT, red squill, strychnine, and zinc phosphide. Bromethalin is a new lethal rodenticide acting on the CNS by uncoupling of oxidative phosphorylation (as defined in Section 9.5.2F). Red squill is a substance of the glycoside family extracted from the bulb of the Mediterranean Sea plant *Urginea maritima*. Strychnine is a highly toxic alkaloid from the Asiatic tree *Strychnos nux vomica*.

15.9.1. Coumarins

Warfarin ($C_{19}H_{16}O_4$; named after the acronym WARF for the U.S. *W*isconsin *A*lumni *R*esearch *F*oundation; Figure 15.3) is the most successful of all known coumarin rodenticides as rats do not develop bait shyness to it. Other known coumarin rodenticides include coumachlor, coumafuryl, coumatetralyl, dicumarol, and the two newer members brodifacoum and bromadiolone. The structures of these rodenticides all bear the nucleus coumarin ($C_9H_6O_2$), which can be found in many plants and *per se* has no anticoagulation activity until after its transformation to the anticoagulant species by fungi or other means. Although coumarin has medical value, it is moderately toxic to the liver and kidneys. Rats and other rodents have the *extra* ability to oxidize coumarin to 3,4-coumarin epoxide, a metabolite that can cause internal hemorrhage in their body ultimately leading to their death.

15.9.2. Indandiones

This class or subgroup refers to all the synthetic anticoagulants derived from 1,3-indandione, which is an isomer of coumarin and therefore has the same molecular formula ($C_9H_6O_2$) as coumarin. The more prominent indandione anticoagulants include pindone, chlorophacinone, and diphacinone. The last two have the ability to uncouple (i.e., to otherwise inhibit) oxidative phosphorylation. This additional ability partially explains the success of the two phacinones as single-dose rodenticides capable of causing lethal neurological and cardiopulmonary injuries in the rat before hemorrhage can take place in its body. As of this time, neither of the two non-anticoagulant injuries mentioned above has been reportedly associated with human poisoning.

15.10. Select Novel/Specialty Pesticides

There are many more novel, loner, and specialty pesticides available in the market today than can be accounted for in this chapter. Only a very few of the more prominent and more intriguing are introduced in this section as a reminder that many more pesticides or pesticide classes are available than those covered in this chapter. Neonicotinoids are a class of newer insecticides worth introducing here because of their widespread applications and low toxicity to mammals. In this section, glyphosate, paraquat, and sodium (mono)fluoroacetate (a.k.a. Compound 1080) are treated as among the loner or specialty group, for lack of a better term. They are included here likewise due to their (current or once) widespread use, but more to their unique toxicological properties.

15.10.1. Neonicotinoids

The mode of pesticidal action of neonicotinoid compounds is similar to that of the natural insecticide nicotine contained in tobacco plants. They all act on the target insect's CNS by causing excitation of its nerves and eventually paralysis and then death. Because these substances bind at a different site referred to as the postsynaptic *nicotinic* acetylcholine receptor, they are not cross-resistant to the CB, OP, and pyrethroid insecticides. As a group, neonicotinoids are effective against sucking insects and the chewing kinds (e.g., beetles, some Lepidoptera, particularly cutworms). Owing to their more favorable (low) toxicological profiles, all neonicotinoids have been registered under U.S. EPA's Conventional Reduced Risk Program.

Imidacloprid ($C_9H_{10}ClN_5O_2$; Figure 15.4) was first marketed in the United States in 1992 and is currently the most widely employed insecticide in the neonicotinoid group. It has a long residual activity and is effective against a wide range of insects including sucking insects, whiteflies, turf insects, and Colorado potato beetle. It can be applied to a wide range of crops and sites such as soils, seeds, pets, field crops, vegetables, pome fruits, and pecans. U.S. EPA (2005b) has qualified the insecticide as a "Group E" (non)carcinogen (i.e., one with no evidence of carcinogenicity to humans or animals). In animals and humans, imidacloprid is quickly and almost completely absorbed from the GI tract and eliminated via urine and feces within 48 hours. Of all the neonicotinoids available, imidacloprid is the most toxic to birds and fishes. Both imidacloprid and another neonicotinoid named thiamethoxam are highly toxic to honeybees and have been linked to the abrupt disappearance of honeybee colonies across the United States, a phenomenon known as colony collapse disorder (a.k.a., honeybee depopulation syndrome) which is alleged to have (indirectly) jeopardized the production of many crops that rely on bees for pollination.

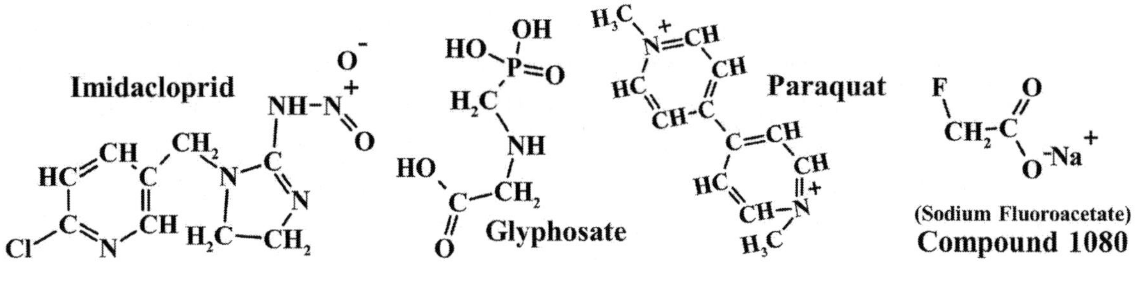

Figure 15.4. Chemical Structures of Four Select Novel/Specialty Pesticides

15.10.2. Glyphosate, Paraquat, and Compound 1080

Glyphosate ($C_3H_8NO_5P$; Figure 15.4) is the common name for N-(phosphonomethyl)-glycine, a nonselective systemic herbicide used to kill weeds, especially perennials. It is the most widely applied herbicide in the United States (US. EPA, 2017), with 200 to 250 million pounds being used each year in the agricultural market sector. Its most common applications include control of broadleaf weeds and grasses grown in areas or fields like hay or pasture, soybeans, cornfields, lawns, turf, rights-of-way, greenhouses, and forest plantings. Many American people are likely more familiar with glyphosate under its trade name Roundup®, which (as of this date) is readily available in stores where gardening equipment and products are sold. Like another herbicide named sulfosate, glyphosate acts by inhibiting the enzyme EPSP (5-*enolpyruvylshikimate*-3-*p*hosphate) synthase responsible for catalyzing the synthesis of the three aromatic amino acids phenylalanine, tryptophan, and tyrosine. The herbicide's use is limited to foliar applications as it will be rapidly and firmly bound to soil particles. Glyphosate, though having a Toxicity Category I (i.e., so classified due to being either severely irritating or highly toxic) for eye irritation, is rated least dangerous in comparison to other herbicides or pesticides. Nonetheless, an *in vitro* study (Benachour and Sralini, 2009) revealed that, even at low doses, various formulations of glyphosate and its metabolic products could induce apoptosis (routine programmed cell death, as briefly described in Chapter 18) as well as necrosis in the umbilical, embryonic, and placental cells.

Paraquat (the trade name of N,N'-dimethyl-4,4'-bipyridinium dichloride, $C_{12}H_{14}Cl_2N_2$; Figure 15.4) is a quaternary nitrogen herbicide widely applied in the United States and the world until recently overtaken by glyphosate. The herbicide is a potent, fast-acting, and nonselective photosynthesis inhibitor, killing green plant tissue on contact. It is highly toxic to humans when ingested, often leading to acute respiratory distress syndrome with no specific antidote. Even a single gulp can cause death from fibrous tissue developing in the human lungs, leading to asphyxiation. The exact mechanism by which paraquat damages the lungs remains unknown. After entering the body, even via the oral or dermal route, it will be distributed to all parts of the body including the liver, the kidneys, and particularly the lungs. Long-term exposure to paraquat can cause chronic pneumonitis. IARC (2017a) has not evaluated paraquat for its carcinogenicity to animals or humans. U.S. EPA (1997c), however, has qualified the herbicide as a Group E (non)carcinogen for lack of evidence of carcinogenicity observed in two animal studies.

Sodium (mono)fluoroacetate ($FCH_2CO_2^-Na^+$; Figure 15.4) occurs naturally as an antiherbivore metabolite in several species of Australian and African plants that have been implicated for the poisoning of livestock grazing on them (U.S. EPA, 1995). The compound, being applied mainly as a rodenticide, can also be produced as a derivative of fluoroacetic acid. This organofluorine derivative is known more commonly as Compound 1080, with the number reportedly coming from an invoice number that the material was assigned during its investigation in the U.S. government laboratories (U.S. EPA, 1995). Compound 1080 is particularly toxic to warm-blooded animals, including humans. Dogs and cats appear to be most susceptible to poisoning by (the Na^+-based) fluoroacetate, a substance similar to acetate ($CH_3CO_2^-$) which plays a key role in cellular metabolism. Fluoroacetate disrupts the Krebs cycle by combining with coenzyme A to form fluoroacetyl CoA which reacts with the enzyme citrate synthase to produce fluorocitrate (Figure 9.3). The resultant fluorocitrate is a lethal metabolite in that it will bind tightly to the enzyme aconitase, thereby halting all other chemical reactions in the Krebs cycle to deprive the affected cells of energy. Such a radical energy deprivation can lead to convulsions and death from respiratory arrest or cardiac failure. Many invertebrates (e.g., aphids, cockroaches, fleas, moths) are also thought to be susceptible to fluoroacetate poisoning (Notman, 1989).

For fear of Compound 1080's harm to humans and nontarget animals, U.S. Congress in 2012 at its 112th Session introduced a bill (assigned with the number H.R. 4214) to ban the substance's use in the nation. That bill, titled "Compound 1080 and Sodium Cyanide Elimination Act", did not receive enough votes from the Session to become law. Five years later, in March 2017 at its 115th Session (which is to end 3 January 2019), U.S. Congress introduced a new bill to ban the use of Compound 1080 again. The new bill (H.R. 1817) is titled "The Chemical Poisons Reduction Act of 2017". Historically, Compound 1080 was banned in 1972 by former President Nixon under pressure from environmentalists who challenged that the poison's use would also kill the endangered species such as grizzly bears and eagles. The 1972 ban lived through two further presidencies until the Reagan Administration, which in mid-July 1985 started permitting again Compound 1080's use in sheep and goat collars to kill coyotes being the predators of concern.

This very brief historical account presented above for Compound 1080 is intended to serve as a reminder that pesticides are indeed economic poisons. It can also be utilized to help explain why health risk assessment (Chapter 23) has a key place in environmental toxicology.

References

Abdul-Hamid M, Moustafa N, Abe Alla Astran MEA, Mowafy L, 2017. Cypermethrin-Induced Histopathological, Ultrastructural and Biochemical Changes in Liver of Albino Rats: The Protective Role of Propolis and Curcumin. *Beni-Suef Univ. J. Basic Appl. Sci.* 6:160-173.

ATSDR (U.S. Agency for Toxic Substances and Disease Registry), 1994. Toxicological Profile for Chlordane. U.S. Department of Health and Human Services, Atlanta, Georgia, USA.

ATSDR (U.S. Agency for Toxic Substances and Disease Registry), 2002a. Toxicological Profile for DDT, DDE, and DDD. U.S. Department of Health and Human Services, Atlanta, Georgia, USA.

ATSDR (U.S. Agency for Toxic Substances and Disease Registry), 2002b. Toxicological Profile for Aldrin/Dieldrin. U.S. Department of Health and Human Services, Atlanta, Georgia, USA.

ATSDR (U.S. Agency for Toxic Substances and Disease Registry), 2003. Toxicological Profile for Pyrethrins and Pyrethroids. U.S. Department of Health and Human Services, Atlanta, Georgia, USA.

ATSDR (U.S. Agency for Toxic Substances and Disease Registry), 2005. Toxicological Profile for Hexachlorocyclohexane. U.S. Department of Health and Human Services, Atlanta, Georgia, USA.

ATSDR (U.S. Agency for Toxic Substances and Disease Registry), 2008. Addendum to the Toxicological Profile for DDT, DDE, and DDD. U.S. Department of Health and Human Services, Atlanta, Georgia, USA.

ATSDR (U.S. Agency for Toxic Substances and Disease Registry), 2013. Addendum to the Toxicological Profile for Chlordane. U.S. Department of Health and Human Services, Atlanta, Georgia, USA.

ATSDR (U.S. Agency for Toxic Substances and Disease Registry), 2015. Toxicological Profile for Hexachlorobenzene. U.S. Department of Health and Human Services, Atlanta, Georgia, USA.

Benachour N, Séralini GE, 2009. Glyphosate Formulations Induce Apoptosis and Necrosis in Human Umbilical, Embryonic, and Placental Cells. *Chem. Res. Toxicol.* 22:97-105.

Carson LR, 1962. *Silent Spring*. Boston, Massachusetts, USA: Houghton Mifflin.

CDPR (California Department of Pesticide Regulation), 2017. Summary of Pesticide Use Report Data. Cal/EPA Department of Pesticide Regulation, Sacramento, California, USA, (data retrieved onsite/online, by year of pesticide use, on 16 May 2017).

Corbett JR, Wright K, Baillie RC, 1984. *The Biochemical Mode of Action of Pesticides*, 2nd Edition. London, UK: Academic Press.

Courtney KD, Gaylor DW, Hogan MD, Falk HL, Bates RR, Mitchell I, 1970. Teratogenic Evaluation of 2,4,5-T. *Science* 168:864-866.

Dymond NL, Swift IM, 2008. Permethrin Toxicity in Cats: A Retrospective Study of 20 Cases. *Aust. Vet. J.* 86:219-223.

Fan WQ, Yanase T, Morinaga H, Gondo S, Okabe T, Nomura M, Komatsu T, Morohashi K-I, Hayes TB, Takayanagi R, Nawata H, 2007. Atrazine-Induced Aromatase Expression Is SF-1 Dependent: Implications for Endocrine Disruption in Wildlife and Reproductive Cancers in Humans. *Environ. Health Perspect.* 115:720-727.

Grossman J, 1995. What's Hiding under the Sink: Dangers of Household Pesticides. *Environ. Health Perspect.* 103:550-554.

Hayden KM, Norton MC, Darcey D, Østbye T, Zandi PP, Breitner JCS, Welsh-Bohmer KA, 2010. Occupational Exposure to Pesticides Increases the Risk of Incident AD: The Cache County Study. *Neurology* 74:1524-1530.

Hayes TB, Khoury V, Narayan A, Nazir M, Park A, Brown T, Adame L, Chan E, Buchholz D, Stueve T, Gallipeau S, 2010. Atrazine Induces Complete Feminization and Chemical Castration in Male African Clawed Frogs (*Xenopus laevis*). *Proc. Natl. Acad. Sci. USA* 107:4612-4617.

Hodgson E, Mailman RB, Chambers JE (Eds.), 1998. *Dictionary of Toxicology*. New York, New York, USA: Grove's Dictionaries Inc.

IARC (International Agency for Research on Cancer), 1979. IARC Monographs on the Evaluation of Carcinogenic Risks to Humans, Volume 20: Some Halogenated Hydrocarbons. Lyon, France: WHO Press.

IARC (International Agency for Research on Cancer), 1987. IARC Monographs on the Evaluation of Carcinogenic Risks to Humans, Supplement 7: Overall Evaluations of Carcinogenicity – An Updating of IARC Monographs Volumes 1 to 42. Lyon, France: WHO Press.

IARC (International Agency for Research on Cancer), 1991. IARC Monographs on the Evaluation of Carcinogenic Risks to Humans, Volume 53: Occupational Exposures in Insecticide Application, and Some Pesticides. Lyon, France: WHO Press.

IARC (International Agency for Research on Cancer), 1999. IARC Monographs on the Evaluation of Carcinogenic Risks to Humans, Volume 73: Some Chemicals That Cause Tumours of the Kidney or Urinary Bladder in Rodents and Some Other Substances. Lyon, France: WHO Press.

IARC (International Agency for Research on Cancer), 2001. IARC Monographs on the Evaluation of Carcinogenic Risks to Humans, Volume 79: Some Thyrotropic Agents. Lyon, France: WHO Press.

IARC (International Agency for Research on Cancer), 2016. IARC Monographs on the Evaluation of Carcinogenic Risks to Humans, Volume 113: Some Organochlorine Insecticides and Some Chlorphenoxy Herbicides. Lyon, France: WHO Press.

IARC (International Agency for Research on Cancer), 2017a. IARC Monographs on the Evaluation of Carcinogenic Risks to Humans, Volumes 1-119: List of Carcinogens. Lyon, France: WHO Press.

IARC (International Agency for Research on Cancer), 2017b (*in preparation*). IARC Monographs on the Evaluation of Carcinogenic Risks to Humans, Volume 117: Pentachlorophenol and Some Related Compounds. Lyon, France: WHO Press.

IOM (U.S. Institute of Medicine), 2011. *Veterans and Agent Orange: Update 2010*. Washington DC, USA: The National Academies Press.

Jamal GA, 1997. Neurological Syndromes of Organophosphorus Compounds. *Adverse Drug React. Toxicol. Rev.* 6:133-170.

Johnson MK, 1975. Organophosphorus Esters Causing Delayed Neurotoxic Effects. Mechanism of Action and Structure/Activity Studies. *Arch. Toxicol.* 34:259-288.

Johnson MK, 1976. Mechanism of Protection against the Delayed Neurotoxic Effect of Organophosphorus Esters. *Fed. Proc.* 35:73-74.

Koldkjaer OG, Wermuth L, Bjerregaard P, 2004. Parkinson's Disease among Inuit in Greenland: Organochlorines as Risk Factors. *Intl. J. Circumpolar Health* 63(Suppl 2):366-368.

Linnett PJ, 2008. Permethrin Toxicosis in Cats. *Aust. Vet. J.* 86:32-35.

Mathur HB, Johnson S, Mishra R, Kumar A, Singh B, 2003. Analysis of Pesticide Residues in Bottled Water – Delhi Region. CSE/PML-6/2002. Centre for Science and Environment, 41, Tughtakabad Institutional Area, New Delhi, India.

Mowry JB, Spyker DA, Brooks DE, McMillan N, Schauben JL, 2015. 2014 Annual Report of the American Association of Poison Control Centers' National Poison Data System (NPDS): 32nd Annual Report. *Clin. Toxicol (Phila.).* 53:962-1147.

Munger R, Isacson P, Hu S, Burns T, Hanson J, Cherryholmes K, Van Dorpe P, Hausler WJ Jr, 1997. Intrauterine Growth Retardation in Iowa Communities with Herbicide-Contaminated Drinking Water Supplies. *Environ. Health Perspect.* 105:308-314.

Murray D, Wesseling C, Keifer M, Corriols M, Henao S, 2002. Surveillance of Pesticide-Related Illness in the Developing World: Putting the Data to Work. *J. Intl. Occ. Environ. Health* 8:243-248.

NEETF (The National Environmental Education & Training Foundation), 2002. Implementation Plan – National Strategies for Healthcare Providers: Pesticide Initiative. NEETF, 1707 H Street, NW, Suite 900, Washington DC, USA.

Notman P, 1989. A Review of Invertebrate Poisoning by Compound 1080. *N. Zeal. Entomologist* 2:67-71.

Ochoa-Acuña H, Frankenberger J, Hahn L, Carbajo C, 2009. Drinking-Water Herbicide Exposure in Indiana and Prevalence of Small-for-Gestational-Age and Preterm Delivery. *Environ. Health Perspect.* 117:1619-1624.

O'Malley M, 2007. Pesticides. In *Current Occupational and Environmental Medicine,* (Ladou J, Ed.), 4th Edition. New York, New York, USA: McGraw-Hill, Chapter 31.

Rauh VA, Garfinkel R, Perera FP, Andrews HF, Hoepner L, Barr DB, Whitehead R, Tang D, Whyatt RW, 2006. Impact of Prenatal Chlorpyrifos Exposure on Neurodevelopment in the First 3 Years of Life among Inner-City Children. *Pediatrics* 118:e1845-e1859 (online journal).

Reigart JR, Roberts JR (Eds.), 1999. Recognition and Management of Pesticide Poisonings, Fifth Edition. EPA #735-R-98-003. Office of Pesticide Programs, Washington DC, USA.

Stevens JT, Sumner DD, 1991. Herbicides. In *Handbook of Pesticide Toxicology* (Hayes WJ Jr, Laws ER Jr, Eds.), Volume 3. San Diego, California, USA: Academic Press, pp.1317-1408.

Sutton NM, Bates N, Campbell A, 2007. Clinical Effects and Outcome of Feline Permethrin Spot-On Poisonings Reported to the Veterinary Poisons Information Service (VPIS), London. *J. Feline Med. Surg.* 9: 335-339.

Tomlin C (Ed.), 2015. *The Pesticide Manual, a World Compendium: Incorporating the Agrochemicals Handbook*, 17th Edition. British Crop Protection Council, Bath, UK: The Bath Press.

Unger MA, Vadas GG, 2017. Kepone in the James River Estuary: Past, Current and Future Trends. Virginia Institute of Marine Science, College of William & Mary, Gloucester Point, Virginia, USA.

U.S. CFR (U.S. Code of Federal Regulations), 2010. Title 40 (Protection of Environment), Part 141 (National Primary Drinking Water Regulations), Appendix A to Subpart O of Part 141.

U.S. EPA (U.S. Environmental Protection Agency), 1975. A Review of Scientific and Economic Aspects of the Decision to Ban Its Use as a Pesticide. EPA-540/1-75-022. Office of Pesticide Programs, Washington DC, USA.

U.S. EPA (U.S. Environmental Protection Agency), 1987. Carcinogenicity Assessment of Aldrin and Dieldrin. EPA/600/6-87/006. Office of Health and Environmental Assessment, Washington DC, USA.

U.S. EPA (U.S. Environmental Protection Agency), 1995. Reregistration of Eligibility Decision (RED) – Sodium Fluoroacetate. EPA-738-R-95-025. Office of Prevention, Pesticides and Toxic Substances, Washington DC, USA.

U.S. EPA (U.S. Environmental Protection Agency), 1997a. Pesticides Industry Sales and Usage – 1994 and 1995 Market Estimates. EPA-733-R-97-002. Office of Prevention, Pesticides and Toxic Substances, Washington DC, USA.

U.S. EPA (U.S. Environmental Protection Agency), 1997b. Reregistration of Eligibility Decision (RED) – Propoxur. EPA-738-F-97-009. Office of Prevention, Pesticides and Toxic Substances, Washington DC, USA.

U.S. EPA (U.S. Environmental Protection Agency), 1997c. Reregistration of Eligibility Decision (RED) – Paraquat Dichloride. EPA-738-F-96-018. Office of Prevention, Pesticides and Toxic Substances, Washington DC, USA.

U.S. EPA (U.S. Environmental Protection Agency), 1998. Pesticide Fact Sheet – Propazine. Office of Prevention, Pesticides and Toxic Substances, Washington DC, USA.

U.S. EPA (U.S. Environmental Protection Agency), 1999. Pesticides Industry Sales and Usage – 1996 and 1997 Market Estimates. EPA-733-R-99-001. Office of Prevention, Pesticides and Toxic Substances, Washington DC, USA.

U.S. EPA (U.S. Environmental Protection Agency), 2000. Pesticide Fact Sheet – Indoxacarb. Office of Prevention, Pesticides and Toxic Substances, Washington DC, USA.

U.S. EPA (U.S. Environmental Protection Agency), 2002. Pesticides Industry Sales and Usage – 1998 and 1999 Market Estimates. EPA-733-R-02-001. Office of Prevention, Pesticides and Toxic Substances, Washington DC, USA.

U.S. EPA (U.S. Environmental Protection Agency), 2003. Interim Reregistration of Eligibility Decision (IRED) for Atrazine. Office of Prevention, Pesticides and Toxic Substances, Washington DC, USA.

U.S. EPA (U.S. Environmental Protection Agency), 2004a. Pesticides Industry Sales and Usage – 2000 and 2001 Market Estimates. EPA-733-R-04-001. Office of Prevention, Pesticides and Toxic Substances, Washington DC, USA.

U.S. EPA (U.S. Environmental Protection Agency), 2004b. Carbaryl IRED Facts [Revised 10/22/04]. Office of Prevention, Pesticides and Toxic Substances, Washington DC, USA.

U.S. EPA (U.S. Environmental Protection Agency), 2005a. Reregistration of Eligibility Decision (RED) for 2,4-D. EPA-738-R05-002. Office of Prevention, Pesticides and Toxic Substances, Washington DC, USA.

U.S. EPA (U.S. Environmental Protection Agency), 2005b. Imidacloprid; Pesticide Tolerances for Emergency Exemptions. *Federal Register* 70:59268-59276.

U.S. EPA (U.S. Environmental Protection Agency), 2006a. Cumulative Risk from Triazine Pesticides. Office of Prevention, Pesticides and Toxic Substances, Washington DC, USA.

U.S. EPA (U.S. Environmental Protection Agency), 2006b. Report of the Food Quality Protection Act (FQPA) Tolerance Reassessment Progress and Risk Management Decision (TRED) for Propazine. EPA-738-R-06-009. Office of Prevention, Pesticides and Toxic Substances, Washington DC, USA.

U.S. EPA (U.S. Environmental Protection Agency), 2007a. Reregistration of Eligibility Decision (RED) for Carbaryl. EPA-738-R07-018. Office of Prevention, Pesticides and Toxic Substances, Washington DC, USA.

U.S. EPA (U.S. Environmental Protection Agency), 2007b. Permethrin Facts. EPA-738-F-09-001. Office of Prevention, Pesticides and Toxic Substances, Washington DC, USA.

U.S. EPA (U.S. Environmental Protection Agency), 2011. Pesticides Industry Sales and Usage – 2006 and 2007 Market Estimates. Office of Chemical and Pollution Prevention, Washington DC, USA.

U.S. EPA (U.S. Environmental Protection Agency), 2016. Atrazine, Simazine, and Propazine Registration Review; Draft Ecological Risk Assessments; Notice of Availability. *Federal Register* 81:36301-36303.

U.S. EPA (U.S. Environmental Protection Agency), 2017. Pesticides Industry Sales and Usage – 2008-2012 Market Estimates. Office of Chemical and Pollution Prevention, Washington DC, USA.

Ware GW, Whitacre DM, 2004. *The Pesticide Book*, 6th Edition. Willoughby, Ohio, USA: MeisterPro Information Resources.

WHO (World Health Organization), 1990. Public Health Impact of Pesticides Used in Agriculture, WHO in Collaboration with UN Environment Programme, Geneva, Switzerland.

WHO (World Health Organization), 2009. WHO Specifications and Evaluations for Public Health Pesticides: Pyrethrum (Pyrethrins). Evaluation Report 32/2009. Geneva, Switzerland.

Yadav SS, Singh MK, Yadav RS, 2016. Organophosphates Induced Alzheimer's Disease: An Epigenetic Aspect. *J. Clin. Epigenet.* 2:1 (online journal).

Yan D, Zhang Y, Liu L, Yan H, 2016. Pesticide Exposure and Risk of Alzheimer's Disease: A Systematic Review and Meta-Analysis. *Sci. Rept.* 6:32222 (online journal).

York G, Mick H, 2008. 'Last Ghost' of the Vietnam War. *The Globe & Mail*, 12 July.

Yu J, Zhu H, Bhat A, El-Sayed H, Gudz T, Gattoni-Celli S, Kindy MS, 2015. Influence of Chlorpyrifos Oxon on the Development and Progression of Alzheimer's Disease in Amyloid Precursor Protein Transgenic Mice. *Neuroimmunol. Neuroinflammation* 2:31-42 (online journal).

Review Questions
1. Define the terms *pest, pesticide*, and *pesticide residues* (as used in this chapter).
2. What is the regulatory mandate of the U.S. Food Quality Protection Act of 1996 to U.S. EPA regarding pesticide risk assessment in the United States?
3. What are (likely) the annual estimates of pesticide usage in the United States and the world?
4. Name four chemical families of pesticides used predominantly or exclusively as insecticides.
5. How many cases of *non*-suicidal, acute severe type pesticide poisoning were estimated to occur around the world each year during the early 1990s?
6. Which member in the organochlorines is the most notorious pesticide in the world? Briefly describe its mode of pesticidal action.
7. Briefly describe the mode of pesticidal action of the chlorinated *cyclodiene* insecticides.
8. Which organochlorine pesticide was associated with the James River pollution in the United States?
9. Which HCH (hexachlorocyclohexane) isomer has been applied not only to protect crop seeds against pests, but also as an active ingredient in shampoos medicated for control of head lice and scabies?
10. What are the common signs and symptoms of *acute* OP (organophosphate) poisoning? Name the OP compound responsible for the Jake leg episode occurring in the United States in 1930.
11. What is the mechanism of insecticidal action of carbamates? And how does this mechanism differ from that of OP insecticides?
12. What are the most documented health effects of pyrethrins, and of pyrethroids? And what are the Type I and Type II symptoms from significant exposure to pyrethroids?
13. Which of the pyrethroids is regarded as the most widely applied insecticide worldwide?
14. What are the subtle reasons for which 2,4-D (and 2,4,5-T to some extent) has recently become the subject of extended investigation?
15. What are some of the potential health effects of atrazine? Briefly explain why, as of today, the herbicide has not been banned from use in cornfields in the United States.
16. What is commonly employed as the antidote for accidental poisoning by coumarin and indandione rodenticides? And briefly explain why or how it can be used biochemically as the antidote.
17. Briefly describe the mode of pesticidal action and toxicity of neonicotinoids.
18. Briefly describe the use and toxicity of the three loner or specialty pesticides covered in this chapter.

CHAPTER 16

Persistent Toxic Substances

16.1. Introduction

For environmental toxicologists, the term *persistent toxic substances* (*PTS*) refers to toxic materials that each have an alarming degradation half-life in a specific environmental medium (e.g., air, water, soils, sediments). These toxic substances collectively represent a huge group of environmental pollutants. Half-life, conventionally denoted by $t_{1/2}$, refers to the time t required for the quantity or concentration of a substance in a medium to diminish to half of its original value and thereby is medium-specific. Various health authorities over the world have adopted numerical persistence criteria for what constitutes an alarming half-life in each of the common environmental media. These criteria are highlighted in Section 16.1.2, following the clarification given below for chemical *vs.* environmental persistence.

16.1.1. Chemical *vs.* Environmental Persistence

Bioaccumulation of persistent toxicants is an environmental phenomenon discussed extensively in Chapter 6. It results in an increase of a pollutant's concentration in a biological organism's tissues that exceeds what is normally expected. On the other hand, a pollutant's persistence in an environmental medium is a measure, or at least a reflection, of its susceptibility to loss or degradation in that medium. In other words, the pollutant's persistence, along with its bioaccumulation potential in the (an) environment, is what makes it ultimately available for environmental exposure. Therefore, parallel to bioaccumulation, persistence is a component more crucial than toxicity in the health risk or ecological impact assessment for environmental toxicants. Underlying this notion is the assertion that a substance's toxicity tends to be more static in nature, whereas in general environmental exposure to the substance is a more dynamic event.

There are two major aspects or quantities of persistence for each substance present in the environment. The first is about its intrinsic chemical persistence and the other, concerning its persistence in the environment. By definition, chemical persistence refers to a substance's ability to remain unchanged in its natural physicochemical state as well as in its chemical composition over time. This ability is nonetheless still influenced considerably by the immediate environmental conditions in which the substance is present.

In contrast, environmental persistence is a term as well as a concept used to imply a constant quantity of a substance in an environmental medium. It can be argued that even an extremely persistent substance would pose no threat of environmental exposure if it were kept at all the time inside a well-sealed, well-insulated, and highly durable container. By convention, a substance's environmental persistence is expressed in terms of its (degradation) half-life in the environmental medium at issue. The use of such a half-life implies first-order kinetics behavior in chemical concentration, a concept borrowed from radioactive decay. One problem with such a simple definition is that many pollutants are present concurrently in more than one environmental medium.

16.1.2. Numerical Persistence Criteria

The numerical criteria used for identifying or qualifying a substance as alarmingly persistent in the environment vary somewhat among health (regulatory) entities in the western countries. As shown in Table 16.1 below, the Canadian Environmental Protection Act of 1999 (CEPA, 2000) considers a substance to be persistent when its half-life in air is more than 2 days (or when it is subject to atmospheric transport from its source to a remote region), *or* when its half-life in water or soils exceeds 180 days, *or* when its half-life in sediments exceeds 364 days.

Table 16.1. Numerical Screening Criteria for Qualifying (Toxic) Substances as Persistent and Bioaccumulative Pollutants in the Environment

Authority[a]	Persistence Half-Life in Days[b]				Bioaccumulativity[c]	
	Air	*Water*	*Soils*	*Sediments*	*BCF(BAF)*	*Log K_{ow}*
UNEP	>2	>60	>180	>180	5,000	5
UNECE	>2	>60	>180	>180	5,000	5
Canada CEPA	>2	>180	>180	>180	5,000	5
U.K. DEFRA	>2	>180	>180	>180	5,000	5
ECHA/European Commission	–	>40 (f) >60 (m)	>120	>120 (f) >180 (m)	2,000	–
U.S. EPA	>2	>60	>60	>60	1,000	–

[a]UNEP (United Nations Environment Programme, 2001); UNECE (United Nations Economic Commission for Europe, 2004); CEPA (Canadian Environmental Protection Act of 1999, 2000); U.K. DEFRA (United Kingdom Department for Environmental, Food, & Rural Affairs, 2002); European Commission (2003); ECHA (European Chemicals Agency, 2016); U.S. EPA (U.S. Environmental Protection Agency, 1999a, 1999b).
[b]synonymous with *degradation* half-life; f ≡ fresh (water); m ≡ marine (water).
[c]BAF (≡ bio*accumulation* factor) ≈ BCF (≡ bio*concentration* factor); K_{ow} ≡ octanol-*water* partition coefficient (*see* Chapter 6 for discussion on estimation of BCF with this partition coefficient).

The United Kingdom government (U.K. DEFRA, 2002) likewise has adopted a similar set of numerical criteria for qualifying toxic materials as PTS. In contrast, the numerical criteria adopted by U.S. EPA (1999a, 1999b) are somewhat more health conservative (Table 16.1). Other nations outside of the western continents tend to follow the criteria set forth by the European Commission. What is certain today is that many health regulatory authorities focus more on water, sediments, and soils, than on air as the environmental medium of concern. Such a bias is not surprising in that atmospheric compartments *per se* are less likely an ideal *direct* environment for either long-term bioaccumulation or long-range transport for most pollutants unless when some grasshopper effect is involved (Chapter 5). Recently, the European Chemicals Agency (ECHA, 2016) has proposed a set of higher numerical persistence and bioaccumulation criteria for substances that the European agency recommends to be treated and regulated as *very* persistent and *very* bioaccumulative. In particular, the ECHA's recent proposal defines that a substance fulfills the *very persistent* criterion if its half-life in soils or sediments is (significantly) longer than 180 days.

16.1.3. Relevance to Long-Range Transport

The issues on bioaccumulation and environmental persistence are closely related to the concern on long-range transport (LRT) of contaminants. Over the years, a number of scholars have shown specific concerns regarding the occurrence of certain pesticides and industrial chemicals in the Arctic. As Matthies and Scheringer (2001) put it, *"These substances have never been emitted in such regions and, thus, must have been transported over long distances from moderate or even tropical climatic zones."*

Both the importance and the relevance of such concerns are on the international level, as evidenced from the once well-publicized workshop held by the International Joint Commission (IJC, 2003) addressing the LRT of toxic substances into and out of the Great Lakes basin. A more recent evidence is the ongoing pledges and numerous efforts made by member states of the 1979 Convention on Long-Range Transboundary Air Pollution (CLRTAP), including notably their scientific assessment of the member region's air pollution trends between 1990 and 2012 (Maas and Grennfelt, 2016). CLRTAP is a treaty entered into force in 1983 by member states within the United Nations Economic Commission for Europe (UNECE) system, with the aim to gradually reduce current air pollution including certainly the long-range transboundary kind. Note that the UNECE system's member states include not only the European nations, but also some countries in North America, Central Asia, and Western Asia.

It is also important to note that contrary to the classic belief, the mode of LRT is no longer restricted to atmospheric. There have been ample data (e.g., AMAP, 1997) showing that nuclear wastes and certain persistent organic pollutants (POPs) can be transported in ocean currents over long distances, such as from reprocessing plants in Europe to the Arctic Ocean. Moreover, as discussed in Chapter 6 on bioaccumulation, at least one case study (Ewald *et al.* 1998) revealed the Pacific salmon's capability of transporting polychlorinated biphenyls (PCBs) and other POPs over a long distance from the ocean back to their spawning lakes. Several other studies also pointed out that with the aid of storms or cyclone activities, even soil dust particles emitted from the Chinese and Mongolian arid regions could be transported over the North Pacific Ocean to as far away as North America (e.g., Takemura *et al.*, 2002; Uno *et al.*, 2009).

16.2. The Stockholm Convention of 2001

Many PTS, including all of those under special global scrutiny, tend to bioaccumulate in living organisms. This explains why PTS are frequently treated loosely as synonymous with the group of environmental contaminants termed *persistent, bioaccumulative, and toxic substances* (PBTs). To date, the PTS or PBTs of global high health concerns have been predominately those termed *persistent organic pollutants* (POPs), the chemical group that has received increasing global attention and scrutiny since the adoption of the international treaty *Stockholm Convention on POPs* in 2001.

Section 16.2.1 below provides a brief account of the Convention's current action (priority) list of POPs as of 2017, followed by Section 16.2.2 highlighting its specific actions and strategies aiming to contain (the pollution of) these POPs in the global environment.

16.2.1. Persistent Pollutants of Global Concerns

From the brief discussion given in Section 16.1.3 on LRT potential for PTS, it is apparent that global efforts are required in order to minimize the presence and the distribution of these pollutants in the global environment. This kind of efforts requires global consensus, which is never an easy task due to the complex political issues involved and the limited resources available across nations. Yet some efforts of such have been proven successful by the United Nations Environment Programme (UNEP), when delegates from 127 nations in May 2001 approved the convention on POPs held in Stockholm, Sweden. As anticipated, the approval underwent a rather lengthy process involving a great deal of negotiations as well as disputes over numerous diverse economic interests and political concerns.

By law, a global agreement must be ratified by 50 nations or more in order for it to become an international treaty. Accordingly, following the approval of the agreement at the Convention, the parties needed to obtain the required ratification from their own governments, a task expected to take a couple of years or longer to accomplish. In the United States, for instance, the agreement was not (ready to be) submitted by then President George W. Bush to the U.S. Senate for ratification until a year later. In any event, soon as the treaty finally entered into force in 2004, it banned outright the use of eight organochlorine (OC) pesticides (aldrin, chlordane, dieldrin, endrin, heptachlor, hexachlorobenzene, mirex, and toxaphene). The Convention has since taken various initiatives to restrict the distribution of DDT, PCBs, as well as the unintentional by-products PCDDs (polychlorinated dibenzo-*para*-dioxins) and PCDFs (polychlorinated dibenzofurans), all of which are also OC substances. This initial group is often referred to as *the dirty dozen*.

By May 2015 (also as of 2017), the amendments to the Stockholm Convention has included 15 new POPs on its approved list either for their elimination or for restriction of their use. For simplicity, these 15 additional POPs are counted off here under six convenient groups as follows: (1) *seven* pesticide-related OC substances, including pentachlorobenzene (PeCB), pentachlorophenol (plus its esters and salts), technical endosulfan (plus its isomers), chlordecone (a.k.a. Kepone being its trade name), as well as three (α-, β-, γ-) isomers of hexachlorocyclohexane (HCH); (2) *two* brominated flame retardants named *hexa*brominated biphenyl (*hexa*BB) and *hexa*bromocyclododecane (HBCD); (3) *two* commercial-based polybrominated diphenyl ethers (PBDEs) named *penta*- and *octa*-brominated diphenyl ether (commercial-based *penta*BDE and *octa*BDE, respectively); (4) *two* perfluorinated compounds named perfluorooctane sulfonyl fluoride (PFOS-F) and perfluorooctane sulfonic acid (PFOS) plus its salts; (5) *one* polychlorinated aliphatic compound named *hexa*chlorobutadiene (HCBD); and (6) *nearly the entire group* of polychlorinated naphthalenes (PCNs), which has 75 theoretically possible congeners.

Most of the OC pesticides on the Convention's current action (i.e., priority) list are described in some detail in Chapter 15 or elsewhere (e.g., pentachlorophenol in Section 5.3). Overviews of the "non-pesticide" POPs, old or new, are given in their own chemical group sections following a brief account of the Convention's programs and strategies adopted to contain the listed POPs in the global environment. The individual overviews are each to start off at the chemical group level in an effort to provide further background and hence better appreciation for the global concerns now in place with the particular pollutant(s) in the group. The chemical groups of the listed POPs that are not intended for use as pesticides are: PFOS/PFOS-F (*perfluorooctane sulfonates/sulfonyl fluoride*); PBBs (*polybrominated biphenyls*); PBDEs (*polybrominated diphenyl ethers*); PBCDs (*polybromi-nated cyclododecanes*); PCBs (*polychlorinated biphenyls*); PCBDs (*polychlorinated butadienes*); PCNs (*polychlorinated naphthalenes*); and PCDDs/PCDFs (*polychlorinated dibenzo-p(ara)-dioxins/polychlorinated dibenzofurans*).

16.2.2. Stockholm Convention's Aims and Actions

The Stockholm Convention is a global treaty with aims to protect human health and the environment from pollution of POPs, of which many are considered carcinogenic, tending to disrupt the endocrine system, or capable of suppressing the immunological system in humans and wildlife. The Convention's practical actions and programs dealing with the POPs on its priority list include, where applicable as by party consensus, the agenda of: planning, coordinating, and implementing the reduction or elimination of the POPs' releases from intentional as well as unintentional production and from stockpiles or wastes. The Convention has the additional obligation and commitment of reducing the POPs' environmental levels over time.

According to the treaty, once any of the POPs becomes a waste, all parties to the Convention are obligated to develop and implement appropriate strategies for identifying stockpiles and articles in use that contain or are contaminated by the pollutant. The parties must manage the stockpiles and wastes in an environmentally sound manner to the extent that the POP's content is eliminated or irreversibly transformed. The parties must also set up strategies for identifying contaminated sites and perform eventual remediation in an environmentally sound manner.

Another international treaty named *The Basel Convention (on the Control of Transboundary Movements of Hazardous Wastes and Their Disposal)* has developed the technical guidelines on waste management for POPs and other hazardous wastes. The Basel Convention, which went into force in 1992, is regarded as the most comprehensive global environmental agreement on hazardous and other wastes. Under these guidelines as part of the cooperative agreement, the Stockholm Convention is responsible for setting levels of destruction and irreversible transformation necessary to ensure the absence of any POP's characteristics.

The Stockholm Convention has another important responsibility of coordinating as well as implementing the Global Monitoring Plan (GMP) to deal with POPs on the action list. Each party to the Convention is, by geographic location, grouped into one of the five regions: Africa; Asia and the Pacific; Central and Eastern Europe; Latin America and the Caribbean; and Western Europe and Others. As part of the treaty, parties from the five regions are required to prepare their own plan on how they will implement their obligations under the agreement and to make efforts in putting their own plan into operation. The GMP thereby represents and requires a collective effort, as its aims are to offer the regions a harmonized organizational framework for collection of comparable monitoring data on the POP levels that are being (or will be) measured in four designated core matrices, which are air, human break milk, human blood, and water. These regional monitoring data are intended for use to identify changes in the POP levels over time, as well as to provide information on the regional and global environmental transport of POPs. The GMP is therefore a key component of the evaluation on the treaty's own effectiveness and success in reducing the pollution of POPs and hence the adverse effects of POPs to humans and the environment.

The first regional monitoring reports for effectiveness evaluation on the treaty were presented to and endorsed by the Conference of the Parties (COPs) at its fourth meeting in May 2009, and served as a baseline for subsequent evaluations. The second regional reports, for which all regional monitoring data were supposedly due by October 2010, were endorsed at the COPs' seventh meeting in May 2015. This second set of regional reports provided some informative changes in concentrations of the POPs placed on the Convention's initial list, as well as the baseline information for the POPs later added to the list.

16.3. Perfluorooctane Sulfonates/Sulfonyl Fluoride

Perfluorooctane sulfonates are each a fully fluorinated anion and thus a member of perfluoroalkyls (which are also broadly referred to as perfluorinated compounds). When the oxygen ion (O^-) in the anion (Figure 16.1) is bonded to a hydrogen (H) atom, the fluorinated sulfonate is called perfluorooctane sulfonic acid (PFOS). PFOS is commonly referred to as *the* perfluorinated sulfonate. Therefore, when the O^- ion in the fluorinated anion is bonded to (i.e., conjugated with) a salt or an ester, the resultant fluorinated sulfonate is often treated as the salt or ester of PFOS or as a PFOS-based compound. Perfluorooctane sulfonyl fluoride (PFOS-F), on the other hand, is not a sulfonate as it possesses the sulfonyl fluoride ($-SO_2-F$) unit in lieu of the $-SO_3^-$ (Figure 16.1). Unlike PFOS, PFOS-F is comparatively not highly persistent in the environment. However, PFOS-F is also put on the Stockholm Convention's action list largely because the substance is used to produce and can be easily degraded to form PFOS. That is, PFOS (and most any other perfluorinated sulfonate compound) is the main derivative of PFOS-F. Note that the fluorinated sulfonates and PFOS-F (as well as PCBDs to be discussed later) are not family members of the polyhalogenated *aromatic* hydrocarbons (commonly known by the acronym PHAHs), as they do not contain any *benzene* ring.

16.3.1. Characteristics, Uses, and Pollution Sources

Owing to its ability to lower the surface tension of water and some other liquids to allow easier spreading, PFOS (perfluorooctane sulfonic acid) is used in a wide variety of applications such as its inclusion as a key component in surfactants, lubricants, food packaging, floor polishes, leather products, paper or textile coating, and fire retardant foams. This fluorosurfactant is also e in large quantities in the photographic and photolithographic industries (as a component in aqueous film forming foam) as well as in the aviation industry (as a component in hydraulic fluids). Much more so than the other groups of POPs discussed below, PFOS is an extremely stable substance in both industrial applications and the environment, mainly owing to the chemical effects of its aggregate

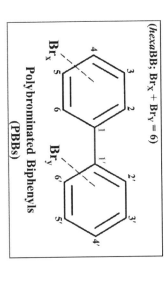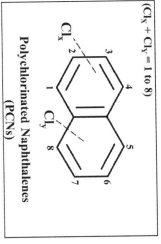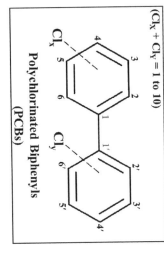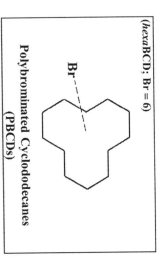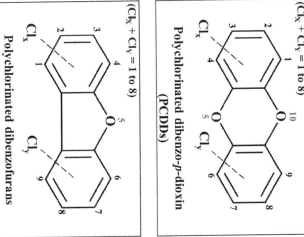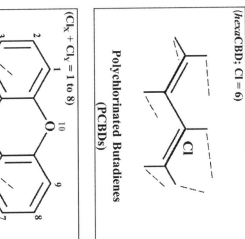

Figure 16.1. General Chemical Structures of Non-Pesticide Persistent Organic Pollutants on the Stockholm Convention's Action List (as of 2017)

strong fluorine-carbon bonds. PFOS was once the active ingredient in numerous stain repellents including the Scotchgard® fabric protector made by 3M Company in the United States.

The environmental fate of PFOS, as well as its toxicity to humans and wildlife, has been reviewed by several health authorities including Health Canada (2006), UNEP (2006a), and U.S. EPA (2016a, 2016b). These reviews collectively point out that, along with perfluoro*octanoic* acid (PFOA), PFOS is among the most common contaminants found in foods and water. PFOA is also a synthetic, highly persistent perfluoroalkyl. It structurally differs from PFOS only in having a carboxylic acid (COOH) unit instead of sulfonic acid (SO_3H). PFOS has been detected worldwide in wildlife such as bald eagle (in mid-western region of the United States), common dolphin (in Mediterranean Sea, Italy), harbor seal (in Wadden Sea, Denmark), and carrion crow (in Tokyo Bay, Japan). In some of these wildlife, the PFOS levels detected in the liver, egg, serum, kidney, and plasma samples were found high enough to cause human health concerns.

The fluorinated sulfonate persists in both the human body and the environment. The anion has not shown any degradation from hydrolysis, photolysis, or biodegradation tested under any environmental condition. The only known condition whereby PFOS can be degraded is via incineration at a very high temperature. The fluorosurfactant fulfills the criteria for bioaccumulation on the basis of its significantly higher concentrations observed in predators on higher trophic levels (e.g., polar bears, seals, minks) than in predators on lower trophic levels.

Unlike the other POPs discussed below, PFOS has a unique bioaccumulation property in that it binds to tissue proteins, instead of accumulating in fatty tissues. Like most other fluorocarbons, the longer C_8F_{17} subunit in PFOS is both hydrophobic and lipophobic, with its shorter sulfonate subunit tending to increase water solubility. PFOS meets the criteria for having the potential of atmospheric LRT. This is evident from monitoring data showing high levels of PFOS found in various remote parts of the northern hemisphere.

16.3.2. Environmental Health Concerns

PFOS (perfluorooctane sulfonic acid) fulfills the general criteria for being a toxic substance (e.g., Health Canada, 2006; UNEP, 2006a; U.S. EPA, 2016b). It displayed toxicity on mammals in subchronic studies. It also showed maternal toxicity with mortality of pups occurring shortly after birth. The fluorinated sulfonate is especially toxic to aquatic organisms, with the lowest no observed effect concentration of 0.25 mg/L being detected in small shrimp-like creatures.

Epidemiological surveys revealed that on average the PFOS serum level was 1,300 ppb (parts per billion) for American workers in certain occupational settings (Olsen *et al.*, 2003), whereas a small segment in the U.S. general population had over 90 ppb (Calafat *et al.*, 2007). On the other hand, a mouse study (Peden-Adams *et al.*, 2008) showed that the PFOS observed in males at serum level of ~90 ppb affected their immunological system, thus raising the concern that highly exposed people are being immunocompromised. In addition, in a study (Peden-Adams *et al.*, 2009) where chicken eggs were dosed with PFOS at 1 mg/kg (ppm) of egg weight, some eggs developed into chickens with serum PFOS at 150 ng/g (ppb) or higher. Effects such as brain asymmetry and decreased immunoglobulin levels were observed in some of those chickens. As of 2017, the World Health Organization's (WHO's) International Agency for Research on Cancer (IARC, 2017) has not classified PFOS or PFOS-F as a potential human or animal carcinogen, but (IARC, 2016a) has listed PFOA as a possible human (Group 2B) carcinogen.

The voluntary phase-out of PFOS production by 3M Company has led to a substantial reduction in the production and hence use of PFOS-related substances. Yet it is likely that the fluorosurfactant is still being actively produced or used in some other nations (e.g., China), inasmuch as the Stockholm Convention has data showing that some other nations continue to detect alarming amounts of PFOS in their environment. Given that PFOS-related substances can be transported in the atmosphere to regions far away from their emission sources, measures taken by single or a few nations are not sufficient or effective to abate the pollution caused by these persistent substances. The Convention hence decided to take regional actions against PFOS, its salts, as well as PFOS-F, and in May 2009 added these substances to the action (priority) list.

16.4. Polybrominated Biphenyls

Polybrominated biphenyls (PBBs), sometimes referred to as poly*bromo*biphenyls, are a family of structurally highly similar brominated hydrocarbons (HCs) with 2 to 10 bromine (Br) atoms attaching to the biphenyl ($C_{12}H_{10}$) nucleus. For completeness, the *mono*brominated homolog as well as its congeners (i.e., those with a single Br atom attaching to the biphenyl) are generally included when characterizing the PBBs. The biphenyl core molecule is simply the bulk portion of the PBB structure without the attachment of any Br atom. Note that the general chemical structure of PBBs depicted in Figure 16.1 can be used to represent any congener of any homolog in the family, simply by designating the desired number of Br atoms to the core molecule by allowing the *sum* of the x and the y number of Br atoms to be between 1 and 10. The sum is thereby *six* for *hexa*brominated biphenyl (*hexa*BB or HBB for short), which is currently the only homolog in the PBB family that has been added to the Stockholm Convention's action list.

From the general structure depicted in Figure 16.1, and with some computation, it can be seen that up to 209 compounds (including the *mono*brominated) are theoretically possible as congeners of the PBB family. Considering the *number* of bromine substituents alone (i.e., regardless of their positions), there are 10 homologous subgroups (i.e., homologs) of PBBs in total, ranging from *mono*- to *deca*-brominated. The *mono*-, *di*-, *tri*-, *tetra*-, *penta*-, *hexa*-, *hepta*-, *octa*-, *nona*-, and *deca*-homologs each can have 3, 12, 24, 42, 46, 42, 24, 12, 3, and 1 possible stereoisomer(s), respectively, thus yielding in total 209 possible congeners (or, less technically, members).

Following the numbering scheme illustrated in Table 16.2, which also reveals the possible sites for halogenation (i.e., for attaching the Br), each of the 209 possible congeners can be identified with a unique number from 1 to 209. The 209 possible PBB congeners are different from one another only in the number of Br atoms as well as in their positions on the biphenyl nucleus. There are no known natural sources for any of these PBB congeners. And the number of these congeners found in commercial PBB mixtures is much smaller than 209.

16.4.1. Characteristics, Uses, and Pollution Sources

Commercial PBB mixtures were widely employed in plastics, electrical equipment, electronic

Table 16.2. Chemical Identities of *Poly*brominated Biphenyls (*PBBs*), *Poly*brominated Diphenyl Ethers (*PBDEs*), and *Poly*chlorinated Biphenyls (*PCBs*)[a]

No.	Position of Halogenation	No.	Position of Halogenation	No.	Position of Halogenation	No.	Position of Halogenation
mono-BB, -BDE, -CB		52	2,2',5,5'	106	2,3,3',4,5	160	2,3,3',4,5,6
1	2	53	2,2',5,6'	107	2,3,3',4',5	161	2,3,3',4,5',6
2	3	54	2,2',6,6'	108	2,3,3',4,5'	162	2,3,3',4',5,5'
3	4	55	2,3,3',4	109	2,3,3',4,6	163	2,3,3',4',5,6
di-BB, -BDE, -CB		56	2,3,3',4'	110	2,3,3',4',6	164	2,3,3',4',5',6
4	2,2'	57	2,3,3',5	111	2,3,3',5,5'	165	2,3,3',5,5',6
5	2,3	58	2,3,3',5'	112	2,3,3',5,6	166	2,3,4,4',5,6
6	2,3'	59	2,3,3',6	113	2,3,3',5',6	167	2,3',4,4',5,5'
7	2,4	60	2,3,4,4'	114	2,3,4,4',5	168	2,3',4,4',5',6
8	2,4'	61	2,3,4,5	115	2,3,4,4',6	169	3,3',4,4',5,5'
9	2,5	62	2,3,4,6	116	2,3,4,5,6	*hepta-BB, -BDE, -CB*	
10	2,6	63	2,3,4',5	117	2,3,4',5,6	170	2,2',3,3',4,4',5
11	3,3'	64	2,3,4',6	118	2,3',4,4',5	171	2,2',3,3',4,4',6
12	3,4	65	2,3,5,6	119	2,3',4,4',6	172	2,2',3,3',4,5,5'
13	3,4'	66	2,3',4,4'	120	2,3',4,5,5'	173	2,2',3,3',4,5,6
14	3,5	67	2,3',4,5	121	2,3',4,5',6	174	2,2',3,3',4,5,6'
15	4,4'	68	2,3',4,5'	122	2,3,3',4',5	175	2,2',3,3',4,5',6
tri-BB, -BDE, -CB		69	2,3',4,6	123	2,3',4,4',5	176	2,2',3,3',4,6,6'
16	2,2',3	70	2,3',4',5	124	2,3',4',5,5'	177	2,2',3,3',4',5,6'
17	2,2',4	71	2,3',4',6	125	2,3',4',5',6	178	2,2',3,3',5,5',6
18	2,2',5	72	2,3',5,5'	126	3,3',4,4',5	179	2,2',3,3',5,6,6'
19	2,2',6	73	2,3',5',6	127	3,3',4,5,5'	180	2,2',3,4,4',5,5'
20	2,3,3'	74	2,4,4',5	*hexa-BB, -BDE, -CB*		181	2,2',3,4,4',5,6
21	2,3,4	75	2,4,4',6	128	2,2',3,3',4,4'	182	2,2',3,4,4',5,6'
22	2,3,4'	76	2,3',4',5	129	2,2',3,3',4,5	183	2,2',3,4,4',5',6
23	2,3,5	77	3,3',4,4'	130	2,2',3,3',4,5'	184	2,2',3,4,4',6,6'
24	2,3,6	78	3,3',4,5	131	2,2',3,3',4,6	185	2,2',3,4,5,5',6
25	2,3',4	79	3,3',4,5'	132	2,2',3,3',4,6'	186	2,2',3,4,5,6,6'
26	2,3',5	80	3,3',5,5'	133	2,2',3,3',5,5'	187	2,2',3,4',5,5',6
27	2,3',6	81	3,4,4',5	134	2,2',3,3',5,6	188	2,2',3,4',5,6,6'
28	2,4,4'	*penta-BB, -BDE, -CB*		135	2,2',3,3',5,6'	189	2,3,3',4,4',5,5'
29	2,4,5	82	2,2',3,3',4	136	2,2',3,3',6,6'	190	2,3,3',4,4',5,6
30	2,4,6	83	2,2',3,3',5	137	2,2',3,4,4',5	191	2,3,3',4,4',5',6
31	2,4',5	84	2,2',3,3',6	138	2,2',3,4,4',5'	192	2,3,3',4,5,5',6
32	2,4',6	85	2,2',3,4,4'	139	2,2',3,4,4',6	193	2,3,3',4',5,5',6
33	2,3',4'	86	2,2',3,4,5	140	2,2',3,4,4',6'	*octa-BB, -BDE, -CB*	
34	2,3',5'	87	2,2',3,4,5'	141	2,2',3,4,5,5'	194	2,2',3,3',4,4',5,5'
35	3,3',4	88	2,2',3,4,6	142	2,2',3,4,5,6	195	2,2',3,3',4,4',5,6
36	3,3',5	89	2,2',3,4,6'	143	2,2',3,4,5,6'	196	2,2',3,3',4,4',5,6'
37	3,4,4'	90	2,2',3,4',5	144	2,2',3,4,5',6	197	2,2',3,3',4,4',6,6'
38	3,4,5	91	2,2',3,4',6	145	2,2',3,4,6,6'	198	2,2',3,3',4,5,5',6
39	3,4',5	92	2,2',3,5,5'	146	2,2',3,4',5,5'	199	2,2',3,3',4,5,5',6'
tetra-BB, -BDE, -CB		93	2,2',3,5,6	147	2,2',3,4',5,6	200	2,2',3,3',4,5,6,6'
40	2,2',3,3'	94	2,2',3,5,6'	148	2,2',3,4',5,6'	201	2,2',3,3',4,5',6,6'
41	2,2',3,4	95	2,2',3,5',6	149	2,2',3,4',5',6	202	2,2',3,3',5,5',6,6'
42	2,2',3,4'	96	2,2',3,6,6'	150	2,2',3,4',6,6'	203	2,2',3,4,4',5,5',6
43	2,2',3,5	97	2,2',3,4',5'	151	2,2',3,5,5',6	204	2,2',3,4,4',5,6,6'
44	2,2',3,5'	98	2,2',3,4',6'	152	2,2',3,5,6,6'	205	2,3,3',4,4',5,5',6
45	2,2',3,6	99	2,2',4,4',5	153	2,2',4,4',5,5'	*nona-BB, -BDE, -CB*	
46	2,2',3,6'	100	2,2',4,4',6	154	2,2',4,4',5,6'	206	2,2',3,3',4,4',5,5',6
47	2,2',4,4'	101	2,2',4,5,5'	155	2,2',4,4',6,6'	207	2,2',3,3',4,4',5,6,6'
48	2,2',4,5	102	2,2',4,5,6'	156	2,3,3',4,4',5	208	2,2',3,3',4,5,5',6,6'
49	2,2',4,5'	103	2,2',4,5',6	157	2,3,3',4,4',5'	*deca-BB, -BDE, -CB*	
50	2,2',4,6	104	2,2',4,6,6'	158	2,3,3',4,4',6	209	2,2',3,3',4,4',5,5',6,6'
51	2,2',4,6'	105	2,3,3',4,4'	159	2,3,3',4,5,5'	—	—

[a] see Figure 16.1, ATSDR (2004, 2017), and Mills *et al.* (2007) for further discussion, which are the primary sources for this table.

products, textiles, and other materials in the early 1970s, predominantly as flame retardants. In the United States, both the production and the use of *hexa*BB were banned shortly after a major agricultural contamination episode took place in the state of Michigan during 1973-1974. That disaster also led to the discontinued production and use of the *octa*brominated biphenyl (*octa*BB) and the *deca*brominated biphenyl (*deca*BB) formulation in 1979.

The massive PBB contamination in Michigan began in September 1973, when a farmer in the state's southern region started noticing his herd of 400 dairy cattle suffering from hair loss, hematomas, and abnormalities in hoof growth, along with significant reductions in milk production and appetite. Exposure of the cattle to PBBs was not identified as the culprit until a year later, after several thousand pounds of PBB powder (containing mainly *hexa*BB) in mislabeled bags were distributed to and utilized by many farms in the state as the livestock feed additive magnesium oxide (MgO). The MgO additive was intended to be mixed with the feed to increase milk production.

16.4.2. Environmental Health Concerns

The health and economic impacts of the PBB contamination in Michigan went far beyond the loss of a herd of 400 cattle. Many farm animals consumed the contaminated feed before the mistake was discovered, including more than a million of chickens, tens of thousands of other cattle, and thousands of pigs and sheep (e.g., Fries, 1985). More than 4,000 people in Michigan were also found exposed to PBBs in 1973 as a result of the disaster. Those dairy farmers exposed to the PBB contaminants were found having significant abnormalities with their immunological system, including decreases in the number and percentage of peripheral blood lymphocytes and in functional response to specific test antigens (Bekesi *et al.*, 1978). A cohort study following 327 girls aged 5 to 24 years for two decades showed that, even after adjustment for potential confounding factors, the breastfed daughters exposed to PBBs *in utero* at or above 7 ppb had an earlier age at menarche compared to the breastfed girls exposed to lower levels of PBBs *in utero* and those not breastfed (Blanck *et al.*, 2000). IARC (2016b, 2017) recently has re-classified all PBB congeners as probable human (Group 2A) carcinogens.

When applied as additives, certain PBB congeners were physically and selectively mixed into electronic products (e.g., computer monitors), instead of chemically bonded to them. Therefore, under normal conditions, these compounds will be more readily released (leached) into the local environment. There is a rising concern with the export of e-waste (electronic waste) to the developing countries for fear of widespread releases of *hexa*BB during recycling operations (e.g., Zhao *et al.*, 2008). PBB homologs that were manufactured for commercial use typically consisted of the highly-brominated congeners such as *hexa*BB and up. Based on a use-lifespan of 5 to 10 years for most electrical and electronic products, it is anticipated that many PBB-containing products now have already been disposed of or are still being disposed of. It is likely though that the *hexa*BB congeners are still being applied to electrical and electronic products in some developing countries. Highly-brominated PBBs are thus still expected to be available in the e-waste sites and around the affected local environments. It was partly due to such environmental health concerns that in 2006, many parties to the Stockholm Convention proposed that commercial *hexa*BB, along with commercial *octa*brominated diphenyl ether (*octa*BDE), be added to the POPs action list. That proposal became a reality on 26 August 2010 (the official date for the amendments to enter into force). On the other hand, as concluded by UNEP (2006b) in profiling the pollutant's health hazard and environmental fate, *hexa*BB satisfies the criteria for being treated as a member of the PBTs (persistent, bioaccumulative, and toxic substances).

16.5. Polybrominated Diphenyl Ethers

Like PBBs, polybrominated diphenyl ethers (PBDEs) are also brominated compounds but each with a diphenyl ether molecule ($C_{12}H_{10}O$), instead of a biphenyl, as their structural nucleus (Figure 16.1). Otherwise, they are structurally very similar to PBBs and likewise have a possible total of 209 congeners as well as 10 homologs. As summarized in Table 16.2 and implicit in the general PBDE structure depicted in Figure 16.1, the 209 congeners each can also be referred to by a unique number between 1 and 209. Note that although each of the 10 homologs generally refers to the isomers within it, its *commercial* term can mean a mixture of isomers from certain other homologs as well. For example, commercial-based *penta*BDE is a mixture of mostly PBDE 99 (a *penta*BDE congener) plus a small quantity of PBDE 47 (a *tetra*BDE congener), whereas commercial-based *octa*-BDE consists of mostly *octa*-homolog congeners (e.g., PBDE 203) mixed with small quantities of *hexa*-homolog (e.g., PBDE 153) and *hepta*-homolog (e.g., PBDE 180) congeners.

16.5.1. Characteristics, Uses, and Pollution Sources

As with the PBB congeners, the PBDE members are part of the specialty group referred to as brominated flame retardants (BFRs). Among the 10 homologs, *penta*-, *octa*-, and *deca*-BDEs are the most utilized. Collectively, the three homologs are widely used as flame retardants contained in a variety of plastics, fabrics, and foams that are components of numerous various consumer products. In particular, *penta*BDE is largely used in flexible polyurethane (e.g., furniture) foams; whereas *deca*BDE is often employed in plastics for television (TV) cabinets, consumer electronics, and wire insulation, as well as in back coatings for upholstery. And *octa*BDE is widely used in plastics for small appliances and personal computers. Inasmuch as PBDEs are commonly used in high-impact polystyrene, epoxy resins, and plastics, they can be found in many e-waste products such as obsolete circuit boards, cables, and TV sets (e.g., Zhao *et al.*, 2008).

The annual global production of PBDEs as flame retardants (plus for minor purposes) has been estimated to exceed 67,000 tons (BSEF, 2000), of which PBDE 209 (the only *deca*BDE isomer) accounts for some 70% and is used substantially in North America. Many PBDE-containing plastics and polyurethane foams were once widely used in electrical and electronic products that now are referred to as end-of-life e-waste. Unlike some other PBDE congeners, PBDE 209 can be degraded rapidly through exposure to light (e.g., ultraviolet radiation) or via biological activity in the environment, with a half-life being in days (Zhao *et al.*, 2008).

PBDEs are mixed with polymers during the production of plastics. Because like PBBs they are not chemically bonded to the plastics, these pollutants too tend to easily leach out of the final consumer products. Accordingly, PBDEs can be found in many homes due to the ubiquity of plastics present in today's modern world. They are different from most other POPs in that their main source is consumer products, whereas those for most other POPs that the general public are exposed to are foods, dust particles, and/or drinking water.

16.5.2. Environmental Health Concerns

Although the application of flame retardant substances preserves lives and properties, it comes with undesired consequences. A number of mammalian studies (e.g., ATSDR, 2017) implicated that these PBDE retardants caused liver and thyroid toxicities. Several others (Eriksson *et al.*, 2001, 2002) found that neonatal exposure of mice to certain PBDE congeners (e.g., PBDE 47, PBDE 99) resulted in adverse effects on spontaneous motor behavior, learning and memory functions, as well as habituation capability that worsened with age. Up to now, IARC (2017) has not listed any PBDE congener as a potential human or animal carcinogen.

There is evidence that PBDE 71 is an endocrine disruptor in rats during their development (Zhou *et al.*, 2002). A fertility study (Harley *et al.*, 2010) implicated that women with high blood levels of PBDEs (particularly the *penta-* and *octa-*homologs) took much longer to get pregnant compared to women with lower levels.

Environmental monitoring programs in various global regions (e.g., Asia, Europe, the Arctic) found trace amounts of PBDEs in human breast milk, fishes, aquatic birds, and elsewhere in the environment. Homologs from *tetra-* to *hexa-*BDEs were those most commonly detected in humans and wildlife. Despite the fact that the exact mechanisms or pathways through which PBDEs got into humans and the environment remain unknown, it is more certain that the main sources of environmental exposure to PBDEs include releases from processing of these ethers into plastics or textiles and from wear and tear of the consumer products being used.

Workers engaging in the production of PBDE-containing materials are likely exposed to highest levels of these brominated substances. There is growing evidence that PBDEs persist in the environment and bioaccumulate in living organisms (e.g., UNEP, 2006c). These POPs tend to accumulate in blood, breast milk, and fatty tissues. Bioaccumulation is therefore of high health concern in such instances, especially for workers in e-waste recycling sites and electronics repair shops. The public are likely exposed to low levels of PBDEs via dietary intake and inhalation. In the United States, near universal exposure to PBDEs was found in the general population, with ~97% of the adult participants in the comprehensive National Health and Nutrition Examination Survey (more known by its acronym NHANES) having detectable levels of PBDEs in their blood (Sjödin *et al.*, 2008). As alluded to earlier, exposure to PBDEs is (more) common in residential places due to the ubiquity of consumer products in modern homes.

Under its Restriction of Hazardous Substances Directive that came into force on 1 July 2006, the European Union restricted the uses of PBDEs and PBBs in electrical and electronic products, with an upper limit of 1 g/kg (0.1%) for the sum of the two chemical groups in the same product. In the United States, *penta-* and *octa-*BDEs are no longer produced. However, millions of pounds of these homologs are expected to remain in American homes and their environment for a long time owing to the continuous extensive use of PBDE-based consumer products.

The *deca*BDE congener is still widely used today, in part because it has a relatively shorter half-life. In the United States, around 50 million pounds of this homolog (with only one congener) are used each year, mostly in TV casings. The usage of *deca*BDE is expected to grow in this nation, as the congener has been approved for use to meet new federal fire safety standards for residential furniture and mattresses. It should be pointed out, though, that *deca*BDE can break down easily into *penta-* and *octa*-BDEs; yet commercial-based *penta-* and *octa*-BDEs have been officially added to the Stockholm Convention's POPs priority list since 26 August 2010.

16.6. Polybrominated Cyclododecanes

Polybrominated (a.k.a. polybromo) cyclododecanes (PBCDs) are still another (i.e., the third) chemical group of BFRs (brominated flame retardants) posing global environmental health threats. As their name implies, PBCDs each have a ring-based cyclododecane ($C_{12}H_{24}$) nucleus, on which one or more of its 24 H atoms are replaced by Br atoms (Figure 16.1). Up to now, *hexa*bromocyclododecane (*H*BCD) is the only homolog in the PBCD family detected in the environment and known to have been actively produced or used in several countries. The six Br atoms in (commercial) HBCD are attached to six of the 12 carbon (C) atoms in the (non-benzene) ring at the 1, 2, 5, 6, 9, and 10 position. With its six Br atoms so positioned, HBCD has 16 possible stereoisomers. The commercial HBCD product is a mixture composed of three main diastereoisomers referenced as α-, β-, and γ-HBCD, with the last form of isomers being 2 to 4 times more abundant than the total of the first two (Heeb *et al.*, 2005; Tomy *et al.*, 2004; UNEP, 2010).

16.6.1. Characteristics, Uses, and Pollution Sources

HBCD (hexabromocyclododecane) is applied predominantly as a flame retardant in extruded (XPS) and expanded (EPS) polystyrene foams that are intended for use as thermal insulation materials in the building and the construction industry. Its secondary applications include uses in high-impact polystyrene for electrical or electronic equipment and in polymer-dispersion back coating agents for upholstered fabrics, furniture, as well as automobile interiors (European Commission, 2008; UNEP, 2010). HBCD is produced mainly in China, Europe, Japan, and the United States. Its annual global production (as well as demand) is reportedly exceeding 20,000 tons, with more than half of the global market volume being used in Europe (UNEP, 2010).

The brominated cyclododecane can be emitted easily into the environment, as it is not bonded chemically to polymers. It is qualified as a persistent and bioaccumulative substance in the environment (ECCC, 2016; UNEP, 2010; U.S. EPA, 2010a) and thus subject to long-range transport. In fact, it is found also widespread in remote regions where HBCD is not produced or (widely) used, such as the Arctic (e.g., Braune *et al.*, 2007; Tomy *et al.*, 2008). Under normal conditions, HBCD is expected to adsorb strongly to soils and aquatic sediments, insomuch as its degradation in sediment cores has been determined to range from years to decades (e.g., Kohler *et al.*, 2008; Minh *et al.*, 2007).

HBCD can be found in various environmental samples such as birds, fishes, marine mammals, soils, and sediments (ECCC, 2016; UNEP, 2010; U.S. EPA, 2010a). The substance is lipophilic, with a log K_{ow} (*octane-water* partition coefficient) of 5.6 at 25° C or 77° F (ECCC, 2016; UNEP, 2010; U.S. EPA, 2010a), and thus has a strong potential to bioaccumulate in humans and wildlife.

In addition, HBCD has shown to biomagnify in human and wildlife food chains (e.g., Fängström *et al.*, 2008; Morris *et al.*, 2004; Tomy *et al.*, 2008). Compared to the other two diastereoisomers, α-HBCD is reportedly more bioaccumulative (e.g., Zhang *et al.*, 2014).

In humans, HBCD can be found in breast milk, fatty tissues, and blood. It has been reported capable of crossing the placenta (ECCC, 2016; UNEP, 2010; U.S. EPA, 2010a). A Flemish dietary study (Roosens *et al.*, 2010) found that children between the ages of three and six had the highest exposure to HBCD, with an estimated average daily intake of 6.6 ng/kg body weight. The primary occupational exposure to HBCD is through inhalation of airborne dusts in workplaces (European Commission, 2008). A more recent study (Yi *et al.*, 2016) showed that up to 70% (500-800) of all workers in the HBCD production and processing industries in China might be at risk of occupational exposure to the flame retardant.

16.6.2. Environmental Health Concerns

HBCD is toxic to humans, wildlife, and particularly aquatic organisms (ECCC, 2016; UNEP, 2010; U.S. EPA, 2010a). Sublethal effects (e.g., oxidative stress, reproductive activity) were observed in fishes (Palace *et al.*, 2008; Ronisz *et al.*, 2004; Zhang *et al.*, 2008).

A study in rats (Ema *et al.*, 2008) revealed various adverse reproductive and developmental effects from exposure to HBCD, such as decrease in ovarian follicles and delays in eye opening in the second generation. A study in mice (Eriksson *et al.*, 2006) observed a number of neurobehavioral effects including reduced habituation and impaired learning. In addition, a study in American kestrels (Fernie *et al.*, 2009) showed that α-HBCD (and certain PBDE congeners) at environmental relevant doses caused eggshell thinning in those birds.

To date, IARC (2017) has not listed HBCD as a potential human or animal carcinogen. However, in response to the other health effects and the environmental impacts at issue, the Stockholm Convention decided in May 2013 to list HBCD for elimination, with specific exemptions for its production and use in EPS and XPS in buildings. The restriction allows member countries to use the exemption for up to five years from time of submission of the exemption request. Japan was reportedly the first country to ban the import and production of HBCD effective May 2014.

16.7. Polychlorinated Biphenyls

As with PBBs and PBDEs, PCBs (polychlorinated biphenyls) are a chemical group of theoretically up to 209 possible congeners, for which there is no known natural source. Structurally and similarly, these 209 possible congeners differ from one another only in the number of Cl atoms as well as their positions on the biphenyl nucleus (as reflected in Figure 16.1 and Table 16.2). About 60% of these congeners could (and still can) be found in some of the PCB mixtures once widely used in electrical and electronic equipment or as plasticizers.

16.7.1. Characters, Uses, and Pollution Sources

Monsanto Corporation was the sole U.S. manufacturer of PCBs from 1929 until the ban of their production (which took into effect) in 1979. The company marketed the product mixtures under the trade name Aroclor followed by a four-digit code (e.g., Table 10.2) to signify the number of carbons and the mass of chlorines contained in each mixture. Owing to the widespread and various applications of these substances in the past and to their notorious persistence in the environment, PCBs still can be found in many places today including particularly the e-waste sites (e.g., Han *et al.*, 2017; Xing *et al.*, 2009). Most capacitors and transformers manufactured prior to 1979 contain large amounts of PCBs. As estimated by the International Programme on Chemical Safety (IPCS, 2003), around 2 million tons of PCBs were produced worldwide between 1929 and their global ban in 2001; and as of 2003, some 10% of this total global production remained in mobile environmental reservoirs. Numerous studies demonstrated that PCBs, as well as several other polychlorinated compounds such as dioxins (i.e., PCDDs and PCDFs), are highly bioaccumulative (*see*, e.g., studies cited in Section 6.3.2 as well as in Tables 6.2 and 6.3).

As can be seen in Figure 16.1, PCBs are structurally and hence in general chemically as well very akin to the PBBs and dioxin compounds. Twelve of the PCB congeners are especially known to have toxic effects very similar to those of dioxins (as discussed in Section 16.10 below) and by convention are referred to as *dioxin-like* PCB congeners. More specifically, the dioxin-like PCBs can bind to the aryl hydrocarbon (Ah) receptors (Section 9.2.3) to cause toxic effects very similar to those induced by dioxins. Accordingly, PCBs are often classified into the "dioxin-like" and "nondioxin-like" subgroups.

PCBs can also be classified into the two subgroups known as *nonplanar* and *coplanar* congeners to align with their dioxin-like properties. This classification practice is brought about by the observation that a PCB congener can cause more health effects when the entire chemical molecule is situated in the same plane (i.e., coplanar). The degree of planarity is determined largely by the number of chlorine substitutions in the *ortho* positions. Note that sites 2, 2′, 6, and 6′ on the biphenyl (Figure 16.1) are called *ortho* positions, as they are closest to the *other* benzene ring; sites 3, 3′, 5, and 5′ are called the *meta* positions. And sites 4 and 4′ are called the *para* positions. The two rings can rotate around the bond connecting them and thus can yield two extreme configurations with one being *coplanar* (i.e., in which the two rings are in the same plane) and the other being *nonplanar* (i.e., in which the two rings are at a 90° angle to each other).

The substitution of the smaller-size, lighter H atoms in the *ortho* positions with the larger-size, heavier Cl atoms would eventually force the two benzene rings to rotate out of the planar configuration. In essence, the benzene rings of non*ortho* substituted PCBs, along with those of the mono-*ortho* substituted, would eventually assume a planar configuration. These PCBs are referred to as non*ortho* (non*ortho*-substituted) or planar PCBs. The rest of the PCB congeners with the two benzene rings not capable of assuming a coplanar configuration are referred to as nonplanar congeners. Coplanar PCBs (e.g., PCB 77, PCB 126, PCB 169) tend to have dioxin-like toxicological properties and in general are regarded as among the most toxic PCB congeners.

16.7.2. Environmental Health Concerns

Although dioxin-like PCBs are generally more potent in causing toxic effects, they normally account for only a small portion of the mass of PCBs found in the environment or in biological samples. The use of the term *nondioxin-like PCBs* is hence not necessarily useful. While the PCB congeners in this larger subgroup are excluded from the toxic equivalency factors (TEF) scheme (*see* Section 16.11 below), they do not truly represent a single subclass of compounds but rather collectively have multiple toxic endpoints with multiple structure-activity relationships (Barnes *et al.*, 1991). There simply has not enough congener-specific research performed to fully characterize all the congeners in this larger subclass. As a point of argument, various PCB congeners were analyzed for their neurotoxic effects on dopamine content in PC12 (rat) cell line (Shain *et al.*, 1991) and on microsomal Ca^{2+}-sequestration in rat cerebellum (Kodavanti *et al.*, 1996), yet by different forms of structure-activity relationships rather than by the degree of their planarity.

PCBs can disrupt hormonal functions and cause developmental as well as thyroid effects. They have been linked to neurological and behavioral problems in children, and to other adverse health effects such as immunological dysfunction, liver damage, skin disorders (including notably chloracne), and cancer. As a group these chlorinated compounds have been listed as a human (Group 1) carcinogen (IARC, 2016b, 2017).

Certain PCB congeners reportedly have metabolites with hormonal activities more potent than those of themselves. Studies supporting this notion included the *in vitro* assays by Andersson *et al.* (1999), in which the estrogenic activities of four structurally diverse PCB congeners and five of their hydroxylated derivatives (OH-PCBs) were investigated. In that series of assays, the various PCB congeners and metabolites were tested for their ability to induce the proliferation of MCF-7 human breast cancer cells as well as for their ability to express the vitellogenin (VTG) gene in rainbow trout hepatocytes. In both cell species, the OH-PCB metabolites showed more hormonally active than their parent PCBs, with one metabolite being almost as potent as the natural estrogens. Another study in human cells (Cheek *et al.*, 1999) found that in examining PCBs and several other OCs (organochlorines) for their binding affinity to the thyroid hormone receptors (and to the thyroid hormone transport proteins), only the OH-PCB metabolites were found bound to the hormone receptors.

Note that the VTG mentioned above is an egg yolk type precursor protein expressed only in the females of almost all oviparous species (e.g., fish) and is normally dormant in the males. Yet when the males are exposed to estrogen mimickers, the VTG gene will be expressed in a dose-dependent manner, thus making the protein expression in a male oviparous a highly effective biomarker of exposure to estrogenic disruptors.

16.8. Polychlorinated Naphthalenes

Polychlorinated naphthalenes (PCNs) are another group of structurally highly similar congeners belonging to the superfamily of polychlorinated aromatic compounds. As with PCBs, they are legacy pollutants and, other than the congeners in their *mono*homolog, have been added to the Stockholm Convention's POPs action list. PCNs and PCBs are regarded as legacy pollutants in that they have remained in the environment for decades, long after they were released from their production sources or emission points. As noted in Section 13.4.1, naphthalene ($C_{10}H_8$) is a fused two-ring aromatic hydrocarbons (HCs) thus with a total of 10 C atoms and eight H atoms. PCNs each possess this naphthalene nucleus on which one or more of the eight H atoms are replaced by

Cl atoms (Figure 16.1). Accordingly, there are theoretically eight possible homologs as well as 75 possible congeners within the PCN family.

16.8.1. Characteristics, Uses, and Pollution Sources

PCN (polychlorinated naphthalene) products are available as oily or waxy solid materials. They were once used in a wide variety of applications including cable insulation, engine and gear oil additives, feedstock for dye production, and as wood preservative. Their applications have been largely phased out worldwide since the early 1980s. High volume productions and uses of PCNs started around 1910 in Europe and the United States, under the commercial names Nibren wax and Halowax, respectively. PCNs have high thermal and chemical stability, with low flammability potential. In the United States, exposure to PCNs was drastically reduced shortly after the enactment of the Toxic Substances Control Act of 1976. This perhaps explains why U.S. EPA has not been more current with its environmental hazard assessment for PCNs since the mid-1970s. Current concerns with PCNs include largely their releases as by-products of waste incineration. While some PCN congeners can be broken down by sunlight and at slow rates by certain types of microorganisms, many others persist in the environment. The reality is that long after some 80 years of use and total global production of several hundred thousand tons, PCN residues were (and are) still found widespread in the global environment (IPCS, 2001).

All homologs in the PCN family, except the *mono*CNs (and perhaps the *di*CNs as well), are regarded as having satisfied the regulatory criteria for pollutants having PBT characteristics (ECCC, 2011; UNEP, 2012a; U.S. EPA, 1975). Many of these homologs have been found in human foods, human fats, fishes, and remote regions such as the Arctic (e.g., ECCC, 2011; UNEP, 2012a). In particular, *hexa*CNs reportedly have been found fairly persistent in the human body, with calculated half-lives of 1.5 to 2.4 years. These half-life estimates were calculated from monitoring results on three Taiwaneses who consumed cooking rice oil contaminated with a mixture of polychlorinated compounds including PCNs (Ryan and Masuda, 1994).

16.8.2. Environmental Health Concerns

According to ECCC (2011), IPCS (2001), UNEP (2012a), and others, the ecotoxicity of PCNs has been studied with several species representing different trophic levels: algae, aquatic plants, invertebrates, fishes, birds, and rats. Studies in rats showed numerous various adverse outcomes from PCN exposure: endocrinal, reproductive, and developmental effects; induction of oxidative stress as well as lipid peroxidation; and decrease in detoxifying activities of certain Phase I enzymes. A study in male rats (Kilanowicz *et al.*, 2012) found that repeated exposure to *hexa*CNs at 0.3 mg/kg body weight impaired long-term memory without signs of overt toxicity.

Adverse health effects associated with occupational exposure to PCNs began to emerge in the 1940s, some 30 years after these substances were first made available for commercial use. The reported effects included largely chloracne, severe skin rashes, and liver diseases that could lead to death. In particular, *penta*- and *hexa*-CNs were found to cause hyperkeratosis (i.e., skin thickening). Moreover, results from a cohort study (Ward *et al.*, 1994) among 9,028 (3,042 female and 5,986 male) workers suggested a link between exposure to PCN and excess malignant neoplasms of the connective tissue. In that cohort study, the association with tumors of the connective tissue was suggested for workers with over 12 months of PCN exposure and 25 years of latency. IARC (2017) has not listed any PCN congener as a potential human or animal carcinogen.

16.9. Polychlorinated Butadienes

In organic chemistry, a diene (C_4H_6) molecule is any aliphatic HC (hydrocarbon) that contains two carbon double bonds, whereas a butadiene (or more specifically 1,3-butadiene) is a simple *conjugated* diene with the two double bonds *adjacent* to each other and therefore with the structure $H_2C=CH-CH=CH_2$. Butadiene is widely employed as a monomer in the making of rubbers. Polychlorinated butadienes (PCBDs), on the other hand, are a class of structurally very similar aliphatic HCs each possessing this butadiene nucleus on which one or more of its six H atoms are replaced by Cl atoms (Figure 16.1). All six homologs of PCBDs have been found in considerable amounts in the environment (ATSDR, 1994, 2012a; IARC, 1999; UNEP, 2012b). However, *hexa*chlorobutadiene (*hexa*CBD or HCBD for short) is currently the only homolog in the PCBD family that has been added to the Stockholm Convention's POPs action list.

HCBD is a colorless liquid at room temperature with a turpentine-like odor. This homolog has a single congener as it is a fully chlorinated butadiene. On the other hand, the *mono*CBD homolog, which is commonly referred to as chlorobutadiene, has two possible congeners since its single Cl atom can bind to either of the two C atoms that are double bonded to each other. Moreover, the 2-chlorobutadiene congener ($H_2C=CCl-CH=CH_2$, i.e., where the Cl atom attaches to the *second* carbon counting from either side) is more known as chloroprene. Chloroprene is the monomer for the making of the polymer polychloroprene, which is a synthetic rubber more commonly known to the public by its trade name Neoprene.

16.9.1. Characteristics, Uses, and Pollution Sources

HCBD (*hexa*chlorobutadiene) mostly occurs as a by-product from the chlorinolysis of butane (C_4H_{10}) derivatives during the productions of tetrachloroethene ($CCl_2=CCl_2$) and carbon tetrachloride (CCl_4). This fully chlorinated butadiene is used mainly as a solvent for chlorine and as an intermediate in the manufacture of rubber compounds (ATSDR, 1994, 2012a; IARC, 1999). HCBD was once utilized as a herbicide until its toxicity to humans has become a high public health concern in recent years.

HCBD has been widely detected in ambient air, water, sediments, foods, and human tissues. As expected, exposure to HCBD occurs mainly due to its production and release as a by-product from the making of chlorinated solvent and related products. This chlorinated aliphatic is a persistent and bioaccumulative substance. According to the U.S. Agency for Toxic Substances and Disease Registry (ATSDR, 1994, 2012a) and UNEP (2012b), a wide range of BCFs (bioconcentration factors; *see* Chapter 6) in marine and freshwater biota (e.g., algae, crustaceans, fishes, molluscs) have been measured or estimated for HCBD, with the highest value being around 17,000 (L/kg, wet weight). Nonetheless, for the biomagnification potential of this fully chlorinated butadiene, the supporting data available thus far have been insufficient or inconclusive (UNEP, 2012b).

16.9.2. Environmental Health Concerns

HCBD (*hexa*chlorobutadiene) is highly toxic to many species of fish and crustaceans (ATSDR, 1994, 2012a; UNEP, 2012b). The acute LC_{50} (i.e., lethal concentration sufficient to kill 50% of a study population) values reportedly ranged from 0.03 mg/L for marine crustacean *Palaemontes pugio* to 4.5 mg/L for the freshwater fish *Poecillia latiphinna* (e.g., IPCS, 1994).

HCBD has shown to produce systemic toxicity in mammalians following exposure via oral, inhalation, and dermal routes (e.g., ATSDR, 1994, 2012a). Adverse effects may include fatty liver degeneration, epithelial necrotizing nephritis, central nervous system depression, and cyanosis. The kidney was the primary target organ observed in a study (Kociba *et al.*, 1977) in which male and female rats were given HCBD in the diet for 2 years at daily doses up to 20 mg/kg of body weight. Effects observed in that chronic study included an increase in relative and absolute kidney weights in males in the highest dose group, and an increase in incidence of renal tubular neoplasms also in males in the highest dose group.

Studies on HCBD toxicity in humans are limited and usually with inconclusive results. For instance, as reported by IPCS (1994) and UNEP (2012b), two Russian studies (Burkatskaya *et al.*, 1982; Krasniuk *et al.*, 1969) observed various adverse health effects in vineyard workers exposed to HCBD, including increased incidence of arterial hypotension, myocardial dystrophy, adverse liver effects, chest pains, upper respiratory tract changes, hand trembling, and nausea. Yet as cautioned by IPCS (1994), co-exposure to other substances cannot be ruled out and therefore results from the two studies are of limited value for health risk assessment.

In terms of carcinogenicity, U.S. EPA (1988) has long classified HCBD as a possible carcinogen (Group C), whereas IARC (1999, 2017) has not listed the aliphatic as a potential human or animal carcinogen.

16.10. Polychlorinated Dioxins/Furans

In environmental toxicology, *dioxins* is a general term referring to the chemical family of polychlorinated dibenzo-*p(ara)*-dioxins (PCDDs) and very frequently including the family of their structural cousins polychlorinated dibenzofurans (PCDFs). This practice owes to the fact that the congeners in the two families are very similar in chemical and toxicological properties. The PCDD and PCDF congeners, along with the dioxin-like PCBs, all share an important common cellular mechanism of action (i.e., activation of the AhR, as illustrated in Figure 9.2) and induce comparable biological and toxic responses. As depicted in Figure 16.1, the skeletal structure (the nucleus) of PCDDs is a dioxin ($C_4H_4O_2$), having one more O (oxygen) atom than the furan (C_4H_4O) nucleus in PCDFs. Unlike the two benzene rings in PCBs, PBBs, or PBDEs, those in PCDDs and PCDFs each have 4, instead of 5, C (carbon) atoms that Cl (chlorine) atoms can attach to. As such, PCDDs and PCDFs each have 75 and 135 theoretically possible congeners, respectively, together yielding a total of 210 possible congeners. PCDDs have 60 fewer possible congeners than PCDFs do because, unlike the furan nucleus, the dioxin nucleus (like the naphthalene nucleus in PCNs) is in a symmetric shape thus resulting in fewer distinct stereoisomers. For the purpose of discussion in this section (and elsewhere in this book), except where necessary to make the distinction, the term *dioxins* includes all the furan congeners (i.e., all the PCDFs) and in certain places also all of the 12 dioxin-like PCBs (*see* Table 16.3).

16.10.1. Characteristics, Uses, and Pollution Sources

Dioxins of global health concern are mostly, if not exclusively, unintentional by-products of those substances used to manufacture certain pesticides and wood preservatives, such as 2,4-D and 2,4,5-T (Chapter 15). However, even prior to industrialization, low levels of naturally occurring dioxins were found in the environment as a result of geological processes or natural combustion (e.g., forest fires). Today, the principal environmental source of dioxins is incineration, although various levels of these OCs have been detected in various environmental media such as plants, foods, animal tissues, water, sediments, and soils.

Dioxins are highly persistent in the environment with half-lives in soils and sediments reportedly ranging from months to years. Because these HC substances are practically neither volatile nor water-soluble, most are contained in soils and sediments serving as environmental reservoirs from which they may be released eventually over a long period. Accordingly, volatilization and particle re-suspension from these environmental reservoirs are still the major potential sources for global distribution of dioxins.

Dietary intake is the main source of exposure to dioxins for the general population, with meat, dairy products, fish, and other seafood accounting for over 90% of the total daily toll. Dioxins are absorbed through the gastrointestinal (GI) tract, skin, and respiratory tract, and then distributed within the body via the bloodstream. Absorption is congener-specific, with the highly-chlorinated homologs having higher absorption rate compared to those containing fewer chlorines. Because of their high lipophilic nature, dioxins tend to accumulate in the fatty tissues and liver. Dioxins are slowly metabolized by oxidation or reductive dechlorination and conjugation. The major routes of their excretion in the human body are via the bile and feces, with small amounts being eliminated in the urine. For most dioxin congeners under normal conditions, their half-lives in the human body reportedly range from 5 to 15 years (e.g., ATSDR, 1998, 2012b).

16.10.2. Environmental Health Concerns

Dioxins can induce the enzymatic activity of Ah (acryl hydrocarbon) hydroxylase in the liver. They can bind to a cytosolic Ah receptor which is capable of regulating the synthesis of a variety of proteins (Figure 9.2). This receptor is present in many human tissues including the lungs, liver, placenta, and lymphocytes. As pointed out by ATSDR (1998, 2012b), although there is sufficient evidence that the receptor is involved in many biological responses to dioxins, the general notion is that its characteristics alone are not sufficient to account for the complexity and broad spectrum of the biological effects that dioxins have reportedly induced.

In animal studies (*see*, e.g., ATSDR, 1998, 2012b), of which many involved oral exposure, numerous types of adverse health effects were observed as induced by dioxins, including hepatic, skin, hematological, neurological, hormonal, GI, immunological, reproductive, and developmental. Several studies (e.g., Marinković *et al.*, 2010) in humans suggested that exposure to dioxins (at high levels) would cause harm especially to children and the developing fetuses.

308 An Introduction to Environmental Toxicology

As many environmental toxicologists would advise, the most potent of all dioxin congeners is 2,3,7,8-tetrachlorodibenzo-*p(ara)*-dioxin (2,3,7,8-TCDD, TCDD, or *the* dioxin for short). TCDD is also called Seveso dioxin, named after the largest dioxins accident occurring in the world's history. This disaster took place on 10 July 1976 involving an explosion in a chemical plant located in a northern Italian town named Seveso. Following the explosion, a huge cloud of dioxins containing TCDD and some other congeners was reportedly seen being drifted over 100 feet (30.5 m) into the sky. The high concern then was that while Seveso was the place most affected by the explosion, its neighboring towns (Cesano Maderno, Desio, and Meda) were also affected, collectively amounting to over 100,000 residents affected. The most evident adverse health effect, ascertained some 17 years later (Bertazzi, 1991), was 193 cases of chloracne. Other reversible, early effects included peripheral neuropathy and excess liver enzyme induction.

For TCDD's carcinogenicity, several epidemiological studies (*see*, e.g., ATSDR, 1998, 2012b; IARC, 2012) revealed a link between exposure to the dioxin and increase in the mortalities from all types of cancers combined as well as from certain individual cancers such as soft-tissue sarcoma, GI tract, respiratory system, and non-Hodgkin's lymphoma. There were also data showing that the PCDD acted as a tumor promoter. Based on this body of evidence, IARC (2012, 2017) has listed TCDD, along with 2,3,4,7,8-penachlorodibenzofuran, as a human (Group 1) carcinogen.

16.11. Toxic Equivalency Factors

Many dioxin mixtures have been found to include not only *the true* dioxins but also some furan and dioxin-like PCB congeners. These chlorinated compounds reportedly all share the common mechanism of toxicity involving activation of the Ah receptor, though with each having its own potency level. To express such a mixture's *overall* potential for inducing the same (or very similar) adverse biological effect(s), WHO with the scientific assistance of two expert groups (*see* van den Berg *et al.*, 1998, 2006) has developed a toxic equivalency (TEQ) concept for the dioxin and dioxin-like congeners as briefly described in the subsection below.

16.11.1. WHO's Concept of Toxic Equivalency

In essence, WHO's TEQ concept weighs the toxicity (potency) of each of the other congeners in the dioxin mixture as a fraction of the toxicity of the most potent 2,3,7,8-TCDD in humans and other mammalians, with the latter congener given a reference value of 1. Each of these other congeners is thereby attributed a specific *toxic equivalency factor* (TEF) equal to or less than 1. The TEF values that WHO has established for the individual dioxin and dioxin-like congeners are reproduced in Table 16.3. Note that as with certain congeners in the PCBs, some PCNs are thought to have dioxin-like toxicological properties as well. Yet at the present time, none of the PCN congeners has been (officially or commonly) included in the TEF system.

To calculate the *overall* (*total*) TCDD-toxic equivalent concentration of a dioxin mixture containing a total of *n* dioxin and dioxin-like congeners, the concentrations of the individual congeners are multiplied by their own specific (assigned) TEF value, and then *added* up in the manner as shown in Equation 16.1.

Table 16.3. Toxic Equivalency Factors Developed by the World Health Organization (WHO) in 1998 and Updated in 2005 for Dioxin and Dioxin-like Compounds[a]

Dioxin or Dioxin-like Compound	Factor by WHO 1998	Factor by WHO 2005
Polychlorinated Dibenzo-p(ara)-Dioxins (PCDDs)		
2,3,7,8-tetraCDD (a.k.a. 2,3,7,8-TCDD)	1.0	1.0
1,2,3,7,8-pentaCDD	1.0	1.0
1,2,3,4,7,8-hexaCDD	0.1	0.1
1,2,3,6,7,8-hexaCDD	0.1	0.1
1,2,3,7,8,9-hexaCDD	0.1	0.1
1,2,3,4,6,7,8-heptaCDD	0.01	0.01
1,2,3,4,6,7,8,9-octaCDD	0.0001	0.0003
Polychlorinated Dibenzofurans (PCDFs)		
2,3,7,8-tetraCDF (a.k.a. 2,3,7,8-TCDF)	0.1	0.1
1,2,3,7,8-pentaCDF	0.05	0.03
2,3,4,7,8-pentaCDF	0.5	0.3
1,2,3,4,7,8-hexaCDF	0.1	0.1
1,2,3,6,7,8-hexaCDF	0.1	0.1
1,2,3,7,8,9-hexaCDF	0.1	0.1
2,3,4,6,7,8-hexaCDF	0.1	0.1
1,2,3,4,6,7,8-heptaCDF	0.01	0.01
1,2,3,4,7,8,9-heptaCDF	0.01	0.01
1,2,3,4,6,7,8,9-octaCDF	0.0001	0.0003
Nonortho-Substituted Polychlorinated Biphenyls (PCBs)		
PCB 77 (3,3',4,4'-tetraCB)	0.0001	0.0001
PCB 81 (3,4,4',5-tetraCB)	0.0001	0.0003
PCB 126 (3,3',4,4',5-pentaCB)	0.1	0.1
PCB 169 (3,3',4,4',5,5'-hexaCB)	0.01	0.03
Monoortho-Substituted Polychlorinated Biphenyls (PCBs)		
PCB 105 (2,3,3',4,4'-pentaCB)	0.0001	0.00003
PCB 114 (2,3,4,4',5-pentaCB)	0.0005	0.00003
PCB 118 (2,3',4,4',5-pentaCB)	0.0001	0.00003
PCB 123 (2,3',4,4',5'-pentaCB)	0.0001	0.00003
PCB 156 (2,3,3',4,4',5-hexaCB)	0.0005	0.00003
PCB 157 (2,3,3',4,4',5'-hexaCB)	0.0005	0.00003
PCB 167 (2,3',4,4',5,5'-hexaCB)	0.00001	0.00003
PCB 189 (2,3,3',4,4',5,5'-heptaCB)	0.0001	0.00003

[a] for humans and other mammalians; adapted from WHO (van den Berg *et al.*, 1998, 2006).

$$\text{Total (Overall) TCDD-based TEQ} = \Sigma\ C_i \times \text{TEF}_i \tag{16.1}$$

where C_i is the concentration of the ith congener in the mixture. Note that this method is for quantifying specifically the toxic effects mediated by activation of the cellular Ah receptor. Other types of adverse health effects induced by dioxins, furans, or dioxin-like PCBs are not intended to be so quantified.

16.11.2. Application of Toxic Equivalency Factor

The TEF approach developed by WHO offers a methodology in which the potential adverse health effects can be quantified for exposure to a complex mixture of dioxin and dioxin-like compounds. However, this approach should be utilized with caution. The WHO methodology estimates the dioxin-based effects of a mixture by assuming dose-additivity and characterizes the mixture in terms of an equivalent mass of TCDD. The reality is that even though the *mixture* may have the toxicological potential of TCDD, neither it as a single (emission) entity nor its individual non-TCDD constituent congeners can be assumed to undergo the same environmental fate as TCDD would, even for exposure assessment purposes. The fate of a *mixture* in its environment is supposed to be the resultant totality of the fates of all its constituent congeners in their own environment. Yet different congeners generally have different physicochemical properties (e.g., vapor pressure, octanol-water partition coefficient, photolysis rate, binding affinity to organic matter). In other words, it is likely that a mixture's actual as well as absolute concentration for environmental exposure would be different from the calculated sum of the relative concentrations of the mixture's constituent congeners. This is because these relative concentrations are the ones actually made up the emission entity to travel through the environmental media with the congeners each on their own being subject to the effects of various meteorological conditions.

With the above-mentioned uncertainties in mind (particularly that on dose-additivity), in June 2005 an expert meeting was held by WHO/IPCS in Geneva, Switzerland, during which the TEF values were re-assessed for dioxin and dioxin-like compounds. As a result of the re-assessment (van den Berg *et al.*, 2006), WHO advised that the 2005 TEF values be used to replace the ones adopted in 1998. U.S. EPA (2010b) is among the first health regulatory entities to support publicly the utilization of these re-assessed consensus TEF values in the risk assessment for TCDD and dioxin-like compounds. The agency nonetheless has advised that the conduct of a sensitivity analysis be included to illustrate the impact that the TEFs may have on the TEQ value.

In practice, the real consequence of these TEF changes on the TEQ for biotic or abiotic samples of dioxin mixtures has not been looked into seriously or sufficiently. Nonetheless, at least one such evaluation analysis (Hong *et al.*, 2009) was performed nearly a decade ago, by applying the data from a major exposure study in which serum, household dust, and soil levels of dioxin and dioxin-like compounds were measured in several regions of Michigan. The mean total TEQ was found to reduce by 26%, 12%, and 14% for the serum, household dust, and soil samples, respectively, when the TEFs used in the evaluation analysis were based on the 2005 values instead of those available in 1998. The resultant reductions were apparently due to the application of a bulk of the TEFs reassigned a down-weighting value.

References

AMAP (Arctic Monitoring and Assessment Programme), 1997. Arctic Pollution Issues: A State of the Arctic Environment Report. AMAP, Oslo, Norway.

Andersson PL, Blom A, Johannisson A, Pesonen M, Tysklind M, Berg AH, Olsson PE, Norrgren L, 1999. Assessment of PCBs and Hydroxylated PCBs as Potential Xenoestrogens: *In vitro* Studies Based on MCF-7 Cell Proliferation and Induction of Vitellogenin in Primary Culture of Rainbow Trout Hepatocytes. *Arch. Environ. Contam. Toxicol.* 37:145-150.

ATSDR (U.S. Agency for Toxic Substances and Disease Registry), 1994. Toxicological Profile for Hexachlorobutadiene. U.S. Department of Health and Human Services, Atlanta, Georgia, USA.

ATSDR (U.S. Agency for Toxic Substances and Disease Registry), 1998. Toxicological Profile for Chlorinated Dibenzo-*p*-dioxins (CDDs). U.S. Department of Health and Human Services, Atlanta, Georgia, USA.

ATSDR (U.S. Agency for Toxic Substances and Disease Registry), 2004. Toxicological Profile for Polybrominated Biphenyls (PBBs). U.S. Department of Health and Human Services, Atlanta, Georgia, USA.

ATSDR (U.S. Agency for Toxic Substances and Disease Registry), 2012a. Addendum to the Toxicological Profile for Hexachlorobutadiene. U.S. Department of Health and Human Services, Atlanta, Georgia, USA.

ATSDR (U.S. Agency for Toxic Substances and Disease Registry), 2012b. Addendum to the Toxicological Profile for Chlorinated Dibenzo-*p*-dioxins (CDDs). U.S. Department of Health and Human Services, Atlanta, Georgia, USA.

ATSDR (U.S. Agency for Toxic Substances and Disease Registry), 2017. Toxicological Profile for Polybrominated Diphenyl Ethers (PBDEs). U.S. Department of Health and Human Services, Atlanta, Georgia, USA.

Barnes D, Alford-Stevens A, Birnbaum L, Kutz FW, Wood W, Patton D, 1991. Toxicity Equivalency Factors for PCBs? *Qual. Assur.* 1:70-81.

Bekesi JG, Holland JF, Anderson HA, Fischbein AS, Rom W, Wolff MS, Selikoff IJ, 1978. Lymphocyte Function of Michigan Dairy Farmers Exposed to Polybrominated Biphenyls. *Science* 199:1207-1209.

Bertazzi PA, 1991. Long-Term Effects of Chemical Disasters: Lessons and Results from Seveso. *Sci. Total Environ.* 106:5-20.

Blanck HM, Marcus M, Tolbert PE, Rubin C, Henderson AK, Hertzberg VS, Zhang RH, Cameron L, 2000. Age at Menarche and Tanner Stage in Girls Exposed *in utero* and Postnatally to Polybrominated Biphenyl. *Epidemiology* 11:641-647.

Braune BM, Mallory ML, Gilchrist HG, Letcher RJ, Drouillard KG, 2007. Levels and Trends of Organochlorines and Brominated Flame Retardants in Ivory Gull Eggs from the Canadian Arctic, 1976 to 2004. *Sci. Total Environ.* 378:403-417.

BSEF (Bromine Science and Environmental Forum), 2000. An Introduction to Brominated Flame Retardants. 37 Square de Meeûs, 1000 Brussels, Belgium.

Burkatskaya EN, Viter VF, Ivanova ZV, Kaskevitch LM, Gorskaya NZ, Kolpakov IE, Deineka KA, 1982. Clinico-Hygienic Data on Working Conditions during Use of Hexachlorobutadiene in Vineyards *Vrach. Delo.* 11:99-102 (in Russian, cited from UNEP, 2012b).

Calafat AM, Wong L-Y, Kuklenyik Z, Reidy JA, Needham L, 2007. Polyfluoroalkyl Chemicals in the U.S. Population: Data from the National Health and Nutrition Examination Survey (NHANES) 2003-2004 and Comparisons to NHANES 1999-2000. *Environ. Health Perspect.* 115:1596-1602.

CEPA (Canadian Environmental Protection Act of 1999), 2000. Persistence and Bioaccumulation Regulations (SOR/2000-107; 29/3/ 2000). *Canada Gazette* Part II, 134(7):607-612.

Cheek AO, Kow K, Chen J, McLachlan JA, 1999. Potential Mechanisms of Thyroid Disruption in Humans: Interaction of Organochlorine Compounds with Thyroid Receptor, Transthyretin, and Thyroid-Binding Globulin. *Environ. Health Perspect.* 107:273-278.

ECCC (Environment and Climate Change Canada), 2011. Risk Management Approach for Polychlorinated Naphthalenes (PCNs). Gatineau, Quebec K1A 0H3, Canada.

ECCC (Environment and Climate Change Canada), 2016. Federal Environmental Quality Guidelines: Hexabromocyclododecane (HBCD). Gatineau, Quebec K1A 0H3, Canada.

ECHA (European Chemicals Agency), 2016. Guidance on Information Requirements and Chemical Safety Assessment – Chapter R.11: PBT/vPvB Assessment (draft V3.0). PO Box 400, FI-00121 Helsinki, Finland.

Ema M, Fujii S, Hirata-Koizumi M, Mastumoto M, 2008. Two-Generation Reproductive Toxicity Study of the Flame Retardant Hexabromocyclododecane in Rats. *Reprod. Toxicol.* 25:335-351.

Eriksson P, Jakobsson E, Fredriksson A, 2001. Brominated Flame Retardants: A Novel Class of Developmental Neurotoxicants in Our Environment? *Environ. Health Perspect.* 109:903-908.

Eriksson P, Viberg H, Jakobsson E, Örn U, Fredriksson A, 2002. A Brominated Flame Retardant, 2,2',4,4',5-Pentabromodiphenyl Ether: Uptake, Retention, and Induction of Neurobehavioral Alterations in Mice during a Critical Phase of Neonatal Brain Development. *Toxicol. Sci.* 67:98-103.

Eriksson P, Fischer C, Wallin M, Jakobsson E, Fredriksson A, 2006. Impaired Behaviour, Learning and Memory, in Adult Mice Neonatally Exposed to Hexabromocyclododecane (HBCDD). *Environ. Toxicol. Pharmacol.* 21:317-322.

European Commission, 2003. Technical Guidance Document on Risk Assessment. EUR 20418 EN/2. Joint Research Centre, Institute for Health and Consumer Protection, European Chemical Bureau, Ispra, Italy.

European Commission, 2008. Risk Assessment: Hexabromocyclododecane. Office for Official Publications of the European Communities, Luxembourg, Luxembourg.

Ewald G, Larsson P, Linge H, Okla L, Szarzi N, 1998. Biotransport of Organic Pollutants to an Inland Alaska Lake by Migrating Sockeye Salmon (*Onchorhynchus nerka*). *Arctic* 51:478-485.

Fängström B, Athanassiadis I, Odsjö T, Norén K, Bergman A, 2008. Temporal Trends of Polybrominated Diphenyl Ethers and Hexabromocyclododecane in Milk from Stockholm Mothers, 1980-2004. *Mol. Nutri. Food Res.* 52:187-193.

Fernie KJ, Shutt JL, Letcher RJ, Ritchie IJ, Bird DM, 2009. Environmentally Relevant Concentrations of DE-71 and HBCD Alter Eggshell Thickness and Reproductive Success of American Kestrels. *Environ. Sci. Technol.* 15:2124-2130.

Fries GF, 1985. The PBB Episode in Michigan: An Overall Appraisal. *Crit. Rev. Toxicol.* 16:105-156.

Han Z-X, Wang N, Zhang H-L, Zhao Y-X, 2017. Bioaccumulation of PBDEs and PCBs in a Small Food Chain at Electronic Waste Recycling Sites. *J. Environ. Forensics* 18:44-49.

Harley KG, Marks AR, Chevrier J, Bradman A, Sjödin A, Eskenazi B, 2010. PBDE Concentrations in Women's Serum and Fecundability. *Environ. Health Perspect.* 118:699-704.

Health Canada, 2006. Perfluorooctane Sulfonate, Its Salts and Its Precursors That Contain the $C_3F_{17}SO_2$ or $C_3F_{17}SO_3$ Moiety. Ottawa, Ontario, K1A 0K9, Canada.

Heeb NV, Schweizer WB, Kohler M, Gerecke AC, 2005. Structure Elucidation of Hexabromocyclododecanes – A Class of Compounds with a Complex Stereochemistry. *Chemosphere* 61:65-73.

Hong B, Garabrant D, Hedgeman E, Demond A, Gillespie B, Chen Q, Chang CW, Towey T, Knutson K, Franzblau A, *et al.*, 2009. Impact of WHO 2005 Revised Toxic Equivalency Factors for Dioxins on the TEQs in Serum, Household Dust and Soil. *Chemosphere* 76:723-733.

IARC (International Agency for Research on Cancer), 1999. IARC Monographs on the Evaluation of Carcinogenic Risks to Humans, Volume 73: Some Chemicals That Cause Tumours of the Kidney or Urinary Bladder in Rodents and Some Other Substances. Lyon, France: WHO Press.

IARC (International Agency for Research on Cancer), 2012. IARC Monographs on the Evaluation of Carcinogenic Risks to Humans, Volume 100F: Chemical Agents and Related Occupations. Lyon, France: WHO Press.

IARC (International Agency for Research on Cancer), 2016a. IARC Monographs on the Evaluation of Carcinogenic Risks to Humans, Volume 110: Some Chemicals Used as Solvents and in Polymer Manufacture. Lyon, France: WHO Press.

IARC (International Agency for Research on Cancer), 2016b. IARC Monographs on the Evaluation of Carcinogenic Risks to Humans, Volume 107: Polychlorinated Biphenyls and Polybrominated Biphenyls. Lyon, France: WHO Press.

IARC (International Agency for Research on Cancer), 2017. IARC Monographs on the Evaluation of Carcinogenic Risks to Humans, Volume 1-119: List of Carcinogens. Lyon, France: WHO Press.

IJC (International Joint Commission), 2003. Long-Range Transport of Toxic Substances into the Great Lakes Basin. IJC's 2003 Great Lakes Conference Workshop, 16-17 September, Ann Arbor, Michigan, USA.

IPCS (International Programme on Chemical Safety), 1994. Hexachlorobutadiene (Environmental Health Criteria 156). World Health Organization, Geneva, Switzerland.

IPCS (International Programme on Chemical Safety), 2001. Chlorinated Naphthalenes (Concise International Chemical Assessment Document 34). World Health Organization, Geneva, Switzerland.

IPCS (International Programme on Chemical Safety), 2003. Polychlorinated Biphenyls: Human Health Aspects (Concise International Chemical Assessment Document 55). World Health Organization, Geneva, Switzerland.

Kilanowicz A, Wiaderna D, Lutz P, Szymczak W, 2012. Behavioral Effects Following Repeated Exposure to Hexachloronaphthalene in Rats. *Neurotoxicology* 33:361-369.

Kociba RJ, Keyes DG, Jersey GC, Ballard JJ, Dittenber DA, Quast JF, Wade CE, Humiston CG, Schwetz BA, 1977. Results of a Two Year Chronic Toxicity Study with Hexachlorobutadiene in Rats. *Am. Ind. Hyg. Assoc. J.* 38:589-602.

Kodavanti PR, Ward TR, McKinney JD, Tilson HA, 1996. Inhibition of Microsomal and Mitochondrial Ca^{2+}-Sequestration in Rat Cerebellum by Polychlorinated Biphenyl Mixtures and Congeners: Structure-Activity Relationships. *Arch. Toxicol.* 70:150-157.

Kohler M, Zennegg M, Bogdal C, Gerecke AC, Schmid P, Heeb NV, Sturm M, Vonmont H, Kohler HE, Giger W, 2008. Temporal Trends, Congener Patterns, and Sources of Octa-, Nona-, and Decabromodiphenyl Ethers (PBDE) and Hexabromocyclododecanes (HBCD) in Swiss Lake Sediments. *Environ. Sci. Technol.* 42:6378-6384.

Krasniuk EP, Ziritskaya LA, Bioko VG, Voitenko GA, Matokhniuk LA, 1969. Health Conditions of Vine-Growers Contacting with Fumigants Hexachlorobutadiene and Polychlorbutan-80. *Vrach. Delo.* 7:111-115 (in Russian, cited from UNEP, 2012b).

Maas R, Grennfelt P (Eds.), 2016. Towards Cleaner Air – Scientific Assessment Report 2016. EMEP Steering Body and Working Group on Effects of the Convention on Long-Range Transboundary Air Pollution, Olso, Norway.

Marinković N, Pašalić D, Ferenčak G, Gršković B, Stavljenić Rukavina A, 2010. Dioxins and Human Toxicity. *Arh. Hig. Rada. Toksikol.* (*Arch. Ind. Hyg. Toxicol.*) 61:445-453.

Matthies M, Scheringer M, 2001. *Editorial*: Long-Range Transport in the Environment. *Environ. Sci. Pollut. Res.* 8:149-149.

Mills SA 3rd, Thal DI, Barney J, 2007. A Summary of the 209 PCB Congener Nomenclature. *Chemosphere* 68:1603-1612.

Minh NH, Isobe T, Ueno D, Matsumoto K, Mine M, Kajiwara N, Takahashi S, Tanabe S, 2007. Spatial Distribution and Vertical Profile of Polybrominated Diphenyl Ethers and Hexabromocyclododecanes in Sediment Core from Tokyo Bay, Japan. *Environ. Pollut.* 148:409-417.

Morris S, Allchin CR, Zegers BN, Haftka JJ, Boon JP, Belpaire C, Leonards PE, Van Leeuwen SP, de Boer J, 2004. Distribution and Fate of HBCD and TBBPA Brominated Flame Retardants in North Sea Estuaries and Aquatic Food Webs. *Environ. Sci. Technol.* 38:5497-5504.

Olsen GW, Burris JM, Burlew MM, Mandel JH, 2003. Epidemiologic Assessment of Worker Serum Perfluorooctanesulfonate (PFOS) and Perfluorooctanoate (PFOA) Concentrations and Medical Surveillance. *J. Occup. Environ. Med.* 45:260-270.

Palace VP, Pleskach K, Halldorson T, Danell RW, Wautier K, Evans B, Alaee M, Marvin C, Tomy GT, 2008. Biotransformation Enzymes and Thyroid Axis Disruption in Juvenile Rainbow Trout (*Oncorhynchus mykiss*) Exposed to Hexabromocyclododecane Diastereoisomers. *Environ. Sci. Technol.* 42:1967-1972.

Peden-Adams MM, Keller JM, EuDaly JG, Berger J, Gilkeson GS, Keil DE, 2008. Suppression of Humoral Immunity in Mice Following Exposure to Perfluorooctane Sulfonate (PFOS). *Toxicol. Sci.* 104:144-154.

Peden-Adams MM, Stuckey JE, Gaworecki KM, Berger-Ritchie J, Bryant K, Jodice PG, Scott TR, Ferrario JB, Guan B, Vigo C, et al., 2009. Developmental Toxicity in White Leghorn Chickens Following *in ovo* Exposure to Perfluorooctane Sulfonate (PFOS). *Reprod. Toxicol.* 27:307-318.

Ronisz D, Farmen FE, Karlsson H, Förlin L, 2004. Effects of the Brominated Flame Retardants Hexabromocyclododecane (HBCD) and Tetrabromobisphenol A (TBBPA), on Hepatic Enzymes and Other Biomarkers in Juvenile Rainbow Trout and Feral Eelpout. *Aquat. Toxicol.* 69:229-245.

Roosens L, Cornelis C, D'Hollander W, Bervoets L, Reynders H, Van Campenhout K, Van Den Heuvel R, Neels H, Covaci A, 2010. Exposure of the Flemish Population to Brominated Flame Retardants: Model and Risk Assessment. *Environ. Intl.* 36:368-376.

Ryan JJ, Masuda Y, 1994. Polychlorinated Naphthalenes (PCNs) in the Rice Oil Poisonings. *Organohalogen Compounds* 21:251-254.

Shain W, Bush B, Seegal R, 1991. Neurotoxicity of Polychlorinated Biphenyls: Structure-Activity Relationship of Individual Congeners. *Toxicol. Appl. Pharmacol.* 111:33-42.

Sjödin A, Wong LY, Jones RS, Park A, Zhang Y, Hodge C, DiPietro E, McClure C, Turner W, Needham LL, Patterson DG Jr, 2008. Serum Concentrations of Polybrominated Diphenyl Ethers (PBDEs) and Polybrominated Biphenyl (PBB) in the United States Population: 2003-2004. *Environ. Sci. Technol.* 42:1377-1384.

Takemura T, Uno I, Nakajima T, Higurashi A, Sano I, 2002. Modeling Study of Long-Range Transport of Asian Dust and Anthropogenic Aerosols from East Asia. *Geophy. Res. Letters.* 29:2158-2161.

Tomy GT, Budakowski W, Halldorson T, Whittle DM, Keir MJ, Marvin C, MacInnis G, Alaee M, 2004. Biomagnification of α- and γ-Hexabromocyclododecane Isomers in a Lake Ontario Food Web. *Environ. Sci. Technol.* 38:2298-2303.

Tomy GT, Pleskach K, Oswald T, Halldorson T, Helm PA, MacInnis G, Marvin CH, 2008. Enantioselective Bioaccumulation of Hexabromocyclododecane and Congener-Specific Accumulation of Brominated Diphenyl Ethers in an Eastern Canadian Arctic Marine Food Web. *Environ. Sci. Technol.* 42:3634-3639.

U.K. DEFRA (U.K. Department for Environmental, Food, and Rural Affairs), 2002. Chemicals Stakeholder Forum Meetings – First Meeting of the UK Chemicals Stakeholders Forum: 2nd October 2000 Criteria for Concern CSF/00/7. London, UK.

UNECE (United Nations Economic Commission for Europe), 2004. Handbook for the 1979 Convention on Long-Range Transboundary Air Pollution and Its Protocols. Section XI (Recent Decisions of the Executive Body), Decision 1998/2 (ECE/EB.Air/60). Geneva, Switzerland, p.299.

UNEP (United Nations Environmental Programme), 2001. Final Act of the Conference of Plenipotentiaries on the Stockholm Convention on Persistent Organic Pollutants (dated 5 June). Geneva, Switzerland, p.41.

UNEP (United Nations Environmental Programme), 2006a. Risk Profile on Perfluorooctane Sulfonate. Report of the Persistent Organic Pollutants Review Committee on the Work of Its Second Meeting (Addendum), Geneva, Switzerland.

UNEP (United Nations Environmental Programme), 2006b. Risk Profile on Hexabromobiphenyl. Report of the Persistent Organic Pollutants Review Committee on the Work of Its Second Meeting (Addendum), Geneva, Switzerland.

UNEP (United Nations Environmental Programme), 2006c. Risk Profile on Pentabromodiphenyl Ether. Report of the Persistent Organic Pollutants Review Committee on the Work of Its Second Meeting (Addendum), Geneva, Switzerland.

UNEP (United Nations Environmental Programme), 2010. Risk Profile on Hexabromocyclododecane. Report of the Persistent Organic Pollutants Review Committee on the Work of Its Sixth Meeting (Addendum), Geneva, Switzerland.

UNEP (United Nations Environmental Programme), 2012a. Risk Profile on Chlorinated Naphthalenes. Report of the Persistent Organic Pollutants Review Committee on the Work of Its Eighth Meeting (Addendum), Geneva, Switzerland.

UNEP (United Nations Environmental Programme), 2012b. Risk Profile on Hexachlorobutadiene. Report of the Persistent Organic Pollutants Review Committee on the Work of Its Eighth Meeting (Addendum), Geneva, Switzerland.

Uno I, Eguchi K, Yumimoto K, Takemura T, Shimizu A, Uematsu M, Liu Z, Wang Z, Hara Y, Sugimoto N, 2009. Asian Dust Transported One Full Circuit around the Globe. *Nature Geosci.* 2:557-560.

U.S. EPA (U.S. Environmental Protection Agency), 1975. Environmental Hazard Assessment Report: Chlorinated Naphthalenes. EPA-560/8-75-001. Office of Toxic Substances, Washington DC, USA.

U.S. EPA (U.S. Environmental Protection Agency), 1988. Evaluation of the Potential Carcinogenicity of Hexachlorobutadiene. EPA/600/8-91/139. Office of Health and Environmental Assessment, Washington DC, USA.

U.S. EPA (U.S. Environmental Protection Agency), 1999a. Persistent Bioaccumulative Toxic (PBT) Chemicals; Lowering of Reporting Thresholds for Certain PBT Chemicals; Addition of Certain PBT Chemicals; Community Right-to-Know Toxic Chemical Reporting. *Federal Register* 64:58666-58753.

U.S. EPA (U.S. Environmental Protection Agency), 1999b. Category for Persistent, Bioaccumulative, and Toxic New Chemical Substances. *Federal Register* 64:60194-60204.

U.S. EPA (U.S. Environmental Protection Agency), 2010a. Hexabromocyclododecane (HBCD) – Action Plan. Office of Pollution Prevention and Toxics, Washington DC, USA.

U.S. EPA (U.S. Environmental Protection Agency), 2010b. Recommended Toxicity Equivalence Factors (TEFs) for Human Health Risk Assessment of 2,3,7,8-Tetrachlorodibenzo-*p*-Dioxin and Dioxin-Like Compounds. EPA/100/R-10/005. Office of the Science Advisor, Washington DC, USA.

U.S. EPA (U.S. Environmental Protection Agency), 2016a. Drinking Water Health Advisory for Perfluorooctane Sulfonate (PFOS). EPA Document No. 822-R-16-004. Office of Water, Washington DC, USA.

U.S. EPA (U.S. Environmental Protection Agency), 2016b. Health Effects Support Document for Perfluorooctane Sulfonate (PFOS). EPA Document No. 822-R-16-002. Office of Water, Washington DC, USA.

van den Berg M, Birnbaum L, Bosveld AT, Brunstrom B, Cook P, Feeley M, Giesy JP, Hanberg A, Hasegawa R, Kennedy SW, *et al.*, 1998. Toxic Equivalency Factors (TEFs) for PCBs, PCDDs, PCDFs for Humans and Wildlife. *Environ. Health Perspect.* 106:775-792.

van den Berg M, Birnbaum LS, Denison M, De Vito M, Farland W, Feeley M, Fiedler H, Hakansson H, Hanberg A, Haws L, *et al.*, 2006. The 2005 World Health Organization Re-evaluation of Human and Mammalian Toxic Equivalency Factors for Dioxins and Dioxin-like Compounds. *Toxicol. Sci.* 93:223-241.

Ward EM, Ruder AM, Suruda A, Smith AB, Halperin W, Fessler CA, Zahm SH, 1994. Cancer Mortality Patterns among Female and Male Workers Employed in a Cable Manufacturing Plant during World War II. *J. Occup. Med.* 36:860-866.

Xing GH, Chan JK, Leung AO, Wu SC, Wong MH, 2009. Environmental Impact and Human Exposure to PCBs in Guiyu, an Electronic Waste Recycling Site in China. *Environ. Intl.* 35:76-82.

Yi S, Liu JG, Jin J, Zhu J, 2016. Assessment of the Occupational and Environmental Risks of Hexabromocyclododecane (HBCD) in China. *Chemosphere* 150:431-437.

Zhang X, Yang F, Zhang X, Xu Y, Liao T, Song S, Wang J, 2008. Induction of Hepatic Enzymes and Oxidative Stress in Chinese Rare Minnow (Gobiocypris rarus) Exposed to Waterborne Hexabromocyclododecane (HBCDD). *Aquat. Toxicol.* 86:4-11.

Zhang Y, Sun H, Ruan Y, 2014. Enantiomer-Specific Accumulation, Depuration, Metabolization and Isomerization of Hexabromocyclododecane (HBCD) Diastereomers in Mirror Carp from Water. *J. Hazard. Mater.* 264:8-15.

Zhao G, Wang Z, Dong MH, Rao K, Luo J, Wang D, Zha J, Huang S, Xu Y, Ma M, 2008. PBBs, PBDEs, and PCBs Levels in Hair of Residents around E-Waste Disassembly Sites in Zhejiang Province, China, and Their Potential Sources. *Sci. Total Environ.* 397:46-57.

Zhou T, Taylor MM, DeVito MJ, Croftonr KM, 2002. Developmental Exposure to Brominated Diphenyl Ethers Results in Thyroid Hormone Disruption. *Toxicol. Sci.* 66:105-116.

Review Questions

1. Define the term *half-life* in relation to environmental persistence.
2. What are the main differences between the two major aspects of persistence for pollutants present in the environment?
3. How is long-range transport potential of pollutants related to their persistence and bioaccumulation potential in the environment?
4. What are the main differences among PTS, PBTs, POPs, and POCs?
5. Which of the following health authorities appear(s) to be more health conservative with respect to their prevention and control of PTS or PBTs? a) UNEP; b) CEPA; c) European Commission; d) U.S. EPA; e) UNECE; f) U.K. DEFRA; g) ECHA.
6. Name the so-termed *dirty dozen* POPs on the Stockholm Convention's initial priority list, and those added to the list between 2004 and 2015 (i.e., as of 2017).
7. Name the global treaty that has *provided* the technical guidelines on waste management for POPs.

8. Briefly describe the programs and strategies being taken by the Stockholm Convention of 2001 for containing the pollution of the POPs placed on its priority/action list.
9. What are the likely sources of environmental exposure to PFOS?
10. How is PFOS structurally different from PFOA and PFOS-F? And how is it biochemically different from the other non-fluorinated POPs in terms of bioaccumulation?
11. What may be the major types of toxic effects of PFOS in humans?
12. How many congeners of PBBs, PBDEs, and PCBs are theoretically possible, and why? Also, why do the *deca*BB, *deca*BDE, and *deca*CB homologs each have only one congener?
13. What are the likely sources of environmental exposure to PBBs worldwide?
14. What may be the major adverse health effects of PBBs on humans, as evident from the massive PBB contamination of livestock feed in Michigan (USA) during 1973-1974?
15. What may be the major adverse health effects of PBDEs on humans?
16. What is commercial-based *penta*BDE commonly used for? And which of the following congener pairs is typically contained in this commercial mixture? a) PBDE 180, PBDE 203; b) PBDE 47, PBDE 99; c) PBDE 47, PBDE 153; d) PBDE 99, PBDE 180; e) PBDE 153, PBDE 203.
17. Which of the following PBDE homologs is still widely produced and used in the United States today? a) *tetra*BDE; b) *penta*BDE; c) *hexa*BDE; d) *octa*BDE; e) *deca*BDE.
18. Among the three main diastereoisomers of hexabromocyclododecane (HBCD) congeners, which is reportedly more bioaccumulative and which is more abundant in the environment?
19. What are the main differences between *coplanar* and *nonplanar* PCB congeners, and between *ortho*-substituted and non*ortho*-substituted PCB congeners?
20. What may be the major adverse health effects of OH-PCBs on humans?
21. What is the likely explanation for U.S. EPA not being current with its environmental hazard assessment for polychlorinated naphthalenes (PCNs)? How many possible congeners can be in the PCN family?
22. Among all the possible *homologs* of polychlorinated butadienes (PCBDs), which one(s) has (have) been added to the Stockholm Convention's action list?
23. What is the widely accepted common mechanism of toxicity shared by both the dioxins and the dioxin-like PCB congeners?
24. Why does the PCDD family have fewer possible congeners than the PCDF family has?
25. What seems to be the (one) major environmental source for dioxins found in these days? And where in today's environment can dioxins be *detected*?
26. What is the main source of exposure to dioxins for the general population?
27. Which congener in the dioxin family is regarded as the most potent? Briefly describe this congener's major adverse health effects on humans.
28. Which of the following pairs of POPs is *least likely* to be found in e-waste? a) HBCD, PFOS-F; b) PBBs, PBDEs; c) PBBs, PCBs; d) PBDEs, PCBs; e) PCBs, PCDFs.
29. What is the *overall* TCDD-toxic *equivalent* concentration of a dioxin mixture in fish tissue containing (ppt ≡ parts per trillion): 10 ppt of TCDD; 20 ppt of 1,2,3,6,7,8-*hexa*CDF; 30 ppt of PCB 113; and 40 ppt of PCB 81?

CHAPTER 17

Biological and Underrated Physical Toxic Agents

ஓ•ஒ

17.1. Introduction

This chapter serves as a reminder that in some parts of the world, there are as many biological and physical toxic agents as there are toxic chemical substances in the environment. Fortunately or not, nowadays many of these nonchemical toxic agents such as malaria and guinea worm parasites are not commonly found in well-developed regions where environmental toxicology practice is more active. Yet perhaps as some form of trade-off, certain other nonchemical hazards such as traffic congestion and noise pollution have been causing environmental health problems predominately in many advanced and developing countries.

In this chapter as due to space limitation, only two underrated physical hazards along with the general biological toxic agents are discussed categorically following the clarifications given on several terms, concepts, and definitions that are deemed crucial to the conception of biological toxic agents. First off, as to be consistent with legal (U.S. Code, 2013) and proper (e.g., Gillard, 2001; Section 1.1.1) usage, the term *toxins* will refer to poisonous, mostly proteinaceous products of the biologic activities of a *living* organism. Furthermore, when the toxins are delivered by an organism to its victim by means of a bite or sting, they are specifically termed *venoms*. In contrast, the term *toxicants* are defined as about all the toxic materials including toxins. Certainly, there are still some people, particularly those in the nonscientific sectors (e.g., media), who would include mercury (Hg) and other chemical agents as toxins found in living organisms.

17.1.1. Concepts of Biological Toxic Agents

The term "*nonchemical agent*", as inferred to in this chapter, also needs clarification. For instance, the most critical constituents in snake venoms are proteolytic enzymes (Section 17.6.1), which literally are all (*bio*)*chemical* substances. The argument here is that the *agent* to which the *exposure* is of immediate concern involves the snake or its bite, not so much its proteolytic enzymes which are nevertheless still biological *in origin* if not in nature. The same argument holds true for the mycotoxin aflatoxin B_1 discussed in Section 17.3.2.

It is also important to realize that biological toxic agents refer to all living matters including organisms *per se* that cause harm, not only the natural toxins that they produce. Although some microbes can produce fatal toxins in humans or other organisms, they or some others can be even more harmful on their own. Research (e.g., Ghoneum and Felo, 2015; HHMI, 2002) has shown that overgrowth of certain types of bacteria (e.g., certain species of *Lactobacillus*) in a body tissue can lead to the development of gastric cancer or other serious disorders (e.g., stomach ulcers) at that very site, signifying the toxic mechanism of *direct* (bacterial) damage (Section 9.1.2).

Furthermore, to avoid confusion, those superficially comparable terms such as *toxins from fish* and *fish toxins* are not used interchangeably in this chapter, as they can mean different things to different people. For instance, many tribal hunters employ various fish toxins, such as fish stupefying plants, to paralyze fish so that their captives would become easier to be caught by hand. In contrast, certain highly potent toxins, such as tetrodotoxin and ciguatoxin (Section 17.4.1), can be found *in* certain species of fish and shellfish.

17.1.2. Infection *vs.* Infectious Disease

Another relevant point for clarification here is that infection and infectious disease do not mean exactly the same thing, but are often loosely used interchangeably to facilitate the discussion only. In reality, infection takes place when a pathogen enters a host's body to start colonizing. In contrast, the disease as a result of the infection occurs only if the microbe starts to multiply aggressively to the level that certain symptoms manifest. The body of most any mammalian host, including that of a human, has high capacity to fight off microbial invasion. Diseases result only when these protective mechanisms are compromised. An infection is thereby the invasion and the colonization by a microbial agent in the host organism, whereas an infectious disease occurs only when the colonization becomes aggressive. In an infection, the pathogen seeks to utilize the resources in the host to multiply. The pathogen can interfere with the normal functioning of the host leading to acute or chronic symptoms, tissue necrosis, loss of an infected limb, or death.

As still another confusion to avoid where practical, some people may argue that a pandemic of infectious disease is of concern more to public health practitioners than to environmental toxicologists. Yet the declaration of a disease pandemic is almost always based on some form of environmental health risk assessment which, as stated in Chapter 3, has preoccupied the field of environmental toxicology for several decades. As also noted in Chapter 3, for these pandemics, both the laboratory confirmation of the infecting microbial agent (or technically referred to as pathogen) and the development of a virus vaccine are directly related to toxicity testing, the role of a toxicologist with the appropriate training.

17.2. Pathogenic Microbial Agents

Infectious diseases as a single entity kill far more people worldwide than any other cause. The microbial agents responsible for diseases of this type are tiny living organisms that are present everywhere in the environment. Infectious diseases are also called communicable or transmissible diseases owing to their potential for transmission from one person or one species to another by a replicating agent (as opposed to a toxin produced by a specific microbe). People can be infected by touching, drinking, eating, or inhaling something contaminated by microbes which are more commonly known as germs to the general public. Germs can also spread through kissing, sexual contact, and animal or insect bites. Most pathogenic agents can be classified into the following four microbe groups: bacteria, viruses, fungi, and protozoa. Pathogenic agents of special or uncommon groups include viroids and prions. Viroids are each composed exclusively of a single piece of circular single-stranded RNA which frequently contains some double-stranded regions.

These RNA (Chapter 18) strands cause mostly plant diseases but recently have been found causing diseases in humans as well. Prions are mis-folded proteins. They have been implicated for causing BSE (bovine spongiform encephalopathy), which is also commonly known as mad-cow disease (Chapter 1). Due to their simplified structures, both prions and viroids are frequently called subviral particles.

In medical microbiology, the causal relationship between a pathogen and an infectious disease is supposed to be confirmed by a set of widely accepted criteria known as the Henle-Koch postulates which specify certain conditions that must be fulfilled (e.g., Evans, 1976). These conditions are: (1) The agent (i.e., the pathogen) must be present in all cases suffering from the disease, but not (sufficiently) in subjects without the disease; (2) the agent must be isolated from the infected host and then grown (successfully) in pure culture *in vitro*; (3) when such a culture is inoculated into a healthy susceptible (animal) host, the disease must be reproducible; and (4) the agent must be recoverable from the experimentally infected (animal) host.

17.2.1. Pathogenic Bacteria

Bacteria are microscopic, single-celled organisms having a shape or an appearance looking like a ball, rod, or spiral. Thousands of different bacterial species are living in virtually every conceivable environment around the world, with some found living even in radioactive wastes. For diagnostic identification purposes and where appropriate, bacterial species are differentiated into two main groups termed *Gram-positive* and *Gram-negative* on the basis of their cell wall's stainability into violet-like color or not, respectively, via a procedure known as the Gram method (e.g., Holt, 1994). The major symptoms of bacterial infection are localized redness, swelling, pains, and discharges in the affected area.

Although a vast majority of the bacteria are harmless to humans and (other) animals, some are highly pathogenic. One bacterial infection with the most disease burden worldwide even today is tuberculosis, caused by the species *Mycobacterium tuberculosis*. According to the recent estimation by the World Health Organization (WHO, 2016), this disease in 2015 killed some 1.4 million people worldwide who were tested negative with human immunodeficiency virus (HIV). Other bacterial diseases of global concern include pneumonia caused by the genera *Streptococcus* and *Pseudomonas*, and foodborne illnesses by the genera *Campylobacter*, *Salmonella*, and *Shigella*. Botulism, tetanus, typhoid fever, syphilis, and diphtheria are examples of serious diseases that are now more or less confined to local regions.

The common pathogenic species of regional or local concerns include: *Escherichia coli (E. coli); Helicobacter pylori (H. pylori); Haemophilus influenzae (H. influenzae)*; and those in the *Staphylococci* (Staph), *Streptococci* (Strep), as well as *Salmonella* genera. In particular, *E. coli* tends to cause gastrointestinal (GI) dysfunctions, as it tends to colonize the GI tract in the human or animal body. This species can also cause food poisoning when transmitted via contaminated food products (e.g., hamburger). *H. pylori* is a main culprit for stomach ulcers. *H. influenzae* is one of the most common bacterial species affecting the human body. The associated symptoms include several types of meningitis and infection of the ear as well as the respiratory tract (without the flu). Children are now often immunized against one of its strains named *H. influenzae* type b.

Many strains of Staph bacteria live harmlessly in or on the human body. However, some others can cause infection and eventually disease. Symptoms from this type of infection (or more correctly diseases) include skin rash, boil, abscess, eczema, and impetigo. Some Staph varieties can cause inflammation of the breast known as mastitis (that releasing the bacteria to the mother's milk) to cause complications for the infant's health. Methicillin-resistant *Staphylococcus aureus*, more often known by its acronym MRSA, gets its name because this Staph species has mutated over time to a different strain ending with a resistance to methicillin as well as numerous other antibiotics used to treat it. MRSA can cause serious skin infection that becomes difficult to treat. On the other hand, a large number of *Salmonella* species are foodborne pathogens that can cause diarrhea and other common symptoms of food poisoning. Undercooked poultry, eggs, and ground beef are common causes (as well as sources) of *Salmonella* infection. Also commonly found in a local or regional environment are several Strep species that can cause the more familiar Strep throat infection and other common respiratory infections (e.g., pneumonia).

17.2.2. Pathogenic Viruses

Most viruses are each about one hundred times smaller than an average bacterium, thus being too small to be seen even with a light microscope. They each consist of the following two or three parts known collectively as virion or viral particle: (1) the genetic material made from either at times DNA (Chapter 18) or mostly RNA (Chapter 18); (2) a protein coat that protects this genetic material; and (3) in some cases a lipid-like envelope surrounding the protein coat when the latter is outside of the living cell. While viruses can replicate only inside the living cells of an organism's body, they are able to infect all parts and all forms of living organisms, from animals and plants of high order to bacteria and archaea. The viral species are reportedly in the millions, of which roughly 5,000 have been investigated in some detail.

Viruses spread in many ways. Plant viruses are typically transmitted from plant to plant by insects such as aphids that feed on sap, whereas animal viruses can be carried by blood-sucking insects commonly referred to as vectors. Influenza viruses in humans are spread largely by sneezes and coughs. The norovirus and rotavirus, which are common causes of viral gastroenteritis (a.k.a. stomach flu, characterized by vomiting and watery diarrhea for up to 1 week), are found in the stool or the vomit of infected people and in contaminated foods or drinks. HIV is one of several viruses transmitted via sexual contact or by exposure to contaminated blood.

A viral infection in humans can cause illness as mild as the common cold and as severe as encephalitis, AIDS (acquired immune deficiency syndrome), and death. In general, viral diseases are systemic, in that they eventually involve many different parts of the body at around the same time. Many viral infections provoke an immunological response capable of eliminating the infecting virus. Immunological responses can also be induced by vaccines which confer an artificially acquired immunity to the specific or a certain type of viral invasion. Some viral pathogens such as those causing AIDS and hepatitis unfortunately can sidestep the immunological response to result in chronic or fatal infectious diseases.

Some viruses do not kill the host cell but alter its biochemical functions instead. Sometimes the infected cell loses its control over normal cell division and becomes cancerous. Some viruses leave their genetic material in the host cell where the material remains dormant for an extended period (to result potentially in a latent infection). When the host cell is sufficiently disturbed, the dormant viral material may begin replicating again and cause disease. Most viruses initially infect one particular type of cells, such as cold viruses infecting predominately cells of the upper respiratory tract. Most viruses also infect a few species of plants or animals only, with some others infecting only people.

The most common viral infections are those of the nose, throat, and upper airways, with symptoms including sore throat, sinusitis, and common cold. Influenza (a.k.a. flu) is a viral respiratory infection tending to cause severe symptoms in infants, older people, and people with other health problems.

Viruses that infect the human nervous system include those causing Japanese, St. Louis, rabies, and several other types of encephalitis. Viral infections can occur around the skin, sometimes resulting in warts or other blemishes. Other types of viral infections commonly found in humans include those caused by the various species of human herpesviruses (HHVs) that normally remain within a host cell in a dormant state. During the host's lifetime, any of these HHVs can become reactivated to cause disease (again).

17.2.3. Pathogenic Fungi

Fungi are a large collection of eukaryotic organisms (i.e., those whose cells contain complex structures enclosed within their membrane) that live in the air, soils, water, or on plants as well as other moist and humid surfaces. Much more so than bacteria, they can be carried by pets or inanimate objects (e.g., combs, brushes, pillows, shoes, towels). Some fungi can reproduce via spores (i.e., tiny reproductive body) in the air. People thus can be exposed by inhaling these spores; or these spores can land on them. As a result, fungal infection frequently start in the lung or on the skin. Fungi can be difficult to get rid of. Their major phyla include yeasts, molds, and mushrooms. Most yeasts (e.g., the genus *Candida*) and some molds (e.g., the genus *Aspergillums*) can be seen only with the aid of a light microscope.

While progressing slowly under normal conditions, fungal infections are rarely serious unless when the host's immunological system is sufficiently compromised, as by disorders (e.g., AIDS) or drugs. In those cases, they may end in serious *bacterial* infections. Most fungal infections seen in humans are caused by a type of fungi called dermophyte tending to infect the top layer of the skin, hair, or nail. The clinical condition induced by fungal infections of the skin is termed ringworm (medically *tinea*). There are various types of ringworms around, including body ringworm (*tinea corporis*), jock itch (*tinea cruris*) around the groin, scalp ringworm (*tinea capitis*), athlete's foot (*tinea pedis*), and nail ringworm (*tinea unguium*). The ringworm typically resembles a rash that forms ring-shaped patches each in pink or red color with a clear center and about one inch in diameter. The rash may itch from slightly to unnerving.

Mycosis is the medical term for infection or disease caused by a fungus. Some of the more serious fungal infections or diseases found in humans include blastomycosis, coccidioidomycosis, paracoccidioidomycosis, and histoplasmycosis. Blastomycosis, caused by the species *Blastomyces dermatitidis* found mostly in soils and decaying wood, is endemic to portions of North America.

Its symptoms include flu-like illness with fever, chills, muscle pains, headaches, and a nonproductive cough resolving in days. Coccidioidomycosis, caused by *Coccidioides immitis* or *posadasii*, is nicknamed California disease or San Joaquin valley fever in the United States. It is endemic to certain regions in the states of Arizona, California, Nevada, New Mexico, Texas, and Utah. The disease is usually not severe, with mostly flu-like symptoms and rashes. Paracoccidioidomycosis, caused by *Paracoccidioides brasiliensis*, is also known as Brazilian or South American blastomycosis, with symptoms including pulmonary infection and skin ulcer. As its nicknames imply, it is endemic to South and Central America. Histoplasmycosis, caused by *Histoplasma capsulatum*, is often called Cave disease, Darling's disease, Ohio valley disease, or reticuloendotheliosis. This disease is common among AIDS patients due to their weakened immunological system, and has symptoms similar to those of blastomycosis. Further characteristics of these various types of fungal infections can be found in the volume by Bologna *et al.* (2007) or by Ryan and Ray (2004).

17.2.4. Pathogenic Parasites

Parasites are tiny organisms that live on or inside another organism with the potential to harm their host. They count on the materials, including cells and tissues, in their host for survival and reproduction, as they are incapable of producing energy or food on their own. The waste products that some parasites release can be highly toxic to their host. Parasitic infections are more common in rural and underdeveloped regions than in industrialized areas. In industrialized areas, infections of this type can still occur in places with poor sanitation or unhygienic practice, such as in some mental institutions and daycare centers. They can also occur in people with a lowered immunological system and in frequent overseas travelers. According to several news reports in the recent past, some American soldiers returning from overseas service had indeed brought with them a number of parasites.

Parasites that infect humans include two prominent subgroups called helminthes and protozoa. Examples of protozoa include those that cause mosquito-borne malaria. Like bacteria, protozoa are microscopic, single-celled organisms. In contrast, helminthes are larvae-producing worms with internal organs consisting of many cells. Members in this second subgroup include the water flea-borne guinea worm (*Dracunculus medinensis*), which is among the longest roundworms (technically termed *nematodes*) infecting humans. It is in this sense that helminthes might (should) not be qualified as *micro*organisms.

The most common infectious protozoa in the world are the genus *Cryptosporidium* and the species *Giardia lamblia, Toxoplasma gondii,* and *Entamoeba histolytica*. These tiny parasites can be transmitted through contaminated foods and water or from person to person, and subsequently throughout the affected body to cause abscesses in the lungs, liver, kidneys, heart, brain, or other tissues. On rare occasions, they can be transmitted through blood transfusions, via injections with a contaminated needle, or from a pregnant woman to her fetus.

Worldwide the most common helminthes found in humans and their pets are roundworms, tapeworms, hookworms, pinworms, and liver fluke. Pinworms (e.g., *Enterobius follicularis*) are among the most common helminthes found in the United States. They make their home in the host's colon, but lay their eggs outside of the host's body. Their transmission can occur through unclean hands and inanimate objects (e.g., bed sheet). The associated symptoms include irritation and scratching in the anal area.

17.3. Toxins from Microorganisms

Covering a subject matter as broad as toxins makes selectivity a necessity in this section. There are more toxins from bacteria studied, followed by those from fungi, than toxins from all other organisms combined. Nonetheless, saxitoxin, brevetoxin, and domoic acid are three infamous toxins produced by algae, not by bacteria or fungi. These three potent toxins are responsible for, specifically and respectively, the symptoms of neurotoxic, paralytic, and amnestic shellfish poisoning. Furthermore, as noted in Section 17.2.4, parasites are known to excrete waste products which can be highly toxic or allergic to their host, amidst the fact that the characteristics of these waste products are not well documented except for a few. One exception is malaria toxin, a glycolipid named glycosylphosphatidylinositol from the protozoan *Plasmodium falciparum*. Malaria toxin is capable of stimulating the production of tumor necrosis factor (TNF) in host cells (e.g., Caro *et al.*, 1996). TNF is a cytokine as well as a general term referring to a superfamily of cytokines. Cytokines are small proteins secreted by specific cells of the immunological system that are able to cause death of tumor cells and systemic inflammation. Overproduction of TNF is reportedly (e.g., Schofield *et al.*, 1993) responsible for the severe, at times life-threatening, pathologies associated with cerebral or complicated malaria.

Toxins produced by viruses are not uncommon, as many viral components and by-products can accumulate in the host cell during the course of virus replication. However, viral toxin can be a confusing or loose term. There are scholars (e.g., DeWitte-Orr and Mossman, 2011) who would treat any double-stranded RNA (dsRNA) as a viral toxin. The genomes (as defined in Chapter 18) of dsRNA are capable of encoding a diverse group of viruses including the families *totiviridae* and *reoviridae*. Virus L-A in the *Saccharomyces cerevisiae* yeast cells is a dsRNA of the *totiviridae* family. It has the ability to encode the cytotoxic proteins named killer toxins K1, K2, K28, and zygocin (e.g., Reiter *et al.*, 2005; Schmitt and Breinig, 2002; Schmitt and Reiter, 2008). In general, the ds-RNA genomes, the viruses encoded by these genomes, and the toxic proteins that the dsRNA encoded may all be referred to as viral toxins.

Under most circumstances, the toxins produced by any type of microorganisms should be treated as significant virulence determinants of microbial pathogenicity, despite the fact that some of them also play a key role in medicine. Potential applications of toxins in medical research include their utilization in the development of novel anti-cancer drugs and as investigation tools in molecular or cellular biology. In the two subsections that follow, as due to space limitation, only certain toxins produced by bacteria and fungi are highlighted.

17.3.1. Toxins from Bacteria

Toxins from bacteria can be broadly divided into two subclasses: *exotoxins* and *endotoxins*. Exotoxins are those actively secreted by the bacteria either inside the host cell or in the cell's external environment. In contrast, endotoxins are part of the bacteria, typically located on their outer membranes, and are not released until the microbes are destroyed by antibiotics or the host's immunological or other defense system. The groups called *enterotoxins*, *neurotoxins*, and *leukocidins* all refer to toxins whose primary adverse action is on or around that implicit target site (i.e., mucous membrane of the intestine, nervous system, white blood cells, respectively). Some toxins from bacteria, such as tetanus toxin and botulin, are the most potent known. The toxicological profiles of tetanus and botulinum toxins, together with those of several prominent ones from other bacterial species, are summarized in Table 17.1.

It is noteworthy that tetanus toxin and botulin are neurotoxins produced by the same Gram-positive bacterial genus *Clostridium*. The species *C. botulinum* and *C. tetani* are producers of the botulin and the tetanus toxin, respectively. *C. botulinum* is an anaerobic bacterium widely distributed in soils, ponds, lake and pond sediments, as well as decaying vegetation. Accordingly, the intestinal tracts of birds, mammals, and fish will occasionally contain the bacteria as a transient. Foodborne botulism, which resembles Staphylococcal food poisoning, is not an infection but an intoxication, in that it results from the ingestion of foods containing the *pre*formed *botulinum* toxin (nicknamed botulin). On absorption in the duodenum and jejunum, the toxin passes into the bloodstream by which it reaches the peripheral neuromuscular synapses and there blocks the release of the neurotransmitter ACh (acetylcholine). This neurotransmitter is required for a nerve to stimulate a muscle (Section 9.2.4). *C. tetani* is commonly found in soils, especially where manure is heavily used, and in the intestinal tracts and feces of various animals. The tetani bacteria produce terminal spores which can get into the human body via a skin wound loaded with the contaminated animal waste, soil, or dust particles. Note that, as an exception to the rule, these bacteria may still stain Gram-negative or Gram-variable despite the fact that they each have a typical Gram-positive cell wall. As with botulism from any source, tetanus is a fatal human disease.

17.3.2. Toxins from Fungi

Many toxic metabolites produced by *micro*fungi tend to colonizing crops. These metabolites are technically termed *mycotoxins*. In other words, toxins found in the *macro*scopic mushrooms are not referred to as such, but simply called toxins from mushrooms. The toxins found in mushrooms include *alpha*-amanitin, coprine, ergotamine, gyromitrin, muscarine, orellanine, phallotoxin, and more. Mycetism is the medical term for poisoning from ingestion of mushroom toxins, with symptoms varying from mild GI discomfort to death. On the other hand, not all *myco*toxins are harmful to humans. Some of their derivatives have been used as antibiotics, growth promoters, and drugs, although some others have been tested for use as warfare agents. As reflected in Table 17.2, six major groups of mycotoxins are deemed highly relevant to environmental health. Under these six groups, aflatoxins, fumonisins, trichothecenes, and zearalenones are either more investigated or with more intriguing toxicities, and thus are specifically discussed below.

Aflatoxins belong to a subgroup of mycotoxins produced by many species of the fungal genus *Aspergillus*, including most notably *A. flavus* and *A. parasiticus*. Although about a dozen kinds or subtypes of aflatoxins are produced in nature, the term *aflatoxins* generally refers to the four kinds named (aflatoxin) B_1, B_2, G_1, and G_2. Aflatoxins are associated largely with agricultural commodities grown in the tropics and subtropics, such as cotton, maize, peanuts, and spices. Aflatoxins B_1

Table 17.1. Toxicological Profiles of Select Major Toxins Found in Certain Pathogenic Bacteria[a]

Toxin	Pathogenic Species	Major Toxic Effects/Specific Health Concerns
Botulinum toxin (botulin) (*neurotoxin*)	*Clostridium botulinum* (Gram-positive, rod-shaped, anaerobic)	Neurologic: blurred vision, numbness around the mouth, weakness of skeletal muscles, respiratory paralysis; in foodborne botulism, the toxin is ingested with food in which the bacterial spores have germinated
Tetanus toxin (*tetanospasmin*; *neurotoxin*)	*Clostridium tetani* (Gram-positive, rod-shaped, endospore-forming, anaerobic)	Pains in and stiffness of jaw, neck, and/or abdominal muscles, with difficulty swallowing; commonly via skin wound loaded with animal waste, soil, or dust particles containing the pathogen as well as the toxin
Clostridium perfringens enterotoxin	*Clostridium perfringens* (Gram-positive, rod-shaped, anaerobic)	Symptoms typically including gangrene, diarrhea, dysentery; possibly hemolytic
Anthrax toxin	*Bacillus anthracis* (Gram-positive, aerobic and anaerobic)	Induction of cytokine release leading to death of target cells; a disease affecting primarily domesticated animals and wildlife
Pertussis toxin	*Bordetella pertussis* (Gram-negative aerobic coccobacillus)	Whooping cough; inhibition of phagocytosis by macrophages and neutrophils; hemolytic as well as leukolytic
Diphtheria toxin	*Corynebacterium diphtheriae* (nonmotile, Gram-positive, rod-shaped, aerobic)	Inhibition of protein synthesis leading to cell death; a serious disease characterized by sore throat and later damage to the brain and heart
Cholera toxin	*Vibrio cholerae* (Gram-negative, straight or curved rods)	A severe contagious disease with symptoms including massive diarrhea, dehydration, and vomiting that collectively may lead to death
Staphylococcus aureus exfoliatin; exotoxin; enterotoxin	*Staphylococcus aureus* (Gram-positive, spherical)	Scalded skin syndrome by exfoliatin; toxic shock syndrome by exotoxin; food poisoning by enterotoxin; otherwise, most strains of the species and most species of the genus are harmless to humans or animals
Streptolysin O (cytolysin); pyrogenic toxin	*Streptococcus pyogenes* (nonmotile, non-spore-forming, Gram-positive)	Lysis of red/white blood cells by Streptolysin O; scarlet fever and systemic toxic shock syndrome by erythrogenic (pyrogenic) toxin
Shiga toxin; shiga-like toxin	*Shigella dysenteriae* (Gram-negative rod); Shigatoxigenic group of *E. coli*	Diarrhea and dysentery, with gastrointestinal and kidney complications; inhibition of protein synthesis within target cells; facilitating cell death
E. coli heat-labile enterotoxin	*Escherichia coli* (a.k.a. *E. coli*; Gram-negative, rod-shaped)	Symptoms similar to cholera; otherwise the intestine of many warm-blooded animals can be colonized by *E. coli* (head of the enterobacteriaceae family which includes *Salmonella*, *Shigella*, and *Yersinia*)
Cytolethal distending toxin	*Salmonella typhi* (Gram-negative, nonspore-forming); certain Gram-negative bacteria (e.g., *H. ducreyi*, *E. coli*)	Cell cycle arrest, cytoplasm distention, and eventually cell death by damage to the DNA strands; some species in the genus *Salmonella* can cause paratyphoid fever, typhoid fever, and the foodborne illness salmonellosis

[a] see, e.g., Brachman and Abrutyn (2009) and Henkel et al. (2010) for further discussion, which are the primary sources for this table.

and B_2 are produced by *A. flavus* and *A. parasiticus*, whereas aflatoxins G_1 and G_2 are produced by *A. parasiticus*. Aflatoxins M_1 is a metabolite of B_1 found in humans and animals, whereas M_2 is a metabolite of B_2 found in milk of cattle grazing on contaminated hay.

Aflatoxins B_1, B_2, G_1, and G_2 are similar to one another in structure and toxicity, with B_1 being the most toxic and among the most potent carcinogens. Aflatoxins B_2 and G_2 are the dihydroxy derivatives of B_1 and G_1, respectively. All four subtypes have been positively correlated to adverse health effects, such as liver cancer, in many animal species. After entering the body, aflatoxin B_1 can be metabolized by the liver to a highly reactive epoxide intermediate, to aflatoxicol of moderate carcinogenicity, or to the less harmful aflatoxin M_1. Aflatoxins B_1, B_2, G_1, and G_2 have been listed as human (Group 1) carcinogens (IARC, 2012, 2017).

Fumonisins, trichothecenes, and zearalenones are other subgroups of mycotoxins produced by several species of the genus *Fusarium*. As listed in Table 17.2, mycotoxins from *Fusarium* also include beauvericins, butenolides, enniatins, equisetins, and fusarins (e.g., Desjardins and Proctor, 2007). These eight subfamilies of *Fusarium* toxins all have a history and tendency of infecting the grains of developing cereals (e.g., wheat, maize).

Fumonisin B_1 is the most prevalent member of the toxin fumonisin subfamily, produced by several species of *Fusarium* molds. The *Fusarium* molds occur mainly in/on maize, wheat, and certain other cereal crops. Contamination of maize by fumonisin B_1 has been reported worldwide on the parts per million (mg/kg) level. Human exposure occurs on levels of μg to mg per day, and is highest in regions where maize products are the dietary staple. Fumonisin B_1, an inhibitor of the enzyme ceramide synthase, is toxic to the liver and kidneys in all animal species investigated. Fumonisin B_2 produced by *F. verticillioides* and *F. moniliforme* is a structural analog of fumonisin B_1 but is more cytotoxic. As with many other members in the fumonisin subfamily, fumonisin B_2 can affect the nervous systems of horses and cause cancer in rodents while tending to contaminate maize (and several other crops).

Trichothecenes are produced by species of the fungal genera *Cephalosporium, Dendrodochium, Myrothecium, Stachybotrys, Trichothecium, Verticimonosporium, Trichoderma,* and most notably *Fusarium*. These mycotoxins are strong inhibitors of protein synthesis as they react with components of the cellular ribosomes (Figure 9.1) where proteins are synthesized. They were reportedly associated with fatal and chronic toxic effects in animals and humans, and can cause rapid irritation to the skin. Historically, large outbreaks of trichothecene-related mycotoxicoses were reportedly linked to the consumption of Japanese rice and Russian wheat grains both infested by species of *Fusarium*.

Zearalenones are potent estrogenic metabolites produced by *F. graminearum* that have not (yet) been shown to correlate well with any fatal toxic effects in humans. They are, however, the primary mycotoxins responsible for infertility, abortion, swelling of uterus, enlarged mammary glands, atrophy of the ovaries, and breeding problems, all predominately or some even specifically in swine. As with many other mycotoxins, zearalenones are heat-stable and are found mostly in maize. Zearalenones are also found in other crops (e.g., wheat, rye, sorghum) over the world, especially in the temperate regions. Their contaminations have reportedly occurred in moldy hay fed to cattle, swine, and sheep.

Table 17.2. Toxicological Profiles of Six Major Common Groups of Mycotoxins Found in Certain Pathogenic Fungi[a]

Mycotoxin	Major Pathogenic Fungal Species	Associated/Affected Commodities	Major Toxic Effects/ Health Concerns
Aflatoxins: B_1, B_2, G_1, G_2	*Aspergillus flavus* and/or *Aspergillus parasiticus*	Maize, cotton, peanuts, pistachios, spices, nuts, and more	Highly carcinogenic (especially to the liver); hepatic aflatoxicosis; suppression of immunological system in animals
Fusarium toxins: fumonisins; trichothecenes; zearalenones; beauvericins; butenolides; enniatins; fusarins; equisetins	Many species of *Fusarium* (e.g., *F. verticillioides*, *F. proliferatum*, *F. oxysporum*)	Distributed mainly in soils; in association with plants or grains of developing cereals (e.g., wheat, maize)	Fumonisins: nervous systems of horses; cancer in rodents. Zearalenones: highly estrogenic causing abortion and infertility specifically in swine. Trichothecenes: potent inhibitors of protein synthesis
Citrinin	Several species of *Aspergillus* and of *Penicillium* (e.g., *P. citrinum*)	Various human foods (e.g., cheese, rice, soy sauce, wheat, barley, corn, rye, food colored with red pigments)	Yellow rice fever in humans; nephrotoxin with hepatoxic/teratogenic activities in many animal species
Ochratoxin (OT) including the three (secondary) metabolites OT_A, OT_B, OT_C	Various species of *Penicillium* (e.g., *P. verrucosum*) and *Aspergillus* (e.g., *A. ochraceus*)	Beverages (e.g., beer, wine), grain, pork products, and dried grapes	OT_A: carcinogen (e.g., in the human urinary tract); nephrotoxin
Ergot alkaloids	In the sclerotia of various species of *Claviceps* (e.g., *C. purpurea*)	Various grass species, cereals, rye, and related plants (e.g., wheat, triticale, barley)	Ergotism (St. Anthony's Fire): vasoconstriction leading to gangrene and loss of limbs; hallucinations; convulsions; and death
Palutin	Certain *Penicillium* (e.g., *P. expasum*), *Aspergillus*, and *Paecilomyces*	Rotting apples, rotting figs, and a variety of moldy vegetables and fruits	Genotoxic; damage to the immunological system in many animal species

[a] see, e.g., Hussein and Brasel (2001) and Richard (2007) for further discussion, which are the main sources for this table.

17.4. Toxins from Fishes and Plants

One major source of food poisoning is from consumption of poisonous fishes. Another major source is from ingestion of poisonous plants. If venomous fishes (e.g., stargazers, scorpionfish, stonefish, lionfish) are included, poisonous fishes will have over a thousand species (Smith and Wheeler, 2006). As alluded to in Section 17.1, the distinction between venomous and poisonous animals is in the way their toxins are delivered to their victims or enemies. Fishes of the venomous type deliver their toxins by means of a sting or a bite, whereas the poisonous type have their toxins consumed by their predators. This section focuses on the latter, which are fewer in species. Worldwide, fish and shellfish poisonings occur more commonly in the South Sea, and only occasionally in the United States (e.g., predominantly in the coastal states such as California, Florida, Hawaii, New York, and Washington).

The list of poisonous plants appears longer, and is not easy to compile in the sense that in many instances one part of them is poisonous whereas another part is edible. Plants contain many classes of biologically active chemical substances such as alkaloids, glycosides, amino acids, and peptides. Some constituents in these various groups (e.g. atropine, digitoxin, colchicine) happen to offer great therapeutic effects in treating human or animal diseases. Yet some others (e.g., jimson weed, nightshade) can produce acute, life-threatening poisonings. Fortunately, among the thousands of plants found in the environment, not many are poisonous or sufficiently poisonous to humans or animals, at least not from dermal contact or inhalation.

The health effects of poisonous plants vary considerably among animals and humans. Timing of ingestion or of contact can be critical. This is because the concentrations of toxic constituents in many plants are seasonal, temporal, and regional. They can vary considerably as a result of certain environmental factors such as drought and flood by altering the soil structure and properties nearby. As highlighted in Section 17.4.2, toxins from plants can be broadly divided into four or five categories according to the body organs or tissues that are affected.

17.4.1. Toxins from Fishes

As noted in Section 17.3, saxitoxin, brevetoxin, and domoic acid are algae-borne toxins. They are known to cause *shellfish* poisoning. There are three toxins from *fishes* that appear even more relevant to public health. These are ciguatoxin, tetrodotoxin, and scombrotoxin.

Ciguatoxin is also an algae-borne toxin. It is produced by *Gambierdiscus toxicus*, a type of dinoflagellates accumulating in big coral reef fishes (e.g., grouper, wrasse, triggerfish, amberjack). The toxin usually accumulates in the skin, head, viscera, and roe of the fish. It cannot be destroyed by heat from cooking. The poisonous effects of ciguatoxin come about from its ability to lower the threshold for opening voltage-gated sodium channels in the synapses of the nervous system. The effects of opening such an ion channel involve depolarization which can cause paralysis, heart contraction, and changing the senses of hearing. As this toxin normally cannot cross the blood brain barrier, it affects the peripheral (rather than the central) nervous system.

Tetrodotoxin is a highly potent neurotoxin with no known antidotes. It blocks action potentials in nerves by binding to the pores of the voltage-gated sodium channels on the biomembranes, thus preventing any affected nerve cells from firing by blocking the channels used in the course of the action. The toxin has been isolated from a variety of animal species, including predominantly puffer fish and occasionally some western newts of the genus *Taricha* and toads of the genus *Atelopus*. Tetrodotoxin is some 100 times more poisonous than potassium cyanide (KCN), an inorganic that has a lethal oral dose of about 200 mg for an adult of average weight. In many cases, the skin and the liver of a puffer fish together contain the neurotoxin at levels sufficient to cause paralysis of the human diaphragm and death from respiratory failure. The symptoms typically develop within 30 minutes of ingestion, but may be delayed by up to a few hours. Yet death has reportedly occurred as fast as 15 minutes from ingestion.

Scombrotoxin, which is composed of histamine and other amines, is frequently implicated for the foodborne illness caused by consumption of spoiled fish. Histamine is a mediator of allergic reactions. The symptoms from the poisoning are thus similar to those seen in a severe allergic response. The illness typically begins minutes to hours after ingestion of the spoiled toxic fish and resembles a histamine reaction, with symptoms including nausea, palpitations, tingling and burning sensations around the mouth, facial flushing, vomiting, sweating, dizziness, and rashes. Some patients complained that the spoiled fish had a peppery or metallic taste. Scombrotoxic food poisoning is about the most common type of seafood poisonings, second only to ciguatera (that caused by ciguatoxin). Seafood poisonings of this type are most commonly reported with the scombridae family (e.g., skipjack, mackerel, tuna, bonito), thereby leading to the name so given to the toxin. The biogenic amine histamine responsible for the various symptoms actually comes from the his*tidine* that is naturally available in various fishes. The conversion from hist*idine* to hist*amine* takes place at temperatures above 16° C (61° F) on air contact. The resultant histamine is not labile to cooking temperatures; so even properly cooked fish can still be affecting.

17.4.2. Toxins from Plants

Many different kinds of substances found in plants can cause GI disturbance (e.g., including diarrhea, nausea, vomiting) due to their ability to irritate the mucous membranes during the course of ingestion. Some have found a place in medicine as mild purgatives, such as the emodin from *Himalayan rhubarb* and *Rhamnus purshiana*. Food plants (e.g., cereal grains, nuts, seeds, beans) with high concentrations of the sugar-binding protein called *lectin* can be harmful if consumed excessively in undercooked form. The adverse effects of lectin on humans may include nutritional deficiencies and allergic reactions. Most of these effects are possibly due to GI distress (e.g., abdominal pain, purging, bloody diarrhea) via interaction of this protein with the gut epithelial cells. Ricin is another protein that can cause GI distress. This toxin is found mostly in castor beans. If ingested, it can cause symptoms that likely begin within 3 hours and include a burning sensation in the mouth and throat, along with GI distress.

Some plant species are known to contain cardiac or cardiotonic glycosides, of which the widely known is from *Digitalis purpurea* (which includes foxglove of the *Plantaginaceae* family). Glycosides are molecules in which a sugar (carbohydrate) unit is bound to a non-carbohydrate moiety. In the lily family, both red squill (*Urginea maritima*) and lily of the valley (*Convallaria majalis*) contain glycosides (named scillaren and convallatoxin, respectively) in their bulbs with actions resembling digitalis. Cardiac glycosides are also a class of medications used to treat heart failure.

However, their overdose can cause serious adverse effects on the heart, stomach, intestines, and nervous system. It is largely and knowingly due to the high potential for such adverse effects that these glycosides have been utilized for arrow poisons.

Cyanogens (those containing the cyano group CN) are constituents of several plant species. One of the widely known cyanogenic glycosides is amygdalin. This glycoside is found in the pits of apples, cherries, and peaches, in related genera of the rose family, and in the highest amounts in the seeds of the bitter almonds *Prunus amygdalus* (which thus gives the glycoside's name). When amygdalin is taken orally, lethal cyanide poisoning can occur because β-glucosidase is one of the enzymes capable of catalyzing the breakdown of the cyanide from amygdalin. This enzyme is present in the human small intestine as well as in a variety of common foods.

Alkaloids are mostly amines containing one or more nitrogen atoms on their cyclic rings. The high concentrations of pyrrolizidine alkaloids found in many plant species (e.g., those in the genera *Crotalaria*, *Heliotropium*, and *Symphytum*) are reportedly responsible for liver damage in the form of cancer or hepatic venoocclusive disease (Schoental, 1968). For kidney damage, one widely known toxin from plants is oxalate. People and many animals can develop kidney stones if they consume food plants (e.g., leeks, spinach, quinoa) high in oxalate. Calcium oxalate is a chemical substance that forms needle-shaped crystals. In plants, the needle-shaped crystals are known as raphides. The poisonous house plant dumb cane contains the toxin that on ingestion can cause mouth and throat irritations with excessive drooling, usually long before the toxin has an opportunity to accumulate in the body sufficient to form kidney stones.

Taxol is a neurotoxin belonging to the class of alkaloids called taxine. It is found in the western yew tree *Taxus breviofolia*. The natural pyrethrins from chrysanthemum can act as neurotoxic alkaloids to cause severe excitation of the nervous system (Section 15.6). Swainsonine is an indolizidine alkaloid found in the Australian plant *Swainsonia canescens* and some locoweed plants in the western United States. In addition to its neurotoxicity, indolizidine can cause abortion and fetal malformation in pregnant livestock grazing on these plants (e.g., Bunch *et al.*, 1992).

Hypericum, *Dieffenbachia*, and *Rhus* are not closely related plants. Yet some species of these genera can cause similar contact dermatitis as an allergic reaction. For example, some people are familiar with dermatitis caused by poison ivy (*R. toxicodendron*) and poison sumac (*R. vernix*). House plants of the genus *Dieffenbachia*, such as dumb cane mentioned earlier, can cause oral irritation, excessive drooling, and localized swelling. In addition, cases of livestock poisoning from *H. perforatum* (a.k.a., St. John's wort) have been reported in the temperate and subtropical regions of North America, Europe, India, Turkey, Russia, and China. The most common adverse effects from this type of livestock poisonings are GI disorders, dizziness, confusion, fatigue, and sedation. On rare occasions, these effects may lead to high levels of photosensitivity that can cause increase in visual sensitivity to light or in skin sensitivity to sunburns.

17.5. Venoms from Arthropods

Arthropods are invertebrates and the largest animal phylum (i.e., division) on the Earth, each with a segmented body called thorax, an abdomen, and six or more jointed legs. The body of each arthropod is covered by a shell or a hard outer skin called exoskeleton. Arthropods frequently encountered by people include ants, bees, beetles, butterflies, crabs, fleas, hornets, lobsters, mosquitoes, scorpions, shrimp, spiders, ticks, wasps, and many more.

The bites by arthropods such as fleas, mites, mosquitoes, and ticks can make many people's life miserable. Certain mosquito species are very dangerous, as they carry diseases such as malaria and dengue fever. Malaria is brought about by the protozoan species *Plasmodium falciparum* parasitizing in female mosquitoes mostly of the *Anopheles* genus. When a female mosquito bites an infected person, the arthropod will inject its saliva containing the malaria parasite into the next victim's body for multiplication in that body's liver. The parasite there then starts to infect the host victim's red blood cells, causing symptoms such as fever, headaches, and in severe cases hallucinations, coma, and death. Dengue fever is caused by dengue virus, characterized by a sudden onset of fever along with headaches as well as joint and muscle pains. Rocky Mountain spotted fever and Lyme disease are infectious diseases brought about by ticks as the vectors.

Despite the fact that as many as 80% of all animals on the planet are arthropods, which are found everywhere, most lack a venom sufficient or sufficiently poisonous to pose threat to human health. The few that can produce a sufficient venom of health concern are highlighted below.

17.5.1. Venoms from Arachnids

Arachnids are a class of arthropods that all have eight legs, such as scorpions and spiders. Among some 40,000 species of spiders identified, only 200 or so are known to have toxic stings. The venom, when injected via a spider's hollow teeth-like small fangs, can rapidly paralyze the victims including humans. Fortunately, most of these some 200 species are not dangerous to humans because their fangs are either fragile or not long enough to penetrate the human skin. The few exceptions include species of the genera *Latrodectus* (the kind of the so-called black widow spiders), *Loxosceles* (the brown recluse spiders), *Phidippus* (the jumping spiders), *Cheiracanthium* (the yellow sac spiders), and *Pardosa* (the wolf spiders). Studies have emerged to confirm that some species of spiders and some species of bacteria share the same or similar toxins. For instance, certain species in the spider genus *Loxosceles* can cause severe necrotic lesions in the human skin due to the presence of their venom enzyme sphingomyelinase D, which is also found in certain species of the bacterial genus *Corynebacteria* that have reportedly caused various illnesses in livestock (e.g., Cordes and Binford, 2006).

The brown recluse spiders are also known as the violin or fiddleback spiders due to their violin shape. Their venoms generally cause some pains, itching, or burning within the first 15 minutes, along with extensive tissue damage over the next two weeks ending with a sunken, open, ulcerated sore to several diameters. The wound has the appearance of a bull's eye, with a center blister surrounded by a red ring and then a blanched whitish ring. Other symptoms include chills, fever, nausea, and hemolytic anemia (a condition where red blood cells are destroyed prematurely).

The black widow spiders are timid and prefer to be in secluded locations (e.g., attics, garages, crawl spaces, sheds) to construct their tangled, crisscross webs. Their bites bring out the appearance of a pale area surrounded by a red ring. Severe muscle pains and cramps can develop in human victims within the first few hours. The cramps are generally first felt around the abdomen, shoulders, back, and thighs. Other symptoms include weakness, headaches, itching, sweating, nausea, breathing difficulty, and hypertension (high blood pressure).

The jumping spiders are the most common biting type reported across the United States, whereas the wolf spiders are found mostly in the state of California. Both groups are large hairy spiders, much like tarantulas of the *Theraphosidae* family, Bites from a jumping spider are painful, itchy, and cause redness as well as swelling. Other symptoms may include fever, headaches, joint and muscle pains, chills, nausea, and vomiting. These symptoms last for a couple of days. Bites from a wolf spider can also cause pains, swelling, and redness. The venoms of the yellow sac spiders, which are so-called due to the yellow to beige color of their abdomen, can cause a small lesion in humans. Its link to a definitive dermonecrosis was challenged not too long ago (Vetter *et al.*, 2006).

Scorpions are predatory arthropods of the *Scorpiones* order within the *Arachnida* class (which spiders also belong to). Their venoms are a mixture of neurotoxins and enzyme inhibitors, with each mixture variety not only causing a different effect but also likely targeting a specific kind of animal victims. Frogs and rabbits are some animals that tend to be victimized by a scorpion's venom. One bark scorpion species named *Centruroides exilicauda* in the western United States and some 25 other species worldwide are known to have poisonous venoms potent enough to harm humans. Most of these venoms, including chlorotoxin produced by Deathstalker scorpions, are similar in toxicity to those from snakes.

17.5.2. Venoms from Insects

Of all the venoms from thousands of the insect species, only those from a few species in the *Hymenoptera* order, such as certain species of bees, hornets, and wasps, will pose some threat to humans. The venoms from these *Hymenopterous* insects are almost all proteinaceous substances (e.g., biogenic amines, peptides, small proteins, enzymes). Most people have only localized reactions to these venoms, amidst the fact that a few may experience serious allergic reactions. Localized, nonallergic reactions range from short-term redness, itching, and burning to massive swelling and itching that last for a couple of weeks. Occasionally, a victim may be found to suffer a life-threatening, systemic allergic reaction to a wasp or bee sting, as the allergic reaction can result in anaphylactic shock within minutes of a sting (as in Type I hypersensitivity reaction with shortness of breath, blockage in the throat, loss of consciousness, and fainting). In the United States, each year around 40 deaths are reported as from anaphylaxis caused by insect stings.

For most people, a wasp sting produces an immediate pain at the sting site. There will be localized reddening, swelling, and itching. Aside from the allergic reaction, the worst risk from insect stings is the less harmful microbial infection that follows. Unlike the honeybees, the common wasps and hornets can insert and withdraw their sting with relative ease, although the amount of venom delivered by a wasp sting is much less than that by a bee. Another feature unique to wasp and hornet stings is a pheromone contained in their venoms that will attract further attacks on the affected victim by those of the same species nearby. Insect stings in nonallergic people, though painful, generally do not cause serious health problems. However, *multiple* insect stings can cause serious complications (e.g., muscle breakdown, renal failure) and even death in those victims.

Fire ants are wingless members of insects belonging to the *Humenoptera* order. Their venoms differ from those of the bees and wasps in that about 95% of the former are non-proteinaceous and contain dialkylpiperidine hemolytic factors. These hemolytic factors can induce the release of histamine and other vasoactive amines from mast cells, resulting in a sterile pustule at the sting site. While these alkaloids *per se* are not immunogenic, venoms from some fire ants do possess certain allergenic proteins capable of causing anaphylaxis in allergic victims.

17.6. Venoms from Reptiles and Amphibians

Reptiles are a class of cold-blooded animals called *Reptilia* in the *Chordata* phylum. Animals in this reptile class include snakes and lizards of the *Squamata* order, crocodiles and alligators of the *Crocodilia* order, as well as turtles and tortoises of the *Testudines* order. Of all the reptiles known to date, snakes are the most notorious for having potent venoms capable of killing humans and large animals. Other groups of reptiles venomous to humans and large animals are limited to a few species of lizards.

Amphibians like frogs, toads, salamanders, newts, and caecilians are in the animal class named *Amphibia*, also belonging to the *Chordata* phylum. Animals in this class are known to metamorphose from a juvenile water-breathing form to either an adult air-breathing form or a form that retains some of their juvenile traits. Some species of amphibians are known being more poisonous to humans and animals than all the venomous lizards and snakes identified.

17.6.1. Venoms from Snakes

Many of the some 3,000 species of snakes identified are nonvenomous or not sufficiently venomous to humans. Of those that are, most are from the *Elapidae* and *Viperidae* families. Cobras, copperheads, mambas, kraits, and coral snakes, along with sea snakes, are venomous elapids occasionally encountered by humans. Venomous viperids familiar to humans include vipers, adders, rattlesnakes, cottonmouths, and bushmasters (e.g., Freiberg and Walls, 1984).

The venoms from snakes are highly modified saliva secreted via their mostly sharp, enlarged, and hollow fangs. Their salivary venoms generally possess one or more of the four distinct types of toxic enzymes: (1) proteases; (2) phosphodiesterases; (3) phospholipases (mostly of the phospholipases-A_2 subtype); and (4) hyaluronidases. Many snake venoms contain additionally the enzymes adenosine triphosphatases (ATPases), which are thought as among the agents responsible for immobilizing the smaller preys by disrupting the supply and release of cellular energy in their body. A variety of other substances such as biogenic amines, lipids, carbohydrates, and metal ions are also present in a snake's saliva. There is some evidence (e.g., Ahmed *et al.*, 2009) that the type of acetylcholinesterase (AChE) found in elapid venoms has the specific effect of disrupting the cholinergic transmission in the prey's central nervous system as well as at its body's neuromuscular junction.

The various types of snake enzymes mentioned above have their own unique venomous properties. Proteases bring about the disruption of peptide and protein bonds in a victim's body tissues, causing the tissues to deteriorate and the blood-vessel walls to rupture. Many of these enzymes thus have their adverse effects mainly on hemostasis and thrombosis (Matsui *et al.*, 2000). Phosphodiesterases, which can break down the 5′-phosphodiester and pyrophosphate bonds in nucleotides and nucleic acids (as defined in Chapter 18), are responsible for the adverse cardiac reactions in the prey, most notably by lowering its blood pressure severely. Phospholipases-A_2 account for a wide range of toxicity, including hemolytic, myotoxic, anticoagulant, neurotoxic, and cardiotoxic effects (Balsinde *et al.*, 2002; Davidson and Dennis, 1990; Nevalainen *et al.*, 2004). Even though phospholipases-A_2 are commonly found in mammalian tissues, their elevated level and hence elevated activity resulting from a snakebite will cause inflammation as well as pains at the site of the bite. Some other subtypes of phospholipases, such as β-bungarotoxin found in venoms from banded kraits, have a subunit capable of destroying sensory and motor neurons (Kwong *et al.*, 1995; Lewis and Gutmann, 2004). Hyaluronidases are the enzymes that catalyze the breakdown of hyaluronic acid, an anionic substance present throughout the human body to help cushion and support joints. Enzymes of this type have the effect of increasing tissue permeability thereby facilitating the absorption of other toxic enzymes into the prey's various body tissues.

17.6.2. Venoms from Lizards

There are some 5,000 species of lizards worldwide. Yet until about a decade ago, only the Gila monster (*Heloderma suspectum*) and the related Mexican beaded (*Heloderma horridum*) species were thought to be (sufficiently) venomous. These two species can be found in Mexico and in the southwestern United States. Studies (e.g., Fry *et al.*, 2006) revealed that lizards of the species *Varanus varius* (of the *Monitor* family) and the species *Pogona barabata* (of the *Agamidae* family) are also venomous. However, none of these new(er) finds has been reported to pose serious threat to humans, possibly due to the fact that their venoms are introduced too slowly by chewing, unlike those injected by snakes. In addition to the several venomous enzymes (e.g., phospholipases, proteases, hyaluronidases) commonly found in snakes, a few previously unnoticed proteinaceous substances have now been identified in venoms from these new finds.

Also intriguing and important to know is the reality that the very largest lizard species, such as the Komodo dragons, can actually pose threat of death to their prey via bacterial infection. That is, amidst the fact that the Komodo dragons have not been considered venomous, the serrations along their teeth are an ideal niche for many species of pathogenic bacteria. To put it another way, if the bite of a Komodo dragon did not get its prey victimized or killed, the infections caused by the bacteria living in its teeth-like fangs ultimately could or would.

17.6.3. Venoms from Amphibians

Most of the venomous amphibians come from the *Salamandridae* family (e.g., the sharp-ribbed newts, the crocodile newts) and from a group of Central American toads (e.g., the harlequin frogs). These amphibians have venomous glands on their flanks positioned adjacent to their rib tips. When picked up by their predators, these amphibians will use their sharp ribs as poisonous spikes by protruding them outwards through their venomous glands. Many of them, such as the Eastern red-spotted newts (*Notophthalmus viridescens*) and the California newts (*Taricha torosa*), possess the potent neurotoxin *tetrodotoxin* found otherwise notably in puffer fish (Section 17.4.1).

The Giant toads (a.k.a. marine toads) and the Colorado River toads are the two venomous species that are most commonly found in the United States. Their venoms are highly poisonous to pets. Dogs, the pets most likely coming in contact with a toad, have a higher risk of dying from contact with a venomous toad if they are left untreated. The skins of these venomous toads collectively provide over 400 different toxic alkaloids including batrachotoxins, histrionicotoxins, pumiliotoxins, and epibatidines. These toxic alkaloids collectively can cause a wide array of adverse effects on humans, including irritation, hallucination, vasoconstriction, cardiac problems, convulsions, and neurotoxic damage. One of the most poisonous frog groups is called poison dart frogs, belonging to the *Dendrobatidae* family.

17.7. Underrated Harmful Physical Agents/Hazards

Harmful agents not chemical or biological in nature or origin are almost always by default treated as physical. Harmful physical agents are sometimes known as physical hazards, in that the latter term embraces also physical risk factors or conditions for the harm at issue. The term *harmful physical hazard* is used mostly by professionals in occupational health and safety, as well as by various sectors (e.g., media, labor unions) and agencies complying with or advocating the worker (employee) right-to-know laws and movements. Many of these entities (e.g., MNDLI, 2017) have limited the physical hazards to heat, noise, non-ionizing radiation (e.g., microwaves), and ionizing radiation (e.g., X-rays), which all have been determined as the general physical agents or phenomena that can cause carcinogenic, mutagenic, reproductive, or other toxic effects particularly on workers. Some health authorities and scholars (e.g., Tweedy, 2005) have extended the short list to include vibration, repetitive motion, and cold stress. Many environmental health scholars, on the other hand, have included certain environmental situations as physical hazards, such as the two cases with noise pollution and traffic congestion to be discussed in this section.

Traffic congestion and noise pollution are environmental as well as physical phenomena causing a wide array of adverse effects on human health, human or animal behavior, and the ecosystem. Another reason for their inclusion in this section is that, to date both phenomena are still two of the prevalent but most underrated environmental health issues around.

The adverse effects of ionizing and non-ionizing radiation are briefly covered in Chapters 14 and 18. For decades now, seemingly very safe low dosages of ionizing radiation have been used in medical and research facilities. Yet huge quantities of harmful radioactive materials from nuclear power plants can be released into the environment by avoidable accidents, such as those due to flawed reactor designs (e.g., as with the 1986 Chernobyl nuclear explosion in Pripyat, Ukraine) or due to serious equipment failures (e.g., resulting from earthquakes or tsunamis, as with the 2011 Fukushima nuclear crisis in Okuma, Japan). Other physical hazards noted earlier in this section are treated as among the more relevant to industrial hygiene and medical physics. For completeness, these other physical hazards are highlighted in Chapter 20 on occupational toxicology.

17.7.1. Traffic Congestion

Traffic congestion generally refers to an adverse environmental condition where the passage of vehicles (or pedestrians) along transportation routes exceeds the available capacity provided by the transportation system in place. This condition is characterized by slower vehicular (or pedestrian) movements and thereby longer trip times. The so-termed traffic jam situation occurs whenever vehicles are fully stopped for an enough time interval. Even individual incidents (e.g., car accident or the sudden braking of one car in an otherwise smooth flow) may cause a chain reaction or a riffle effect leading to a traffic jam.

The health and economic impacts of traffic congestion on a community can be substantial. Traffic delays can result in late arrival for many important events such as employment, business meetings, medical appointments, and education. Idling in traffic and frequent braking can cause more wear and tear on vehicles. In addition, road rage may result with increases in frustration and stress of the drivers and riders. Yet more importantly, traffic situations of this type will lead to more emissions of nitrogen oxides (NO_x), carbon monoxide (CO), and other air pollutants into the atmosphere. For year 2005, such emissions in the United States were reportedly associated with approximately 3,000 premature deaths (Levy *et al.*, 2010).

In particular, studies have shown that traffic congestion is a significant contributor to poor health in affected infants (Currie and Walker, 2009) and to a surge in asthma rates in a Latino community (NRDC, 2004). Another study conducted in Germany (Peters *et al.*, 2004) has implicated an increase in the risk of myocardial infarction (i.e., heart attack) for every hour a driver or a rider will be stuck in traffic.

17.7.2. Noise Pollution

Noise is the term used to refer to any unpleasant or annoying sound, the intensity of which is conventionally measured in decibel (dB) units on a logarithmic scale. In general, a normal conversation between two persons measures about 60 dB; and loud singing within 3 feet measures about 75 dB. One hazard with loud noise is acoustic trauma to the human ears when they are subjected to noise at 85 dB or higher without respite. Noise at around this level is equivalent to that from an automobile or a motorcycle running within about 30 feet. By noise pollution, it means an excessive amount of environmental noise of sufficient duration that comes with significant adverse impacts on human or animal health. Vehicles and industrial engines are the major sources of noise pollution, accounting for up to 90% of the total in certain urban areas (Section 3.1). Depending on the efficiency in urban planning, some cities are more affected than others by the loud and rhythmical sounds generated from transportation means and construction works.

Noise pollution has direct impacts on human health, including both physiological and psychological effects. Nuisance noise of even medium intensity can be responsible for emotional stress, anxiety, insomnia, hypertension, and panic attacks. This type of environmental pollution can lower people's sensitivity to sounds leading to the premature aging of their auditory system. Problems such as aggression, frustration, and stress are some psychological effects that can be caused by nuisance noise. According to the U.S. National Institute on Deafness and Other Communication Disorders (NIDCD, 2008), approximately 26 million American adults at ages 20 to 69 (i.e., about 17% of the total population in this age group) have high frequency of hearing loss that might have been induced by exposure to loud noise at work or in recreational activities.

There is strong speculation, if not substantial evidence, that noise pollution can increase the mortality among animal species and affect the natural occurring phenomena that govern their world. For instance, with noise pollution, birds may find themselves disturbed during expression with one another for mating desires or may have navigation problems due to the unnatural sound level present.

Worldwide, the concerns with noise pollution and the needs for acoustic control have been addressed in numerous presentations given annually at the INTER-NOISE Congresses, often under a sensational theme such as in 2012 being *Quieting the World's Cities*. These congresses are the largest international conferences from various regions on noise control engineering and have been held at venues around the world since the early 1970s.

Over the years, noise control measures and regulations in various forms have been adopted in or within many countries including Australia, China, Demark, France, Japan, Spain, and more. For instance, two important measures being implemented by the Council of Paris in France are reducing speed limits and cutting back on the number of streets that trucks can use. Japan's national capital Tokyo, on the other hand, amended its local rules in 2015 to exempt only the sound of children playing in daycare centers, even at levels exceeding 45 dB, as noise pollution in the residential areas. In the United States, the control measures and standards for noise emission are specifically justified under the Noise Control Act of 1972. Under this act, U.S. EPA is responsible for coordinating all federal programs relating to noise research and noise control.

References

Ahmed M, Rocha JBT, Morsch VM, Schetinger MRC, 2009. Snake Venom Acetylcholinesterase. In *Handbook of Venoms and Toxins of Reptiles* (Mackessy SP, Ed.). Boca Raton, Florida, USA: CRC Press, Chapter 9 (pp.207-220).

Balsinde J, Winstead MV, Dennis EA, 2002. Phospholipase A2 Regulation of Arachidonic Acid Metabolism. *FEBS Lett.* 531:2-6.

Bolognia JL, Jorizzo, JL, Rapini RP (Eds.), 2007. *Dermatology*. Philadelphia, Pennsylvania, USA: Elsevier Health Sciences.

Brachman PS, Abrutyn E (Eds.), 2009. *Bacterial Infections of Humans – Epidemiology and Control*, 4th Edition. New York, New York, USA: Springer Science+Business Media.

Bunch TD, Panter KD, James LK, 1992. Ultrasound Studies of the Effects of Certain Poisonous Plants on Uterine Function and Fetal Development in Livestock. *J. Anim. Sci.* 70:1639-1643.

Caro HN, Sheikh NA, Taverne J, Playfair JH, Rademacher TW, 1996. Structural Similarities among Malaria Toxins Insulin Second Messengers, and Bacterial Endotoxin. *Infect. Immun.* 64:3438-3441.

Cordes MHJ, Binford GJ, 2006. Lateral Gene Transfer of a Dermonecrotic Toxin between Spiders and Bacteria. *Bioinformatics* 22:264-268.

Currie J, Walker R, 2009. Traffic Congestion and Infant Health: Evidence from EZPass. NBER Working Paper No. 15413. National Bureau of Economic Research (NBER), Inc., 1050 Massachusetts Avenue, Cambridge, Massachusetts, USA.

Davidson FF, Dennis EA, 1990. Evolutionary Relationships and Implications for the Regulation of Phospholipase A2 from Snake Venom to Human Secreted Forms. *J. Mol. Evol.* 31:228-238.

Desjardins AE, Proctor RH, 2007. Molecular Biology of Fusarium Mycotoxins. *Intl. J. Food Microbiol.* 119: 47-50.

DeWitte-Orr SJ, Mossman KL, 2011. The Antiviral Effects of Extracellular dsRNA. In *Viruses and Interferon: Current Research* (Mossman K, Ed.). Norfolk, UK: Caister Academic Press, Chapter 1.

Evans AS, 1976. Causation and Disease: The Henle-Koch Postulates Revisited. *Yale J. Biol. Med.* 49:175-195.

Freiberg M, Walls JG, 1984. *The World of Venomous Animals*. Neptune, New Jersey, USA: TFH Publications.

Fry BG, Vidal N, Norman JA, Vonk FJ, Scheib H, Ramjan SFR, Kuruppu S, Fung K, Hedges SB, Richardson MK, *et al.*, 2006. Early Evolution of the Venom System in Lizards and Snakes. *Nature* 439:584-588.

Ghoneum M, Felo N, 2015. Selective Induction of Apoptosis in Human Gastric Cancer Cells by Lactobacillus kefiri (PFT), a Novel Kefir Product. *Oncol. Rep.* 34:1659-1666.

Gillard J, 2001. The Definition of Toxin. *Emer. Med. News* 23:53-53.

Henkel JS, Baldwin MR, Barbieri JT, 2010. Toxins from Bacteria. In *Molecular, Clinical, and Environmental Toxicology Volume 2: Clinical Toxicology* (Luch A, Ed.). *Experientia Supplementum* 100:1-29.

HHMI (Howard Hughes Medical Institute), 2002. Research News: *Excessive Growth of Bacteria May Also Be Major Cause of Stomach Ulcers*. HHMI, 4000 Jones Bridge Road, Chevy Chase, Maryland, USA, 15 January.

Holt JG (Ed.), 1994. *Bergey's Manual of Determinative Bacteriology*, 9th Edition. Philadelphia, Pennsylvania, USA: Lippincott Williams & Wilkins.

Hussein HS, Brasel JM, 2001. Toxicity, Metabolism, and Impact of Mycotoxins on Humans and Animals. *Toxicology* 167:101-134.

IARC (International Agency for Research on Cancer), 2012. IARC Monographs on the Evaluation of Carcinogenic Risks to Humans, Volume 100F: Chemical Agents and Related Occupations. Lyon, France: WHO Press.

IARC (International Agency for Research on Cancer), 2017. IARC Monographs on the Evaluation of Carcinogenic Risks to Humans, Volume 1-119: List of Carcinogens. Lyon, France: WHO Press.

Kwong PD, McDonald NQ, Sigler PB, Hendrickson WA, 1995. Structure of *Beta* 2-Bungarotoxin: Potassium Channel Binding by Kunitz Modules and Targeted Phospholipase Action. *Structure* 3:1109-1119.

Levy JI, Buonocore JJ, von Stackelber K, 2010. Evaluation of the Public Health Impacts of Traffic Congestion: A Health Risk Assessment. *Environ. Health* 9:65 (online journal).

Lewis RL, Gutmann L, 2004. Snake Venoms and the Neuromuscular Junction. *Semin. Neurol.* 24:175-179.

Matsui T, Fujimura Y, Titani K, 2000. Snake Venom Proteases Affecting Hemostasis and Thrombosis. *Biochem. et Biophy. Acta (BBA) – Protein Struc. & Mol. Enzym.* 1477:146-156.

MNDLI (Minnesota Department of Labor and Industry), 2017. An Employer's Guide to Developing a Hazard Communication or Employee Right-To-Know Program. Occupational Safety and Health Division, 443 Lafayette Road North, St. Paul, Minnesota, USA.

Nevalainen TJ, Peuravuori HJ, Quinn RJ, Llewellyn LE, Benzie JAH, Fenner PJ, Winkel KD, 2004. Phospholipase A2 in Cnidaria. *Comp. Biochem. Physiol.* 139(Part B):731-735.

NIDCD (National Institute on Deafness and Other Communication Disorders), 2008. NIDCD Fact Sheet: Noise-Induced Hearing Loss. NIH Pub. No. 08-4233. NIDCD Information Clearinghouse, 1 Communication Avenue, Bethesda, Maryland, USA.

NRDC (Natural Resources Defense Council), 2004. Hidden Danger: Environmental Health Threats in the Latino Community (principal authors: Quintero-Somaini A, Quirindongo M). 40 West 20th Street, New York, New York, USA.

Peters A, von Klot S, Heier M, Trentinaglia I, Hörmann A, Wichmann HE, Löwel H, 2004. Exposure to Traffic and the Onset of Myocardial Infarction. *NEJM* 351:1721-1730.

Reiter J, Herker E, Madeo F, Schmitt MJ, 2005. Viral Killer Toxins Induce Caspase-Mediated Apoptosis in Yeast. *J. Cell Biol.* 168:353-358.

Richard JL, 2007. Some Major Mycotoxins and Their Mycotoxicoses – An Overview. *Intl. J. Food Microbiol.* 119:3-10.

Ryan KJ, Ray CG (Eds.), 2004. *Sherris Medical Microbiology*, 4th Edition. New York, New York, USA: McGraw Hill.

Schmitt MJ, Breinig F, 2002. The Viral Killer System in Yeast: From Molecular Biology to Application. *FEMS Microbiol. Rev.* 26:257-276.

Schmitt MJ, Reiter J, 2008. Viral Induced Yeast Apoptosis. *Biochim. Biophys. Acta.* 1783:1413-1417.

Schoental R, 1968. Toxicology and Carcinogenic Action of Pyrrolizidine Alkaloids. *Cancer Res.* 28:2237-2246.

Schofield L, Vivas L, Hackett F, Gerold P, Schwarz RT, Tachado S, 1993. Neutralizing Monoclonal Antibodies to Glycosylphosphatidylinositol, the Dominant TNF-Alpha-Inducing Toxin of *Plasmodium falciparum*: Prospects for the Immunotherapy of Severe Malaria. *Ann. Trop. Med. Parasitol.* 87:617-626.

Smith WL, Wheeler WC, 2006. Venom Evolution Widespread in Fishes: A Phylogenetic Road Map for the Bioprospecting of Piscine Venoms. *J. Heredity* 97:206-217.

Tweedy JT, 2005. *Healthcare Hazard Control and Safety Management*, 2nd Edition. Boca Raton, Florida, USA: CRC Press, Chapter 4 (p.111).

U.S. Code (United States Code), 2013. Title 18 (Crimes and Criminal Procedure), Chapter 10 (Biological Weapons), Section 178 (Definitions). Office of the Law Revision Counsel, U.S. House of Representative, http://uscode.house.gov/ (still effective as of 19 August 2013, retrieved 12 December 2016).

Vetter RS, Isbister GK, Bush SP, Boutin LJ, 2006. Verified Bites by Yellow Sac Spiders (Genus *Cheiracanthium*) in the United States and Australia: Where Is the Necrosis? *Am. J. Trop. Med. Hyg.* 74:1043-1048.

WHO (World Health Organization), 2016. Global Tuberculosis Report 2016. Geneva, Switzerland.

Review Questions

1. What are the main technical differences between a toxicant and a toxin or a venom?
2. What are biological toxic agents?
3. Give one example of toxins that can harm fish, and three examples of toxins that can be found in various species of fish.
4. What are the main technical differences between microbial infection and infectious disease?
5. Name the four main groups of pathogenic microbial agents discussed in this chapter.
6. What are prions and viroids? And what is the general term used to refer them as a special pathogenic group?
7. What are the pathogenic bacteria that are currently of global (*vs.* regional or local) concern?
8. Briefly describe the characteristics of a virus.

9. Name four fungal infections that appear more serious (harmful) than the rest, and list the pathogenic fungi that are responsible for them.
10. What are some of the most common infectious protozoa found in the world?
11. What are some of the most common helminthes found in humans?
12. Briefly describe the characteristics of viral toxins.
13. Name three toxins produced by the bacterial genus *Clostridium*.
14. What are the major symptoms or toxic effects of diphtheria, and of shiga toxins?
15. How are aflatoxins M_1 and M_2 produced? And is aflatoxin M_1 more carcinogenic than aflatoxin B_1?
16. Name four algae-borne toxins that are commonly found in seafood. What are their main toxic effects on humans?
17. Name the mycotoxin that has toxic effects mostly in or unique to swine.
18. Name the one species of scorpions that is considered to have sufficient venom to cause harm to a person living in the western United States.
19. Briefly characterize the symptoms caused by (the venoms of) black widow spiders.
20. Which insect order is responsible for most of the venoms that pose a serious threat to humans? Give a few examples of the venomous insects from this animal order.
21. Match each of the toxins found in plants (left side) to its own *specific, prominent* toxic effect on humans (right side).

    (1) taxol (a) cardiotoxicity
    (2) oxalate (b) hepatotoxicity
    (3) pyrrolizidine alkaloid (c) nephrotoxicity
    (4) toxin from *R. vernix* (d) GI distress
    (5) ricin (e) dermatitis
    (6) toxin from foxglove (f) neurotoxicity

22. Briefly characterize the venoms commonly found in snakes.
23. What are the two species of lizards that are found venomous to people living in Mexico or the southwestern United States?
24. Which animal family is found to have most of the venomous amphibians? And what is the specific neurotoxin that may be found in California newts?
25. What are the four main categories of harmful physical agents or hazards that most professionals in occupational health and safety focus on?
26. What are the major adverse health effects of noise pollution?
27. What are the major health and economic impacts of traffic congestion on a community?

CHAPTER 18

Environmental Mutagenesis/Carcinogenesis

18.1. Introduction

Mutagenesis is the process involving the formation of genetic mutations (i.e., changes in the structure or sequence of DNA's genetic bases) and their progression in a cell's genetic materials. Carcinogenesis is the process whereby normal cells are transformed to tumor cells which are further developed into an abnormal mass of tissue known as tumor with the potential of becoming a cancer. The terms *mutagenicity* and *carcinogenicity* refer to the ability or tendency to induce mutation and cancer (including tumor), respectively. The common risk factors relevant to most mutagenic or carcinogenic effects include one or more of the following: age; gender; race; lifestyle; family medical history; diet; occupational setting; and infection. As discussed in Chapter 10, these factors are also associated with the development of many other diseases.

The main reason why the pathocellular processes mutagenesis and carcinogenesis are frequently discussed side by side, as in this chapter, is that mutagenicity and carcinogenicity are closely interrelated. Over the years, studies have shown strong positive correlation between mutagens (i.e., agents or conditions capable of causing mutation) and carcinogens (i.e., agents or conditions capable of causing tumor or cancer). One widely referenced study in this correlation series is the work by McCann *et al.* (1975), in which 90% (156 out of 174) of the carcinogens under analysis showed mutagenic when they were subjected to the sensitive, short-term *Salmonella* microsome assay developed by Ames *et al.* (1973). With some caveats, the positive correlations compiled later by the U.S. National Research Council (NRC, 1983) ranged from 50% to over 90%.

18.1.1. DNA, RNA, Gene, and Chromosome

The general term for DNA (deoxyribonucleic acid) and RNA (ribonucleic acid) is nucleic acid, which typically consists of hundreds to thousands of nucleotides. Each nucleotide of DNA or RNA is made of one sugar-phosphate backbone binding to either one purine base (adenine [A] or guanine [G]) or one pyrimidine base (cytosine [C] or thymine [T]). The purines and pyrimidines are also known as nitrogenous bases as they each contain some nitrogen (N) atoms (Figure 18.1). The sugar-phosphate backbone includes either the sugar *ribose* (as on RNA) or *deoxyribose* (as on DNA) and one or more phosphate (PO_4^{3-}) groups (Figure 18.1).

DNA is a double-helix (double-stranded) chain of units carrying the genetic materials in a cell, and is responsible for self-replication and the synthesis (encoding) of RNA. As depicted in Figure 18.2, the two strands of DNA are held together by weak hydrogen bonds between the purine and pyrimidine bases. RNA is a constituent of all cells and of many viruses, consisting of normally a single strand with the bases [A], [G], [C], and [U] ($\equiv$ uracil, in lieu of [T]) bonded to the ribose.

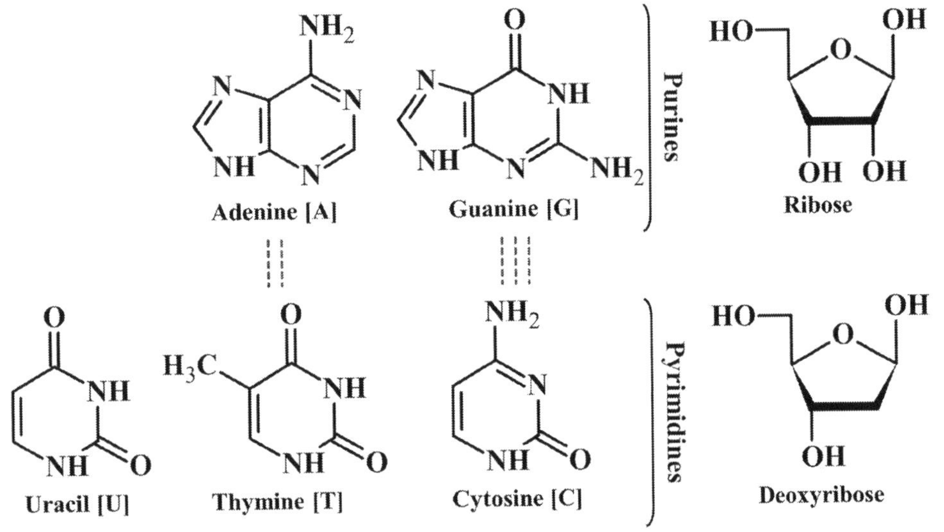

Figure 18.1. Chemical Structures of the Purines, Pyrimidines, Ribose, and Deoxyribose on Nucleic Acids
(*each dotted line signifies one hydrogen bonding between the normal pair of bases*)

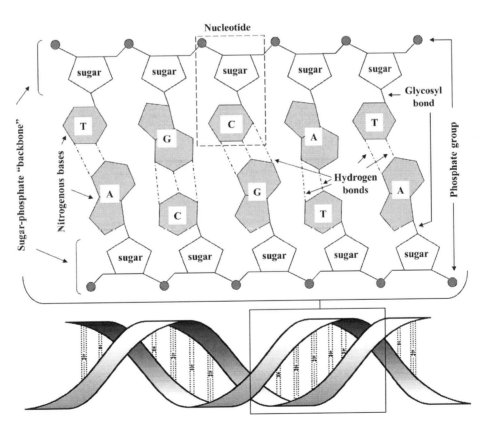

Figure 18.2. Double-Helix (Double-Stranded) Structure of DNA (Deoxyribonucleic Acid)
[Sugar ≡ Deoxyribose; A ≡ Adenine; G ≡ Guanine; C ≡ Cytosine; T ≡ Thymine]

Through certain RNA (i.e., mRNA) acting as a messenger, DNA's base sequence and structure are determinants of protein synthesis and of the transmission of genetic data that it encodes.

The term *genome* denotes the entire (set of) hereditary materials (e.g., including the mitochondrial DNA) in a cell as well as in the organism. It is inscribed in the DNA or, for many types of viruses, in the RNA. The portion of the genome that encodes an RNA and hence a protein is referred to as a gene. The gene that encodes a specific protein (including a specific enzyme) is composed of trinucleotide base units (e.g., [G][G][A], [A][A][C]) termed *codons*, with each encoding a single amino acid (which is the building block of a protein as well as an enzyme).

A gene is thereby a linear sequence on the DNA molecule that encodes a specific form or type of RNA (and hence mostly a specific protein or a certain kind of proteins) that has a specific biochemical role in the organism. An allele is a variant of this physical hereditary unit. An *onco*gene is a gene capable of transforming normal cells into the tumor or cancer kind, whereas a *proto-*oncogene is a gene having the potential to become an oncogene.

Each chromosome is a single piece of long, continuous, highly coiled strand of DNA molecules plus certain proteins. In eukaryotes (i.e., organisms whose cells contain complex structures enclosed within their membranes), chromosomes are housed in the cell nucleus and are packaged by the special proteins *histones* into a condensed structure termed *chromatin*, thereby enabling a very long strand of DNA molecules to fit inside the highly crowded cell nucleus. The genetic materials contained in chromosomes are those that determine an organism's every trait from hair and eye color to sex and behavior. In human cells, the nuclei each contain 22 pairs of non-sex chromosomes termed *autosomes* and 1 pair of sex chromosomes known as XX chromosomes in females and XY chromosomes in males.

Chromosomes must be replicated, divided, and passed on successfully to the daughter cells in order to ensure survival of their progeny and genetic diversity. These essential elements in cell division, or oftentimes referred to as vectors of heredity, may exist as either duplicated or unduplicated. When a chromosome replicates itself at the early stages (e.g., prophase) of cell division, the two identical pieces are termed *chromatids* and are joined together at their most condensed region termed *centromere*. Once the two chromatids have been separated from each other at the later stages (e.g., anaphase) of cell division, they each become a twin daughter chromosome. In humans, certain solid tumors (those without cysts or liquid areas) and leukemia are linked to specific chromosome alterations which, as in gene mutations, can transform certain proto-oncogenes to active oncogenes.

18.1.2. Characteristics of Tumor and Cancer

In the medical literature, neoplasm is the more technical or professional term for tumor; and neoplasia is the technical or professional term for the abnormal proliferation of cells leading to an abnormal mass of tissue (i.e., tumor). Straightly speaking, neoplasm (and hence tumor) is not synonymous with cancer. A neoplasm can be benign, premalignant, or malignant. In contrast, a cancer is supposedly always regarded as malignant and, in a few cases, does not form a solid tumor. For example, leukemia is a cancer of the blood or bone marrow characterized by an abnormal increase of blood cells, usually of leukocytes (i.e., white blood cells).

Cancer is medically treated as a malignant tumor in that it is the kind characterized not only by uncontrolled cell division and growth, but also by its invasive nature and tendency to intrude on or destroy neighboring tissues. In the more severe cases, it also has the capability to spread to more distant tissues via the bloodstream or lymphatic system. Pathocellular spread of this type is medically termed *metastasis* (further discussed in Section 18.3.2).

18.2. Environmental Mutagenesis

Mutagenesis can either occur spontaneously *in vivo* or be induced by mutagenic factors, conditions, or agents largely from the environment. The mutagenicity involved may include a number of autosomal dominant disorders which are genetic diseases capable of being passed down from *one* (and hence *dominant*) parent having the abnormal gene on one of his or her 22 pairs of autosomes. Serious consequences such as sickle-cell anemia can result if the mutation leads to the replacement of a hydro*phobic* amino acid (e.g., valine) for a hydro*philic* one (e.g., glutamic acid), or vice versa, in the affected hemoglobin. Sickle-cell anemia is a genetic blood disorder characterized by red blood cells that take on a rigid, sickle shape. It is a serious or even fatal disease in that red blood cells in sickle shape are very fragile and tend to rupture long before the end of their normal lifespan of approximately 120 days in humans. Nevertheless, it should be mindful that not all genetic mutations are bad. Now and then, a gene mutation can lead to a cell or a species with a greater ability to survive certain physiological hardship or to cope with the stress.

18.2.1. Concepts of Mutagenesis

In addition to induction by environmental mutagens (Section 18.2.4), mutagenesis can occur naturally such as due to spontaneous lesion, integration of transposable genetic elements, or errors in DNA replication. An error in DNA replication can occur when an illegitimate nucleotide pair forms in the course of the replication. Spontaneous lesions are those damages to DNA that occur naturally, such as from cleavage of the purine (adenine [A] or guanine [G]) at the DNA backbone or from removal of an amino group (NH_2) in one of the four distinct nitrogenous bases on the DNA. The cleavage and the removal involved are referred to as depurination and deamination, respectively. There also exists a series of genetic elements that can transpose from one position on a chromosome to another position on the same or a different (e.g., nearby) chromosome. These elements are called transposons if their transposition is through direct DNA transfer, or called retrotransposons if via RNA intermediates.

Although mutation rates vary considerably across species, in most cases they are very low. The estimate for humans has been at about one mutation in every 33 million nucleotides per generation (Xue *et al.*, 2009). Unfortunately, there exist the so-called hotspots on a DNA molecule, such as at the unusual base *5-methyl*cytosine (*5-methyl*-[C]), where mutations can be up to 100 times more frequent than the norm. These hotspots are vulnerable to an array of mutagenic agents including many of those listed in Table 18.1. The DNA (base) sequence of a gene can be altered in a number of ways. Oftentimes for simplicity, the mechanisms involved are classified into two main types: (1) point or intragenic (gene) mutation; and (2) chromosome aberration or alteration.

18.2.2. Point Mutation and Intragenic Mutation

Point and intragenic mutations are the two subtypes of gene mutation occurring in the base sequence of a gene, which unlike chromosome aberrations cannot be seen microscopically. Point mutation involves the replacement of a single DNA base, a subtype that can affect vital cellular functions. For example, sickle-cell anemia is caused by a point mutation in the β-hemoglobin gene that converts the codon [G][A][G] into [G][U][G], leading to the inscription of the amino acid valine instead of glutamic acid. This kind is called *base-pair* substitution in that the nucleotide on the opposite complementary DNA strand is also replaced accordingly. The base replacement in the opposite nucleotide becomes necessary because in the DNA nucleotide, purine [A] (adenine) always pairs with pyrimidine [T] (thymine) by means of weak hydrogen bonding (Figure 18.2), whereas purine [G] (guanine) always pairs with pyrimidine [C] (cytosine).

Intragenic mutation is a special form of point mutation involving *insertion* or *deletion* of a single base pair, which frequently produces an incorrect gene product leading to potentially a more detrimental effect on the biosynthesized protein (which can be an enzyme with a significant biological function). This form is also called frameshift mutation in that while the nucleotides are still read in triplets, they are in different frames as a result of the insertion or deletion.

18.2.3. Chromosome Aberration

Chromosome aberration brings about *structural* or *numerical* alterations of chromosomes. Numerical change that involves one or more extra or missing chromosomes is termed *aneuploidy*. For example, one of the most common aneuploidies that infants can survive with is trisomy 21, which means that these children each have an extra, third copy of autosome 21 (i.e., the 21st autosome, with the longest being named the first). These children not only suffer from mental retardation but also allegedly look like people of a certain ethnicity. This condition is medically known as Down (or Down's) syndrome as it was first formally reported in 1866 by an English physician named John L. Down. Another example of aneuploidies is Turner syndrome, which attributes to a *female* human with only one sex chromosome. This genetic disorder is characterized by short stature, broad chest, low hairline, low-set ears, and webbed necks. Turner syndrome is sometimes referred to as gonadal dysgenesis in that most victims would experience gonadal dysfunction with a nonfunctional ovary leading to sterility from absence of menstrual cycle.

The type or form of toxicity causing changes in chromosome structure is termed *clastogenicity*. Major types of structural changes in chromosomes include *deletion, duplication, inversion*, and (reciprocal) *translocation* of genes on chromosomes. These four subclasses occur mostly at the meiotic stage of cell division. Meiosis is a complex process in which the number of *sex* chromosomes per cell is cut in half. This process involves the sex chromosomes exchanging segments with one another via the event called crossover. If the event loses its fidelity, the structure of these chromosomes will be altered.

Chromosome deletion refers to the loss of one or more genes on a chromosome (e.g., genes A*B*CDE → ACDE), such as in children suffering from the *cri du chat* syndrome due to a missing part of autosome 5. The syndrome includes intellectual disability, delayed development, microcephaly, and weak muscle tone. It gets its name from the characteristic cry of affected infants sounding like a cat's due to problems with the larynx and the nervous system. Chromosome duplication (e.g., ABCDE → ABC*CD*D*E*) results from replication of one or more segments of a chromosome. An example of chromosome duplication disorders in humans is Charcot-Marie-Tooth neuropathy, characterized by loss of muscle tissues and touch sensation in the feet and legs, yet in the advanced stages also in the hands and arms.

Chromosome inversion (e.g., ABCDE → AB*DC*E) can result from re-attachment of a chromosome segment to the original chromosome but in a reverse order, such as when caused by a mutagen or an error at the meiotic stage. As a case example (e.g., Webb *et al.*, 2008), an inverted region on autosome 17 was reportedly linked to several Pick complex diseases (e.g., frontotemporal dementia) and other neurological disorders including corticobasal degeneration and progressive supranuclear palsy. Chromosome translocation (e.g., $A_1B_1C_1D_1E_1 \rightarrow A_1B_1C_2D_2E_1$, where genes C_2 and D_2 are from *another* nearby chromosome) can result from the attachment of a chromosomal segment to a non-homologous chromosome. Both of the last two subclasses of chromosome aberration affect a gene's activity and regulation by altering its position on a chromosome. Accordingly, these two subclasses tend to cause more detrimental effects. Burkitt's lymphoma (Burkitt, 1958; Liu *et al.*, 2007) and Mantle cell lymphoma (e.g., Li *et al.*, 1999) are the two types of cancer reportedly caused by chromosome translocation.

18.2.4. Environmental Mutagens

Most of the mutagens of concern are environmental in origin. As expected, these mutagens can be broadly subsumed under the three major common source categories: biological, chemical, and physical. Examples of the various types of mutagens representing the three source groups are given in Table 18.1, of which only certain abiologic ones are elaborated on here as due to space limitation. Examples of physical mutagens include ultraviolet (UV) radiation, ionizing radiation, and mineral fibers. These various physical kinds act on the DNA gene sequence via different modes. Ionizing radiation can come from X-rays or gamma rays and from the decay of uranium. Muller (1927) was the first to discover that X-ray caused mutations in fruit flies. Mutagens of this kind literally can pass through an organism's body to the chromosomes in its cells to directly corrupt the DNA's proper base sequence there. UV radiation (e.g., sunlight) can cause portions of DNA to bond to one another when they should not. This will cause the DNA sequence to be misread leading to mutation. For instance, UV light can cause two adjacent pyrimidine bases to form a dimer, such as with a [T] (thymine) covalently bonded to an adjacent [T] to cause the misreading of the true DNA base sequence. Certain natural mineral fibers, such as the long-shaped asbestos, can interfere with chromosome distribution during cell division to cause genomic or chromosome aberration (Jensen *et al.*, 1996; Nelson and Kelsey, 2002).

Many chemical agents can alter the gene sequence by binding to the DNA in a cell. Examples of chemical mutagens include nitrogen mustards, nitrous acid, hydroxylamine, proflavine, vinyl chloride, 5-bromouracil (5-BU), benzo[α]pyrene (upon metabolic activation), aflatoxin B_1 (upon metabolic activation), and heterocyclic amines. Many of these chemical substances can be found at some level in various environments. For example, nowadays 5-BU is often utilized as an experimental mutagen. Nitrogen mustards are now more utilized as cytotoxic chemotherapy agents in medicine. The major precursors of nitrous acid are nitrites which have been employed heavily as preservatives in foods (e.g., hot dogs, luncheon meats, smoked fish). Proflavine has been applied as a surface disinfectant. Vinyl chloride has been employed predominantly as an intermediate to form PVC (polyvinyl chloride) in the plastics industry. Hydroxylamine has been used as an antioxidant for fatty acids. Aflatoxin B_1, produced by the fungal genus *Aspergillus*, tends to grow on spice, cereal, and nut type crops. Benzo[α]pyrene is a five-ring PAH (polycyclic aromatic hydrocarbon) found in tobacco smoke, coal tar, and automobile exhaust fumes. Heterocyclic amines are frequently found in (over-)cooked meat.

Table 18.1. Select (Environmental) Agents Known or Suspected to Cause Mutation in Human or Some Other Mammalian Cells[a]

Type/Subgroup	Examples of Mutagens	Mode/Site of Mutagenic Action
Physical		
Ionizing Radiation	X-rays; gamma rays; α- or β- particles; radionuclides (e.g., isotopes of uranium)	By causing irreparable DNA damage usually from exposure at chronic or high levels
Ultraviolet Radiation	UV-A wavelength; UV-B wavelength; sunlight	By causing typically adjacent pyrimidine (thymine or cytosine) bases to covalently bond together (thereby forming pyrimidine dimers); also by inducing oxidative damage to DNA (particularly by UV-A)
Biological		
Viruses	Adenoviruses (DNA viruses); human papillomaviruses (DNA viruses); retroviruses (RNA viruses)	By inducing gene mutations like the way mutagenic bacteriophages will; by forming gross chromosome alterations; by inducing reverse transcription by retroviruses to replicate DNA
Bacteria	*Helicobacter pylori*	By causing inflammation-induced DNA damaging activity
Chemical		
Alkylating agents	Nitrogen mustards; cisplatin sodium azide; melphalan; nitrosoureas	Primarily by adding molecular components to DNA bases
Cross-linking agents	Melphalan; cisplatin	By creating covalent bonds with DNA bases
DNA-adductors	Benzo[α]pyrene; aflatoxin B_1	By forming stable DNA adducts (particularly with the guanine base)

[a]from various sources (and further review of references that these sources cited) including a number of hand/textbooks in mutagenesis, carcinogenesis, and related subjects (e.g., genetics, molecular biology).

Mutagens can also be divided into different categories according to their effects on DNA replication. Some (e.g., 5-BU) act as base analogs to replace the true nitrogenous bases on the DNA strand during replication. Some others react with DNA to cause structural changes, such as by forming adducts with DNA (e.g., as in the case with the epoxide metabolite of benzo[α]pyrene or of aflatoxin B_1) and by intercalating (i.e., wedging) between two nitrogenous bases on the DNA (e.g., as in the case with proflavine). The last two cases can lead to miscopying of the template strand when the affected DNA is replicated. Still some others work indirectly by causing the cells to synthesize substances that have the direct mutagenic effect. To some scholars, mutagens of this *biosynthesized* kind might not be treated as environmental in origin.

Until more recently, the mutagenicity of environmental agents was largely determined by the *Salmonella* microsome *in vitro* assay. This relatively low-cost test utilizes several strains of the bacterial species *Salmonella typhimurium* that each carry a defective gene which otherwise is responsible for encoding the essential amino acid *histidine*, by utilizing the ingredients provided in the culture medium. Many chemical substances have the ability to induce a reverse mutation on this defective gene so that the gene can regain its normal function to enable the bacterium strain to grow on a medium lacking histidine. Those chemical substances that have been tested positive (i.e., to have such an ability) are qualified as (potential) mutagens.

In the *Salmonella* assay known also as the Ames test, as named after its developers (Ames *et al.*, 1973), a mixture of *hepatic* microsomes (which are rich in *liver* enzymes) is purposely added to the culture medium as an enhancer of the intended reverse (i.e., backward) mutation. This is because certain substances, such as benzo[α]pyrene and aflatoxin B_1, are not mutagenic *per se* until they have been metabolically activated. Given that *S. typhimurium* is not meant to be a perfect model for the human body as it is simply a bacterium, the Ames test now is but one of several methods employed to determine the mutagenicity of a suspect agent. These other testing methods include a variety of *in vitro* and *in vivo* assays utilizing mammalian cell lines as culture media, such as the *in vitro* and *in vivo* micronucleus test, the mouse lymphoma (thymidine kinase gene mutation) assay, the bone marrow metaphase analysis, and the transgenic animal models. Details and references for these other testing methods can be found in a harmonization project paper issued by the World Health Organization (WHO) on mutagenicity testing (Eastmond *et al.*, 2009).

18.3. Environmental Carcinogenesis

Carcinogenesis, as well as tumorigenesis, is a pathocellular process involving erratic cell division which otherwise occurs at a normal pace in almost all cells. A basic knowledge of cell (division) cycle is therefore essential to the understanding of carcinogenesis. The cell cycle represents a repeating series of biological events within a cell that leads to the cell's division and replication. In an autosomal (also called somatic) cell with a nucleus (as in the eukaryotes), the cell cycle can be broadly divided into four distinct as well as technical phases: (1) the *first g*rowth G*1* phase; (2) the *s*ynthesis S phase; (3) the *second g*rowth G*2* phase; and (4) the *m*itosis M phase.

The first three phases G1, S, and G2 collectively are also referred to as the *interphase*, during which the non-gamete (i.e., the somatic) cell grows and accumulates nutrients required for DNA replication as well as for chromatid duplication in the S phase. Further cell growth for mitosis takes place in the G2 phase which represents the last stage of the interphase. The M phase itself involves two tightly coupled events: mitosis and cytokinesis. In *mitosis*, the chromosomes in a *somatic* cell are each divided between the two identical daughter cells being formed, whereas in cytokinesis the cell's cytoplasm is divided in half to complete the formation of the two daughter cells proper. Initiation of each of the four phases is contingent on the proper progression and completion of the previous phase. Following a cell division, each of the daughter cells begins the interphase of her own.

Meiosis is a special type of cell division involving the formation of only *gamete* (i.e., sperm or egg) cells. These sex cells each have to undergo the *meiotic* division process twice, though with only one round of DNA replication, in order for their daughter cells each to end up having half of the number of chromosomes that they (i.e., the parent sex cells) each have. Meiosis does not lead to a cell cycle in the way that mitosis does, as fertilization of two opposite sex cells is required to extend the genetic life of *each* of the two opposite sex cells. The preparatory steps that lead to meiosis include only the first two stages in the interphase (i.e., the G1 and the S phase) of the *mitotic* cell cycle.

Cell cycle is by no means an ever-ongoing biological or cellular process. There are a number of signal transduction pathways or systems, commonly known as checkpoints, in a cell cycle that play a key role in upholding the fidelity of DNA replication as well as the genetic stability in cells. For instance, one checkpoint is there to prevent cells from entering mitosis if they fail to replicate all their chromosomes. Another checkpoint is there to either stall or arrest a critical stage of the cell cycle in an effort to facilitate DNA repair, whenever it senses an event leading to DNA damage or misalignment of the replication structure. In general, those checkpoints that function in response to moderate DNA damage will activate the p53 protein to block or stall the cell cycle. When the DNA damage becomes substantial enough, the p53 protein in turn will activate genes that induce the regular process of programmed cell death which is known technically as *apoptosis*. Apoptosis is an important process in that it helps maintain genetic stability by destroying cells that are unlikely repairable or that represent a threat to the integrity of a multicellular organism.

18.3.1. Concepts of Carcinogenesis

A fundamental principle underlying most theories of carcinogenesis as well as tumorigenesis is the alteration of DNA's base sequences. Extensive alteration of the DNA's base sequences will lead to altered base sequences in the mRNA (*m*essenger RNA) and subsequently to the synthesis of abnormal proteins, of which many are important enzymes. The functions of the so biosynthesized enzymes consequently can become so abnormal that cell proliferation subject to their catalytic regulations either becomes out of control or continues indefinitely.

The most accepted theory of carcinogenesis today is that mutations of the genetic materials in normal cells will cause an upset of the normal balance between cell proliferation and apoptosis, eventually leading to uncontrolled cell division and proliferation. The uncontrolled and often rapid proliferation of cells then leads to the formation of a tumor, which may turn into the malignant kind known as cancer.

More than one kind of mutations is thought necessary for activation of carcinogenesis. Only mutations in genes playing a key role in the cell cycle, DNA repair, and cell death are likely to cause cells to lose control of their proliferation. The current school of thought is that a series of mutations involving at least three types of genes is generally required for cells to start dividing erratically. The three gene types of most relevancy are tumor suppressor genes, DNA repair genes, and proto-oncogenes. Tumor suppressor genes will encode proteins (including enzymes) or anti-proliferation signals that function to suppress mitosis and cell growth. Proto-oncogenes will encode proteins that promote cell growth. DNA repair genes, on the other hand, will encode enzymes whose normal functions are to identify and correct errors that arise when cells replicate their DNA prior to cell division. More specifically, for tumor cells to form, a mutation is needed to inactivate one or more tumor suppressor genes so that cells are allowed to proliferate at abnormal rates. Another required mutation is one that inactivates one or more DNA repair genes to cause repair failure. Still another mutation is needed to activate proto-oncogenes into oncogenes which are the type more ready to synthesize hormones and proteins (enzymes) that promote uncontrollable cell proliferation. The final outcome of this set of mutations is tumor or cancer formation.

18.3.2. Mechanism of Carcinogenesis

At the mechanistic level involving molecular and cellular changes, carcinogenesis is viewed by many in the scientific sectors (e.g., Abel and DiGiovanni, 2011; Dong *et al.*, 1988; Hofseth *et al.*, 2017; Weinberg, 2013; Weiss, 2004) as a multistage process involving broadly the *initiation*, *promotion*, and *progression* stages of normal cells into tumor or cancer cells (Figure 18.3). It is thought that the transition from one of these stages to another, likely necessarily in that order, is inducible by a wide array of environmental and endogenous agents, while subject to various genetic regulations and biochemical influences. Yet from a genetic perspective, carcinogenesis should or could still be characterized as an accumulation of mutations in the tumor suppressor genes, DNA repair genes, and proto-oncogenes, as discussed in the preceding subsection.

Certain endogenous and exogenous substances are known capable of initiating the carcinogenic (as well as tumorigenic) process by yielding or becoming highly reactive species that have the ability or tendency to bind covalently to cellular DNA. These agents are referred to as procarcinogens. There are other agents that can cause DNA damage directly without their undergoing any chemical or metabolic activation. These agents are called ultimate or genotoxic carcinogens. In either case, if the DNA damage is irreparable, it will lead to irreversible genetic mutations. Other characteristics of the initiation stage include the requirement of fixation and the high tendency of having an additive as well as a non-threshold effect. For the *irreversible* initiation process to take its full force and course, the damaged or affected DNA segment needs to be placed securely (i.e., fixed) into the daughter genome throughout the DNA replication.

The promotion stage is where one or more other agents, factors, or conditions stimulate the proliferation and the clonal expansion of the initiated cells to yield a massive production of their daughter cells. Many of these promoting agents (e.g., tobacco smoke, alcohol) or factors (e.g., lack of physical activity, health condition), also called promoters or more technically epigenetic carcinogens, are found extrinsic to the host. The effects that they promote oftentimes exhibit a threshold and tend to be dose-dependent and thereby likely *reversible*. These agents or factors may pose a relatively low risk for causing a tumor when the dose and the frequency of exposure to them are insufficiently low. An essential condition for this stage to take its course is the setting of a proper mitogenic environment (i.e., that conducive of mitosis). For this second mechanistic stage to have its full force and effect, the environment requires the presence of continuous stimulation which will then increase the risk of inducing further genetic changes on the initiated cells.

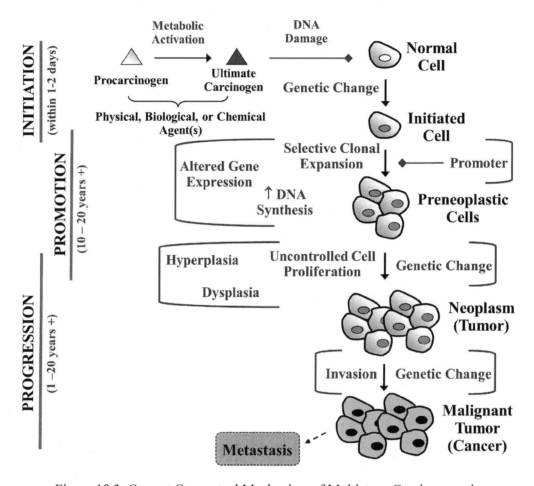

Figure 18.3. Current Conceptual Mechanism of Multistage Carcinogenesis

During tumor progression, preneoplastic cells will develop into a tumor by undergoing further proliferation and expansion of the successful clones (which are each a cluster of cells derived from the same parent cells). In this final stage of carcinogenesis (or more correctly tumorigenesis), the preneoplastic cells become increasingly resistant to apoptotic stimuli and other negative regulatory controls. The progression is thought to be *irreversible*, with the involved proliferation and expansion being conceived as primarily passive and spontaneous. In a sense, the progression from preneoplastic cells into a tumor is a chain of stepwise pathocellular changes, involving at least the hyperplastic and the dysplastic subphase. This early stage of tumor progression is referred to as the malignant conversion stage by some scholars (e.g., Hofseth *et al.*, 2017). In the hyperplastic phase, the preoplastic cells in a local region of the affected tissue divide in an uncontrolled manner leading to an excess of cells which all still have the normal appearance. Yet further progression with the hyperplastic cells will result in an abnormal growth not only in size but also in shape and appearance. At this point of progression, the now dysplastic cells may become disorganized but not yet invasive. Toward the very late progression stage, however, the tumor may become malignant or more so if its cells have the ability or tendency to invade surrounding tissues and spread to regions outside of the affected tissue (e.g., Weinberg, 2013).

As hinted in Section 18.1.2, the part of the progression that leads to the spread of cancerous cells to more distant regions in the body is medically termed *metastasis*. This substage represents the most fearsome aspect of cancer development as it signals a very late stage disease involving highly complicated treatment with poor outcomes. Metastasis occurs most commonly by way of the bloodstream or the lymphatic system. Occasionally, it can occur by local extension from the tumor to somewhat more distant tissues. The cells in a (primary) tumor by nature adhere to one another as well as to a mesh of proteins that fill the space between them. Therefore, to begin metastasis, the cancerous cells must be capable of breaking away from the (nonmalignant) tumor. In most instances, the loosened cells then proceed to make their way into the bloodstream which provides them with a means for their transport to (almost) all other parts of the body, as well as with the nutrients and energy required for their growth.

Not all cells in a tumor are able to metastasize (i.e., spread). For those that are able to, the extent of their dissemination is determined in part by the host's physiological conditions that may or may not be conducive for certain physiological inhibitors to kick in to suppress the invasive activity. That is, these cancerous cells must be able to fight off the host's numerous defense systems before they can re-attach themselves in a new location. Such a metastatic process also depends on the complex interaction of many factors pertaining to the nature of the primary cancer, including its type, maturity, and location.

The new cancer developed from metastasis is medically referred to as secondary or metastatic cancer, in that its cells all appear and behave much more like those in the primary cancer (as well as tumor) than in tissues at the invaded location. For instance, if breast cancer metastasizes to the brain, the secondary cancer is made up of abnormal breast cells, not of cells in or around the brain. In essence, metastasis is characterized by invasive activity and cell resemblance, in addition to the host's physiological conditions.

18.3.3. Environmental Carcinogens

Over the years, a vast number of chemical, physical, and biological agents found in the environment have been determined or suspected as carcinogenic to humans or other mammalians. For some of these environmental agents, their carcinogenicity potential has been evaluated extensively by the International Agency for Research on Cancer (IARC), which is a very authoritative as well as a highly influential extension of WHO that strives to promote intergovernmental collaboration in cancer research and prevention.

IARC's main objectives include coordinating and conducting epidemiological as well as laboratory studies relevant to the causes of human cancers. The agency also has a strong commitment in developing sound strategies for cancer prevention. IARC maintains a series of monographs on the carcinogenic risks to humans that are brought about from exposure to select chemical, biological, and physical agents (supposedly) of high health concerns. These agents (including in the form of exposures) are evaluated by IARC in terms of the evidence available for human exposure and carcinogenicity (e.g., IARC, 2015). After evaluation, these agents are each classified into one of the five categories of carcinogenicity potential listed in Box 18.1 below.

Box 18.1. Classification of Carcinogenicity Potential as Developed and Set Forth by the International Agency for Research on Cancer (e.g., IARC, 2015)

Group 1:	Carcinogenic to humans.
Group 2A:	Probably carcinogenic to humans.
Group 2B:	Possibly carcinogenic to humans.
Group 3:	Not classifiable as to the agent's carcinogenicity to humans.
Group 4:	Probably not carcinogenic to humans.

In their simplest terms, Group 1 in Box 18.1 is used for those agents with sufficient evidence of carcinogenicity in humans. Group 2A is used for those with limited evidence of carcinogenicity in humans but sufficient evidence of carcinogenicity in experimental animals, whereas Group 2B is for those with limited evidence of carcinogenicity in humans and less than sufficient evidence of carcinogenicity in experimental animals. Group 3 is used for agents with *both* inadequate evidence of carcinogenicity in humans *and* inadequate or limited evidence of carcinogenicity in experimental animals. Lastly, Group 4 (the fifth category) is used for agents with solid or sound support pointing to the lack of carcinogenicity in both humans and experimental animals.

For illustration as well as didactic purposes, a list of select agents/exposures covering all these five categories of carcinogenicity potential is given in Table 18.2. Note that a few individual government agencies, notably U.S. EPA, have opted to adopt a somewhat different categorization scheme to rate the carcinogenicity potential for the agents under their own cancer risk assessment.

18.4. DNA Damage and Repair

DNA damage is one of the several crucial underlying causes of genetic mutation leading to the development of tumor or cancer. Its repair is thereby a pivotal point of mutagenesis, and hence of carcinogenesis or tumorigenesis as well, that deserves further discussion in this chapter. DNA damage occurs in living cells at very high frequency, owing to the enormous factors, agents, and conditions present in the environment as well as the high volume of metabolic processes occurring spontaneously inside most any cell. It has estimated (Vilenchik and Knudson, 2000) that in human cells, the spontaneous formation of DNA damage on average occurs at a daily rate of roughly 19,000 molecular lesions per cell. Fortunately or not, this still constitutes only a very small fraction of the human genome's approximately 6 billion nitrogenous bases. And in many instances, the damage can be repaired through genetic information stored in the intact opposite strand of the

Table 18.2. Human Carcinogenicity Potential of Select Agents or Exposures as Determined and Classified by IARC[a]

Agent/Exposure (Carcinogen)	Carcinogenicity Potential[b]	IARC Volume(s)[a]
Physical		
Ionizing radiation: all types	1	100D
Ultraviolet radiation: UV-A, UV-B, UV-C	1	100D, 118
Fluorescent lighting	3	55
Biological		
Aflatoxins (B_1, B_2, G_1, G_2)[c]	1	56, 82, 100F
Hepatitis B and C viruses (infection with)	1	59, 100B
HIV type 1 (infection with)	1	67, 100B
Helicobacter pylori (infection with)	1	61, 100B
Salted fish, Chinese style	1	56, 100E
Human papillomavirus type 68 (infection with)	2A	100B
HIV type 2 (infection with)	2B	67
Human papillomavirus type 26 (infection with)	2B	100B
Hepatitis D virus (infection with)	3	59
Chemical		
Asbestos: all forms	1	14, Sup 7, 100C
Benzene	1	29, Sup 7, 100F
Benzo[α]pyrene	1	92, Sup 7, 100F
Chromium VI compounds	1	49, Sup 7, 100C
Diethylstilbestrol (DES)	1	21, Sup 7, 100A
Dioxin/TCDD (2,3,7,8-tetrachlorodibenzo-*p*-dioxin)	1	69, Sup 7, 100F
Ethanol in alcoholic beverages	1	96, 100E
Formaldehyde	1	62, 88, Sup 7, 100F
Polychlorinated biphenyls (PCBs)	1	18, Sup 7, 107
Vinyl chloride	1	97, Sup 7, 100F
Diazinon	2A	112
Nitrogen mustard	2A	9, Sup 7
Carbon tetrachloride	2B	20, Sup 7, 71
Perfluorooctanoic acid (PFOA)	2B	110
Hair coloring products (personal use of)	3	57, 99
Caffeine; tea	3	51
Toluene; xylenes	3	47, 71
Vitamin K substances	3	76
Caprolactam	4	39, Sup 7, 71

[a] International Agency for Research on Cancer (*see* IARC, 2017 and the IARC website for access to each monograph volume listed in this table); an effort has been made here, though through a somewhat arbitrary selection process, to cover all types of agents/exposures and all carcinogenicity potential categories.

[b] as listed in Box 18.1, Group 1 ≡ carcinogenic to humans; Group 2A ≡ probably carcinogenic to humans; Group 2B ≡ possibly carcinogenic to humans; Group 3 ≡ not classifiable as to the agent's carcinogenicity to humans; Group 4 ≡ probably (or likely) not carcinogenic to humans.

[c] note that aflatoxins are treated as biological (*vs.* chemical) agents for the argument given in Section 17.1.1.

DNA's double helix. Moreover, most cells have a feedback system in place that, following DNA damage, several checkpoints are activated to block or stall the cell cycle in an effort to allow time for the affected cells to repair the damage before they continue to divide. Checkpoints responsive to DNA damage typically occur at the cell cycle G1/S and G2/M boundaries (e.g., Barnum and O'Connell, 2014; Houtgraaf *et al.*, 2006).

18.4.1. Causes of DNA Damage

In a broad sense, DNA damage is caused either by certain highly bioactive endogenous substances such as reactive oxygen species (ROS) produced from normal metabolic processes, or by certain external agents in the environment such as chemicals, viruses, bacteria, and UV radiation. The various types or forms of DNA damage commonly found in cells include: modification or loss of DNA base; DNA replication error; crosslinks between DNA's two strands or between DNA and proteins (including enzymes); and DNA strand breakage.

The glycosyl bond linking a DNA base to the sugar deoxyribose (Figure 18.2) is labile under physiological stress, thus easily resulting in the loss of the base. All four types of bases on the DNA (i.e., adenine [A], guanine [G], cytosine [C], thymine [T]) are susceptible to numerous modifications at various positions by UV radiation as well as by a wide variety of chemical and biological agents. For instance, the primary amino groups (NH_2) in the DNA bases are relatively unstable. They can be converted to a carbonyl group (C=O). One of the most frequent base modifications is therefore the loss of an amino group (with the removal reaction being termed *deamination*), such as with a cytosine [C] being converted to a uracil [U]. On the other hand, several ROS (e.g., superoxide $O_2\cdot$, hydroxyl radical $HO\cdot$, singlet oxygen $^1\Delta_g O_2$) can alter the DNA bases, such as in the oxidation of thymine [T] to thymine glycol.

Other major sources of DNA damage include the generation of mismatches and the minor insertions or deletions of bases during DNA replication. Mismatches of the normal bases can occur due to a failure of proofreading during DNA replication, such as the incorporation of uracil [U] (normally found in RNA only) in place of [T].

Covalent linkages can be formed between bases on the same DNA strand (thus called *intrastrand* crosslink) or between bases on the opposite strand (*interstrand* crosslink). DNA topoisomerases are enzymes that facilitate DNA replication through winding and unwinding DNA's complex double helix. These enzymes (proteins) too can form covalent linkages between themselves and their DNA substrates during the course of their catalytic action. These types of crosslinkage can all cause blockage of DNA replication, leading to replication arrest and cell death unless the crosslink can be repaired timely.

Several chemotherapeutic drugs employed for anti-cancer treatment can crosslink with DNA, such as the alkylating agent nitrogen mustard to form an *inter*strand crosslink by acting on the opposite strand at the N7 position of guanine [G] (i.e., at this base's only nitrogen (N) atom as shown on the upper left of the molecule in Figure 18.1). Another example is the platinum-based cisplatin which can act on the N7 position of an adjacent [G] to form an *intra*strand crosslink. Psoralen is a phytochemical used with UV-A light to treat psoriasis, eczema, and vitiligo. It has both the ability to absorb UV photons and a strong tendency to intercalate with DNA base pairs. Upon activation by UV-A radiation, this phytochemical can form covalent crosslinks between the pyrimidines located opposite to each other on the double strands.

Breaks or breakage in the sugar-phosphate backbone can involve just one of the two DNA strands (i.e., resulting in a single-stranded breakage, SSB) or both strands (i.e., a double-stranded breakage, DSB). The two kinds of strand breakage can be induced by ionizing radiation and certain anticancer (e.g., camptothecin) or antibiotic (e.g., bleomycin) agents. In addition, both SSB and DSB can be formed during normal DNA metabolism by DNA topoisomerases and DNA nucleases, as well as during DNA repair processes though at a much lower frequency.

18.4.2. Mechanisms of DNA Repair

DNA repair generally refers to an *enzymatic* defense system whereby a cell can enzymatically identify and correct damage to the DNA molecules. This system, present in all biological organisms tested today, is essential for the genetic integrity of the organism, considering that a failure to repair DNA damage can result in a severe genetic mutation. In mammalians, DNA repair is accomplished via broadly two types (modes) of enzymatic defense mechanisms: (1) repair mechanisms; and (2) damage tolerance mechanisms. The repair mechanisms all involve removal of DNA damage via a series of enzymatic events, whereas the damage tolerance mechanisms all circumvent the damage enzymatically without fixing it.

Perhaps the most frequent cause of point mutation in humans is the spontaneous alkylation of cytosine [C] (e.g., by addition of a methyl group CH_3^- to the base) followed by its deamination into a thymine [T]. Fortunately, this type of base modification can be readily repaired by a series of enzymes under the so-termed *base excision repair (BER) mechanism*. First, the damaged or mismatched base is removed by the enzyme DNA glycosylase. The related phosphodiester bond (that linking two adjacent sugars via a phosphate group on the same DNA molecule) is then cut off by an enzyme named (DNA) AP endonuclease (where AP ≡ *ap*urinic or *ap*yrimidinic) after recognizing the missing "tooth" (i.e., the missing base). The cleaved part is subsequently resynthesized by a DNA polymerase of the kind capable of catalyzing the polymerization of DNA into a strand. Lastly, a DNA ligase is there to perform the final nick-sealing step.

Another closely related repair mechanism is *nucleotide excision repair (NER)*, which recognizes and repairs various bulky helix-distorting lesions (e.g., those induced by UV radiation). A typical NER involves over 20 enzymes to recognize and excise the damage to a DNA oligonucleotide of about 30 bases in length. As with BER, NER also requires enzymes to activate as well as to catalyze the repair and ligation steps. A specialized form of NER known as transcription-coupled repair recognizes the DNA lesions differently by deploying NER enzymes to the damaged genes (in the nucleotides on the affected strand) that are being actively transcribed.

Mismatch repair (MMR) is an enzymatic mechanism used in DNA replication and recombination to correct errors that resulted in mispaired nucleotides or bases. In this repair, some of the enzymes involved in BER and NER may be required, in addition to those specific for recognizing and excising the mismatch.

DNA damage due to SSB, and particularly to DSB, is often highly destructive to the cell in that such damage is more likely to cause genome rearrangements. The repair of SSB generally calls for the same enzyme systems that are used in BER or NER. For the DSB repair, typically three repair submechanisms are involved: (1) homologous recombination (HR); (2) non-homologous end joining (NHEJ); and (3) microhomology-mediated end joining (MMEJ). Both MMEJ and NHEJ require enzymes that recognize and then bind to the broken ends to bring them together for ligation. MMEJ differs from NHEJ mainly in its using its *own* short (around 5 to 25) base-pair microhomologous sequences as a template for aligning the broken strands before joining. In HR, the broken ends are repaired using the genetic sequence on the intact sister chromatid or homologous chromosome as a template. On the other hand, some cells are capable of removing and repairing certain types of DNA lesion by chemically reversing the damage without requiring a template. This process is known as direct chemical reversal.

In any event, many cells also have the ability to proceed the DNA replication by utilizing the damaged strand as a template though in an error-prone process known as translesion DNA synthesis (TLS). TLS is a (DNA) damage tolerance or lesion bypass process in which the lesion is not repaired by the regular type of DNA polymerases, but is bypassed by the specialized type called TLS (DNA) polymerases. These TLS polymerases allow the DNA replication machinery to replicate by *traversing* the DNA lesion. Some of the DNA lesions that reportedly can be so circumvented include *AP* sites (i.e., those *without* a purine or a pyrimidine) and thymine [T] dimers (e.g., in response to UV radiation). Along with some general discussion of DNA damage, the functions of TLS polymerases and their role in this type of damage tolerance process have been reviewed extensively in a number of excellent articles (e.g., Goodman and Woodgate, 2013; Knobel and Marti, 2011; Prakash *et al.*, 2005; Sale, 2013; Vaisman and Woodgate, 2017; Waters *at al.*, 2009).

References

Abel EL, DiGiovanni J, 2011. Multistage Carcinogenesis. In *Chemical Carcinogenesis* (Penning TM, Ed.), New York, New York, USA: Humana Pressm, Chapter 2.

Ames BN, Durston WE, Yamasaki E, Lee FD, 1973. Carcinogens Are Mutagens: A Simple Test System Combining Liver Homogenates for Activation and Bacteria for Detection. *Proc. Natl. Acad. Sci. USA* 70: 2281-2285.

Barnum KJ, O'Connell MH, 2014. Cell Cycle Regulation by Checkpoints. *Mthds. Mol. Biol.* 1170:29-40.

Burkitt D, 1958. A Sarcoma Involving the Jaws in African Children. *Brit. J. Surg.* 46:218-223.

Dong MH, Redmond CK, Mazumdar S, Costantino JP, 1988. A Multistage Approach to the Cohort Analysis of Lifetime Lung Cancer Risk among Steelworkers Exposed to Coke Oven Emissions. *Am. J. Epidemiol.* 128:860-873.

Eastmond DA, Hartwig A, Anderson D, Anwar WA, Cimino MC, Dobrev I, Douglas GR, Nohmi T, Phillips DH, Vickers C, 2009. Mutagenicity Testing for Chemical Risk Assessment: Update of the WHO/IPCS Harmonized Scheme. *Mutagenesis* 24:341-349.

Goodman MF, Woodgate R, 2013. Translesion DNA Polymerases. *Cold Spring Harb. Perspect. Biol.* 5: a010363 (online journal).

Hofseth LJ, Weston A, Harris CC, 2017. Chemical Carcinogenesis, In *Holland-Frei Cancer Medicine* (Bast RC Jr, Croce CM, Hait WN, Hong WK, Kufe DW, Piccart-Gebhart M, Pollock RE, Weichselbaum RR, Wang H, Holland JF, Eds.), 9th Edition, Hoboken, New Jersey, USA: John Wiley & Sons, Chapter 23.

Houtgraaf JH, Versmissen J, van der Giessen WJ, 2006. A Concise Review of DNA Damage Checkpoints and Repair in Mammalian Cells. *Cardiovasc. Revasc. Med.* 7:165-172.

IARC (International Agency for Research on Cancer), 2015. IARC Monographs on the Evaluation of Carcinogenic Risks to Humans: Preamble (amended in 2006, updated in 2015). Lyon, France: WHO Press.

IARC (International Agency for Research on Cancer), 2017. IARC Monographs on the Evaluation of Carcinogenic Risks to Humans, Volume 1-119: List of Carcinogens. Lyon, France: WHO Press.

Jensen CC, Jensen LCW, Rieder CL, Cole RW, Ault JG, 1996. Long Crocidolite Asbestos Fibers Cause Polyploidy by Sterically Blocking Cytokinesis. *Carcinogenesis* 17:2013-2021.

Knobel PA, Marti TM, 2011. Translesion DNA Synthesis in the Context of Cancer Research. *Cancer Cell Intl.* 11:39 (online journal).

Li JY, Gaillard F, Moreau A, Harousseau J-L, Laboisse C, Milpied N, Bataille R, Avet-Loiseau H, 1999. Detection of Translocation t(11;14)(q13;q32) in Mantle Cell Lymphoma by Fluorescence *in situ* Hybridization. *Am. J. Pathol.* 154:1449-1452.

Liu D, Shimonov J, Primanneni S, Lai Y, Ahmed T, Seiter K, 2007. t(8;14;18): A 3-Way Chromosome Translocation in Two Patients with Burkitt's Lymphoma/Leukemia. *Mol. Cancer* 6:35 (online journal).

McCann J, Choi E, Yamasaki E, Ames BN, 1975. Detection of Carcinogens as Mutagens in the *Salmonella*/ Microsome Test: Assay of 300 Chemicals. *Proc. Natl. Acad. Sci. USA* 72:5135-5139.

Muller HJ, 2007. Artificial Transmutation of the Gene. *Science* 46:84-87.

Nelson HH, Kelsey KT, 2002. The Molecular Epidemiology of Asbestos and Tobacco in Lung Cancer. *Oncogene* 21:7284-7288.

NRC (U.S. National Research Council), 1983. *Quantitative Relationship between Mutagenic and Carcinogenic Potencies: A Feasibility Study*. Washington DC, USA: National Academies Press, Chapter 2.

Prakash S, Johnson RE, Prakash L, 2005. Eukaryotic Translesion Synthesis DNA Polymerases: Specificity of Structure and Function. *Annu. Rev. Biochem.* 74:317-353.

Sale JE, 2013. Translesion DNA Synthesis and Mutagenesis in Eukaryotes. *Cold Spring Harb. Perspect. Biol.* 5:a012708 (online journal).

Vaisman A, Woodgate R, 2017. Translesion DNA Polymerases in Eukaryotes: What Makes Them Tick. *Crit. Rev. Biochem. Mol. Biol.* 52:274-303 (online journal).

Vilenchik MM, Knudson AG Jr, 2000. Inverse Radiation Dose-Rate Effects on Somatic and Germ-Line Mutations and DNA Damage Rates. *Proc. Natl. Acad. Sci. USA* 97:5381-5386.

Waters LS, Minesinger BK, Wiltrout ME, D'Souza S, Woodruff RV, Walker GC, 2009. Eukaryotic Translesion Polymerases and Their Roles and Regulation in DNA Damage Tolerance. *Microbiol. Mol. Biol. Rev.* 73:134-154.

Webb A, Miller B, Bonasera S, Boxer A, Karydas A, Kirk C. Wilhelmsen KC, 2008. Role of the Tau Gene Region Chromosome Inversion in Progressive Supranuclear Palsy, Corticobasal, Degeneration, and Related Disorders. *Arch. Neurol.* 65:1473-1478.

Weinberg RA, 2013. *The Biology of Cancer*, 2nd Edition. New York, New York, USA: Garland Science (Taylor & Francis Group), primarily Chapters 2 and 11.

Weiss RA, 2004. Multistage Carcinogenesis. *Br. J. Cancer* 2004:1981-1982.

Xue Y, Wang Q, Long Q, Ng BL, Swerdlow H, Burton J, Skuce C, Taylor R, Abdellah Z, Zhao Y, *et al.*, 2009. Human Y Chromosome Base-Substitution Mutation Rate Measured by Direct Sequencing in a Deep-Rooting Pedigree. *Curr. Biol.* 19:1453-1457.

Review Questions

1. Briefly explain or justify why in many instances the two pathocellular processes *carcinogenesis* and *mutagenesis* are discussed side by side.

2. Briefly describe the main differences among DNA, RNA, codon, genome, gene, and chromosome.

3. Briefly describe the current concepts of mutagenesis.

4. Match *each* attribute or term listed in the left column to *only one* set of chemical substances or genetic materials listed in the right column that the attribute or term ascribes to.

    (1) chromatin (a) deoxyribose, adenine
    (2) centromere (b) sugar, sugar
    (3) glycosyl bond (c) guanine, cytosine
    (4) phosphodiester bond (d) phosphate, sugar, base
    (5) nucleotide (e) chromatid, chromatid
    (6) hydrogen bond (f) chromosome, histone

5. The five genes, denoted by letters A through E and contained in a segment of a normal chromosome, appear in the following order: ABCDE. Match *each* gene arrangement shown in the left column to *only one* clastogenic cause listed in the right column.

    (1) → $A_1B_1C_2D_2E_2$ (a) duplication
    (2) → ABDCE (b) deletion
    (3) → ABCCDE (c) inversion
    (4) → ABCE (d) translocation

6. What is a frameshift mutation? And how is it related to a point mutation?

7. What is an aneuploidy? Name the two diseases covered in this chapter that are related to this condition.

8. Briefly describe the four distinct phases of a typical cell division cycle (in an eukaryote).

9. Why is the concept of reverse (backward) mutation so crucial to the *Salmonella* assay? And what is the purpose for this *in vitro* assay to add a mixture of liver microsomes to the culture medium?

10. What is likely to happen (pathologically) when a point mutation causes the conversion of the codon [G][A][G] to [G][U][G] in the *beta*-hemoglobin gene?

11. Match *each* agent listed in the left column to *only one* site/mode of mutagenic action listed in the right column that the agent is associated with or responsible for.

    (1) *Helicobacter pylori* (a) covalent bonding with DNA bases
    (2) retrovirus (b) inflammation-induced DNA damage
    (3) benzo[α]pyrene (c) formation of stable DNA adducts
    (4) *beta*-particle (d) reverse transcription to DNA
    (5) melphalan (e) addition of molecules to DNA bases
    (6) nitrogen mustard (f) irreparable DNA damage

12. Briefly describe the main differences between mitosis and meiosis in cell division.

13. What are the current concepts of carcinogenesis?

14. Briefly describe the three main mechanistic stages that are currently accepted by many scholars as involved in carcinogenesis.

15. Name five agents that are human carcinogens and three that are *possible* human carcinogens, as classified by IARC.

16. What are the three main characteristics of metastasis? And how does it usually occur?
17. Briefly explain the importance of DNA damage checkpoints and of DNA repair, both in relation to mutagenesis and carcinogenesis.
18. Briefly describe the main types of DNA damage that commonly occur.
19. How would nitrogen mustard and cisplatin biochemically act in terms of their capacity of crosslinking with a DNA molecule?
20. Briefly describe the main differences among the following DNA repair mechanisms: base excision repair (BER); nucleotide excision repair (NER); single-stranded breakage (SSB) repair; and mismatch repair (MMR).
21. Name three (sub)mechanisms available for repairing double-stranded breakage (DSB).
22. Give an example of the damage tolerance processes as an organism's enzymatic defense mechanism in dealing with DNA lesions.

CHAPTER 19

Reproductive Toxicity and Endocrine Disruption

19.1. Introduction

The pertinence between human reproductive health and endocrine disruption is best appreciated starting with a brief review of the endocrine-reproductive system, which accordingly is presented shortly in Section 19.2. This physiological system is actually composed of the endocrine system and the developmental-reproductive system. In this chapter as well as in many places in the literature, the two subsystems are treated as one in the sense that neither one can be fully appreciated without referencing the other.

The endocrine system in the human body is also referred to as the endocrine network, as it is about the physiological functions of a network of ductless glands along with the hormones that they produce. Hormones are chemical messengers that an organism's body deploys to regulate or influence its many crucial daily physiological functions, including those related to the body's development, reproduction, and behavior. The thyroid gland, for instance, is a crucial component of the human endocrine network as, through its hormones, it affects many crucial daily physiological functions such as body metabolism, body temperature, and heart rate.

The developmental-reproductive system, on the other hand, revolves around a process that is regarded as a physiological cycle extremely vital on the population and species level. The cycle starts from the fertilization of an egg for the life of an individual and then back to the union of the individual's gamete (e.g., egg) with a gamete (e.g., sperm) of another individual of the opposite sex for the life of a third individual, and so on. During this physiological cycle, many environmental toxicants can cause reproductive disorders by their own effects, or via their disruption on the endocrine system. Naturally, those environmental toxicants whose effects rest on endocrine disruption are called environmental endocrine disruptors (EEDs). Many EEDs identified or suspected today tend to affect the developmental-reproductive cycle, as their effects are primarily estrogenic, androgenic, or thyroidal in nature (Section 19.2.2). Many of them are natural or synthetic chemicals. For this large subgroup, they are commonly referred to as endocrine-disrupting chemicals (EDCs). Toxicants that cause birth defects are specifically termed *teratogens*.

As noted above, not all (environmental) reproductive toxicants including teratogens have their adverse health effects exerted via endocrine disruption. It is actually true that not all endocrine disruption effects are confined to the developmental-reproductive system, as virtually every part or system in the body is responsive to hormonal action. In fact, many EEDs have been linked specifically to the nervous or immunological system. However, such specificity is perhaps overstated in that most, if not all, reproductive and developmental processes can still be adversely affected if the nervous system is compromised (*see* Section 19.2.2).

19.1.1. Impacts and Causes of Human Birth Defects

Birth defects are congenital abnormalities of a newborn's structure, physiological function, or body metabolism present at birth and can occur in virtually any part of the fetal body. As further discussed in Section 19.4.1, structural malformations are those in which a specific body part is missing or malformed. In contrast, congenital metabolic defects are those in which an inborn error or disorder occurs in the fetal body's biochemical system.

Each year approximately 8 million babies are born with birth defects worldwide, of which 40% die before age 5 and another 40% are disabled for life (Christianson *et al.*, 2006). In the United States, each year around 120,000 babies (or about 3% of all newborns) are diagnosed with one or more birth defects (CDC, 2008). There are thousands of different kinds or forms of birth defects documented (Weinhold, 2009), ranging from minor and treatable to severe and fatal. Among the more severe kinds, many lead to permanent mental or physical disabilities and collectively are one of the leading causes of infant deaths in the United States and worldwide, particularly during their first year of life (e.g., Mathews and MacDorman, 2008; Russo and Elixhauser, 2007). The health and economic impacts of the more common and severe types of birth defects are devastating. The more severe types oftentimes cause life-long disability and require extensive medical treatment. In the United States, the estimated hospital costs for birth defects in 2004 amounted to $2.6 billion (Russo and Elixhauser, 2007).

More recent statistics (Ferrero *et al.*, 2016) have confirmed that about two-thirds of birth defects have no apparent known cause, thereby making the aforesaid decade-old morbidity statistics likely still current or valid today. After all, there cannot be any effective approach to preventing or reducing birth defects of unknown cause. The remaining one-third are thought to be caused by genetic factors or environmental agents, or some interplay of the two. Environmental causes are found to take their adverse effects mostly during pregnancy: maternal use of drugs or alcohol; maternal exposure to physical hazards (e.g., radiation) or toxic chemicals; and maternal infections (e.g., with rubella, syphilis, or Venezuelan equine encephalitis).

19.1.2. Concerns with Human Reproductive Disorders

Reproduction is the crux of every organism's survival as a species. Any massive severe effect on this physiological process can have a serious consequence to a population, including its distinction. Disorders or health problems from reproductive effects can occur at several stages during the organism's lifespan. In most mammalians, some of these disorders involve the reproductive system of either sex directly. Others involve a relevant body system or biochemical process, or may manifest many years after exposure to the cause or even in a later generation. Overall, the effects can manifest as abnormalities or disorders in any critical stage of reproduction, including gamete production, menstrual cycle, sexual behavior, fertilization, pregnancy, and parturition.

Aside from birth defects being treated as a distinct adverse effect category on its own, the most common reproductive disorders in humans include infertility, ovarian cysts, and erectile dysfunction (ED). In the United States, infertility means for a woman age 34 or younger not being able to get pregnant after one year of unprotected intercourse. For an American woman over age 34, the wait period is shortened to six months for making the infertility determination, as after this age she is expected to start having fewer healthy eggs available for fertilization. Women who get pregnant but are unable to stay pregnant may also be treated as infertile.

A closely related problem is failure in pregnancy, which is the result of a process that involves mostly the union of a healthy ovum with a healthy sperm or the implantation (attachment) of a fertilized egg to the inside of the uterus. The failure can occur if there are problems with the above or other steps involved in the process. According to the statistics for 2006 to 2010, more than 6 million (over 10%) of American married women at age 44 or younger had difficulty getting pregnant or staying pregnant (NHSR, 2013). Ovarian cysts and ED are two major reproductive conditions that can adversely affect fertilization or pregnancy. These two reproductive disorders are specifically discussed later in Section 19.4.2.

19.1.3. Concepts of Endocrine Disruption in Humans

Historically, the medical tragedy allegedly alerting some relevance of endocrine disruption to human health was the prescription of diethylstilbestrol (DES) to several millions of pregnant American women during the late-1930s to mid-1970s. The drug was prescribed to those women primarily as an agonist of their natural sex hormone estrogen for prevention of miscarriage. In the mid-1970s, DES was banned for such use not so much for lack of substantial efficacy data, but more for an increase in a rare vaginal clear cell carcinoma observed in 1971 in a significant number of female offspring who were exposed to the synthetic estrogen *in utero*. The DES saga, however, did not appear to bear as much relevance to endocrine disruption as it should, as the term *endocrine disruption* was not coined until about two decades later at a multidisciplinary conference convened in 1991. That 1991 conference, held at the Wingspread Conference Center in Racine, Wisconsin (USA), was led by Theo Colborn, Ph.D. then working for the World Wildlife Fund US. The conference's focus was primarily on issues related to transgenerational health impacts. Yet the concept consensus on endocrine disruption and its scientific discussion at the conference were found so intriguing that they were quickly turned into a journal volume (Colborn and Clement, 1992) in the following year.

Four years later, jointly with two new colleagues, Dr. Colborn wrote a book to give a fuller account of the issues on endocrine disruption. That book, titled *Our Stolen Future* (Colborn *et al.*, 1996) with a foreword by then U.S. Vice-President Al Gore, is currently (as of 2017) available in 14 languages. For many years since the book's first publication, the concept of endocrine disruption has been accepted amidst some controversies, as some scholars still believe that the fairly low ambient levels of EDCs (endocrine-disrupting chemicals) that the public are mostly exposed to are harmless (*see*, e.g., discussion in Vandenberg *et al.*, 2009). Yet in spite of such controversies, the concept on the whole has continued to gain momentum as well as support from proceedings of multiple scientific and medical conferences on the subject matter. A case in point is the extensive global effort made not long ago by a group of international experts working for the United Nations Environment Programme and the World Health Organization (UNEP/WHO, 2013). That global effort was about updating the scientific knowledge and key concerns on endocrine disruptors. In particular, those experts have reassured the scientific community with data (e.g., Vandenberg *et al.*, 2010) that some endocrine disruptors, like most hormones, can indeed act at fairly low doses.

19.2. The Endocrine-Reproductive System

As noted at the beginning of this chapter, the human endocrine-reproductive system is composed of the endocrine system and the developmental-reproductive system. These two subsystems are highly interactive and closely interconnected. The endocrine-reproductive system is essentially a physiological cycle on the species level that becomes functional and interactive fairly early in both the human embryo and the mother, typically by the first trimester of pregnancy. For example, in about four weeks following conception, the human embryo will produce hormones to stop the mother's menstrual cycle.

In this section, as a quick reference for further discussion, an overview is given on the human developmental-reproductive cycle, followed by a brief account of the endocrine system and then a synopsis of the hormones that the endocrine network produces.

19.2.1. The Human Developmental-Reproductive Cycle

In humans (and other mammalians), the reproductive cycle starts with gametogenesis. More specifically, the cycle starts with spermatogenesis for males and oogenesis for females. In the female, oogenesis is the process involving the formation of primary oocytes from the primordial germ cells termed *gonocytes* via mitosis, leading to the production and development of a mature ovum. Such a developmental process takes place during the female's fetal period and ceases at birth (Figure 19.1). A mature oocyte is commonly called an egg or, more technically, an ovum. In the male, spermatogenesis is the parallel process leading to the production and development of mature sperms. Like the eggs, these sperms start with gonocytes during the male's fetal period. After birth, these cells are transformed to spermatogonia and then to spermatocytes. A mature spermatocyte is commonly known as a sperm or, more technically, a spermatozoon.

Fertilization calls for not only the availability of a healthy ovum and a healthy sperm, but also the effective delivery of the sperm and a conducive environment for fertilization. The fertilized ovum (i.e., now called the conceptus or zygote) is then proliferated, implanted in the uterus, and later develops to full term after undergoing the embryonic and then the fetal stage. The relatively short interval from fertilization of an ovum to its implantation in the uterus is termed the *germinal* stage or *predifferentiation* period. The embryonic stage involves four precise, sequential cellular processes (or substages), proceeding in the following order: *cell proliferation, cell differentiation, cell migration*, and *organogenesis* (Figure 19.1).

At the embryonic stage, cell proliferation is the process in which cells of the fertilized ovum that have begun to multiply during the predifferentiation period continue to do so. Cell differentiation involves the formation of specialized cells to acquire specific structural, functional, and biochemical properties. Cell migration is the third substage in which the specialized cells are orchestrated to move in a specific direction to a particular location. Organogenesis is the final and critical process in the embryonic period whereby the main structures and organs are formed. This final substage is the period in which the embryo is most susceptible or vulnerable to the effects of environmental teratogens. In humans, this period generally begins in the fifth week and ends in the fourteenth week of the gestation period. Not all embryonic tissues or organs are susceptible to teratogenic injuries at the same time during this period.

366 An Introduction to Environmental Toxicology

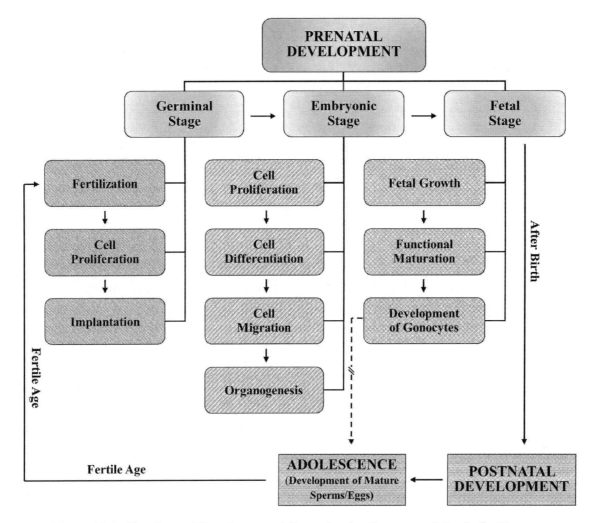

Figure 19.1. The General Developmental-Reproductive Process and Cycle for Humans

After organogenesis, the embryo undergoes a period of fetal development prior to parturition. This fetal stage is where the organs of the embryo, which is now more appropriately called *fetus*, grows to full term leading to *functional* maturation. Teratogens are less likely to cause *gross structural* malformations during this fetal stage. Another likewise resistant period is the earlier germinal (predifferentiation) period, at which time teratogens tend to either cause death of the fertilized egg by killing most if not all of its cells or have no other apparent toxic effect on it. The overall developmental-reproductive cycle for humans is outlined schematically above in Figure 19.1.

19.2.2. The Human Endocrine System

Every cell, tissue, organ, and function of the human body are regulated or affected practically every moment by its two highly-specialized physiological (as well as anatomical) systems. These are the nervous system and the endocrine system. The nervous system coordinates rapid and precise responses to stimuli through action potentials. Action potential is an energy concept measuring a momentary change in electrical potential that occurs when a cell or tissue has been activated by a stimulus. The physiological functions performed by the nervous system are much more immediate, such as the control of body movement and breathing. Further discussion on this energy concept and the neurophysiological system is beyond the purview of this chapter as well as this book. Those who have an interest in this area are referred to textbooks on general physiology or neurophysiology.

The endocrine system, on the other hand, maintains homeostasis and longer-term control of body functions by means of chemical signals. It works in parallel with the nervous system to control growth and maturation along with homeostasis. This system is a collection of ductless glands that secrete hormones essential or relevant to the body's physiological functions. The signals from these chemical messengers are passed predominately via the bloodstream to arrive at a target organ, where there are cells possessing the proteinaceous receptors that act much like lock holes which only certain keys can fit into. Exocrine glands that secrete substances that are passed outside of the body are *ducted* structures, such as the familiar salivary gland, sweat gland, and digestive gland, which by definition are not components of the *endo*crine network.

Compared to the nervous system, the endocrine network operates in a less rapid but longer-lasting manner by synthesizing and releasing the required hormones supposedly at the appropriate time and in the proper amount. These chemical messengers (further discussed in Section 19.2.3), through the proper transfer of information and instructions from one set of cells to another, regulate or at least influence the body's growth, development, tissue function, metabolism, mood, behavior, sexual function, and much more. In women, some of these messengers specifically support pregnancy and other reproductive processes. When the glands in the endocrine system or the hormones that they secrete function improperly, a variety of health problems will arise.

The major ductless glands that make up the endocrine system in humans are the *hypothalamus, pituitary, pineal body, thyroid, parathyroid, adrenals, pancreas*, and the *testes* or *ovaries* (Figure 19.2). By anatomical design, part of the pancreas is exocrine in that it is connected to the digestive system and secretes digestive enzymes into the intestine. Note that endocrine glands are not the only ones to secrete hormones in the human body. Some nonendocrine organs, such as the brain, placenta, brain, heart, lungs, liver, kidneys, and skin, are likewise capable of producing and releasing certain hormones.

Anatomically, the hypothalamus is a collection of specialized cells located in the lower center part of the brain. This gland is the primary link between the endocrine system and the nervous system via the pituitary gland. The pituitary gland, located at the base of the brain just beneath the hypothalamus and under the latter's control, is no bigger than the size of a pea. These two glands together control many other endocrine (and hence hormonal) functions. The pituitary is often referred to as the "master gland", and is divided into the anterior and the posterior lobe. Nerve cells in the hypothalamus control the pituitary gland by producing substances that either stimulate or suppress the latter's hormone secretion.

In particular, the hypothalamus and the pituitary gland together secrete a number of hormones that are crucial to the female menstrual cycle, pregnancy, birth, and lactation. The pituitary gland-based hormones include the follicle-stimulating hormone (FSH) and the luteinizing hormone (LH). The functions of FSH include stimulating the development and maturation of a follicle in one of the woman's ovaries, whereas those of LH include bursting of that follicle (or otherwise known as undergoing ovulation) and forming a corpus luteum from the remains of the follicle. One non-sex hormone secreted by the posterior pituitary is antidiuretic hormone, which helps prevent excess water excretion by the kidneys.

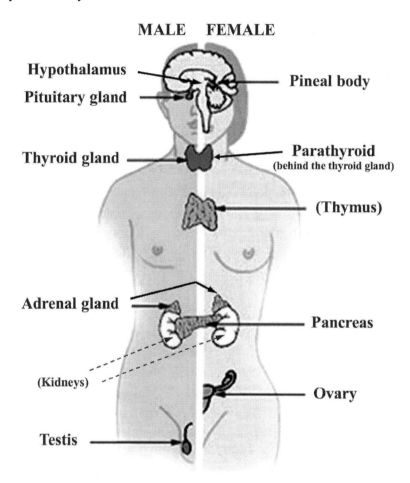

Figure 19.2. The Human Endocrine System (*image modified and adapted from the U.S. National Cancer Institute public domain*)

The pineal body, also known as the pineal gland, is located near the center of the human brain. It is stimulated by nerves from the eyes. The pineal gland secretes the hormone melatonin when the surrounding environment is dark such as at night, thereby secreting more in winter when the nights are longer. The hormone makes the individual feel sleepy and affects the individual's reproductive, thyroid, and adrenal cortex functions. Seasonal affective disorder syndrome (SADS) is a condition in which too much melatonin is released, causing profound depression, sadness, fatigue, inactiveness, over-sleeping, and thus likely weight gain as well. As expected, treatment of SADS typically consists of exposure to bright lights for several hours each day to retard melatonin production. The functions of the pineal gland have been implicated in a number of health disorders including cancer, sexual dysfunction, hypertension (high blood pressure), and epilepsy.

The thyroid, located in the lower neck, is shaped like a bow tie and secretes predominantly the hormones thyroxine and triiodothyronine. These two thyroid hormones together control the rate at which cells burn body fuels from food to produce energy. Accordingly, as the level of any of the two hormones increases in the bloodstream, so will the speed at which certain biochemical reactions occur in the body. Some other thyroid hormones like calcitonin play a key role in children in terms of their bone growth and the development of their brain as well as their nervous system. Calcitonin is a polypeptide of 32 amino acids that has the ability to decrease calcium (Ca^{2+}) levels by suppressing the release of Ca^{2+} from the huge reservoir in the bones. Locating behind the thyroid are four pea-size glands named parathyroids, which function together to release the parathyroid hormone (PTH). PTH, made of 84 amino acids, can counteract the effect of calcitonin by stimulating the release of Ca^{2+} from the bones into the bloodstream. It also regulates phosphate (PO_4^{3-}) homeostasis by increasing the secretion or the renal excretion of PO_4^{3-}.

The two adrenal glands are triangular in shape, with each being situated on top of a kidney. The adrenal glands each have two main parts, each of which produces its own set of hormones leading to a different set of hormonal functions. The outer portion, called adrenal cortex, produces hormones such as corticosteroids which regulate the sexual functions, the metabolic processes, the immunological system, the body's response to stress, as well as the salt and water balance in the body. Some of these corticosteroids are aldosterone, cortisol, and adrenal androgens. The inner portion of the adrenal gland, called adrenal medulla, produces epinephrine (a.k.a. adrenaline) and some other catecholamines which are a family of neurotransmitters. Epinephrine increases heart rate and blood pressure when the body experiences a sudden and substantial stress.

Again, the pancreas has two distinct types of functions. It serves as a ducted gland secreting digestive enzymes into the small intestine via the pancreatic duct. It also serves as a ductless gland, with its specialized cells called islets of Langerhans secreting the hormones insulin and glucagon to regulate sugar levels in the blood. The islets consist of two types of cells termed *alpha cells* and *beta cells*. The alpha cells secrete glucagon, which guides the liver to take carbohydrate (sugar) molecules out of storage to raise the blood sugar level when the level becomes low. The beta cells are responsible for the secretion of insulin. If a person's body does not make sufficient insulin, or if there is a reduced response of the target cells in the liver, the blood sugar may rise out of control to cause *diabetes mellitus*.

The gonads are the female's ovaries and the male's testes, which all are commonly known as the sex or reproductive organs. In addition to producing gametes (i.e., sperms or ova), they secrete certain hormones. The secretion of these sex hormones is controlled by pituitary gland hormones including predominately FSH and LH. Although both sexes make some of each of these sex hormones, the (male) testes secrete predominately androgens, of which testosterone is the principal member. In contrast, the (female) ovaries make estrogens and progesterone in varying amounts depending on where in her menstrual cycle the woman is at. In a pregnant woman, the fetus's placenta also secretes hormones to biochemically support the pregnancy.

Production of testosterone in a male begins during fetal development, continues for a short period after birth, nearly ceases during childhood, and resumes at puberty. This sex hormone is responsible for several growth and sexual-related functions: growth and development of the male reproductive structures; increased skeletal and muscular growth; enlargement of the larynx along with voice change; growth of body hair; increased sexual drive; and others.

The estrogens and progesterone contribute to the development and functions of the female reproductive organs and sex characteristics. At the onset of puberty the estrogens, of which estradiol is the predominant member, promote a number of crucial physiological processes: development of the breasts; distribution of fats in the hips, legs, and breasts; maturation of the reproductive organs (e.g., uterus, vagina). Progesterone, the predominant member of the subclass called progestogens, then causes the uterine lining to thicken in preparation for pregnancy.

From the short description of the endocrine system given above, it becomes clear that adverse health effects can be induced by an undesired interference with or disruption of the production, release, or use of hormones throughout the body. Also apparent is that not all endocrine disruption is necessarily detrimental, as reflected in the intended use of the now banned DES. However, within the context of this chapter, the focus is on *undesired* endocrine disruption.

19.2.3. Hormones (The Chemical Messengers)

It is noteworthy here that the shape of each hormone molecule is specific and can be recognized by its target cells only. The binding sites on the target cells are termed *hormone receptors* which are proteinaceous in nature. Much of the hormonal regulation depends on feedback loops to maintain balance and homeostasis. *Steroids*, *peptides*, and *amines* are the three general groups of hormones classified on the basis of their chemical structure, which is the more conventional practice. Depicted in Figure 19.3 are the chemical structures of nine prominent hormones selected to represent the three groups.

Steroid hormones are lipids derived from cholesterols through a series of biochemical reactions. These steroids include the male sex hormones androgens and the female sex hormones estrogens. Testosterone and estradiol, which are similar in structure (Figure 19.3), are the principal member of androgens and of estrogens, respectively. These sex hormones are secreted by the gonads, placenta, and adrenal cortex. Other examples of the steroid group are androstenedione, corticosterone, glucocorticoid, and progesterone. Defects along the series of biochemical reactions often lead to hormonal imbalances with serious consequences. Once synthesized, steroid hormones are released into the bloodstream and not usually stored in or by the cell.

Most hormones are *peptides* which are secreted largely by the pituitary, parathyroids, stomach, heart, liver, and kidneys. These hormones, such as insulin (Figure 19.3), are synthesized as precursor molecules and processed by the cell's endoplasmic reticulum and Golgi (*see* Figure 9.1 for structural location) where they are stored in secretory granules. When needed, these granules are released into the blood. Different hormones can be produced from the same precursor molecule by cleaving it with a different enzyme.

Amine hormones are derived from single amino acids, such as tryptophan and tyrosine. While secreted primarily by the thyroid and adrenal medulla, they are stored mostly as granules in the cytoplasm until when needed. Some notable amines, as included in Figure 19.3, are melatonin, thyroxine, triiodothyronine, epinephrine, and norepinephrine. Except for melatonin derived from tryptophan, the other four amines are produced from tyrosine.

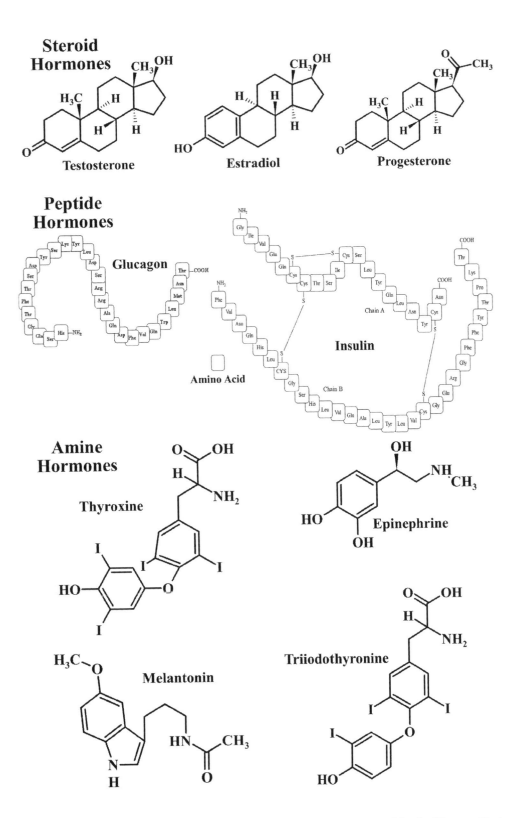

Figure 19.3. Chemical Structures of Nine Select Hormones Found in the Human Body
(*Three Steroids, Two Peptides, and Four Amines*)

19.3. Endocrine/Hormonal Disruption

In practice, the environmental health concerns on endocrine disruption come down to essentially two pivotal points, with both revolving around the disruption's effect potential: (1) low threshold effects with ubiquitous exposure; and (2) a wide array of persistent health effects. People are exposed to a vast number of EDCs found in many of the everyday stuffs that they consume or encounter. Even at low doses, exposure to them can result in the disruption of the body's delicate hormonal functions leading to a host of adverse health effects. This is not an overstatement as even a tiny alteration in hormone levels can trigger the body's endocrinal response.

There is evidence (Franczak et al., 2006), for instance, that a single low oral prepubertal exposure to the AhR (aryl hydrocarbon receptor) agonist 2,3,7,8-TCDD was sufficient to hasten a rat's reproductive senescence. Studies (e.g., Mackay and Lazier, 1993; Pakdel et al., 1991) also showed that a single dose of an estrogen was sufficient to cause persistent activation of the hormone's receptors, which can act as DNA-binding transcription factors to affect gene expression. Moreover, estrogenic substances like DES were shown able to cause carcinogenic effects persisting into the daughter's cells to manifest only after puberty. And as alluded to in the preceding sections, the adverse health effects of endocrine disruption are not limited to the numerous types of developmental-reproductive disorders discussed earlier. They include those that involve the nervous or immunological system, the gut, the liver, the kidneys, and more, as the endocrine system also works closely with these other body tissues, organs, and systems.

19.3.1. Modes and Mechanisms of Endocrine Disruption

In toxicology, endocrine disruption is generally treated as a mode of biochemical action which, when sufficient, can lead to one or more adverse health effects. In other words, endocrine disruption is not necessarily an immediate functional toxicological endpoint. There are basically two types of adverse endocrine disruption, each of which involves broadly two different modes of action. One type of disruption is, directly or indirectly, on the structure or the function of endocrine glands and the target cells. The other type is, directly or indirectly, on the metabolism or the function of hormones that the glands produce. In both types, the disruption can lead to either *activation* or *inhibition* of the natural hormone's normal functions. Collectively, the four modes of endocrine disruption can cause: (1) the damage to or modification of the endocrine network including the target receptors; and (2) the damage to or binding of the natural hormones.

The endocrine glands as target organs can be impaired directly via certain toxicological events or mechanisms of action. On the other hand, such impairment can be a secondary adverse response due to reactions or actions occurring elsewhere inside or outside of the endocrine axis. In this sense, endocrine toxicity and endocrine disruption may be treated as two loosely interchangeable terms. Even with an endocrine gland being a toxicological target, the major concern is still the secretion of improper amounts of hormones.

Agents that have been reportedly found to cause primary endocrine toxicity include nicotine on the adrenal, nitrogen mustards on the ovary, and estrogens on the pituitary. An example of a secondary endocrine toxicity is the development of castration cells in the pituitary as a result of primary or direct testicular toxicity (Harvey et al., 1999). As another example for the secondary kind,

DES has been banned for use as a synthetic estrogen by pregnant women since 1971 primarily due to its carcinogenicity to the ovary of their offspring.

The biosynthesis of hormones can be impaired by the ability of an EDC to inhibit a specific enzymatic reaction during the production process, or by the intruder's ability to regulate at the DNA transcription or translation stage. The antisteroid drug aminoglutethimide, the antifungal drug ketoconazole, and the sex pheromone cyanoketone are three of the handful substances identified (over two decades ago) to have an inhibitory effect on the biosynthesis of steroid hormones (e.g., U.S. EPA, 1997). Overall, the EDCs collectively can exert their disruption on a natural hormone's functions in various ways. For example, some of these xenobiotics have the potential to mimic natural hormones in the body and thereby can bind to the receptors intended for the natural hormones. When the receptors mistreat the mimicker as the natural hormone, they respond biochemically and functionally as they would to the natural hormone.

In mimicking the natural hormones, some EDCs can act as inhibitors by reducing the number of target receptors, whereas some others can cause the body into over-responding to the stimulus when more receptors are activated. Still some others, such as the pesticides lindane and atrazine (Chapter 15), can affect the metabolic pathway of certain sex steroid hormones (e.g., estradiol, testosterone, progesterone). There are also other EDCs that can activate enzymes to speed up the metabolism of certain hormones. For example, the testes contain enzymes specific for metabolizing estrogens (Toppari, *et al.*, 1996). These enzymes break down estrogens rapidly to a form that can no longer bind to the receptors. Either way, the metabolism and actions of some hormones can be modified by certain exogenous substances. Such a disruption can cause the natural hormone not able to bind to the target receptor at the right moment or in the proper manner.

In essence, the modes of endocrine or hormonal disruption involve basically the following: (1) binding of antagonistic and agonistic receptors; and (2) exertion of adverse effects on the biosynthesis, release, transport, storage, and clearance of natural hormones (e.g., Kavlock, *et al.*, 1996). In all cases, hormonal functions can be altered. And when the alteration is severe, some serious or even fatal health effects can result. One key mechanism of toxic action involved in endocrine disruption is the disruption of receptor functions, as discussed in general terms in Chapter 9 and more specifically in this chapter.

19.3.2. Types of Endocrine Disruptors

Despite the fact that a host of chemicals are considered having endocrine-disrupting potential, to date there is still no international consensus on a list officially accepted as EDCs (endocrine-disrupting chemicals). UNEP/WHO (2013) and U.S. EPA (2009, 2013) did provide explicitly or implicitly their own list of suspected or confirmed EDCs for further action or more analysis purposes. Some substances included on one of the two lists did not appear on the other. In the meantime, many of the commonly considered EDCs are listed online by the *OurStolenFuture.org*, a web home reportedly (initially) for the book authors of *Our Stolen Future* (Section 19.1.3) as well as for (now) tracking the most recent scientific development in endocrine disruption.

Actually, the notion that some xenobiotics can mimic certain natural hormones is not something new. The estrogenic effects of some DDT analogues were described in the ovariectomized rat by Fisher *et al.* (1952) well over six decades ago, and confirmed within twenty years later by Bitman *et al.* (1968) specifically for the *o,p'*-DDT isomer. And by the 1990s, two studies (Høyer *et al.*, 1998; Hunter *et al.*, 1997) were conducted to investigate the estrogenic potential of several organochlorines (e.g., DDT, DDE, dieldrin, PCBs) in breast cancer patients, as by that time lifetime exposure to estrogens was a well-accepted risk factor for breast cancer.

There are at least three conventional ways to categorize the EDCs considered to date. In some documents, they are arranged according to their adverse effects confined to a specific endocrine gland, such as labeling them as androgenic, estrogenic, or thyroidal. In some other documents, these environmental toxicants are classified on the basis of their general use or chemical features, such as putting them into the pesticide or metal group. Still in some others, they are grouped according to the mode of their disruption or the type of their disruption effect involved, such as citing them and their actions as agonistic, antagonistic, reproductive, or alteration of gene expression. Considering that none of the above categorization schemes is completely effectual on its own, the select EDCs in Table 19.1 are listed by using all three categorization schemes to some degree.

19.4. Developmental-Reproductive Effects in Humans

Reproductive toxicants are any agents that impair the reproductive capabilities in individuals or a population. As a special group being treated on their own, many teratogens interfere with proper growth or health of the fetus, acting at any time point from conception to birth. Agents that impair the normal growth of a child from birth to puberty are referred to commonly, if not specifically, as developmental toxicants but in many instances subsumed under reproductive toxicants. Some of these agents can have a beneficial effect on other occasions, such as aspirin, dental X-ray, and vitamin A. The best approach to defending against toxicants of this type is hence by knowing when to avoid what. As noted earlier, not all adverse developmental-reproductive effects are caused by endocrine disruption. Such effects from other causes can be equally or at times even more devastating. Accordingly, they are further discussed in a broader context in this section.

The sources of exposure to reproductive toxicants are broad and vary depending on the agent and the setting involved. Harmful exposures to reproductive toxicants can come from consumption of contaminated foods and water, as well as from being around workplaces and other areas where the air is contaminated. Of particular importance to newborns and infants is that they can be exposed in the womb or via breast milk. Paternal or maternal exposure prior to conception or during pregnancy can lead to adverse health effects on the offspring. Overall, these various exposure sources collectively can cause a wide array of reproductive and developmental effects from minor to life-threatening. The more serious or fatal effects include fetal death, congenital abnormalities, infertility, and damage to reproductive structures. Naturally, these reproductive toxicities can be seriously affected by such critical factors as amount of exposure, timing of exposure, and sex of the exposed individual.

19.4.1. Birth Defects and Environmental Teratogens

As noted in Section 19.1.1, several thousands of different kinds or forms of birth defects have

Reproductive Toxicity and Endocrine Disruption

Table 19.1. Select Common (Suspected) Endocrine Disrupting Chemicals and Their (Suspected) Major Endocrinal Effects[a]

Endocrine Disruptor	Endocrinal Effect(s)[b]	Endocrine Disruptor	Endocrinal Effect(s)[b]
Food Additives			
4-Hexyl resorcinol	Estrogenic	Nonylphenol	Estrogenic
Butylated hydroxyanisole (BHA)	Estrogenic	perfluorooctane sulfonate (PFOS)	Reproductive/thyroidal
Propyl gallate	Estrogenic	*Pesticides*	
Metals		Alachlor	Thyroidal
Arsenic	Glucocorticoid	Aldicarb	Reproductive
Cadmium	Estrogenic	Aldrin, dieldrin	Estrogenic
Lead	Reproductive	Atrazine	Pituitary/testosterone
Mercury	Reproductive/thyroidal	Carbaryl	Estrogenic/progesterone
Persistent Organics		Chlordane	Testosterone/progesterone
Hexachlorobenzene (HCB)	Thyroidal	Cypermethrin	Reproductive
Hydroxylated-PCBs (OH-PCBs)	Estrogenic	DDT[c]	Estrogenic/androgenic
Polybrominated biphenyls (PBBs)	Estrogenic/thyroidal	Dicofol	Estrogenic
Polybrominated diphenyl ethers (PBDEs)	Thyroidal	Endosulfan	Estrogenic
Polychlorinated biphenyls (PCBs)	Estrogenic/androgenic/thyroidal	Ethylene thiourea	Estrogenic
Polychlorinated dioxins/furans	Reproductive	Heptachlor, heptachlor-epoxide	Thyroidal/reproductive
Phthalates		Iprodione	Androgenic (testosterone)
Butyl benzyl phthalate (BBP)	Estrogenic	Kepone (chlordecone)	Estrogenic
di-Ethylhexyl phthalate (DEHP)	Estrogenic/androgenic	Lindane[c]	Estrogenic/androgenic
Diethyl phthalate (DEP)	Estrogenic	Malathion	Thyroidal
di-*n*-Butyl phthalate (DBP)	Estrogenic/androgenic	Methoxychlor	Estrogenic
Other (Organic) Substances		Mirex	Antiandrogenic/thyroidal
Benzo[α]pyrene	Androgenic	Permethrin	Estrogenic
Bisphenol A	Estrogenic	Toxaphene	Estrogenic/thyroidal
Diethylstilbestrol (DES)	Estrogenic	Tributyltin	Reproductive
		Vinclozolin	Androgenic

[a] as *suspected or considered* by UNEP/WHO (2013), U.S. EPA (2009, 2013), or *http://www.ourstolenfuture.org* (see text), except for propyl gallate (Amadasi et al., 2009) and 4-hexyl resorcinol (Amadasi et al., 2009); the notion of commonness is largely based on their mention in the literature.
[b] glucocorticoid (i.e., a steroid hormone) may cause alteration of gene expression; reproductive effects may include reduced sperm count, infertility, ovarian cysts, erectile dysfunction, and/or other related outcomes.
[c] DDT ≡ dichlorodiphenyltrichloroethane; lindane ≡ γ-hexachlorocyclohexane.

been identified or suspected (Weinhold, 2009). Among these, 45 were treated by the U.S. Centers for Disease Control and Prevention (CDC, 2006) as responsible for causing about 3% of some 4 million babies born in the United States each year with major structural birth defects. Out of the 45 major types, CDC selected 18 that the agency determined as having highest public health concerns and thereby placed for further prevalence surveillance during the three study years from 1999 through 2001. Table 19.2 is a summary of the CDC findings on the nation's average annual prevalence (i.e., average annual number of total *existing* cases across the nation) for each of the 18 most prominent types of *structural* birth defects.

Table 19.2. Average National Annual Prevalence on 18 Most Prominent Types (in Six Groups) of Structural Birth Defects in the United States, 1999-2001

Group and Type of Birth Defects	National Estimates[a,b]	
	Prevalence Rate	Annual Cases
Eye Defects	*2.08*	*834*
Anophthalmia or microphthalmia	2.08	834
Cardiovascular Defects	*16.25*	*6,527*
Truncus arteriosus (a.k.a. common truncus)	0.82	329
Transposition of great arteries	4.73	1,901
Tetralogy of Fallot	3.92	1,574
Atrioventricular septal defect	4.35	1,748
Hypoplastic left heart syndrome	2.43	975
Orofacial Defects	*16.87*	*6,776*
Cleft palate without cleft lip	6.39	2,567
Cleft lip with or without cleft palate	10.48	4,209
Gastrointestinal Defects	*7.18*	*2,883*
Esophageal atresia/tracheosophageal fistula	2.37	952
Rectal and large intestinal atresia or stenosis	4.81	1,931
Musculoskeletal Defects	*14.45*	*5,799*
Reduction defect, upper limbs	3.79	1,521
Reduction defect, lower limbs	1.90	763
Gastroschisis	3.73	1,497
Omphalocele	2.09	839
Diaphragmatic hernia	2.94	1,179
Chromosomal Defects	*17.39*	*6,916*
Down syndrome (trisomy 21)	13.65	5,429
Trisomy 13	1.33	528
Trisomy 18	2.41	959

[a]per 10,000 live births; adapted from Table 1 in the mortality and morbidity weekly report (*MMWR*) issued by the U.S. Centers for Disease Control and Prevention (CDC, 2006).

[b]projected by CDC from the average annual prevalence rates estimated from 11 participating states (Alabama, Arkansas, California, Georgia, Hawaii, Iowa, Massachusetts, North Carolina, Oklahoma, Texas, Utah); adjusted for either maternal age (for chromosomal defects) or race-specific distribution (for all other birth defects) of live births in the United States during 1999-2001.

Table 19.2 shows that for the three years (1999-2001) under study, the most common group of major structural defects at birth was chromosomal defects which affected about 6,900 newborns in each of the three years. Within that group, the most predominant structural defect reported was Down syndrome, a condition involving some degree of mental retardation and affecting nearly 5,500 newborns in each of the three years. The group with the second highest annual prevalence was orofacial defects, which consisted of predominantly cleft palate and cleft lip and collectively affected nearly 6,800 newborns annually during the three years. Cleft palate and cleft lip are defects involving the improper formation of the mouth roof and the lip, respectively. The national annual prevalence estimates for some of these birth defects were updated with data from 2004 through 2006 (Parker *et al.*, 2010). The updated annual estimate for Down syndrome was 14.5 (per 10,000 live births), up by 6.6% from the earlier estimate of 13.7.

Metabolic birth defects as a group are equally common, affecting roughly 1,000 (or 1 in 4,000) newborns in the United States (Heese and Zori, 2009; March of Dimes, 2002), with each involving typically a missing or an improperly formed enzyme. Although most affected newborns show no visible abnormalities, some can suffer from a life-threatening metabolic disorder, such as the genetic conditions Tay-Sachs disease (TSD) and phenylketonuria (PKU). Newborns with TSD are without the enzyme hexosaminidase A, which is responsible for the degradation of gangliosides (a subtype of glycolipids). As the fatty gangliosides accumulate in the brain, they affect the baby's sight, hearing, movement, and mental development. Babies born with PKU lack the (or proper form of) enzyme named phenylalanine hydroxylase, which metabolizes the amino acid phenylalanine present in most foods. Despite the fact that phenylalanine is an essential amino acid for building proteins in the body, without special diet treatment it will build up in the bloodstream to harmful levels to cause mental retardation and other serious health problems. All states and territories in the United States currently screen for PKU in babies, on the notion that if detected early this metabolic disorder can be prevented by feeding the child a special diet.

A wide range of genetic disorders and environmental agents can cause birth defects in humans. Listed in Table 19.3 are the more specific teratogenic effects caused by some of the more prominent agents or genetic disorders, including those noted in this chapter (e.g., DES, PKU) and elsewhere in this book (e.g., methylmercury). As reflected in Table 19.3, one common birth defect shared by several of the agents and disorders listed is microcephaly, a condition in which the head or cranial capacity is abnormally small. The high incidences of this condition recently observed in Brazil were reportedly linked to the Zika pandemic starting there in 2015 (Chapter 1).

19.4.2. Reproductive Effects and Environmental Toxicants

Examples of environmental reproductive (including developmental) toxicants, along with their more prominent effects on humans, are listed in Table 19.4. Some of these agents damage specifically spermatogenesis or cause testicular atrophy in males, whereas some others affect specifically the oocytes in females. In both cases, many of their effects involve impairment of the reproductive functions and are mediated via activities of the endocrine or the nervous system.

As noted in Section 19.1.2, in addition to infertility, the two most common reproductive disorders found in the United States (and in many parts of the world) are ED (erectile dysfunction) and ovarian cysts. Ovarian cysts are (follicle) sacs filled with fluid on or within the ovaries and are very common in women of childbearing age (ACOG, 2009). These cysts can rupture, resulting in significant symptoms including menstrual irregularities, painful bowel movements, painful intercourse, and pelvic pains. Fortunately or not, statistics show that many women tend to experience little or no pain or discomfort from ovarian cysts that they have in their lifetime. In addition, practical effective treatment may involve simply shrinking or removing the cyst if it does not go away on its own.

Table 19.3. Teratogenic Effects of Select Agents or Causes in Humans[a]

Agent/Cause	Common or (Potential) Specific Birth Effect(s)
Alcohol	Microcephaly (abnormally small head); mental retardation
Androgen	Masculinization of external female genitalia
Cocaine	Neurobehavioral abnormalities; microcephaly; pregnancy loss
Diethylstilbestrol (DES)	*At birth*: abnormal enlargement of the clitoris in female newborns; *years later*: adenocarcinoma of the cervix or vagina of female offspring; *in general*: structural or functional disorders of the genital organs of male offspring
Diphenylhydantoin	Microcephaly; cleft palate (abnormal development of the mouth's roof); mental retardation
Lithium	Ebstein anomaly (malformation of the heart)
Metabolic imbalance (folic acid deficiency, phenylketonuria)	Spina bifida (incomplete development of the spinal cord or its coverings); anencephaly (abnormal formation of the brain and the skull bones); mental retardation
Methylmercury	Cerebral palsy; microcephaly; blindness; cerebellar hypoplasia (underdevelopment of the cerebellum)
Radiation	Embryonic death; leukemia; microcephaly; skeletal and genital anomalies
Retinoid (including vitamin A)	Malformations of brain, ears, and eyes; heart defects; mental retardation
Syphilis	Abnormal teeth and bones, mental retardation
Thalidomide	Phocomelia (reduced or absent limbs)
Trimethadione	Developmental retardation, dysmorphic facial features
Valproic acid	Spina bifida
Zika virus	Microcephaly

[a] from various sources (and further review of references that these sources cited) including largely several hand/textbooks in teratogens, teratogenicity, birth defects, and related subjects (e.g., reproductive and developmental toxicology).

Table 19.4. Select Environmental Reproductive (and Developmental) Toxicants of Potential Concern to Men and/or Women of All Ages[a]

Environmental Toxicant(s)	Common or (Potential) Specific Reproductive Effect(s)	Common Source(s) or Exposure Site(s)
Benzo[α]pyrene	Damage to the oocytes	Charcoaled meat; tobacco smoke
Cadmium	Cause of prostate cancer	A widely used metal
Carbon disulfide	Impotence; abnormal sperm count and morphology	Viscose rayon; chemical production; fumigant
DBCP (1,2 dibromo-3-chloropropane)	Infertility due to azoospermia and oligospermia	Pesticide application
DDT (dichlorodiphenyl-trichloroethane)	Affecting the development of conceptus	Pesticide application
Endosulfan	Cause of testicular atrophy	Pesticide application
Ethylene oxide	Chromosome aberration; spontaneous abortions	Healthcare products; industrial use; food sterilization
Glycol ethers	Spermatogenic	A group of widely used solvents
Kepone (chlordecone)	Decreased libido; decreased sperm count, motility, and morphology	Pesticide application
Lead (and some of its compounds)	Decreased sperm count and motility; spontaneous abortions; increased neonatal mortality; menstrual disorders	Smelting; battery; lead-based paint
Methoxychlor	Increased weight of the uterus	Pesticide application
Methyl methanesulfonate	Affecting spermatids and spermatozoa	Widely used for cancer treatment and as a research chemical
Nicotine	Affecting the development of conceptus	Cigarette smoke
Nitrogen mustards	Damage to the oocytes	Used as chemotherapeutic drugs
PCBs (polychlorinated biphenyls)	Menstrual disorders; stillbirth; malformations	Contaminated seafood; e-waste recycling centers
Vinyl chloride	Chromosome aberration; miscarriage; sperm abnormalities; stillbirth	During manufacturing and processing of polyvinyl chloride

[a] from various sources (and further review of references that they cited) including largely several hand/textbooks in reproductive and developmental toxicology or related subjects (e.g., teratogenesis), as well as the toxicological profiles on toxicants that the U.S. Agency for Toxic Substances and Disease Registry has prepared.

The most common type of ovarian cysts is functional cysts which generally form during the menstrual cycle and consist of mainly two kinds from two causes: (1) follicle cysts; and (2) corpus luteum cysts. Follicle cyst forms when the follicle holding the egg fails to break open, as often caused by the pituitary gland not releasing LH (sufficiently) to signal the release of the egg. Corpus luteum is what is left of the follicle after the latter has ruptured to release the egg. At times, the opening of the short-lived corpus luteum is sealed off and the fluid then builds up in the follicle sac to form a cyst. Otherwise, a healthy corpus luteum would produce the hormone progesterone to make the uterine lining thickened for implantation to ensure a healthy pregnancy.

For men, the most common reproductive disorder is ED, also commonly known as impotence. This disorder is characterized by an inability to get an erection or sustain it long enough for sexual intercourse. Studies (e.g., Capogrosso *et al.*, 2013; Laumann *et al.*, 1999; NIH, 1993; Selvin *et al.*, 2007) have suggested that more than 10 million American men have ED problems. ED can be brought about by interruption in the processes responsible for generating an erection. The causes underlying such an interruption include: psychological factors such as stress, guilt, and depression; disruptions in neural activity; smoking; health conditions (e.g., diabetes, alcoholism, hypertension); and exposure to toxicants that cause damage to the nerves, arteries, and other relevant tissues. Some of these agents or factors can reduce the health or the number of sperm cells.

Many environmental agents can exert their adverse effects on either the reproductive functions or the reproductive system of either sex. Examples of reproductive functional disorders include: impotence; hypogonadism (a condition impairing the functional activity of the gonad which produces the sex hormone testosterone in males and estradiol in females); ectopic pregnancy (a condition in which a fertilized ovum is implanted on tissues other than the uterine wall); low sexual desire; and premature ejaculation.

The reproductive system of either sex *per se* can be impaired by a vast number of environmental toxicants. Each genital system represents a network of organs that are supposed to work together to effect reproduction. These reproductive organs, as briefly outlined below, are vulnerable to the exposure of the numerous various agents present in the environment.

The direct function of the human male reproductive system is to provide the sperm for fertilization of a female's ovum. The male's reproductive system consists of several organs located largely outside of his body around his pelvic region. His major reproductive organs include: *the testes* (which are housed inside the scrotum and produce sperms); *the epididymis* (a tightly coiled tube connecting the efferent ducts from each testicle to its vas deferens); *the seminal vesicles* (which holds the fluid that mixes with sperms to form semen); *the prostate gland* (which secretes the fluid that is one of the components of semen); *the vas deferens* (which produces the ejaculatory fluid); and *the penis* with the urethra for copulation and deposition of sperms.

The human female reproductive system is likewise a network of genital organs located around a female's pelvic region, but primarily inside her body. Her principal reproductive organs include: *the vagina* (a tubular tract serving as the receptacle for the sperm); *the uterus* (which holds the developing fetus); and *the ovaries* (which produce the ova). Her two breasts may be treated as reproductive organs during the nursing stage of reproduction. Some literature may further include *the fallopian (uterine) tubes* (where fertilization and thereby embryogenesis normally occur) and *the cervix* (which should be healthy as it is the neck-like passage forming the lower part of the uterus and is leading to the upper end of the vagina).

References

ACOG (American College of Obstetricians and Gynecologists), 2009. Patient Education Pamphlet AP075 – Ovarian Cysts. ACOG, 409 12th Street, SW, PO Box 96920, Washington, DC, USA.

Amadasi A, Mozzarelli A, Meda C, Maggi A, Cozzini P, 2009. Identification of Xenoestrogens in Food Additives by an Integrated *in silico* and *in vitro* Approach. *Chem. Res. Toxicol.* 22:52-63.

Bitman J, Cecil HC, Harris SO, Fries GF, 1968. Estrogenic Activity of o,p'-DDT in the Mammalian Uterus and Avian Oviduct. *Science* 162:371-372.

CDC (U.S. Centers for Disease Control and Prevention), 2006. Improved National Prevalence Estimates for 18 Selected Major Birth Defects – United States, 1999-2001. *MMWR* (CDC Morbidity and Mortality Weekly Report) 54:1301-1305.

CDC (U.S. Centers for Disease Control and Prevention), 2008. Update on Overall Prevalence of Major Birth Defects – Atlanta, Georgia, 1978-2005. *MMWR* 57:1-5.

Capogrosso P, Colicchia M, Ventimiglia E, Castagna G, Clementi MC, Suardi N, Castiglione F, Briganti A, Cantiello F, Damiano R, *et al.*, 2013. One Patient out of Four with Newly Diagnoses Erectile Dysfunction Is a Young Man – Worrisome Picture from the Everyday Clinical Practice. *J. Sex Med.* 10:1833-1841.

Christianson A, Howson CP, Modell B, 2006. The March of Dimes Global Report on Birth Defects: The Hidden Toll of Dying and Disabled Children. March of Dimes Birth Defects Foundation, White Plains, New York, USA.

Colborn T, Clement C (Eds.), 1992. *Chemically Induced Alterations in Sexual and Functional Development: The Wildlife/Human Connection.* Princeton, New Jersey, USA: Princeton Scientific Publishing.

Colborn T, Dumanoski D, Peterson J, 1996. *Our Stolen Future: Are We Threatening Our Fertility, Intelligence, and Survival? A Scientific Detective Story.* New York, New York, USA: Penguin Books.

Ferrero DM, Larson J, Jacobsson B, Di Renzo GC, Norman JE, Martin JN Jr, D'Alton M, Castelazo E, Howson CP, Sengpiel V, *et al.*, 2016. Cross-Country Individual Participant Analysis of 4.1 Million Singleton Births in 5 Countries with Very High Human Development Index Confirms Known Associations but Provides No Biological Explanation for 2/3 of All Preterm Births. *PloS One* 11:e0162506 (online journal).

Fisher AL, Keasling IIII, Schueler FW, 1952. Estrogenic Action of Some DDT Analogues. *Proc. Soc. Exp. Biol. Med.* 81:439-441.

Franczak A, Nynca A, Valdez KE, Mizinga KM, Petroff BK, 2006. Effects of Acute and Chronic Exposure to the Aryl Hydrocarbon Receptor Agonist 2,3,7,8-Tetrachlorodibenzo-p-Dioxin on the Transition to Reproductive Senescence in Female Sprague-Dawley Rats. *Biol. Reprod.* 74:125-130.

Harvey PW, Rush KC, Cockburn A, 1999. Endocrine and Hormonal Toxicology: An Integrated Mechanistic and Target Systems Approach. In *Endocrine and Hormonal Toxicology* (Harvey PW, Rush KC, Cockburn A, Eds.). New York, New York, USA: John Wiley & Sons, Chapter 1.

Heese BA, Zori RT, 2009. Molecular Biology: Genomics and Proteonomics. In *Civetta, Taylor, & Kirby's Critical Care* (Gabrielli A, Layon AJ, Yu M, Eds.), 4th Edition. Philadelphia, Pennsylvania, USA: Lippincott Williams & Wilkins, Chapter 51.

Høyer AP, Grandjean P, Jørgensen T, Brock JW, Hartvig HB, 1998. Organochlorine Exposure and Risk of Breast Cancer. *Lancet* 352:1816-1820.

Hunter DJ, Hankinson SE, Laden F, Colditz GA, Manson JE, Willett WC, Speizer FE, Wolff MS, 1997. Plasma Organochlorine Levels and the Risk of Breast Cancer. *NEJM* 337:1253-1258.

Kavlock RJ, Daston GP, DeRosa C, Fenner-Crisp P, Gray LE, Kaattari S, Lucier G, Luster M, Mac MJ, Maczka C, et al., 1996. Research Needs for the Risk Assessment of Health and Environmental Effects of Endocrine Disruptors: A Report of the U.S. EPA-Sponsored Workshop. *Environ. Health Perspect.* 104: 715-740.

Laumann EO, Paik A, Rosen RC, 1999. Sexual Dysfunction in the United States: Prevalence and Predictors. *JAMA* 281:537-544.

Mackay ME, Lazier CB, 1993. Estrogen Responsiveness of Vitellogenin Gene Expression in Rainbow Trout (*Oncorhynchus mykiss*) Kept at Different Temperatures. *Gen. Comp. Endocrinol.* 89:255-266.

March of Dimes, 2002. Birth Defects: Strategies for Prevention and Ensuring Quality of Life. Testimony Given on 26 July by Dr. Nancy Green, Medical Director of the March of Dimes Birth Defects Foundation before the Subcommittee on Children and Families, U.S. Senate Health, Education, Labor and Pensions Committee (U.S. Senate Hearing 107-592).

Mathews TJ, MacDorman MF, 2008. Infant Mortality Statistics from the 2005 Period Linked Birth/Infant Death Data Set. *Natl. Vital Statistics Reports* 57(2 July 30):1-32.

NHSR (National Health Statistics Reports), 2013. Infertility and Impaired Fecundity in the United States, 1982-2010: Data from the National Survey of Family Growth (reported by A. Chandra, C.E. Copen, and E.H. Stephen). No. 67 (August 14). NHSR, U.S. Centers for Disease Control and Prevention, Hyattsville, Maryland, USA.

NIH (U.S. National Institutes of Health), 1993. Impotence. Consensus Conference. NIH Consensus Development Panel on Impotence. *JAMA* 270:83-90.

Pakdel F, Féon S, Le Gac F, Le Menn F, Valotaire Y, 1991. *In vivo* Induction of Hepatic Estrogen Receptor mRNA and Correlation with Vitellogenin mRNA in Rainbow Trout. *Mol. Cell. Endocrinol.* 75:205-212.

Parker SE, Mai CT, Canfield MA, Rickard R, Wang Y, Meyer RE, Anderson P, Mason CA, Collins JS, Kirby RS, et al., 2010. Updated National Birth Prevalence Estimates for Selected Birth Defects in the United States, 2004-2006. *Birth Defects Res. (Part A. Clin. Mol. Teratol.)* 88:1008-10016.

Russo CA, Elixhauser A, 2007. Hospitalizations for Birth Defects, 2004. Statistical Brief #24. U.S. Agency for Healthcare Research and Quality, Rockville, Maryland, USA.

Selvin E, Burnett AL, Platz EA, 2007. Prevalence and Risk Factors for Erectile Dysfunction in the US. *Am. J. Med.* 120:151-157.

Toppari J, Larsen JC, Christiansen P, Giwercman A, Grandjean P, Guillette LJ Jr, Jégou B, Jensen TK, Jouannet P, Keiding N, et al., 1996. Male Reproductive Health and Environmental Xenoestrogens. *Environ. Health Perspect.* 104(Suppl 4):741-803.

UNEP/WHO (United Nations Environment Programme/World Health Organization), 2013. State of the Science of Endocrine Disrupting Chemicals – 2012. Geneva, Switzerland.

U.S. EPA (U.S. Environmental Protection Agency), 1997. Special Report on Environmental Endocrine Disruption: An Effects Assessment and Analysis. EPA/630/R-96/012. Risk Assessment Forum, Washington DC, USA.

U.S. EPA (U.S. Environmental Protection Agency), 2009. Final List of Initial Pesticide Active Ingredients and Pesticide Inert Ingredients to Be Screened under the Federal Food, Drug, and Cosmetic Act. *Federal Register* 74:7579-17585.

U.S. EPA (U.S. Environmental Protection Agency), 2013. Endocrine Disruptor Screening Program: Final Second List of Chemicals and Substances for Tier 1 Screening. *Federal Register* 78:35922-35928.

Vandenberg LN, Maffini MV, Sonnenschein C, Rubin BS, Soto AM, 2009. Bisphenol A and the Great Divide: A Review of Controversies in the Field of Endocrine Disruption. *Endocrine Rev.* 30:75-95.

Vandenberg LN, Colborn T, Hayes TB, Heindel JJ, Jacobs DR, Lee DH, Shioda T, Soto AM, vom Saal FS, Welshons WV, *et al.*, 2010. Hormones and Endocrine-Disrupting Chemicals: Low-Dose Effects and Non-monotonic Dose Responses. *Endocrine Rev.* 33:378-455.

Weinhold B, 2009. Environmental Factors in Birth Defects. *Environ. Health Perspect.* 117:A440-A447.

Review Questions

1. Briefly explain why thyroid is treated as a crucial component of the human endocrine system.
2. What are endocrine-disrupting chemicals (EDCs)?
3. It has estimated that worldwide each year approximately _____ babies are born with birth defects and die before age 5: a) 1,000,000; b) 2,000,000; c) 3,000,000; d) 4,000,000.
4. List some of the major environmental causes of congenital abnormalities.
5. Approximately how many American couples are affected by infertility?
6. How was the use of diethylstilbestrol (DES) (supposed to be) relevant to the concept of endocrine disruption?
7. What are the main differences between the functions of the nervous system and those of the endocrine system (in humans)?
8. Briefly describe the terms *gametogenesis*, *spermatogenesis*, and *oogenesis*.
9. Besides infertility, what are the most common reproductive disorders occurring in the United States?
10. Which of the following phases (substages) in the embryonic stage is most susceptible to the structural effects of teratogens? a) cell proliferation; b) cell differentiation; c) cell migration; d) organogenesis.
11. Which of the following glands is stimulated by nerves from the eyes to secrete a hormone responsible for the seasonal affective disorder syndrome? a) thyroid; b) hypothalamus; c) adrenal; d) pineal.
12. Which of the following in the body regulates or influences the release of the hormones thyroxine and triiodothyronine? a) thyroid gland; b) pituitary gland; c) parathyroid; d) hypothalamus.
13. What are hormones? And what are their three main groups classified by chemical structure?
14. Why is it important not to overlook the exposure of EDCs even at very low dose levels?
15. Briefly describe the two different types of adverse endocrine disruption in terms of biochemical action.
16. Briefly characterize the basic modes of endocrine disruption.
17. Name two common (or suspected) EDCs whose endocrinal effects are thyroidal and estrogenic.
18. Name the three chromosomal defects collectively having one of the highest, if not the highest, average national annual prevalence rates of congenital abnormalities in the United States.
19. What are functional cysts, as experienced by many women in their lifetime?
20. What would/could happen to the health of (untreated) newborns with PKU (phenylketonuria) and those with TSD (Tay-Sachs disease)?
21. Which of the following is apparently the (more) common birth defect that each of several known teratogenic agents can cause? a) spina bifida; b) microcephaly; c) Down syndrome; d) cleft palate.
22. Name a fumigant or pesticide that can cause or lead to: a) impotence; b) a decrease in the development of conceptus; c) a decrease in libido as well as in sperm count.

CHAPTER 20

Occupational Toxicology/Workplace Hazards

20.1. Introduction

Occupational diseases are those resulting from work-related exposure, such as from exposure to certain metals, fibers, dusts, pesticides, and organic solvents released during industrial processes. Diseases under this category have gained public attention since the late 18th or early 19th century, when the Industrial Revolution Period started involving many large-scale dramatic innovations in agriculture, manufacturing, and transportation initially in Britain. Diseases linked to this type of exposure sources continue to be of great significance to date, inasmuch as enormous amounts of metals, inorganic compounds, and complex organic mixtures are still being utilized in industry today. It is interesting to know, though, that a few of the widely known classic occupational diseases did not take place in an industrial setting. For instance, epithelioma (a form of cancer located in the skin) of the scrotum was first recognized as a frequent occupational hazard peculiar to chimney sweeps back in 1775 by a London physician named Percival Pott.

Another point noteworthy is that outbreaks of many infectious diseases also frequently occur in workplaces, such as the classic case with the 1976 episode of a serious type of pneumonia (lung infection) caused by the bacterium *Legionella pneumophila*. That 1976 episode took place at a hotel convention for the American Legion held in Philadelphia, Pennsylvania being the workplace, where the source of the bacteria was never confirmed but suspected to be via the water supply or air conditioning system at the hotel. The type of pneumonia involved later was characterized as the severe form of legionellosis and now is commonly known as Legionnaires' disease.

20.1.1. Classic Industrial/Occupational Diseases

Historically, lead (Pb), white phosphorus (P), and fine silica (SiO_2) dust particles were among the handful toxicants contributing to the classic industrial or occupational diseases that first received public attention during the Industrial Revolution Period (e.g., Cheremisinoff, 2001). Silicosis is a serious form of the restrictive lung disease known as pneumoconiosis that results from chronic exposure to silica dust particles. The disease was commonly observed among British miners working in the 19th century. Also frequently reported around that period were cases of painful phossy jaw (i.e., exposed bone necrosis exclusively in the jaws) seen among workers exposed to white phosphorus used to manufacture matches. A third classic is potter's disease, that involving neurological disorders experienced by potters working with lead glazes in the ceramic industry. Actually, lead poisoning cases were observed in British miners long before 1800 (Carter, 2004). In some literature, silicosis is also referred to as potter's disease or potter's rot among workers in the pottery industry, as silica is a key ingredient of clays and glazes used for pottery.

20.1.2. Uniqueness of Occupational Toxicology

Occupational toxicology, the subject matter of this chapter, has the objective to prevent and control occupational diseases with the ultimate goal of effecting worker health. It is unique from other subdivisions of environmental toxicology in having its focus on two distinct basic principles as well as practices: (1) the special need for exposure limits; and (2) the reliance on workplace or worker monitoring. Industrial workplaces are engaged in the production, processing, transport, or utilization of a variety of toxic substances (e.g., pesticides, paints, metals, solvents) that people in a modern society economically cannot afford to eliminate completely. It thus becomes more practical for such places to protect the health and safety of their workers by assessing and setting safe legal standards of occupational exposure. To ensure that employers comply with the limits of permissible exposure, it is also necessary for the laws and regulations to find ways to monitor the workplace, the workers, or both at least periodically for the exposure potential of concern.

20.1.3. Occupational Health and Safety Laws

In many parts of the world, it was more due to the public's concerns on occupational injuries and diseases that prompted the passage of legislations for worker health and safety. In the United States, contrary to general misconception, the first federal legislation for worker health and safety was not the U.S. Occupational Safety and Health Act (OSH Act) passed in 1970. Rather, it was the Federal Employers Liability Act passed during the Progressive Era being (more or less) the first. Historically, U.S. Congress passed that law in 1908 to help and protect railroad workers injured on the job. Two years later in further response to a series of highly publicized tragedies of mine explosions and collapses, U.S. Congress established the U.S. Bureau of Mines with the agency's mission being to improve safety in mining through research and training (though with no authority to regulate mine safety). At around the same time, backed by labor unions, several states passed workers compensation laws in an effort to discourage employers from letting their employees to work in an unsafe place or setting.

Then came the mid-1960s, a period when public awareness of the pollution impacts of many notorious chemicals was at its peak leading to a politically powerful environmental movement. To address these concerns, U.S. Congress eventually passed a comprehensive occupational health and safety bill that was signed into law on 29 December 1970 by then President Richard Nixon. That legislation is known as the now widely received OSH Act of 1970.

Over the years, similar worker health and safety laws also have been enacted in many other nations. For example, in 1986 South Australia (a large state of Australia) passed its Occupational Health, Safety and Welfare Act to safeguard the safety and welfare of its workers. In 1993, the Republic of South Africa passed its Occupational Health and Safety Act to ensure the health and safety of its workers in relation to the use of tools, equipment, and machinery. Still another example is China's Occupational Disease Control Act, which came into force in May 2002.

Yet perhaps with only a few exceptions, the European Union (EU) has set the most comprehensive and stringent occupational health and safety standards in the world. The EU has adopted many of its occupational health and safety legislations via a series of directives, including notably the framework directive (Directive 89/391/EEC) which was brought into effect by the Council of

European Communities. The framework directive has since laid down many principles of occupational health and safety as a binding commitment for the EU member states. Subsequent EU directives based on this set of principles then offer the specifics for numerous relevant issues such as noise, pregnancy, and the application of chemicals in various work settings.

20.2. U.S. Legislation/Agencies for Occupational Health

Laws and regulations for occupational health and safety vary considerably among provinces, states, nations, and regions. Yet their central themes are similar and consistent. They all have the ultimate goal of developing standards to protect workers against injuries and illnesses from occurring in workplaces. Laws and regulations of this type have been dealt with or discussed extensively in a number of excellent publications (e.g., DOL, 2009; Kloss, 2005; Lewis and Thornbury, 2010). It is beyond this chapter's purview to address the complexities of this type of laws and their differences across jurisdictions. Due to space limitation, this section affords only a brief account of the OSH Act (of 1970) and its two major establishments, with the aim to exemplify both the scope and the level of national as well as global concerns on occupational health and safety.

20.2.1. U.S. Occupational Safety and Health Act

In the United States, the OSH Act is the principal federal law governing occupational health and safety primarily for the private sector. This statute, signed into law on 29 December 1970, has its focus on ensuring that employers provide a working environment free from recognized hazards. Under the act, the hazards subject to federal regulatory actions include those associated with mechanical dangers, heat stress, excessive noise levels, exposure to toxic chemicals, and unsanitary conditions.

The specifics regarding the OSH Act's scope and legal intent can be found in Title 29 of the *U.S. Code of Federal Regulations* (*CFR*), Chapter 15. The federal statute was passed to ensure safe and healthy working conditions for non-federal government workers, by authorizing enforcement of standards developed under the act, by assisting and encouraging the states in their own efforts to ensure similar safe and healthy working conditions, and by providing for research, training, information, and education in occupational health and safety or related issues.

The act established not only the U.S. Occupational Safety and Health Administration (OSHA), which is a prominent agency component of the U.S. Department of Labor, but also the highly regarded U.S. National Institute for Occupational Safety and Health (NIOSH). NIOSH is organized as an arm to the U.S. Centers for Disease Control and Prevention (CDC), which is within the U.S. Department of Health and Human Services.

Many Americans are likely more familiar with OSHA's mission being to protect the nation's workers from occupational hazards and injuries by promulgating safety and health standards. Yet very few realize that it is NIOSH that carries out the research work to develop *"information on safe levels of exposure to toxic materials and harmful physical agents and substances."* Through the joint efforts of its several functional units, such as the Toxicology/Molecular Biology Branch, the Biomonitoring/Health Assessment Branch, and the Chemical Exposure/Monitoring Branch,

NIOSH provides the nation (and other countries) with some of the most relevant databases for the study and practice of occupational toxicology.

20.2.2. U.S. Occupational Safety and Health Administration

The federal OSHA's mission is to prevent as well as to reduce occupational injuries, illnesses, and fatalities by promulgating and enforcing standards for worker health and safety. This federal agency is headed by a Deputy Assistant Secretary of Labor, with its responsibility covering workplaces in mostly the private sector.

The OSH Act permits the states to develop their own plans as long as they provide worker protection equivalent to that offered under federal OSHA regulations and cover also local public sector workers. In return, a portion of the cost of the approved state program is to be paid for by the federal government. To date, some 20 states and one territory (Puerto Rico) have been operating their own plans which cover both the private and the local public sector. In addition, there are currently four states and U.S. Virgin Islands that have been operating their plans for their government workers only. In this group of five, protection of worker health and safety for the private sector remains under the federal OSHA's jurisdiction. In 2000, the U.S. Postal Act made the U.S. Postal Service the only quasi-government entity to fall under the purview of OSHA jurisdiction.

OSHA helps employers and employees reduce injuries, illnesses, and deaths in workplaces by means of three strategies as well as directions: enforcement, assistance, and cooperation. More specifically, the agency operates under the policy and direction that its regulations be followed, that outreach and training to employers and employees be provided, and partnerships as well as alliances through voluntary programs be cooperated with. Below are a few of the numerous regulatory milestones that OSHA has achieved over the years in providing health and safety protection for American workers:

- Permissible exposure limits (PELs) – promulgated for protecting workers against the adverse health effects of exposure to hazardous agents. PELs are regulatory limits on a toxicant's concentration in the air or its amount in a physical environment. They cover several hundreds of agents; and most are based on standards recommended by other organizations (*see* Section 20.3.1).

- Personal protective equipment (PPE) requirements – requiring that employers conduct a hazard assessment of their workplace in order to provide the appropriate PPE to their workers. The PPE required typically includes one or more of the following: respirator, coveralls, and gloves when handling hazardous agents; In addition, goggles, headgear, and earplugs are required in (almost) all industrial and construction sites.

- Right-to-know standard – developed under the principle that workers have a right as well as a need to know about the hazards occurring in their workplace.

- Bloodborne pathogens (BBP) standard – promulgated with the intent and effort to protect healthcare and other workers from occupational exposure to potentially infectious materials present in the blood (as in a hospital setting).

♦ Exposure to asbestos standard – promulgated for: (1) worker protection from exposure to asbestos in the general industry (including a PEL as well as provisions for medical examinations); (2) appropriate PPE/engineering controls; (3) proper exposure monitoring; (4) acceptable hygiene facilities/practices; and (5) effective recordkeeping.

20.2.3. U.S. National Institute for Occupational Safety and Health

While having its headquarters situated in Washington DC, NIOSH has scattered tactfully its research laboratories and regional offices across the nation in several cities including: Anchorage (Alaska), Atlanta (Georgia), Cincinnati (Ohio), Denver (Colorado), Morgantown (West Virginia), Pittsburgh (Pennsylvania), and Spokane (Washington). This federal institute is primarily a professional organization with a diverse staff of some 1,300 scientists from a variety of disciplines including biostatistics, chemistry, epidemiology, engineering, industrial hygiene, medicine, safety, and toxicology. It was established under the OSH Act to help ensure that American people have the right to a safe and healthy workplace by offering research, information, education, and training related to occupational health and safety. Today, NIOSH has become the national as well as the world leader in the prevention of work-related illnesses, injuries, and deaths.

NIOSH has three overarching goals as well as strategies: (1) to conduct research leading to the prevention and reduction of work-related illnesses and injuries; (2) to promote safe and healthy working conditions through interventions, recommendations, and capacity development; and (3) to foster safe and healthy working conditions at the global level through international collaborations. These strategies are supported and guided by NIOSH's program portfolio which has organized the institute's efforts into about 10 Sector Programs representing various available industrial sectors (e.g., construction, transportation, services, healthcare and social assistance, mining). Its program portfolio further subdivides these efforts into some 24 cross sectors according to adverse health outcomes, statutory programs, and global collaborations (e.g., engineering control, respiratory diseases, surveillance, exposure assessment, hearing loss prevention).

Unlike its partner OSHA (or to some people, its counterpart), NIOSH is not a regulatory entity as it does not promulgate any safety or health standard. Instead, under the OSH Act, NIOSH is authorized to: (1) "*develop recommendations for health and safety standards*"; (2) "*develop information on safe levels of exposure to toxic materials and harmful physical agents and substances*"; and (3) "*conduct research on new safety and health problems.*" The federal institute may also perform onsite investigations (e.g., Health Hazard Evaluations) to analyze the toxicity of materials used in workplaces, and offer funds for research conducted by other government agencies or private organizations via contracts, grants, and other arrangements.

In addition, pursuant to the authority by the Mine Safety and Health Act of 1977, NIOSH may provide services relevant to worker health and safety in mining operation as follows: (1) to administer a medical surveillance program for miners, including chest X-rays for detection of pneumoconiosis in coal miners; (2) to develop health standard recommendations for the Mine Safety and Health Administration (MSHA); (3) to conduct onsite inspections in mines similar to those authorized for the general industry under the OSH Act; and (4) to certify PPE and hazard measurement instruments.

Over the years, NIOSH has made numerous accomplishments for worker health and safety. Among the many, two are especially noteworthy. One of them is the *Pocket Guide to Chemical Hazards* and the other, *Criteria Documents*. Each *Criteria Document* generally contains a critical review of: (1) the available technical information and scientific data relevant to the prevalence of the hazards in a workplace; (2) the existence of the safety and health risks from the occupational exposure; and (3) the adequacy of analytical methods employed to identify and control the workplace hazards.

The *Pocket Guide to Chemical Hazards* is designed as an abridged source of general industrial hygiene information for workers, employers, and occupational health and safety professionals. It details key information and data in abbreviated tabular form for collectively over 650 chemicals and compound groupings (e.g., inorganic tin compounds, manganese compounds) found in workplaces. The information contained in the pocket guide is there intended to help users recognize and control occupational chemical hazards. The chemicals and compound groupings contained in the more recent revisions include the ones for which NIOSH has set recommended exposure limits (RELs) and those with permissible exposure limits (PELs) found in the OSHA General Industry Air Contaminants Standard (29 *U.S. Code of Federal Regulations* 1910.1000).

Historically, the pocket guide was the result of the joint effort initiated in 1974 by NIOSH and OSHA in developing a series of occupational health regulations for substances with existing PELs. That joint effort was labeled the Standards Completion Program, involving the cooperative efforts of several contractors as well as staff units from various divisions within NIOSH and OSHA. The joint program initially drafted approximately 380 substance-specific standards with supporting technical information and recommendations needed for promulgating new occupational health and safety regulations. The pocket guide was developed to make the information in the draft standards more readily available to the workers, the employers, and the occupational health and safety professionals. It is now revised periodically (though at a slow pace) to reflect new data on both the changes in exposure standards and the toxicities of workplace hazards.

In addition to the pocket guide and *Criteria Documents*, NIOSH's helpful scientific efforts can be further evidenced from its other publications, such as the *Alerts, Current Intelligence Bulletins (CIB), Fact Sheets*, and *Hazard IDs*. These other publications are likewise informative and useful, with many of them being available online at NIOSH's website. For example, although not as current as its title implies, a *CIB* reports new data on a known workplace hazard, draws attention to a formerly unrecognized workplace hazard, or presents information and recommendations on hazard control. The *Alerts* are issued to request urgent assistance in preventing, (re)solving, or controlling newly recognized workplace hazards. The *Fact Sheets* contain recommendations from research conducted in-house for the prevention of work-related hazards. And the *Hazard IDs* are each a brief, user-friendly document summarizing the results of the institute's studies as well as analyses on or for a specific worksite. This brief document also identifies current or new workplace hazards and offers the supposedly best recommendations for their control or prevention.

Another major program that NIOSH takes on is developing and periodically updating RELs for hazardous substances or conditions found in workplaces. To develop these RELs, the institute reviews thoroughly all types of available information relevant to the hazards, including chemical, biological, physical, medical, engineering, and trade. It then recommends proposals for appropriate preventive measures to mitigate or eliminate the adverse health effects caused by these workplace hazards. Afterwards, these proposals are transmitted to OSHA or MSHA, where applicable, for consideration to promulgate the required standards.

20.3. Relevant Concepts for Occupational Toxicology

In response to the unique special need for worker exposure limits (Section 20.1.2), the PEL (permissible exposure limit) standard or its equivalent, is widely used in many countries to protect their workers. In the United States, PEL is a legally enforceable standard promulgated by OSHA for exposure to a workplace hazard. For chemical substances, this legal standard is expressed either in parts of substance per million of air by volume (ppm), or in milligrams of substance per cubic meter of air (mg/m^3). For airborne fiber dusts such as those of asbestos, it is expressed as fibers per cubic centimeter (f/cc) or per milliliter (f/ml) of air. Units of measure for physical agents (e.g., lifting, noise, heat stress) are specific to the agent or exposure of concern (e.g., number of lifts per hour, sound level in decibels, temperature limit).

Many PELs adopted by OSHA for inhalation exposure are equivalent to or based on the threshold limit values (TLV®s) published (practically annually since 1946) by the American Conference of Governmental Industrial Hygienists (e.g., ACGIH®, 2017), which is a non-governmental, non-profit scientific association. The TLV®s published by ACGIH® represent non-consensus occupational health standards asserting that "*Nearly all workers may be repeatedly exposed day after day for a working lifetime without adverse effect.*" Both OSHA's PELs and the TLV® estimates are health-based, in that they are assessed and derived in terms of relevant toxicity test results observed in experimental animals along with limited epidemiological or clinical data. In many instances, OSHA also takes into heavy consideration the RELs published by NIOSH in promulgating many of the enforceable PELs. It is nonetheless somewhat confusing or ironic to find that the RELs are prepared by NIOSH for a 10-hour workday, whereas the PELs are set by OSHA for 8 hours as a workday.

20.3.1. Exposure Limit Values

In addition to the PELs promulgated by OSHA, other similar occupational exposure limits have been implemented by the Netherlands, New Zealand, and United Kingdom governments, such as the maximum allowable concentrations (MACs), workplace exposure standard (WES) values, and workplace exposure limits (WELs), respectively. Chemical substances listed under the above occupational exposure standards all include pesticides, metals, organic solvents, fibers, and dusts. For many of these chemical substances, as due to lack of relevant data and/or (sufficiently) high health concerns, values are set for only the first of the following three air concentration-based categories of (permissible or recommended) occupational exposure limits.

- ♦ TWA – this exposure limit refers to the *t*ime-*w*eighted *a*verage air concentration for a routine 8- or 10-hour workday in a 40- or 50-hour workweek.

- STEL – this exposure limit refers to the *s*hort-*t*erm *e*xposure *l*imit to which workers may not be exposed for more than (typically) *15 minutes* at any time during a workday; this air concentration is set with the intent to avoid workers suffering from severe adverse health effects such as acute irritation, narcosis, and irreversible tissue damage.

- PEAK – this exposure limit refers to the peak, maximum, or ceiling air concentration that should not be exceeded during any part of the working exposure period.

20.3.2. Biological Exposure Index Values

In addition to the PELs or the kind, health authorities in various countries along with ACGIH® have published or adopted a list of biological exposure index values (BEIVs). These index values are intended as guidance references in assessing the results of biological monitoring (a.k.a. biomonitoring) for certain chemical substances in workers. For example, included in (many of) these BEIV lists is the reference value set for the activity of the enzyme acetylcholinesterase (AChE) in red cells. The AChE inhibition activity (Chapter 15) in plasma or whole blood is a highly sensitive indicator of exposure to organophosphate pesticides (e.g., parathion). Other examples include the reference values for blood levels of lead (Pb) and of total inorganic mercury (Hg), both of which are good indicators of the extent of exposure to the two heavy metals (whose toxicological properties are briefly characterized in Chapter 14).

Basically, the available BEIVs represent the levels of biomarkers (i.e., determinants or bioindicators) that are most likely to be observed in relevant specimens (e.g., urine, blood) collected from supposedly healthy workers who have been exposed to the toxicants implicated by the biomarkers, to the same extent as these workers with inhalation exposure at the TWA under normal conditions. The exceptions are for those substances for which the TWAs are set for use to protect against non-systemic effects (e.g., localized irritation) or when inhalation is not the principal or only route of daily exposure.

By definition, BEIVs are not meant for non-systemic effects. On the other hand, for systemic effects of those exception substances, biomonitoring should be more superior and thereby more appropriate due to the potential for significant absorption or uptake via additional routes of entry. As with environmental exposure in general, exposure in the workplace can occur via any or all of the three main routes: inhalation; dermal contact; and ingestion (oral). Results from biomonitoring of workers thus can be used to assist in determining toxicant absorption not only via inhalation but also through the skin and the gastrointestinal tract. More specifically, BEIVs can be utilized to account for the exposures to a substance from all routes, whereas the TWAs are limited to inhalation exposure to the same substance. Biomonitoring therefore can serve at least as a complement to exposure assessment by air sampling in the workplace.

Despite the advantages stated above, the application of BEIVs and the interpretation of biomonitoring data must be treated with caution. For one thing, individuals in the same working environment may not be equally affected by (or even equally exposed to) the same (level of the) toxicant. The differences can be due to age, gender, body build, medication, disease state, diet, and other affecting factors or conditions (as discussed in Chapter 10). In addition, there can be subtle or profound differences in occupational exposure factors, such as work-rate intensity and duration, humidity, temperature, work practice, and time elapsed since the last exposure, all of which have some or strong influence on the interpretation of biomonitoring results (e.g., ACGIH®, 2017; WSNZ, 2016). Such uncertainties appear less relevant to the TWAs because both the interpretation and the implications of a substance's air concentration in a workplace tend not to be affected as much by the physiological and environmental factors mentioned above.

20.4. Occupational Toxic Agents/Workplace Hazards

For didactic purposes, Table 20.1 provides a representative list of OSHA's PELs (permissible exposure limits), NIOSH's RELs (recommended exposure limits), and the WES (workplace exposure standard) values adopted by WorkSafe New Zealand (WSNZ). WSNZ has governmental duties and functions similar to those of OSHA. One reason for the inclusion of these various occupational exposure limits in this table is to bring out the reality that some of them are inconsistent, inappropriate, outdated, or probably overlooked. For example, both the PEL list and the REL list currently include aldrin and DDT, whereas the WES list does not. As stated in Chapter 16, the two pesticides are among the dirty dozen that have been placed on the Stockholm Convention's initial action list for global elimination or use restriction.

Four major types (classes) of toxicants are included in Table 20.1. They are pesticides, metals, organic solvents, and fibers/dusts. Of these four, pesticides as a class appear to be most related to mild and severe *acute* poisoning from workplace exposure. According to a survey (Jeyaratnam, 1990) conducted in and for the Asian region almost thirty years ago, each year around 25 million agricultural workers in countries in this region might suffer at least one episode of mild or acute pesticide poisoning. Despite the fact that the survey provided arguably outdated statistics, there is no known evidence showing that either the agricultural work practice or the pesticide usage in any of the Asian nations under survey has improved or altered to the point to have drastically reduced the incidence rates there for the recent years.

20.4.1. Pesticides

Each year approximately 1 billion pounds of pesticide active ingredients in some 16,000 pesticide products are used in the United States (NIOSH, 2006; *see* also Table 15.1). Pesticides can be highly beneficial economic poisons. When utilized properly, they would provide significant economic benefits to a population, including increase of crop yields and preservation of produce. However, as discussed in Chapter 15, pesticides have the high potential for causing serious harm to people and the ecosystem. This is especially the case for workers handling pesticides or otherwise having direct contact with these agrochemicals. Agricultural applicators, field reentry workers, structural pest control operators, homeowner users, and other handlers are at a higher risk for exposure to the various forms of pesticides that are applied as fungicides, herbicides, insecticides, rodenticides, sanitizers, and more.

Each year approximately 15,000 of some 2.5 million agricultural workers in the United States are reported by physicians to have experienced some form of acute pesticide poisonings (Blondell,

Table 20.1. Permissible Exposure Limits (PELs), Recommended Exposure Limits (RELs), and Workplace Exposure Standard (WES) Values for Select Toxicants[a]

Group	Toxicant(s)	PEL	REL	WES
Pesticides (mg/m^3)[b]	2,4-D (2,4-dichlorophenoxyacetic acid)	10	10	10
	Aldrin, including its metabolite dieldrin	0.25	0.25	–
	Carbaryl	5	5	5
	DDT (dichlorodiphenyltrichloroethane)	1	0.5	–
	Diazinon	–	–	0.1
	Lindane	0.5	0.5	0.1
	Malathion (as dust for PEL)*	*15	10	10
	Methoxychlor (as dust for PEL)*	*15	–	10
	Parathion	0.1	0.05	–
	Pyrethrum	5	5	5
	Sodium (mono)fluoroacetate (Compound 1080)	0.05	0.05	0.05
Metals (mg/m^3)[b]	Arsenic, soluble organic compounds	0.5	–	0.05
	Beryllium, including its compounds	0.002	–	0.002
	Cadmium, including its compounds	0.005	–	0.01
	Chromium, elemental	1	0.5	0.5
	Chromium (III)	0.5	0.5	0.5
	Chromium (VI)	0.005	0.0002	0.05
	Copper fume	0.1	0.1	0.2
	Lead, including its inorganic compounds	0.05	0.05	0.1
	Mercury, alkyl (organo)	0.01	0.01	0.01
	Nickel, elemental	1	0.015	1
	Nickel, soluble compounds	1	0.015	0.1
	Nickel carbonyl (not specified for WES)*	0.001	0.007	*–
	Selenium compounds	0.2	0.2	0.1
Organic solvents (ppm)[b]	Benzene (in general industry for PEL)*	*1	0.1	1
	Carbon tetrachloride	10	–	0.1
	Ethanol (ethyl alcohol)	1,000	1,000	1,000
	Ethylene dichloride	50	1	5
	Formaldehyde	0.75	0.016	0.5
	Methyl n-butyl ketone (2-hexanone)	100	1	5
	Methylene chloride (dichloromethane)	25	–	50
	Toluene	200	100	50
	Trichloroethylene	100	25	50
	Xylenes (o-, m-, p- isomers)	100	100	50
Fibers/dusts (f/cc; mg/m^3)[b]	Asbestos, all forms (f/cc)	0.1	0.1	0.1
	Cotton dust (mg/m^3), in construction areas*	*1	<0.2	0.2
	Silica, crystalline (mg/m^3), respirable	10	0.05	0.1
	Synthetic mineral fibers[c] (f/cc), respirable	[c]500	[c]500	1

[a] PELs from U.S. Occupational Safety and Health Administration (OSHA, 2016, 2017a) and WES values from WorkSafe New Zealand (WSNZ, 2016) are time weighted averages (TWAs) each for up to 8 hours per day; RELs from the NIOSH *Pocket Guide to Chemical Hazards* (CDC, 2016) are TWAs each for up to 10 hours per day.

[b] mg/m^3 ≡ milligrams of substance per cubic meter of air; ppm ≡ parts of (substance's) vapor or gas per million parts of air by volume; f/cc (≈ f/ml) ≡ fibers (≈ particles) per cubic centimeter (≈ per milliliter) of air.

[c] currently (as of 2017), synthetic mineral fibers are treated as nuisance dust (particles) for PELs/RELs in the United States.

1997; CDC, 2014; Reigart and Roberts, 1999; U.S. EPA, 2010). It is actually not surprising to see such a large number of annual cases reported, considering that occupational exposure to pesticide residues can occur anytime during formulation or handling when the pesticide used can contaminate the workplace due to spilling, leaking, or discharging from the mixing/loading or the processing system. Exposure to pesticide residues can also occur when fieldworkers harvest treated crops. In short, worker exposure to pesticides in agricultural applications can indeed be a common cause of acute poisoning or health problem.

Surveillance for illnesses and injuries related to worker exposure to pesticides (or any other class of toxicants) therefore becomes a critical health and safety agendum, as it can offer worker protection by analyzing the magnitude or the underlying causes of overexposure to pesticides in a workplace. The results can also be used to alert any toxic effect of the pesticide that might not have been determined (or "caught") during the premarket approval process. In the United States, NIOSH has been conducting surveillance for occupational pesticide-related illnesses and injuries via the *S*entinel *E*vent *N*otification *S*ystem for *O*ccupational *R*isks (SENSOR)-Pesticides program. The program involves the participation of 13 (as of 2017) state health agencies to employ a standard set of variables along with standard case definitions to collect and analyze illness and injury data from various sources. The information is later transmitted to the program headquarters at NIOSH, where it is compiled and put into a national database. Together with U.S. EPA, NIOSH provides technical support to all and funding to some of the participating states.

Government officials and researchers both from and outside of NIOSH have been publishing findings and related implications from analyzing information compiled in the SENSOR database. Their findings have led to issues and concerns that include eradication of invasive species, pesticide poisoning in schools, and residential use of total release foggers (which are canister type devices used to get rid of fleas or ticks by releasing a pesticide mist).

20.4.2. Metals

As alluded to in Chapter 14, most elemental metals are not synthetic elements but occur naturally in the environment. Unfortunately, many are also toxicants frequently found in workplaces, as they have been widely utilized or processed in numerous various industries since the 19th century. In very small amounts, many metals are actually essential for human life. However, in large quantities all will become toxic. Some metals or their compounds can build up in the human body and thereby can eventually become a significant health hazard to workers.

In recent years, toxic metallic products are increasingly being utilized in a wide range of applications, including fabrication, electroplating, smelting, and welding. Consequently, thousands of metalworkers are at risk of contracting fatal respiratory diseases from fumes and dusts that are unavoidable by-products released in workspaces. Beryllium (Be), in particular, is among the most widely used toxic industrial metals in the United States, where the nationwide workforce in this sector is estimated at around 21,000 workers (ATSDR, 2002, 2015). Of this workforce, some 12% eventually will become sensitized and develop allergic type response to the metal.

A similar health concern is that the lungs of a machinist can be severely damaged by inhalation of numerous toxic metals, including arsenic (As), cadmium (Cd), chromium (Cr), cobalt (Co), lead

(Pb), manganese (Mn), mercury (Hg), and nickel (Ni). Respiratory disorders that result from chronic exposure to these metals (including beryllium) and their alloys usually develop slowly. Initial symptoms may include coughing, shortness of breath, fever, fatigue, weight loss, irritation of the airways, and even asthma. Over a long enough period, however, this type of ongoing exposure can prove to be severe or fatal.

Metal fume fever is the most common acute respiratory illness experienced by welders and other metalworkers. This type of illness, occurring most frequently in poorly ventilated areas in a workplace, is typically caused by exposure that arises through hot metalworking processes, such as smelting and casting of zinc alloys, or welding of galvanized metals. The fumes of high occupational health concern are those of zinc oxide (ZnO) and magnesium oxide (MgO), but fumes of copper (Cu), iron (Fe), and Cd also have been implicated. In fact, acute exposure to high levels of Cd fume can result in more serious health outcomes such as pulmonary edema or even death, before the worker will develop metal fume fever.

The symptoms associated with metal fume fever are nonspecific and are generally flu-like including fever, chills, headaches, nausea, fatigue, thirst, muscle/joint pains, and chest soreness. Also frequently reported by these patients are an irritated or hoarse throat and a metallic or sweet taste in their mouth (that would likely distort the taste of food and cigarettes). The fumes of certain other toxic metal compounds are also known to cause more than metal fume fever. For example, nickel carbonyl (as being a nickel compound) has been classified as a human (Group 1) carcinogen (IARC, 2012, 2017), in addition to being an irritant to the eyes and the skin.

20.4.3. Organic Solvents

According to NIOSH (CDC, 2013a), millions of American workers are exposed to organic solvents everywhere every day. Organic solvents are a huge group of liquid organic substances that each have the ability to dissolve certain solids, gaseous solutes, and other liquids to form a solution. Substances in this group have variable lipophilicity and volatility that accordingly can lead to a wide array of health problems, including adverse effects on the central or peripheral nervous system, impairment of reproductive or respiratory functions, damage to the liver or kidneys, and development of cancer or dermatitis.

Organic solvents are hydrocarbon (HC) substances that can be broadly divided into two sub-families: (1) the aliphatic-chain type, each without a benzene-like ring (e.g., cyclohexene, *n*-hexane, 2-hexanone); and (2) the aromatic kind, each *with* one or more benzene-like rings (e.g., benzene, naphthalene, xylene isomers). These aliphatics and aromatics each may contain one or more substituted halogens (e.g., Br, Cl, F) in place of hydrogen (H) atoms and accordingly may be referred to as halogenated HC compounds, such as chlorobenzene (C_6H_5Cl), CFCs (chlorofluorocarbons), methylene chloride (CH_2Cl_2), and trichloroethylene ($ClCH=CCl_2$). Alcohols, aldehydes, esters, ethers, glycols, ketones, and pyridines are some of the organic solvent compounds from substitutions for one or more H atoms on the HC chain.

Millions of workers in the United States and in many other countries are exposed to organic solvents because these substances are employed everywhere every day to dissolve fats, oils, plastics, resins, and rubbers, which all are omnipresent in high volumes. Organic solvents are useful in a wide variety of products such as paints, adhesives, degreasing agents, cleaning agents, and glues, as well as in the production of dyes, plastics, textiles, pesticides, and pharmaceuticals. The industries processing or manufacturing these numerous various types of products collectively represent the bulk of the workforce in many countries, mostly second only to agriculture.

Organic solvents came around in the second half of the 19th century during the coal tar industry era. Their widespread and diverse applications have since grown strikingly in both the developed and developing regions. Reports of their toxicities, including predominately neurological effects, began to emerge in the early 1900s when chlorinated solvents became available. Although thousands of organic solvents are being used today, only a small number of them have been (fully) tested for neurotoxicity or other adverse health effects.

Workers can be exposed to organic solvents not only from their workplace or being near there. They can be exposed to these substances if they come in contact with contaminated water, soils, air, or foods. Ambient and indoor air, drinking and shower water, as well as foods are common sources of exposure to environmental toxicants in general, but to organic solvents in particular owing to their widespread use coupled with generally higher solubility and volatility.

As evidenced from the numerous NIOSH publications noted in Section 20.2.3, organic solvents have long been recognized to cause damages to multiple body tissues and organs in addition to the nervous system. It is also a known fact to many toxicologists that exposure to organic solvents can cause hematological disorders (e.g., anemia, leukemia), liver disorders (e.g., fatty liver), or renal diseases (e.g., chronic glomerulonephritis). A number of animal and epidemiological studies have implicated that chronic exposure to certain organic solvents (e.g., benzene as discussed in Chapter 13) can cause tumors in certain body organs, including the kidneys, liver, and blood.

20.4.4. Fibers/Dusts

A variety of inorganic materials are made into fine fibers for use to strengthen and insulate building and other structures. The fibrous materials used generally are from glass, rock, silica, and alumina (Al_2O_3). The resultant fibers, which were once called *man-made mineral fibers* (MMMFs) or synthetic vitreous (i.e., with glass-like appearance) fibers, are now more commonly or technically known as *synthetic mineral fibers* (SMFs). Some of these end products are composed of a mixture of the fibers in various shapes and sizes.

In recent years, SMFs have been extensively utilized as alternatives to asbestos in insulation and fire-retardant products. They are recently also applied extensively as reinforcement materials in cement and plastic products. Worldwide, SMF products are used broadly as thermal and acoustic insulation materials in commercial and residential buildings. In the United States, over 200,000 workers are exposed to SMFs in manufacturing or end-use applications (OSHA, 2017b). SMFs are generally classified into the following three source or use categories:

- Fiberglass (e.g., glasswool, glass filaments) – those utilized in automobiles, reinforced plastics, textiles, and as electrical insulation.
- Mineral wool (e.g., rockwool, slagwool) – those utilized in limpet and formed insulation materials, such as acoustic insulation and fire-rating materials.

♦ Refractory ceramic fibers – those utilized for high-temperature (up to 1,400° C or 2,552° F) insulation applications (e.g., insulation blanket) and fire protection materials.

All three types of SMFs have been suspected to cause lung cancer and other adverse respiratory effects since the 1970s, when they became increasingly utilized to replace asbestos. Asbestos is a group of six naturally occurring fibrous silicate materials also used predominantly for insulation applications (Chapter 4). By the 1960s, there were already several epidemiological studies linking elevated incidences of pulmonary fibrosis and cancer to inhalation of crocidolite and chrysotile. The amphibole-shaped crocidolite and the serpentine-shaped chrysotile are two of the six members of asbestos. The widespread utilization of SMFs as replacements naturally brought about similar concerns that they too might cause cancer and other adverse effects to or in the respiratory system. These concerns came around largely due to the similarities between SMFs and asbestos in both their appearance and industrial applications. Today, a large body of evidence from occupational and laboratory studies is available linking a variety of adverse health effects to SMF exposure. Both IARC (2002, 2017) and U.S. EPA (1992) have classified only refractory ceramic fibers, but not the other two types (reportedly for lack of sufficient data), as possible human (Group 2B and Group C, respectively) carcinogens.

In general, short-term exposure to SMFs can result in skin, eye, and/or upper respiratory tract irritation. The skin and eye cases often occur in workers having direct contact with SMF products for the first time or in those workers with a short lapse from exposure. The symptoms generally involve reddening, burning, itching, and inflammation around the finger nails. The cases with respiratory tract come about largely from inhalation to very high levels of SMFs. Long-term exposure to SMFs was reportedly linked to slightly increased incidences of lung cancer among exposed workers in earlier SMF industries (ATSDR, 2004; U.S. EPA, 1992). OSHA recently has recommended the use of a dust mask for persons working with fiberglass products.

Dusts as a related occupational hazard consist of any tiny solid particles, not necessarily fibers, that are carried by air currents. MSHA defines dusts as finely divided particles that may become airborne from the original state without any chemical or physical alteration other than fracture. These tiny particles are generally formed by a disintegration or fracture process, such as grinding, crushing, or impact. Agriculture, construction, and mining are among the few industries contributing the most to high levels of various workplace dusts in the air.

As mentioned in Chapter 12, various dusts can be classified by size into the respirable and inhalable groups. Yet in terms of their composition, workplace dusts are generally divided into the fibrogenic and the nuisance type. Fibrogenic dust particles, such as those of free crystalline silica or asbestos which have fiber-like tendencies, are biologically toxic. And if retained in the lungs long enough, they could form fibrogenic scar tissues and impair lung functions.

In contrast, nuisance or inert dust particles can be defined as those containing less than 1% quartz. Quartz is a hard mineral composed of silica (SiO_2) in the silicon-oxygen tetrahedron (SiO_4) shape. Owing to their low content of silicates, nuisance dust particles have little or no history of causing any significant adverse effect on the lung. Any reaction that may occur from nuisance dust particles is potentially reversible. Nevertheless, excessive levels of nuisance dust particles in the workplace can reduce visibility there (e.g., with FeO dust), can cause unpleasant deposits in the eyes, ears, and nasal passages (e.g., with Portland cement dust), and can induce injury to the skin or the mucous membranes by chemical or mechanical action.

Silicosis, that being the prominent form of the black lung disease medically termed *pneumoconiosis*, is caused by inhalation of the respirable crystalline silica dust particles. In the United States, around 2 million workers remain potentially exposed to this type of dust particles (OSHA, 2016). Silicosis is the most common occupational lung disease in the world, particularly in the developing regions. According to a fact sheet published by the World Health Organization (WHO, 2000), China reported over 24,000 deaths due to silicosis each year between 1991 and 1995, mostly among older workers. Also stated in the fact sheet was WHO's projection that in the United States, among the million or so workers (e.g., sandblasters) who were occupationally exposed to free crystalline silica dust particles, about 60,000 would eventually develop silicosis.

Apparently because of rising health concerns over pneumoconiosis in general, many developed countries have banned the use of asbestos in new constructions. Yet ironically or not, along with some developing countries (e.g., Indonesia, India), the United States continues to allow the use of these fibrous silicate minerals in new construction projects, though now with a lower federal PEL of 10 $\mu g/m^3$ imposed for the respirable fraction of silicate dust (OSHA, 2016, 2017a).

20.4.5. Other Groups/Kinds of Workplace Hazards

In addition to the four classes of toxicants highlighted in Table 20.1 and discussed in the preceding subsections, there are other groups that are likewise ubiquitous in workplaces and at times as threatening to occupational health and safety. One example that comes to mind is metalworking fluids (MWFs), to which workplace exposure can occur via inhalation or dermal contact to result in asthma, lung diseases, skin disorders, and/or cancer (NIOSH, 1998). MWFs are complex mixtures of petroleum oils applied during machining and grinding to prolong a tool's life by protecting the work piece's surfaces. Approximately one million American workers engaging in machine finishing, machine tooling, and similar metalworking operations are potentially exposed to MWFs (CDC, 2013b; Kreiss and Cox-Ganser, 1997; Zacharisen *et al.*, 1998).

Physical and biological hazards are likewise commonly found in workplaces. OSHA's Hazard Communication Standard (29 *CFR* 1910.1020), which went into effect in 1985, is the centerpiece of a powerful American ideology known as the worker right-to-know movement. In most literature, such a regulation continues to be treated more as a requirement for *chemical* manufacturers and employers to relate information to their workers concerning the hazards of *chemical* products in their workplace. Yet as misleading as some of the terms used might seem to be, the hazard materials subject to such communication, as mandated by the federal and state laws, should include information concerning *physical* and *biological* hazards as well.

For example, the Employee Right-To-Know Act passed by the Minnesota state legislature in 1983 does include infectious agents in hospitals and clinics. It also covers heat and noise as additional potential physical hazards. Another case in point is the New Jersey state law on occupational health and safety, under which workers have the rights to receive monitoring records for exposures not only to chemicals, but also to noise, radiation, heat/cold stress, vibration, and molds.

Heat is an occupational hazard because excessive heat from working in places such as around boilers, ovens, furnaces, and open fields can result in dehydration, heat rash, and heat stroke. Similarly, excessive cold from working in a place with air temperature below the freezing point, such as when taking inventory in a walk-in freezer for long hours, can result in frostbite, chilblains, or hypothermia. Chilblain is a general skin condition characterized by an inflammation of the skin, accompanied by burning and itching, when exposed to very cold temperatures. Hypothermia is a condition of abnormally low body temperature that can fatally affect normal metabolism and body functions. Vibration exposure too can be a physical hazard to workers engaging in jobs with vibrating machinery and equipment, such as when constantly operating a chainsaw or jackhammer. Vibration can have serious effects on the tendons, muscles, bones, joints, and other body parts including the nervous system, frequently leading to pains, tingling, and loss of sensation in the affected area. And excessive noise is not uncommon in many occupational settings. It can cause hearing impairment and other health problems (Chapter 17).

Furthermore, ionizing radiation (e.g., X-ray, uranium isotopes) can also be exposed to in workplaces such as healthcare facilities, mining areas, and nuclear reactor plants. Non-ionizing radiation (e.g., microwave, infrared, visible light) too can be found in many occupational settings such as installing telephone cables, paving asphalt roadways, and working on farms. The two types of radiation collectively can cause a wide array of adverse health effects. Common health effects associated with ionizing radiation include cancer, damage to the eyes or the skin, sterility, cataracts, and blood disorders. Although non-ionizing radiation carries less energy and thus less health risks compared to ionizing radiation, it still can cause severe effects on workers from high levels of exposure. For example, people who constantly work outdoors are most susceptible to ultraviolet radiation, to which chronic exposure can cause not only photochemical cataracts but also skin cancer (e.g., ICNIRP, 2007; Martin and Sutton, 2015).

As noted in Section 20.1, the bacterium *Legionella pneumophila* can cause the severe form of legionellosis in a workplace. To people in some sectors, it may be debatable whether the American Legion's 1976 convention held in Philadelphia (Pennsylvania), where the first reported episode of Legionnaires' disease took place, should be treated as a workplace. Regardless, the 2005 outbreak in Norway (Nygård *et al.*, 2008) is by all standards qualified as occurring in an occupational setting. In the Norway outbreak, more than 50 persons reportedly became ill (with 10 deaths) from Legionnaires' disease reportedly caused by the bacteria growing in a lignin type spray dryer scrubber placed in the Borregaard chemical plant located in Sarpsborg, a municipality near the city of Fredrikstad.

Many other infectious agents can be found in workplaces as well, especially in hospitals and clinics where healthcare and other workers may be exposed to the agents via inhalation or dermal contact. Healthcare workers may be exposed to infectious agents not only through accidental contact with contaminated blood specimens, a high health concern reflected in OSHA's BBP standard noted in Section 20.2.2, but also more commonly through inhalation of contaminated air a the workplace. SARS (severe acute respiratory syndrome) may serve as a rather convincing practical case example of airborne infection involving a significant number of employees working in clinics and hospitals.

The way in which SARS spreads is mainly by close person-to-person contact with the respiratory secretions or body fluids of a SARS patient (e.g., CDC, 2004). This respiratory disease, as briefly introduced in Chapter 1, was notorious for its global pandemic occurring during the nine months from November 2002 through early July 2003. This relatively short-lived pandemic involved over 8,000 human cases, more than 700 human deaths, and some 30 nations around the world (WHO, 2003).

Among all the global SARS cases confirmed by WHO, many were healthcare workers. The first outbreak of SARS reportedly occurred in southern China in November 2002. When the local health authority there notified WHO about the outbreak, 105 of the 305 reported cases (and 5 deaths), or about 30%, were healthcare workers. A group of medical investigators (Ho *et al.*, 2003) later found that hospital workers accounted for 25% of the cases in Hong Kong and were the first to contract SARS from a few infected patients before the disease got spread to the entire community. The investigators further noted in their study report that Canadian hospital workers had even a higher risk, accounting for 65% of all the SARS cases reported in that nation.

Another practical case example is with Ebola, which like SARS is a deadly infectious disease. As noted in Chapter 1, during the two-year global outbreak of Ebola beginning in early 2014, three of the four cases diagnosed in the United States were healthcare workers.

References

ACGIH® (American Conference of Governmental Industrial Hygienists), 2017. *TLVs® and BEIs® Based on Documentation of the Threshold Limit Values on Chemical Substances and Physical Agents & Biological Exposure Indices*, 7th Edition. ACGIH®, Cincinnati, Ohio, USA.

ATSDR (U.S. Agency for Toxic Substances and Disease Registry), 2002. Toxicological Profile for Beryllium. U.S. Department of Health and Human Services, Atlanta, Georgia, USA.

ATSDR (U.S. Agency for Toxic Substances and Disease Registry), 2004. Toxicological Profile for Synthetic Vitreous Fibers. U.S. Department of Health and Human Services, Atlanta, Georgia, USA.

ATSDR (U.S. Agency for Toxic Substances and Disease Registry), 2015. Addendum to the Toxicological Profile for Beryllium. U.S. Department of Health and Human Services, Atlanta, Georgia, USA.

Blondell JM, 1997. Epidemiology of Pesticide Poisonings in the United States, with Special Reference to Occupational Cases. *Occup. Med.* 12:209-220.

Carter T, 2004. British Occupational Hygiene Practice 1720-1920. *Ann. Occup. Hyg.* 48:299-307.

CDC (U.S. Centers for Disease Control and Prevention), 2004. Fact Sheet: Basic Information about SARS. U.S. Department of Health and Human Services, Atlanta, Georgia, USA.

CDC (U.S. Centers for Disease Control and Prevention), 2013a. All Workplace Safety & Health Topics – Organic Solvents (webpage last updated 30 December 2013). https://www.cdc.gov/niosh/topics/organsolv/ (retrieved 30 May 2017).

CDC (U.S. Centers for Disease Control and Prevention), 2013b. All Workplace Safety & Health Topics – Metalworking Fluids (MWFs) (webpage last updated 16 August 2013). https://www.cdc.gov/niosh/topics/metalworking/ (retrieved 10 June 2017).

CDC (U.S. Centers for Disease Control and Prevention), 2014. All Workplace Safety & Health Topics – Agricultural Safety (and Injury Prevention) (webpage last updated 15 December 2014). https://www.cdc.gov/niosh/topics/aginjury/ (retrieved 26 April 2017).

CDC (U.S. Centers for Disease Control and Prevention), 2016. All Workplace Safety & Health Topics – NIOSH Pocket Guide to Chemical Hazards (NPG) (downloadable PDF version, webpage last updated 18 May 2016). https://www.cdc.gov/nio-sh/npg/ (retrieved 15 May 2017).

Cheremisinoff NP, 2001. *Practical Guide to Industrial Safety: Methods for Process Safety Professionals.* New York, New York, USA: Marcel Dekker, Chapter 1.

DOL (U.S. Department of Labor), 2009. *Employment Law Guide: Laws, Regulations, and Technical Assistance Services.* Washington, DC, USA.

Ho AS, Sung JJY, Chan-Yeung M, 2003. An Outbreak of Severe Acute Respiratory Syndrome among Hospital Workers in a Community Hospital in Hong Kong. *Ann. Intern. Med.* 139:564-567.

IARC (International Agency for Research on Cancer), 2002. IARC Monographs on the Evaluation of Carcinogenic Risks to Humans, Volume 81: Man-Made Vitreous Fibres. Lyon, France: WHO Press.

IARC (International Agency for Research on Cancer), 2012. IARC Monographs on the Evaluation of Carcinogenic Risks to Humans, Volume 100C: Arsenic, Metals, Fibres, and Dusts. Lyon, France: WHO Press.

IARC (International Agency for Research on Cancer), 2017. IARC Monographs on the Evaluation of Carcinogenic Risks to Humans, Volumes 1-119: List of Carcinogens. Lyon, France: WHO Press.

ICNIRP (International Commission on Non-Ionizing Radiation Protection), 2007. Protecting Workers from Ultraviolet Radiation. ICNIRP, Helmholtz Centre Neuherberg, German Radiation Protection Agency, Oberschleissheim Munich, Bavaria, Germany.

Jeyaratnam J, 1990. Acute Pesticide Poisoning: A Major Global Health Problem. *World Health Stat. Q.* 43: 139-144.

Kloss D, 2005. *Occupational Health Law.* Oxford, UK: Blackwell Science.

Kreiss K, Cox-Ganser J, 1997. Metalworking Fluid-Associated Hypersensitivity Pneumonitis: A Workshop Summary. *Am. J. Ind. Med.* 32:423-432.

Lewis J, Thornbury G, 2010. *Employment Law and Occupational Health – A Practical Handbook.* Oxford, UK: Wiley-Blackwell.

NIOSH (U.S. National Institute for Occupational Safety and Health), 1998. What You Need to Know about Occupational Exposure to Metalworking Fluids. NIOSH Pub. No. 98-116. U.S. Department of Health and Human Services, Atlanta, Georgia, USA.

NIOSH (U.S. National Institute for Occupational Safety and Health), 2006. Pesticide-Related Illness and Injury Surveillance: A How-To Guide for State-Based Programs. NIOSH Pub. No. 2006-102. U.S. Department of Health and Human Services, Atlanta, Georgia, USA.

Nygård K, Werner-Johansen Ø, Rønsen S, Caugant DA, Simonsen Ø, Kanestrøm A, Ask E, Ringstad J, Ødegård R, Jensen T, *et al.*, 2008. An Outbreak of Legionnaires Disease Caused by Long-Distance Spread from an Industrial Air Scrubber in Sarpsborg, Norway. *Clin. Infect. Dis.* 46:61-69.

OSHA (U.S. Occupational Safety and Health Administration), 2016. Occupational Exposure to Respirable Crystalline Silica. *Federal Register* 81:16285-16890.

OSHA (U.S. Occupational Safety and Health Administration), 2017a. Chemical Sampling Information, by Name A-Z Search (no information on webpage update). https://www.osha.gov/dts/chemicalsampling/toc/toc_chemsamp.html (retrieved 5 May 2017).

OSHA (U.S. Occupational Safety and Health Administration), 2017b. Safety and Health Topics: Alphabetical Listing of Topics – Synthetic Mineral Fibers (no information on webpage update). https://www.osha.gov/SLTC/syntheticmineralfibers/in-dex.html (retrieved 3 June 2017).

Reigart JR, Roberts JR (Eds.), 1999. Recognition and Management of Pesticide Poisonings, Fifth Edition. EPA #735-R-98-003. Office of Pesticide Program, Washington DC, USA.

Taylor DK, 2015. Non-Coherent Optical Radiation Sources. In *Practical Radiation Protection in Healthcare* (Martin CJ, Sutton DG, Eds.), 2nd Edition. Oxford, UK: Oxford University Press, Chapter 22.

U.S. EPA (U.S. Environmental Protection Agency), 1992. Integrated Risk Information System (IRIS) on Refractory Ceramic Fibers. Office of Research Development, Washington DC, USA.

U.S. EPA (U.S. Environmental Protection Agency), 2010. Funding Opportunity Announcement: Pesticide Safety Program for Agricultural Workers and Farmworker Children. Funding Opportunity No. 2010-02. Office of Pesticide Programs (Field and External Affairs Division), Washington DC, USA.

WHO (World Health Organization), 2000. Fact Sheet No. 238 (May 2000): Silicosis. Geneva, Switzerland.

WHO (World Health Organization), 2003. Summary of Probable SARS Cases with Onset of Illness from 1 November 2002 to 31 July 2003. Geneva, Switzerland.

WSNZ (WorkSafe New Zealand), 2016. Workplace Exposure Standards and Biological Exposure Indices, Eighth Edition. Wellington 6011, New Zealand.

Zacharisen MC, Kadambi AR, Schlueter DP, Kurup VP, Shack JB, Fox JL, Anderson HA, Fink JN, 1998. The Spectrum of Respiratory Disease Associated with Exposure to Metal Working Fluids. *J. Occup. Environ. Med.* 40:640-647.

Review Questions

1. Briefly describe the two unique basic principles as well as practices that occupational toxicology has its focus on.
2. Name three examples of classic *industrial* diseases covered in this chapter.
3. Briefly describe the functions and organizational structure of NIOSH.
4. What was the first federal legislation related to occupational health and safety in the United States?
5. Over the years, how has the European Union's Framework Directive affected or directed the occupational health and safety regulations and standards adopted by its member states?
6. Briefly describe the different statuary obligations that OSHA and NIOSH each have in safeguarding the health and safety of American workers.
7. How does OSHA's Hazard Communication Standard affect or influence the health and safety of workers in the United States?
8. Why is NIOSH's *Pocket Guide to Chemical Hazards* such an important document to both the workers and the occupational health and safety professionals in the United States?
9. In what ways is an illness surveillance program an important tool for advancing or promoting occupational health and safety?
10. How does NIOSH carry out its SENOR-Pesticides program in the United States?
11. Briefly characterize the symptoms and causes of the illness condition known as metal fume fever.
12. Briefly describe the regulatory standard referred to as *Permissible Exposure Limit*.
13. Briefly characterize the following concepts (terms) in relation to occupational exposure limits: PEAK, STEL, and TWA.
14. Which of the major chemical classes of toxicants as well as hazards, as covered in this chapter, appears most related to acute poisoning from worker exposure?

15. What is the most common occupational lung disease in the world?
16. Based on the occupational exposure limit values listed in Table 20.1, rank the following pesticides from having the highest to the lowest *potency*: a) DDT; b) parathion; c) pyrethrum; d) sodium fluoroacetate; e) 2,4-D.
17. How are the BEIVs related to their corresponding TWAs for substances or compound groups having both of these estimates provided by a health authority or regulatory agency?
18. Why or how should the biological monitoring results be interpreted with caution when checking them against/to a BEIV for potential exposure to a specific workplace hazard?
19. Briefly explain why so many workers are exposed to organic solvents each year in many countries.
20. List and briefly characterize the three general source/use categories of SMFs. And which of the three apparently has been proven as most carcinogenic to humans (as of 2017)?
21. Which of the following two types of workplace dust particles tend to be more harmful to humans? a) fibrogenic; b) nuisance. And why?
22. Name five types of physical hazards that are commonly found in workplaces.
23. Name four occupations as common sources of potential exposure to ionizing radiation, and another four for potential exposure to non-ionizing radiation.
24. Give two case examples of infectious agents covered in this chapter that had outbreaks occurring in a workplace.
25. Why do healthcare workers, compared to the general public, tend to be more susceptible to SARS or Ebola type infection?

CHAPTER 21

Food Toxicants and Toxic Household Substances

21.1. Introduction

Food and household products are closer to home than any other kind or form of purchasable goods. Household products are consumer goods that often cause health concerns to the public, especially those that can harm children and the elderly. On the other hand, a vast number of harmful foreign substances are found in foods that people consume every day. Some of these harmful substances are added to the food product intentionally or as a result of contamination. Food toxicants of lingering concern to environmental toxicologists may fall under the three major source categories: (1) direct or intentional food additives; (2) indirect or unintentional food additives; and (3) food contaminants. Note that here the term *food additive* may not have the same legal connotation worldwide. However, at the minimum, the term should be employed to refer to any added substance either not normally consumed as a food by itself, or not used as an ingredient of a food item (FAO/WHO, 1994).

According to a research team (Scallan *et al.*, 2011) affiliated with the U.S. Centers for Disease Control and Prevention (CDC), each year some 48 million American people get sick, 128,000 are hospitalized, and about 3,000 die as a result of foodborne illness. For household products, the poisoning statistics are as disturbing. The U.S. Consumer Product Safety Commission (CPSC, 2015) estimated that in 2014, emergency rooms in clinics and hospitals across the United States treated nearly 67,000 children <5 years old for accidental poisoning occurring at home. And the top 10 household products found responsible for these cases included blood pressure medications, bleach, and laundry packets.

The acute poisoning statistics mentioned above did not include adverse health effects from chronic exposure that might lead to severe or fatal damage, such as cancer or early (premature) death. To put it another way, in terms of food or household product safety, the scope of public health concern goes far beyond what the above statistics have inferred.

21.1.1. Concerns with Food Toxicants

In the United States, as authorized by the (Federal) Food, Drug, and Cosmetic (FD&C) Act, the federal safety regulation for most types of foods in the nation is the responsibility of the U.S. Food and Drug Administration (FDA). The federal statute was enacted in 1938 after an improperly prepared sulfanilamide antibacterial drug took the life of more than 100 people. With several amendments passed over the years, including in the form of the Food Quality Protection Act (FQPA) of 1996, the FD&C Act completely overhauled the nation's health regulatory system. Among other provisions, the law empowers FDA to promulgate food (as well as cosmetic and drug) safety and health standards, to conduct factory inspections, and to call for safety evidence for new food additives to be put on the market.

Foods may also be contaminated by biological agents, environmental toxicants, or toxins present within a food proper. Symptoms of acute food poisoning usually involve, at the minimum, nausea, vomiting, or diarrhea. Some foodborne toxins, such as those found in certain seafood, can affect the nervous system (and hence are commonly referred to as neurotoxins). Many foreign substances are also present in foods due to environmental pollution or to faulty handling of foods. These substances are generally referred to as food contaminants, as they serve no purpose either in the food product or in its processing.

There are foreign substances that may become part of a food product as a result of their contact with or migration into the food proper during packaging, holding, or processing. These substances are commonly referred to as *indirect* or *unintentional* food additives. There are also many substances intentionally added to foods to accomplish an intended effect, such as to increase a food's shelf life or to enhance its appeal to consumers. Still some substances are added to make a food more tractable for bountiful or consistent production. These added substances are generally referred to as *intentional* or *direct* food additives, amidst the recent trend that some of them have been showing up with questionable or (more) unfavorable toxicity.

21.1.2. Concerns with Toxic Household Substances

In the United States, the federal safety regulation for certain types of consumer products is the responsibility of CPSC, as authorized under the federal Consumer Product Safety Act (CPSA) of 1972. This federal statute empowers CPSC to promulgate health and safety standards as well as advisories for (certain types of) consumer products, to pursue recalls for those that present unacceptable health or safety risks to consumers, and to ban any of the more than 15,000 kinds of consumer products (including household products) that are under its jurisdiction if there is no feasible alternative. Consumer products not under CPSC's regulations are those expressly fall within the jurisdictions of other federal agencies, such as foods, drugs, most cosmetics, medical devices, pesticides, tobacco products, boats, motor vehicles, explosives, and firearms.

Over-the-counter (OTC) medicines, personal care products, cleaning agents, and other organic compounds are the four major source categories of toxic household substances that reportedly cause more harm to young children, pregnant women, and the elderly. With toxic household substances, a particular underrated health concern is the common misconception that OTC medicines are absolutely safe for use by the general public, under the notion that they are all allowed by law to be sold without medical advice. Yet what remains a serious health concern, particularly for long-term health effects, is the potential for adverse drug (chemical) interaction between two or more OTC medicines or between an OTC and a prescription drug, which are commonly taken by the same (especially elderly) person at around the same time.

21.2. Toxic Substances in Food Products

As noted earlier, food toxicants can be broadly subsumed under three major source categories:

(1) intentional or direct food additives; (2) unintentional or indirect food additives; and (3) food contaminants. Figure 21.1 below presents a graphic overview of the three major categories, along with their subcategories intended to highlight more specifically the numerous various sources involved. Following the graphic presentation are separate brief accounts of the general aspects of these various source categories, including the toxicological concerns on certain food toxicants selected as specific or didactic examples.

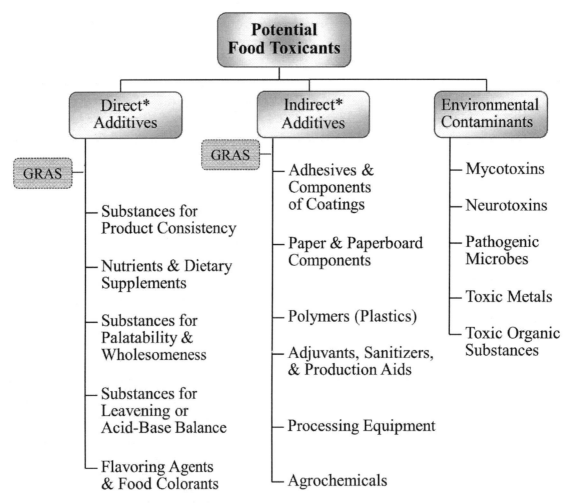

Figure 21.1. Major Source Categories of Potential Food Toxicants in the United States
(*subject to premarket review/approval by the U.S. Food and Drug Administration, except for those food additives placed on the generally recognized as safe [GRAS] list)

21.2.1. Direct Food Additives

According to an FDA (1992) document, this category includes several types of additives that are generally referred to by their functions: emulsifiers; stabilizers; anticaking agents; thickeners; preservatives; antioxidants; bleaching and maturing agents; buffering and sequestering agents; spices; vitamins and minerals; natural and synthetic flavoring boosters; and food colorants. Many consumers doing the cooking are fairly familiar with the functions of these additives and their purposes. In essence, emulsifiers are utilized to give foods a consistent texture and prevent them from separating. Stabilizers and thickeners are applied to give foods a smooth uniform texture. Preservatives are used to retard food spoilage caused by air or microorganisms. Anticaking agents are added to foods to prevent lumping. Antioxidants are a special kind of preservatives that are used mainly to prevent oils and fats in foods from becoming rancid. Spices and flavoring agents are added to enhance a food's taste. Food colorants are used to enhance the appearance of foods to satisfy consumer expectations. Vitamins and minerals are added to foods to make up for those known to be insufficient in a diet or lost in the processing.

In the United States, any *new* additive to be included in a food product must be approved by FDA as a new food ingredient. The approval is based on a favorable premarket review of extensive scientific data on safety and toxicity. Such a premarket safety evaluation generally requires, in addition to clinical observations whenever available, a series of animal studies involving about eight categories relevant to the analysis of health effects: toxicokinetics; acute toxicity; short-term (subchronic) toxicity; long-term (chronic) toxicity; teratogenicity; reproductive toxicity; carcinogenicity; and mutagenicity. As food safety evaluation needs to rely on a benchmark (i.e., a qualified safe level) for dietary intake of the new ingredient, the safety measure termed *acceptable daily intake* (ADI) or its equivalent (e.g., *tolerance level*) has been adopted by food safety sectors worldwide. These ADI levels are typically determined in relation to the no observed [adverse] effect level (NO[A]EL) derived from (primarily) animal toxicity studies. Further discussion on these health risk assessment issues and criteria is given in Chapter 23.

It should be noted that some direct (and less so, indirect) additives have been accepted by the U.S. legislation as "generally recognized as safe" (GRAS) as far back as 1958. GRAS exemptions are granted for substances that are generally recognized or affirmed as safe by a panel of experts qualified by their scientific training and experience in evaluating the safe use of these or similar substances. Currently, more than a couple thousands of substances are placed on the GRAS list, including many commonly available substances such as acetic acid, calcium carbonate, carbon dioxide, cocoa butter substitute, ethyl alcohol, hydrogen peroxide, lactic acid, malt syrup, rapeseed oil, red algae, vitamin A, vitamin D, wheat, wheat gluten, and many more. The use of a number of GRAS substances is now being challenged, however, largely due to the emergence of more or new (sometimes questionable) toxicity data on these substances in recent years. As a recent case in point (and noted in Section 4.2.2), the dietary source of artificial trans fats in processed foods sold in the United States is predominantly hydrogenated oils, which FDA in 2015 decided to remove from the GRAS list. FDA (2015) also announced that artificial trans fats would have to go away from the American diet by 2018.

Food emulsifiers, also called food emulgents, are molecules whose one end is water-loving (hydrophilic) and the other end is fat-loving (hydrophobic). Adding molecules of this kind to a food material will make it possible for the water and oil molecules in the mixture to become finely dispersed in each other, thereby creating a stable, homogenous, smooth emulsion (of which milk is a classic example). Egg yolk, containing the emulgent lecithin, is frequently applied as a food emulsifier, in spite of the fact that it is one of the common causes of food allergies in children. Some emulsifiers such as calcium and magnesium stearates (salts of certain fatty acid) can also act as anticaking agents. A few other emulsifiers such as sorbitan monostearate and sorbitan tristearate can also be utilized as stabilizers.

The more commonly used natural raw materials for food emulsifiers include soybean lecithin and sunflower lecithin. Lecithin, a mixture of phospholipids and found in all living cells, can be utilized to keep cooking oil blended with vinegar in salad dressings. The production of basic emulsifiers involves trans-esterification of triglycerides (a type of lipids consisting of three fatty acid groups that are also found in the human blood) with glycerols to form monoglycerides. The monoglycerides in turn can be esterified with other substances, such as citric acid and lactic acid, to improve their emulsifying strength. Although most food emulsifiers including the various esters of monoglyceride are of low toxicity, significant amounts of aluminum are reportedly found in them. Aluminum has been suspected to cause Alzheimer's disease (Section 14.3.1).

A nutrient is a substance that an organism's body relies on for development, growth, metabolism, or health maintenance and that the organism must take in from its environment. This substance is taken in to build and repair tissues, to regulate body functions, or to provide a source for energy. Organic nutrients include proteins (as well as their building blocks amino acids), lipids, carbohydrates, and vitamins. Inorganic compounds such as oxygen, water, and dietary minerals (including certain metals) may also be considered as nutrients.

Under the U.S. Dietary Supplement Health and Education Act (DSHEA) of 1994, dietary supplements sold in the United States are defined as edible products each containing an ingredient intended to supplement a diet. The ingredient may be one or any combination of the following: vitamins; minerals; herbs or other botanicals; amino acids; enzymes; organ tissues; and metabolites. These supplements can be extracts or concentrates and may be available in various forms such as tablets, capsules, powder, and liquid. They can be made available in other forms (e.g., a bar); but in that case, the information on their labels must not represent them as a conventional food or a sole item of a diet. Whatever their form may be, DSHEA places dietary supplements in a special category under the general umbrella of foods and mandates that these items be labeled as dietary supplements.

The main concern with the dietary supplements is their misuse or overuse, as such abuses can bring in a host of side effects. For instance, excess levels of vitamin A over 15,000 international units (IU) may lead to hepatotoxic effects as well as undesired changes in vision, hair, and skin. Adverse health levels of vitamin D may result from intakes greater than 2,000 IU daily and can induce hyperkalemia or soft tissue calcification. Intakes of vitamin E over 800 IU daily may lead to untoward effects such as headaches, vomiting, fatigue, and nausea. Moreover, taking vitamin C more than the daily recommendation of 100 mg per kg of body weight may retard metabolic activities or cause stomach aches and diarrhea.

Likewise, minerals as a group can cause many side effects if not used wisely. For example, in large or repeated doses, calcium can cause osteoporosis. Fluorine (usually available in the form of fluoride) can lead to skeletal or dental fluorosis. Iron can cause deficiency in zinc. Excess intake of macronutrients can also cause a number of untoward health effects. At the least, the presence of a large quantity of one macronutrient (e.g., lipid) as an energy source can induce adverse effects indirectly by causing *either* nutritional deficiencies in (one or more of) the other macronutrients (e.g., carbohydrate) *or* an interference with their normal functions and utilization. In addition to vitamin and nutrient toxicities caused by overdose, dietary supplements may interact with one another or with prescription drugs to induce adverse effects due to chemical interaction.

Preservatives are substances added to maintain the palatability and wholesomeness of food. They retard food spoilage caused by air and microorganisms. As noted earlier, antioxidants are preservatives used largely to prevent fats and oils in baked goods and other oily foods from becoming rancid. They also retard cut-fresh fruits (e.g., apples, peaches) from turning brownish when exposed to air. Preservatives such as butylated hydroxyanisole (BHA), butylated hydroxytoluene (BHT), sodium nitrate, sodium nitrite, and propyl gallate are commonly added to foods to uphold their quality, with some also serving as antioxidants. As listed in Table 19.1, BHA and propyl gallate are (potential) endocrine disruptors. There is some evidence (Pop *et al.*, 2013; Wada *et al.*, 2004) that BHT, the chemical cousin of BHA, is a weak endocrine disruptor.

Sodium bicarbonate (baking soda) and active dry yeast are two common leavening agents that produce gas bubbles to cause biscuits, cakes, and similar baked products to rise during baking. There are also leavening agents that can help modify the acidity of foods for proper flavor or taste. For example, fumaric acid, lactic acid, phosphoric acid, sodium aluminum phosphate, sodium aluminum sulfate, and tartrates may be added to adjust a baked product's acidity. Some of these agents reportedly have the potential to cause side effects. In particular, phosphoric acid, which is used in many soft drinks, has been linked to lower bone density (i.e., osteoporosis) in epidemiological studies. Sodium aluminum phosphate, commonly found in processed foods such as cheese and pickles, can be a rich source for aluminum found in the body. The toxicity of aluminum has remained controversial (Section 14.3.1), but any such excess dietary intake certainly could and should be avoided. Moreover, very high levels of lactic acid can cause (lactic) acidosis, a serious physiological condition with abnormally low pH in the blood and body tissues, though dietary intake alone is not likely able to account for such a high toxicity level involved.

Some substances are used to simulate natural flavors, such as benzaldehyde (C_6H_5CHO) for almond flavor even though the ADI for this flavorant might be as low as 4 mg/kg (e.g., Andersen, 2006). Some others, such as monosodium glutamate (MSG), are added to intensify food flavor and taste. One side effect of MSG ingestion is the sudden onset of an asthma-like attack, with symptoms including headaches, heart palpitations, chest pains, and shortness of breath.

In the United States, the most common artificial *primary* colorants used in foods include allura red AC (a.k.a. FD&C red No. 40), brilliant blue FCF (FD&C blue No. 1), and tartrazine (FD&C yellow No. 5). Primary colorants are referred to those from which secondary colorants are formulated. Studies have linked excessive consumption of certain artificial colorants to a number of adverse effects, such as tartrazine yellow on the reproductive functions of male mice (Mehedi *et al.*, 2009) and allura red on the behavioral activities in young rats (Vorhees *et al.*, 1983).

In the European Union (EU), since July 2010 most foods containing the synthetic colorants mentioned above (and others as well) have been required to add a product label statement warning consumers that the food *"may have an adverse effect on activity and attention in children"*. The health authorities of Austria, Finland, France, and the United Kingdom have gone further. The four EU members, along with Norway, have actually banned the use of all artificial food dyes.

21.2.2. Indirect Food Additives

Unintentional or indirect food additives are substances present mostly in food-contact articles that have the potential to migrate into the food proper being packaged, stored, or processed. These substances are often found at least in some trace amount in the final food product, all being part of the packaging materials or processing equipment that have migrated into the food proper. Accordingly, as depicted in Figure 21.2, the major sources of these substances include the following: adhesives and components of coating; paper and paperboard components; adjuvants, production aids, or sanitizers; and polymers (e.g., mostly plastics). Also included as indirect additives are growth promoters and other drugs used during the raising of food animals. These drug residues are in a different subcategory on their own not involving food-contact type articles.

Under FDA's Threshold of Regulation program, substances that come in contact with foods are exempted from being listed as indirect food additives if they migrate into foods at levels resulting in no appreciable risk to human health. FDA (1995) has outlined four "*not's*" criteria for what qualifies as the threshold of no appreciable human health risk in handling indirect food additives. First, migration of the food-contact substance at issue is *not* expected to result either in a dietary concentration above the benchmark threshold of 0.5 ppb (parts per billion) adopted by FDA for this purpose, or in a dietary intake above 1% of the ADI equivalent calculated for the additive. Second, the substance has *not* been shown or suspected to be a human or an animal carcinogen. Third, under its intended use conditions, the additive (e.g., a preservative residing in the packaging) must *not* produce a technical effect (e.g., retarding decomposition by microbial growth) in the food into which it migrates. The fourth and final criterion is that the additive's use must *not* have shown any significant adverse impact on the environment.

Per Title 21 of the *U.S. Code of Federal Regulations* (Section 175.105 – Adhesives), several phthalates, of which some are (suspected) endocrine disruptors (Table 19.1), have FDA approval for use as adhesives and components of coating in food processing and packaging materials. As a result, some phthalates may be ingested from foods (Castle *et al.* 1990; Hauser *et al.*, 2004; Page and Lacroix, 1995). BPA (bisphenol A), which is also considered as an endocrine disruptor (Table 19.1), is a key building block of polycarbonate plastic and epoxy resins used for coating the interior surfaces of food cans, beverage cans, and plastic bottles. BPA has been found leachable from such interior surfaces, including notably those of common baby bottles (Biles *et al.*, 1997; Gibson, 2007; Munguia-Lopez *et al.*, 2002). Amidst such rising health concerns among authorities (e.g., CEPA, 2010; FDA, 2010), Canada was the first nation to list BPA as a toxic substance. And on 17 July 2012, FDA made it official to ban BPA-based baby bottles and sippy cups.

Paper materials are used every day for packaging or holding foods in a variety of ways. Substances in paper plates, paper cups, cartons, wrappers, and boxes can leach into foods during storage, preparation, and service activities. These substances include polystyrene and many VOCs (volatile organic compounds) such as chloroform, benzene, dichloromethane, carbon tetrachloride, and trichloroethylene. In particular, dioxins and the kind can become a large component of paper plates as their one major source is from chlorination (as in bleaching) of wood pulp. Many of the substances mentioned above have been found harmful to humans when exposed to at sufficiently high levels (*see*, e.g., Chapters 13 and 16).

Polymers are long-chain giant organic molecules assembled from many smaller ones called monomers. A common name for most synthetic polymers is plastics. Some plastics are especially ubiquitous to consumers, such as: *polyethylene terephthalate*, as used in two-liter beverage bottles; *high-density polyethylene*, as used in milk jugs and food containers; *low-density polyethylene*, as used in film applications for meat and poultry wrapping; *polypropylene* (of normal density), as used in candy packaging; and *polystyrene*, as used in deli food containers and foam cups. Due to their high chemical inertness and insolubility in water, plastics generally have low toxicity in their finished state; and they will pass through the gastrointestinal system without inducing any noticeable adverse health effect. However, plastics frequently embedded with a variety of toxic additives such as BPA and phthalates. These plasticizers are often added to brittle plastics to improve the latter's flexibility for food packaging. Another concern is that plastic monomers, such as propylene and ethylene, can be harmful to humans. These monomers may remain trapped as unbound residues in polymer plastics that they were used to build.

Per Title 21 of the *U.S. Code of Federal Regulations* (Part 178), adjuvants are agents added to a food-contact article to facilitate the action of the article's principal ingredient(s), such as toluene being utilized as a blowing agent adjuvant in the production of foamed polystyrene. Sanitizers are agents generally used to remove unpleasant or infective features by controlling microbial growth. These sanitizers include hydrogen peroxide (H_2O_2) solution (which may be used to sterilize polymeric food-contact surfaces) and lithium hypochlorite (LiClO) solution (which may be used on food processing equipment, utensils, and other food-contact articles). Production aids are agents used to offer a processing environment conducive to the production of the food-contact article. For example, both polyethylene glycol (PEG) and hydrogenated castor oil may be used in the production of articles or components of articles authorized for food-contact use. And pentachlorophenol (PCP) may be used to preserve wooden articles intended to be used in packaging, transporting, or holding raw agricultural products. While the definitions of adjuvants and production aids may be overlapping, none of the examples given above (including for sanitizers) can or should be treated as absolutely harmless to humans at high levels of exposure.

The use of a thin dense chromium coating and a polytetrafluoroethylene (PTFE) coating can make the food-processing equipment last longer and cleaned faster. PTFE, more known by the DuPont brand name Teflon®, is a synthetic fluoropolymer with numerous applications. It is polymerized using PFOA (perfluorooctanoic acid) as a surfactant (Chapter 16). The supposedly nontoxic PTFE is a stable compound but begins to decompose after the cookware's temperature rises to about 350° C (662° F). Its degradation by-products can cause flu-like symptoms in humans; and some of them may be carcinogenic.

Drug residues in food animals are likewise of high health concern insomuch as many food animals need to be treated with drugs during their lifetime to ensure a continuing, wholesome, and affordable food supply to the public. Although several hundreds of drugs are used for this purpose, U.S. National Research Council (NRC, 1999) and several other entities have them all conveniently subsumed under five or six major use categories as listed below in Table 21.1. The NRC report addresses not only the benefits from using these drugs in food animals, but also the associated risks of human diseases (e.g., development of antibiotic resistance, cancer, drug residue allergy).

Table 21.1. Major Categories of Drugs Used in Food Animals[a]

Category	Example of Application
Topical antiseptics (e.g., buffered iodine, neomycine)	As those used to treat infections, wounds, and abrasions of surface skin or hoofs
Ionophores (e.g., monensin)	As those lipid-soluble molecules used to improve feed efficiency and as an aid to prevent coccidiosis
Anabolic steroid growth promoters (e.g., trenbolone acetate, zeranol)	As those protein hormones used to promote growth
Peptide production enhancers (e.g., rBST)	As those genetically-engineered hormone-like peptides such as recombinant bovine somatotropin (rBST) used to increase milk production in dairy cattle
Antiparasite drugs (e.g., ivermectin)	As those used to treat parasite diseases caused by gastrointestinal roundworms and sucking lice and mange mites on cattle and swine
Antibiotics (e.g., oxytetracycline, tetracycline)	As those used to control overt or occult (sub-clinical) diseases and to treat microbial infections

[a]see, e.g., NRC (1999) for further discussion, which is the primary source for this table; note that some of the drug examples given in this table may no longer or may not be allowed in some countries.

21.2.3. Food Contaminants

Food contaminants include a wide array of chemical substances and pathogenic microbes present in various forms or types of food products. Of all the food contaminants found, mycotoxins have one of the most serious consequences in terms of public health and agroeconomics. These mycotoxins can contaminate numerous various agricultural commodities before harvest or under post-harvest conditions. As noted in Chapter 17, the most notorious mycotoxins are the aflatoxins produced by the fungal species *Aspergillus flavus* and *Aspergillus parasiticus*, which tend to grow in drought-stressed corn and groundnuts under warm and humid climates.

Food infection is caused by the presence of bacteria or other microbes in a host organism's body after consumption. In contrast, food intoxication refers to the ingestion of toxins contained in the food, which can happen even when the microbes that produced the toxin (e.g., exotoxins produced by bacteria) are no longer present or capable of causing infection. Despite the term food intoxication often being treated loosely as synonymous with *food poisoning*, most food poisonings are caused directly by a variety of pathogenic bacteria, viruses, or parasites contaminating the food, not by their specific toxins. *Staphylococcus*, *Salmonella*, and *Clostridium* are among the common bacterial genera causing food poisoning in the United States. On the other hand, even when hepatitis A virus seems to be a more familiar disease to most people, the most prominent viral contaminant found in American foods is norovirus, which has been estimated to cause annually over 50% of all foodborne illnesses in the United States (Scallan et al., 2011).

The toxins from microbes can accumulate within certain tissues of predacious aquatic creatures which may become a source of seafood poisoning for organisms on the higher trophic levels in a food web. These toxins include tetrodotoxin, saxitoxin, ciguatoxin, and domoic acid toxin, all of which affect primarily the nervous system (Chapter 17). Tetrodotoxin and saxitoxin abusively block the sodium channels whereas ciguatoxin opens them. Domoic acid stimulates the excitatory amino acids at certain (e.g., glutamate) receptors. Ingestion of scombrotoxin in fish can cause illness resembling a histamine attack.

Fish and shellfish as sources account for a significant portion of foodborne illnesses reported across the world. In general, three types of diseases can result from consumption of contaminated seafood: allergy, infection, and intoxication. These days, certain fish species have become a popular food in the United States owing to a better appreciation of their health benefits. Consequently, fishing stocks in the nation are now reportedly at an all-time low.

Examples of contaminants with relatively less acute and more subtle symptoms when exposed to at low levels are certain POCs (persistent organochlorine compounds) and certain toxic metals (e.g., mercury) present in contaminated fish or other foods. Agrochemicals are substances utilized in agricultural practice and animal husbandry with the intent to raise farm yields at the lowest cost possible. These substances, of which many are organic compounds, include pesticides (e.g. insecticides, herbicides), plant growth regulators, and veterinary drugs (e.g., Table 21.1). Through environmental pollution, many of these contaminants can spread over a variety of media to end in the foods consumed by people. Toxic metals and pesticides as food contaminants have contributed to public's uneasiness over the pollution boom in the past half century, beginning in the mid-1960s when the publication of *Silent Spring* helped launch the environmental movement (Chapter 3). Pesticides in foods are predominantly residues from applications on or around growing crops, more so than from post-harvest applications on stored agricultural commodities. In contrast, toxic metals contaminate foods nearly at all stages along the food production line. The general toxicological properties of toxic metals and pesticides are discussed in Chapters 14 and 15, respectively. Overall, food contaminants in these two groups, along with those in the other groups discussed earlier in this subsection, collectively contribute to a wide array of public health problems.

21.3. Toxic Substances in Household Products

Many of the active or inert ingredients in household products sold in the United States (and other parts of the world) are not harmless, as evident from the mandate that they all come with a Material Safety Data Sheet (MSDS) per federal Hazard Communication Standard (29 *U.S. Code of Federal Regulations*, 1910.1200). These MSDS, or their equivalent likewise required in other nations, all contain a part on toxicity information for the material at issue. For example, cocamide *d*iethanol*a*mine (a.k.a. cocamide DEA) is widely used as a foam stabilizer in hand soaps, shampoos, and other bath products. The MSDS specifies that the stabilizer can cause irritation to the skin, eyes, and respiratory tract. A mouse study (NTP, 1999) also found kidney and liver tumors in the test animals following a two-year long repeated application of DEA to their skins.

Of all the substances contained in household products, as many as 150 have been linked to various allergies, asthma attacks, birth defects, tumors, and psychological abnormalities. As noted in Chapter 4, the toxic substances found in household cleaners are reportedly three times more likely to cause cancer than outdoor air pollution. Furthermore, indoor air in homes has been found to have five times higher toxic chemical concentrations compared to outdoor air. And according to a report cited by U.S. EPA (1989; 2015), studies from the United States and Europe observed many people in industrialized countries spending over 90 percent of their time indoors.

Figure 21.2 below presents a graphic overview of four categories of toxic household products commonly found in homes. Also included in the figure are their individual subcategories with the intent to highlight more specifically the numerous various sources of toxic household substances. As with the food toxicants, following the graphic presentation are separate brief accounts of the general aspects of the various product (source) categories. Likewise, these brief accounts include the toxicological concerns on certain substances selected as specific or didactic examples.

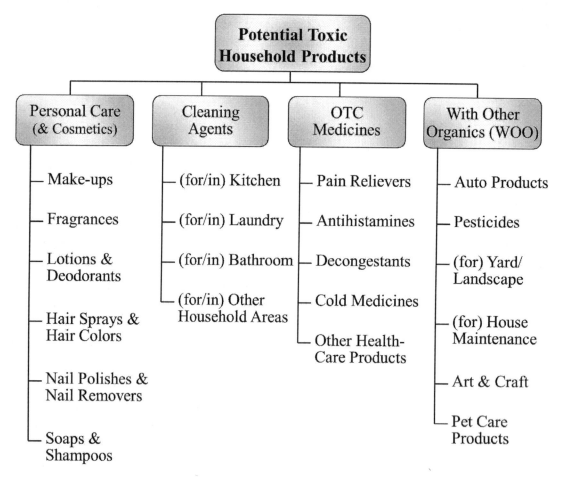

Figure 21.2. Major Categories of American Household Products in Which Potentially Toxic Substances Can Be Found (OTC ≡ Over-the-Counter; WOO ≡ Products with Other Organic Substances in Them)

21.3.1. Substances in Personal Care Products

Products in this category represent a huge and highly diverse collection of consumer stuffs such as facial tissues, toothpastes, cleansing pads, fragrances, make-ups, eye liners, gloss lipsticks, deodorants, colognes, personal lubricants, mouthwashes, shampoos, skin creams, toilet papers, and many more. Along with cocamide DEA introduced earlier, the substances highlighted below represent merely the more prominent among the numerous various ingredients contained in these personal care products. These select substances are considered posing higher health threats to the public especially if exposed to at sufficiently high levels repeatedly.

Sodium lauryl sulfate (SLS) is an anionic surfactant used in many cleaning and hygiene products (e.g., shampoos, soaps, toothpastes). The MSDS lists the surfactant as mutagenic for bacteria and yeasts. A preliminary clinical investigation suggested that SLS in toothpastes could cause the recurrence of canker sores (Herlofson and Barkvoll, 1994). According to the *Cosmetic Ingredient Review* (CIR, 1983) published by the U.S. Personal Care Products Council, studies showed that SLS had a high dermal absorption rate and maintained residual levels in major organs such as the liver, lungs, and brain. These findings hence pose serious concerns regarding the surfactant's potential health threat from its application in personal care products. The review noted that when rats in a study were exposed to a formulation containing 15% ammonium lauryl sulfate (a compound identical to SLS in structure except for the cation), 4 of the 20 test animals experienced eye damage, along with depression, labored breathing, severe skin irritation, or death.

Sodium laureth sulfate (SLeS), a chemical cousin of SLS, is an inexpensive as well as a highly effective foaming agent. It is thus likewise commonly used in soaps, shampoos, toothpastes, and many other personal care products. Although SLeS is somewhat less irritating than SLS, it cannot be metabolized by the liver. Its toxic effects are thereby more long-lasting. Some cosmetic materials containing SLeS were found to have been contaminated with low levels of the carcinogen 1,4-dioxane (Black *et al.*, 2001).

Polyethylene glycol (PEG) and its various available forms are used in a large variety of products from cleansing (e.g., caustic spray-on oven cleaner), medical (e.g., laxative), to personal care (e.g., toothpaste). Certain PEGs of high molecular weight have been utilized successfully as a dietary preventive agent against colorectal cancer in test animals (Corpet *et al.*, 2000). However, many PEGs were found containing potential toxic impurities such as 1,4-dioxane and the neurotoxicant ethylene oxide (CIR, 1999).

Propylene glycol (PG) is a common moisturizer ingredient found in mouthwashes, cosmetics, shampoos, and toothpastes, in addition to being utilized as a food additive and in antifreeze. It has been linked to liver and kidney problems in laboratory animals, and to common skin rashes and lesions in humans. The MSDS warns against dermal contact with the substance due to its ability to quickly penetrate the skin, as it can then cause systemic effects leading to brain, liver, and kidney problems.

Mineral oils including baby oil are produced from petroleum for use in numerous moisturizing materials. These oils can interfere with the skin's ability to exchange carbon dioxide for oxygen in the air, by forming an impermeable film over the skin pores. Because of this effect, they promote acne and other skin disorders. Mineral oils have been linked to early aging. Any product containing mineral oils may be contaminated by certain PAHs (polycyclic aromatic hydrocarbons), of which many are potential carcinogens.

Isopropyl (rubbing) alcohol is a solvent and denaturant commonly found in hand lotions, hair color rinses, fragrances, and other cosmetics. The solvent is oxidized by alcohol dehydrogenase in the liver into acetone, a metabolite that like the solvent itself is a central nervous system (CNS) depressant. Repeated inhalation of isopropyl alcohol at high concentrations can cause headaches, dizziness, damage to the liver and kidneys, narcosis, and coma.

Fragrances are a collection of over 3,000 mostly synthetic ingredients used in many deodorants, shampoos, sunscreens, and products for body, skin, or baby care. As many of these ingredients are petroleum by-products, some are carcinogenic while many others are toxic. Symptoms associated with their uses as reported to the FDA to date have included asthma attack, headaches, dizziness, violent coughing, and skin allergic reactions as well as skin rashes. According to a recent study (Steinemann, 2016), as many as one in three Americans have experienced migraine headaches, respiratory difficulties, and/or other health problems when exposed to fragranced consumer products. There were findings (e.g., Fisher, 1998; FPIN, 2002) suggesting that sick building syndrome could be developed or exacerbated by the chemical mixtures in indoor air that had been contaminated by the ingredients in perfumes and colognes worn by co-workers. In fact, the American Lung Association started in 2013 to offer the public with a sample fragrance-free policy to be instated in workplaces. And the Office of Information Technology at the University of Colorado at Boulder is among the fast growing number of places that have initiated or promoted a working environment with fragrance-free buildings.

Formaldehyde (CH_2O) is a colorless, pungent-smelling gas at ambient temperature (Chapter 13). Imidazolidinyl urea ($C_{11}H_{16}N_8O_8$) and DMDM hydantoin (1,3-*di*methylol-5,5-*di*methylhydantoin, $C_7H_{12}N_2O_4$) are two of the common CH_2O-releasing preservatives available today. Nearly all brands of skin care, hair care, antiperspirants, and nail polishes found in stores contain these or other CH_2O-releasing ingredients. Formaldehyde can cause watery eyes, burning sensations in the eyes, nose, and throat, as well as nausea, coughing, and breathing difficulties in some people exposed to air levels above 0.1 ppm (parts per million). At higher levels, formaldehyde can trigger asthma and allergic reactions. Formaldehyde has been found to cause cancer in humans and animals (Chapter 13; ATSDR, 1999, 2010; CPSC, 1997; IARC, 2012, 2017).

FD&C type colorants are used in many cosmetics and other personal care products, in addition to foods and drugs. Some of these color pigments can induce skin sensitivity and irritation in humans. Absorption of some of them can cause oxygen depletion in the body leading to even death. There is, nonetheless, a rising controversy over the application of colorants in personal care products, partly due to the many inconsistent findings on their more serious toxic effects observed in animal studies. Yet a subtle argument for their application in cosmetics (even in lipsticks) is that the principal route of their absorption is through the skin, not via the faster route of ingestion like for those colorants contained in foods.

21.3.2. Substances in Cleaning Agents

Cleaning agents can be highly toxic if they are not handled properly. Laundry detergents and oven cleaners are the two most common examples. Other examples include carpet and upholstery shampoos, furniture polishes, toilet bowl cleaners, and dishwasher detergents. Children are at a higher risk when playing on floors contaminated by chemical residues from application of household cleaners. These youngsters are usually among the first to breathe the toxic fumes generated by these cleaning agents. Yet their immunological and nervous systems, as well as many of their other body organs, are not fully developed.

Laundry detergents contain phosphorus (P), ammonia (NH_3), phenol (C_6H_5OH), enzymes, and numerous other substances. These ingredients collectively can cause a wide array of acute (and at times also chronic) adverse health problems (e.g., rashes, itches, burns, allergies, sinus headaches). In particular, ammonia is both a highly volatile inorganic gas and a very potent irritant to the skin, eyes, and respiratory tract. Phenol is an organic compound, which in vapor form is corrosive to the skin, eyes, and respiratory tract. On prolonged contact, this organic can cause the skin to burn and break out in hives.

Oven cleaners are among the most toxic products used in homes. They contain ammonia and lye, as well as their lingering fumes that can burn the skin, eyes, and lungs. Lye's chemical name is sodium hydroxide (NaOH), which is also known as caustic soda and by itself already a highly corrosive substance.

Many carpet and upholstery shampoos are designed with the additional utility of removing stains. They fulfill this added objective by including highly toxic substances such as ammonium hydroxide (NH_4OH) and PCE (perchloroethylene). As noted in Chapter 13, PCE (a.k.a. PERC) is a carcinogenic solvent that can additionally cause damage to the kidneys, liver, and nervous system. NH_4OH, like NaOH, is not only a strong corrosive agent but also a potent irritant to the skin, eyes, and respiratory tract.

Many dishwasher detergents contain chlorine (Cl) specifically at a high concentration. Chlorine is a potent bleaching agent and a strong disinfectant. Its harmful effects will be intensified when its fumes are heated, as in or around a hot shower. As per product label warning, consumers handling chlorine products need to use goggles or face masks, protective gloves, and proper ventilation. Furthermore, mixing chlorine with ammonia or acid toilet bowl cleaners will easily produce fumes that can be lethal.

Air fresheners are designed to interfere with a person's sense of smell by including a nerve-deadening agent or by coating nasal passages with an oil film such as methoxychlor ($C_{16}H_{15}Cl_3O_2$) which is a toxic organochlorine (pesticide) tending to accumulate in fatty tissues. Other common toxic ingredients found in air fresheners include p-dichlorobenzene (e.g., used as the active ingredient of mothball), naphthalene, and formaldehyde.

Many toilet bowl cleaners are acidic as they typically contain hydrochloric acid (HCl) and hypochlorite (ClO^-) bleach, both of which are highly corrosive to the skin, eyes, and respiratory tract. If accidentally ingested as by naïve toddlers, these cleaner products would cause vomiting, pulmonary edema, coma, or death.

Furniture polishes may contain naphtha (i.e., petroleum distillates) which can cause irritation of the skin, eyes, and throat, as well as dermatitis and chronic respiratory problems. These products may also contain nitrobenzene ($C_6H_5NO_2$), which can be easily absorbed through the skin and can then cause fatigue, shortness of breath, cyanosis, and even coma.

21.3.3. Substances in Over-the-Counter Medicines

Over-the-counter (OTC) medicines used in homes include mostly pain relievers, antihistamines, decongestants, and cold medicines, all of which come with side effects. Pain relievers available to consumers without prescription include the ones with acetaminophen used as the active ingredient and a number of the anti-inflammatory kind. OTC medicines in this group are supposed to be safe to use as long as they are not taken at an excess dose or for an excessively long period. Otherwise, the most common side effects from taking them are gastritis and ulcers.

Other OTC pain-relieving substances are largely topicals. They are predominantly creams that can be rubbed on or around a painful area of the body. Some of these creams such as capsaicin (a.k.a., hot pepper) are proven helpful and can be used by patients having musculoskeletal pains. These substances may also be used as substitutes for stronger drugs which can come with more or more serious side effects.

Antihistamines are intended to relieve or prevent mild (to moderate) allergy symptoms which may include skin rashes, itching, stuffy or runny nose, nausea, and watery eyes. Two generations of OTC antihistamines have been made available to date, with doxylamine and brompheniramine generally representing the first generation whereas cetirizine and loratadine representing the second. When the body is exposed to allergens, it releases the organic nitrogen molecules known as histamines ($C_5H_9N_3$) which will cause the body's cells to swell and leak fluid upon contact, leading to a sequence of allergic reactions. The most severe allergic reaction is known as anaphylaxis, which can be life-threatening as it can cause the body to go into shock due to sudden drastic drop in blood pressure coupled with severe airway restriction. Antihistamines are designed to block histamines from attaching to the cells in the body and consequently from causing allergy symptoms. Some of these OTC medicines can make a person feel drowsy, thereby affecting the patient's sense and ability to drive safely or think clearly. In certain cases, antihistamines can cause headaches, nausea, blurred vision, dry mouth, restlessness, and trouble peeing.

The vast majority of nasal decongestants (e.g., ephedrine, pseudoephedrine) act by enhancing vasoconstriction of blood vessels in the nose, throat, and paranasal sinuses, to result in reduced inflammation (i.e., reduced swelling) and reduced mucus formation in these areas. Common side effects with decongestants include hypertension (high blood pressure), anxiety, dizziness, insomnia (sleeplessness), excitability, and nervousness.

In addition to nasal decongestants, cough suppressants and expectorants are among the few types of ingredients found either alone or in combination in many OTC cough and cold medicines. Cough suppressants act by suppressing the cough reflex in the throat and lungs, so that the mucus or irritation there will not trigger coughing. Expectorants act by loosening thick mucus, making it easier to be coughed up and out. The side effects with these two types of ingredients are usually minimal but can include constipation, headaches, skin rashes, mild drowsiness, confusion, mild dizziness, and stomach pains.

Yet in all cases whenever possible, all these OTC medicines should not be taken along with other medications or with substances such as alcohol that jointly can cause adverse drug interaction. Many people have heard how older folks complain about all the pills that they need to take simultaneously. On the other hand, there have been studies (e.g., Patterson and Jeste, 1999) showing that a considerable number of older people are addicted to various prescription drugs (including OTC medicines) and alcohol, while many others misuse them.

Drug-drug or drug-alcohol interaction is a biochemical reaction (Section 10.4) that indeed can result in severe health consequences. For example, acetaminophen (e.g., the active ingredient in Tylenol®) may cause liver damage in people having excessive daily consumption of alcohol over a long period. Alcohol can also aggravate CNS depression in people taking antidepressants (e.g., Elavil, Prozac, Wellbutrin) or sedatives (e.g., Secobarbital, Phenobarbital, Valium). Drug-drug interaction can lead to severe side effects such as excessive sedation, coma, and even death, despite the general observation that in many cases the side effects from the individual drugs alone are mild or unnoticeable.

21.3.4. Other Major Relevant Organic Substances

Other harmful or potentially harmful organic substances commonly found in homes include those contained in: gasoline (e.g., for lawn mower operation); paints and paint-related products; floor and furniture polishes; inks; degreasers; pesticides; and batteries. Paints, paint strippers, and varnishes all contain organic solvents such as benzene, methylene chloride, or toluene. Gasoline and other fuel products typically contain additional organic solvents as additives, such as cyclohexane, hexane, one or more (other) members from the so-called BTEX group (i.e., *b*enzene, *t*oluene, *e*thylbenzene, *x*ylene isomers), and sometimes ethanol.

The various kinds of pesticide products that are commonly found in homes include, but are not limited to: cockroach sprays and baits; insect repellents for personal use; rat and other rodent poisons; flea and tick sprays; pet collars; kitchen, laundry, or bathroom disinfectants and sanitizers; products that eliminate mold and mildew; garden and lawn care products (e.g., weed killers); and swimming pool disinfectants.

Some of these organic compounds found in homes are highly flammable, corrosive, or toxic (for some of the toxicities involved, *see* Chapters 13 and 15). As so specifically and repeatedly urged by CPSC and U.S. EPA on their websites, household products of this type should be stored per label instructions and out of the reach of children as well as pets. Effective measures should include having all potentially toxic household products locked in a garden shed, in a cabinet free of food items, or in a utility area with sufficient ventilation.

21.4. Didactic Cases with Food and Household Products

In recent years, there have been serious or special public health concerns with various contamination issues involving food and household products. These concerns and issues include, but are not limited to, those with the BPA (bisphenol A) leaching from baby bottles, the PTS (persistent toxic substances) residues found in fishes worldwide, the metal lead coated on children's toys and toy jewelry, and the triclosan used as antibacterial agent in personal care products. The contamination issues and health problems with the above four and other chemical entities are highlighted elsewhere in this book. In this section, as part of the learning lessons of contemporary environmental health issues, elaborations are given on the relevant incidences and events specifically for the PTS, lead, and triclosan involved. This section as well as this chapter then ends with offering a practical approach for the mitigation and prevention of this kind of contaminations or incidences.

21.4.1. Persistent Toxic Substances in Seafood

As noted in Chapter 16, many PTS of global health concern are POCs (persistent organochlorine compounds). Between the 1990s and the early 2000s, a number of POCs were analyzed for their residue levels in fishes from localities across various countries. It turned out that, as summarized in Table 6.2 (for the 1990s) and Table 6.3 (for the early 2000s), the fish samples from each of the localities under study had tissue residue levels far exceeding U.S. EPA's screening values for at least one of the POCs analyzed. In particular, an extensive collaboration study by Hites *et al.* (2004) showed significant residue levels of several POCs detected in farmed and wild salmons of various species from around the globe.

The collaboration study analyzed more than two metric tons of farmed and wild salmons from around the world for PCBs (polychlorinated biphenyls) and other POC contaminants. The analysis found significantly higher residue levels of these contaminants in farmed salmon species than in their wild counterparts. The study also observed a significantly greater contaminant load in salmons raised in Europe than in North or South America. The investigators were concerned that consumption of farmed salmon might pose health risk to the point that it would detract from the basic beneficial effects of fish consumption. Their concern should not be underrated or overlooked. As they put it, the annual global production of farmed salmons has increased about 40-fold since some 50 years ago, all because salmons from farms in northern Europe, North America, and Chile are now available to consumers year round at more affordable prices.

21.4.2. Lead on Children's Toy Jewelry

For the past ten years or so, a series of acute lead poisoning cases has been linked to children's toy jewelry and toys sold in the United States. Many of these jewelry and toys were manufactured overseas where labor costs were more affordable. Some of these products were found to have been coated with relatively high contents of lead (Pb) on their surfaces. Further investigations by CPSC for these cases led to a number of nationwide product recalls.

Of particular concern at the national level were two recall cases involving two children exposed to two unsuspected objects, with both cases happening within the past decade or so. The first case occurred in the state of Oregon in 2003 (e.g., VanArsdale *et al.*, 2004). It involved a four-year-old boy with intermittent diarrhea, abdominal pains, and vomiting lingering for weeks. The boy was first misdiagnosed by his physician as having viral gastroenteritis. An abdominal radiograph performed on a later visit revealed a metallic object in the boy's stomach, without evidence of obstruction. An endoscopy led to the retrieval of a U.S. coin and a medallion pendant from the young patient's stomach. Then a subsequent measurement of venous blood lead level (BLL) showed an extremely elevated content of 123 µg/dL in the boy's blood (i.e., well over 10 times the level of concern currently set at around 10 µg/dL).

The medallion, which the boy obtained from a toy vending machine, was reportedly imported from India. It contained 38.8% (388 mg/g) Pb, 3.6% antimony (Sb), and 0.5% tin (Sn) by weight (of the extracted), as measured and reported by the Oregon state's Department of Environmental Quality Laboratory. Other medallions obtained from toy vending machines shortly afterward were all found containing a similar content of lead. The Oregon state health officials thus notified CPSC for a nationwide investigation, which soon resulted in a national voluntary recall of 150 million pieces of the imported metallic toy jewelry sold in vending machines (CDC, 2006).

The other recall case involved some 300,000 heart-shaped charm bracelets available during the three-month period between March and May 2004. The charm bracelets were each offered as a gift with a purchase of children's footwear in certain styles manufactured by Reebok International. In 2006, Reebok received a report about a boy in Minneapolis, Minnesota dying from lead poisoning after swallowing a piece off his charm bracelet (CDC, 2006).

The little patient, who was also four years old but with a medical history of microcephaly and developmental delay, was brought to an emergency room (ER) with a complaint of vomiting. Again, as in the previous case, the boy was misdiagnosed with a probable viral gastroenteritis and accordingly was sent home after receiving an antiemetic. When the boy returned to the ER two days later with a poor oral intake and intractable vomiting, he was admitted to the hospital and received an IV (intravenous) fluid replacement. The next day, when the boy was being transferred to the radiology department, he had a seizure which led to a respiratory arrest. After resuscitation, the boy was placed on a ventilator. Various tests were then performed on the boy in the following day, including one showing a BLL of 180 µg/dL and another revealing no blood flow to the boy's brain. The boy was pronounced dead on the fourth day of hospitalization. Abdominal radiographs revealed a foreign heart-shaped object in his stomach. When the ingested charm piece was measured for Pb (lead) content, it was found to contain 99.1% Pb by weight (of the extracted).

In reviewing these two cases where young children were the victims, it is important to realize again that they are more sensitive and more susceptible to chemical exposure compared to adults. Lead is a potent neurotoxicant that can cause intellectual impairment and death particularly among young children. This is because young children are in the most critical phase of human development. Their frontal lobes are particularly vulnerable to the effects of lead poisoning. Lead neurotoxicity in children can result in disruption of vital functions, attention, behavioral conduct, and impulse control, all of which may not be fully manifested until late childhood especially when the exposure level is not sufficiently high.

21.4.3. Triclosan in Antibacterial Products

Triclosan ($C_{12}H_7Cl_3O_2$) is a lipophilic polychloro phenoxy phenol (used to be) commonly utilized as an active ingredient in many antibacterial products. Due to its widespread use in products ranging from hand and body soaps to plastics, alarming levels of this antimicrobial agent have been found in ground and surface waters (e.g., Loraine and Pettigrove, 2006; Servos *et al.*, 2007) and in the urine of nearly 1,900 (75%) of the 2,517 participants tested in a national survey (CDC, 2010). Studies showed that triclosan caused endocrine disruption in amphibians (Veldhoen *et al.*, 2006) and allergies in humans (Clayton *et al.*, 2011). A literature review (Aiello *et al.*, 2007) concluded that consumer soaps containing triclosan as an antiseptic active ingredient were no more effective than plain soaps in preventing infectious illnesses, and that the antimicrobial agent could even induce the development of bacterial strains resistant to antibiotics.

Triclosan can promote the emergence of antibiotic-resistant bacteria because its mode of action and its target site are similar to those of many antibiotics. In other words, the bacteria that became resistant to triclosan would likely become resistant to many antibiotics as well, thereby making the latter also less effective. Triclosan can bioaccumulate in fatty tissues owing to its high lipophilicity which allows it to have an easy entry into the human body. Recent findings that triclosan might serve as a production source for several dioxin congeners have caused additional public health concerns (e.g., Buth *et al.*, 2010), as some dioxins have been found carcinogenic or highly toxic to humans and animals (Chapter 16). As noted in Section 4.2.1A, FDA (2016) recently has issued its ruling that effective 6 September 2017, hand and body soaps can no longer be allowed on the market as OTC consumer products if they contain triclosan (and/or some other similar substances) as an active ingredient. As of 2017, triclosan is still allowed to be used as an antibacterial active ingredient in toothpastes and loads of other consumer products.

21.4.4. Self-Mitigation and Self-Prevention

Most human exposures to harmful food and household products, including those like problem toys not among the major categories listed in Figure 21.2, are highly preventable. For potentially harmful household products and other consumer goods, the most effective mitigation measure appears to be *self*-prevention coupled with common sense. It is under this notion that CPSC has urged parents and caregivers to follow the 10 poison prevention tips that the commission (e.g., CPSC, 2003) periodically publicizes as effective prevention measures. The 10 prevention tips, as reproduced below, are simply a set of common sense-based housekeeping principles.

1. Keep all products locked up from children, out of sight and out of reach.

2. Use child-resistant packaging properly by closing the container securely after each use or (alternatively) choose child-resistant unit packaging which (that) does not need to be re-secured.

3. Call the 800 hotline (as available on the product label or from local poison centers) immediately in case of poisoning.

4. When products are in use, keep children in sight, even if the adult must take them along when answering the phone or doorbell.

5. Keep items in original containers.

6. Leave the original labels on all products, and read the label (the instructions) before using.

7. Do not put decorative lamps and candles that contain lamp oil (in a place) where children can reach them. (Note: lamp oil can be highly toxic if ingested.)

8. Always turn the light on when giving or taking medicine so that the patient or caregiver can see what he/she is taking or giving. Check the dosage every time.

9. Avoid taking medicine in front of children.

10. Clean out the medicine cabinet periodically and safely dispose of unneeded and outdated medicines.

The manufacturers or distributors need to do their share as well. In fact, it is a federal law in the United States, such as under FIFRA (*Federal Insecticide, Fungicide, and Rodenticide Act*) Section 25 (c)(3), that they distribute certain household (pesticide) products in an effective child-resistant packaging. There has been a strong appeal for them to promote more effective senior-friendly packaging of household products, along with more effective safety and use instructions.

For prevention of exposure to food toxicants, again by far the most effective strategy or measure should still be the consumer's self-awareness and self-prevention. This is because in most instances, ultimate prevention of food poisoning or food intoxication is considered more practical and more effective at the individual level than either at the community level or by means of forceful regulatory intervention.

Using the earlier case with POC-contaminated salmons (Section 21.4.1) as an example, the initial step of self-prevention is for the consumer to make every attempt to purchase a younger salmon to eat since compared to an older salmon, a younger one has less lifetime to bioaccumulate the POCs in its body. Prior to cleaning the (younger) fish thoroughly, the consumer should remove its guts, as many POCs tend to concentrate not only in a fish's fat but also in its organs including especially its liver, stomach, and intestines.

Lipophilic substances like POCs are stored primarily in the fatty tissues which are located mainly along the fish's back as well as its belly and dark meat area. The consumer thus should trim the fat, remove the skin, and cut away the fatty dark meat. Skinning the fish will take away the thin layer of fat under the skin. The final step is to cook the fish in a way that would allow getting the fat dripped away or drained off. This last step can be achieved effectively with most cooking methods (e.g., baking, broiling, steaming, grilling). Data gathered by U.S. EPA (2000) showed that up to 60% of the POCs was reduced by the way in which the fish's fat was dripped away or drained off. A subsequent study (Hori *et al.*, 2005), carried out in Japan for fish contents of specifically dioxin and dioxin-like compounds, continued to demonstrate acceptable reductions of POCs at up to 31% by various cooking methods. These lower reduction yields nevertheless might have been due to the different fish species and/or cooking methods employed in the Japanese study.

References

Aiello AE, Larson EL, Levy SB, 2007. Consumer Antibacterial Soaps: Effective or Just Risky? *Clin. Infect. Dis.* 45(Suppl 2):137-147.

Andersen A, 2006. Final Report on the Safety Assessment of Benzaldehyde. *Intl. J. Toxicol.* 25 (Suppl 1): 11-27.

ATSDR (U.S. Agency for Toxic Substances and Disease Registry), 1999. Toxicological Profile for Formaldehyde. U.S. Department of Health and Human Services, Atlanta, Georgia, USA.

ATSDR (U.S. Agency for Toxic Substances and Disease Registry), 2010. Addendum to the Toxicological Profile for Formaldehyde. U.S. Department of Health and Human Services, Atlanta, Georgia, USA.

Biles JE, McNeal TP, Begley TH, 1997. Determination of Bisphenol A Migrating from Epoxy Can Coatings to Infant Formula Liquid Concentrates. *J. Agric. Food Chem.* 45:4697-4700.

Black RE, Hurley FJ, Havery DC, 2001. Occurrence of 1,4-Dioxane in Cosmetic Raw Materials and Finished Cosmetic Products. *J. AOAC Intl.* 84:666-760.

Buth JM, Steen PO, Sueper C, Blumentritt D, Vikesland PJ, Arnold WA, McNeill K, 2010. Dioxin Photoproducts of Triclosan and Its Chlorinated Derivatives in Sediment Cores. *Environ. Sci. Technol.* 44:4545-4551.

Castle L, Jickells SM, Gilbert J, Harrison N, 1990. Migration Testing of Plastics and Microwave-Active Materials for High-Temperature Food-Use Applications. *Food Addit. Contam.* 7:779-796.

CDC (U.S. Centers for Disease Control and Prevention), 2006. Death of a Child after Ingestion of a Metallic Charm – Minnesota, 2006. *MMWR* (CDC Morbidity and Mortality Weekly Report) 23:1-2.

CDC (U.S. Centers for Disease Control and Prevention), 2010. National Report on Human Exposure to Environmental Chemicals – Triclosan. Fact Sheet. U.S. Department of Health and Human Services, Atlanta, Georgia, USA.

CEPA (Canadian Environmental Protection Act of 1999), 2010. Regulatory Impact Analysis Statement (SOR/DORS/2010-194; 13/10/2010). *Canada Gazette* Part II, 144(21):1807-1818.

CIR (Cosmetic Ingredient Review), 1983. Final Report on the Safety Assessment of Sodium Lauryl Sulfate. *J. Amer. College Toxicol.* 2:127-181.

CIR (Cosmetic Ingredient Review), 1999. Final Report on the Safety Assessment of PEG-2, -3, -5, -10, -15, and -20 Cocamine. *Intl. J. Toxicol.* 18:43-50.

Clayton EM, Todd M, Dowd JB, Aiello AE, 2011. The Impact of Bisphenol A and Triclosan on Immune Parameters in the US Population, NHANES 2003-2006. *Environ. Health Perspect.* 119:390-396.

Corpet DE, Parnaud G, Delverdier M, Peiffer G, Tache S, 2000. Consistent and Fast Inhibition of Colon Carcinogenesis by Polyethylene Glycol in Mice and Rats Given Various Carcinogens. *Cancer Res.* 60: 3160-3164.

CPSC (U.S. Consumer Product Safety Commission), 1997. An Update on Formaldehyde, 1997 Revision. Washington DC, USA.

CPSC (U.S. Consumer Product Safety Commission), 2003. National Poison Prevention Week Warns New Parents to Lock Up Medicines and Household Chemicals. Release #03-092. Washington DC, USA.

CPSC (U.S. Consumer Product Safety Commission), 2015. Unintentional Pediatric Poisoning Injury Estimates for 2014 (Memorandum prepared by staff members A. Qin and A. Layton, 18 December 2015). Washington DC, USA.

FAO/WHO (Food Agriculture Organization of the United Nations/World Health Organization), 1994. Food Additives. Codex Alimentarius, Vol. XIV. Rome, Italy.

FDA (U.S. Food and Drug Administration), 1992. Food Additives. FDA/IFIC Brochure: January 1992. Rockville, Maryland, USA.

FDA (U.S. Food and Drug Administration), 1995. Food Additives; Threshold of Regulation for Substances Used in Food-Contact Articles. *Federal Register* 60:36582-36596.

FDA (U.S. Food and Drug Administration), 2010. Update on Bisphenol A for Use in Food Contact Applications: January 2010. Silver Spring, Maryland, USA.

FDA (U.S. Food and Drug Administration), 2015. Final Determination Regarding Partially Hydrogenated Oils. *Federal Register* 80:34650-34760.

FDA (U.S. Food and Drug Administration), 2016. Safety and Effectiveness of Consumer Antiseptics; Topical Antimicrobial Drug Products for Over-the-Counter Human Use. *Federal Register* 81:61106-61130.

Fisher BE, 1998. Scents & Sensitivity. *Environ. Health Perspect.* 106:A594-A599.

FPIN (Fragranced Products Information Network), 2002. Fragrances: The Health Risks. Columbia, Missouri, USA.

Gibson RL, 2007. Toxic Baby Bottles – Scientific Study Finds Leaching Chemicals in Clear Plastic Baby Bottles. Environmental California Research & Policy Center, 3435 Wilshire Boulevard, Suite 385, Los Angeles, California, USA.

Hauser R, Duty S, Godfrey-Bailey L, Calafat AM, 2004. Medications as a Source of Human Exposure to Phthalates. *Environ. Health Perspect.* 112:751-753.

Herlofson BB, Barkvoll P, 1994. Sodium Lauryl Sulfate and Recurrent Aphthous Ulcers: A Preliminary Study. *Acta Odontol. Scand.* 52:257-259.

Hites RA, Foran JA, Carpenter DO, Hamilton MC, Knuth BA, Schwager SJ, 2004. Global Assessment of Organic Contaminants in Farmed Salmon. *Science* 303:226-229.

Hori T, Nakagawa R, Tobiishi K, Iida L, Tsutsumi T, Sasaki K, Toyoda M, 2005. Effects of Cooking on Concentrations of Polychlorinated Dibenzo-p-Dioxins and Related Compounds in Fish and Meat. *J. Agric. Food Chem.* 53:8820-8828.

IARC (International Agency for Research on Cancer), 2012. IARC Monographs on the Evaluation of Carcinogenic Risks to Humans, Volume 100F: Chemical Agents and Related Occupations. Lyon, France: WHO Press.

IARC (International Agency for Research on Cancer), 2017. IARC Monographs on the Evaluation of Carcinogenic Risks to Humans, Volumes 1-119: List of Carcinogens. Lyon, France: WHO Press.

Loraine GA, Pettigrove ME, 2006. Seasonal Variations in Concentrations of Pharmaceuticals and Personal Care Products in Drinking Water and Reclaimed Wastewater in Southern California. *Environ. Sci. Technol.* 40:687-695.

Mehedi N, Ainad-Tabet S, Mokrane N, Addou S, Zaoui C, Kheroua O, Saidi D, 2009. Reproductive Toxicology of Tartrazine (FD and C Yellow No. 5) in Swiss Albino Mice. *Amer. J. Pharmacol. Toxicol.* 4:130-135.

Munguia-Lopez EM, Peralta E, Gonzalez-Leon A, Vargas-Requena C, Soto-Valdez H, 2002. Migration of Bisphenol A (BPA) from Epoxy Can Coatings to Jalapeño Peppers and an Acid Food Stimulant. *J. Agric. Food Chem.* 50:7299-7302.

NRC (U.S. National Research Council), 1999. *The Use of Drugs in Food Animals – Benefits and Risks.* Washington DC, USA: National Academy Press.

NTP (U.S. National Toxicology Program), 1999. Toxicology and Carcinogenesis Studies of Diethanolamine (CAS No. 111-42-2) in F344/N Rats and B6C3F1 Mice (Dermal Studies). Research Triangle Park, North Carolina, USA.

Page BD, Lacroix GM, 1995. The Occurrence of Phthalate Esters and Di-2-Ethylhexyl Adipate Plasticizers in Canadian Packaging and Food Samples in 1985-1989: A Survey. *Food Addit. Contam.* 12:129-151.

Patterson TL, Jeste DV, 1999. The Potential Impact of the Baby-Boom Generation on Substance Abuse among Elderly Persons. *Psychiatr. Serv.* 50:1184-1188.

Pop A, Berce C, Bolfa P, Nagy A, Catoi C, Dumitrescu I-B, Silaghi-Dumitrescu LA, Loghin F, 2013. Evaluation of the Possible Endocrine Disruptive Effect of Butylated Hydroxyanisole, Butylated Hydroxytoluene and Propyl Gallate in Immature Female Rats. *Farmacia* 61:202-211.

Scallan E, Hoekstra RM, Angulo FJ, Tauxe RV, Widdowson MA, Roy SL, Jones JL, Griffin PM, 2011. Foodborne Illness Acquired in the United States – Major Pathogens. *Emerg. Infect. Dis.* 17:7-15.

Servos MR, Smith M, Mcinnis R, Burnison BK, Lee B-H, Seto P, Backus S, 2007. The Presence of Selected Pharmaceuticals and the Antimicrobial Triclosan in Drinking Water in Ontario, Canada. *Water Quality Res. J. Canada* 42:130-137.

Steinemann A, 2016. Fragranced Consumer Products: Exposures and Effects from Emissions. *Air Qual. Atmos. Health* 9:861-866.

U.S. EPA (U.S. Environmental Protection Agency), 1989. Report to Congress on Indoor Air Quality, Volume II: Assessment and Control of Indoor Air Pollution. EPA 400-1-89-001C. Office of Air and Radiation, Washington DC, USA.

U.S. EPA (U.S. Environmental Protection Agency), 2000. Guidance for Assessing Chemical Contaminant Data for Use in Fish Advisories: Volume 2. Risk Assessment and Fish Consumption Limits – Third Edition. EPA 823-B-00-008. Office of Water, Washington DC, USA.

U.S. EPA (U.S. Environmental Protection Agency), 2015. Indoor Air Pollution: An Introduction for Health Professionals. Washington DC, USA (downloadable PDF version, webpage last updated 28 September 2015). http://www.epa.gov/iaq/pubs/hpguide.html (retrieved 18 July 2017).

VanArsdale JL, Leiker RD, Kohn M, Merritt TA, Horowitz BZ, 2004. Lead Poisoning from a Toy Necklace. *Pediatrics* 114:1096-1099.

Veldhoen N, Skirrow RC, Osachoff H, Wigmore H, Clapson DJ, Gunderson MP, Van Aggelen G, Helbing CC, 2006. The Bactericidal Agent Triclosan Modulates Thyroid Hormone-Associated Gene Expression and Disrupts Postembryonic Anuran Development. *Aquatic Toxicol.* 80:217-227.

Vorhees CV, Butcher RE, Brunner RL, Wootten V, Sobotka TJ, 1983. Developmental Toxicity and Psychotoxicity of FD and C Red Dye No. 40 (Allura Red AC) in Rats. *Toxicology* 28:207-217.

Wada H, Tarumi H, Imazato S, Narimatsu M, Ebisu S, 2004. In Vitro Estrogenicity of Resin Composites. *J. Dent. Res.* 83:222-226.

Review Questions

1. Briefly explain the major health concerns with toxic household substances.
2. Briefly explain the major health concerns with food toxicants.
3. What are the general source categories of food toxicants?
4. Are substances on the GRAS list required to undergo premarket approval by FDA? And if yes, why? And if no, why not?
5. Match *each* of the characteristics, sources, or effects in the right column to *only one* of the food additives in the left column that are potentially harmful when consumed excessively.

    (1) vitamin D   (a) substance for wholesomeness
    (2) lecithin   (b) on the GRAS list
    (3) BHA   (c) substance for product consistency
    (4) tartrazine   (d) flavoring agent
    (5) vitamin C   (e) from plastic
    (6) polyethylene terephthalate (f) antioxidant
    (7) monosodium glutamate   (g) food colorant

6. Briefly describe FDA's four criteria set forth in its Threshold of Regulation program for use to determine the threshold of no appreciable human health risk (from exposure to indirect food additives).
7. Name four indirect food additives commonly found in paper materials used for packaging or holding food products.
8. Name four polymers commonly found as indirect food additives.
9. Name the six major categories of drugs commonly used to treat food animals.

10. Which group of food contaminants has one of the serious consequences in terms of agroeconomics and public health? And why?
11. Name four neurotoxins commonly found in seafood worldwide.
12. What are the general source categories of toxic household substances?
13. Name six potential toxic ingredients commonly found in personal care products.
14. What are the OTC antihistamines mostly used for? And what are their common side effects?
15. Which of the following pairs includes the two most common examples of potentially toxic cleaning agents? a) dishwasher detergents, toilet bowl cleaners; b) oven cleaners, air fresheners; c) toilet bowl cleaners, laundry detergents; d) laundry detergents, oven cleaners.
16. What are the four BTEX organic solvents commonly found in gasoline?
17. Give five use groups of pesticide products that are commonly found in many (American) homes.
18. What appears to be the understated or underrated concern with the use of OTC medicines?
19. What may be a major side effect when a person takes pain relievers containing acetaminophen as the active ingredient (e.g., in Tylenol®), along with excessive (daily) consumption of alcohol over a long period?
20. What illness or symptom would acute lead poisoning at its first stage be likely misdiagnosed with?
21. Are farmed salmons across the various countries more likely to be contaminated with POCs, compared to their wild counterparts? Give a (scientific) justification for the answer.
22. What are the potential problems or concerns with using the antimicrobial agent triclosan?
23. For exposure to food toxicants or toxic household substances, what type or form of mitigation and prevention measures appears to be most effective or practical?
24. What are the basic steps that can be taken to minimize the dietary exposure to POC residues (suspected as) present in a fish?

CHAPTER 22

Human Health Aspects of Ecotoxicology

ॐ•ॐ

22.1. Introduction

Despite the argument given in Chapter 1 that environmental toxicology and ecotoxicology are two separate branches of toxicology, they do have certain things in common. There are numerous aspects of ecotoxicology that have strong implications for human health. In this chapter, such strong implications from several aspects in three subdivisions of ecotoxicology are discussed in their individual sections that follow shortly. Each of the three sections also includes the subdivision's general practice and development with the aim to provide the basics for a fuller appreciation of its health implications. The three select subdivisions are *aquatic toxicology, wildlife toxicology*, and *hazardous waste toxicology*. These three subdivisions are deemed most relevant to environmental toxicology owing to their strong implications for environmental health. The pertinence and significance of the three subdivisions to environmental toxicology as well as to human health are highlighted first in the rest of this Introduction section as a prelude. It is intended and hoped that with the highlights and discussions so presented, this chapter can help bridge the pathway leading to a better appreciation of the key aspects shared by the two branches of toxicology.

22.1.1. Relevance of Aquatic Toxicology

In its simplest term, aquatic toxicology is concerned with adverse effects of toxicants on aquatic organisms and on the ecosystem where these biota inhabit. This subdivision of ecotoxicology thus has a focus on water contamination and its ecological impacts. Topics and issues covered in aquatic toxicology in general are similar to those in the toxicology for humans or other non-aquatic species. Accordingly, they include: the fate and transport of aquatic pollutants; the disposition, including toxicodynamics and toxicokinetics, of environmental toxicants in aquatic organisms; the assessment and modeling of the effects of aquatic pollution on aquatic biota; and the analysis of risks to aquatic ecosystems. As for any other types of ecosystems or species of living organisms, the effects of toxicants on aquatic organisms may range from those at the biochemical, molecular, and cellular level to those at the individual and population or species level.

With respect to human health, a major contribution from aquatic toxicology is the relatively simple toxicity tests developed over the years to assure high quality of water for drinking and other uses (Section 22.2.2). Water quality assurance is crucial for supply of healthy seafood to consumers. In the United States, the annual seafood consumption recently has reached 14.5 pounds per capita, which is about 9% of the per capita in Hong Kong or 3.5% of that worldwide (NMFS, 2015). Moreover, by applying the results from these various aquatic toxicity tests, several health regulatory achievements have been made in the United States and worldwide (Section 22.2.3).

22.1.2. Relevance of Wildlife Toxicology

For wildlife toxicology, the scope and focus are similar to those of aquatic toxicology, except with the wildlife species being broadened to include all undomesticated organisms. Wildlife toxicology therefore covers topics similar to those covered by aquatic toxicology, except for its focus being more on non-aquatic species. Pollution of concern in wildlife toxicology tends to be terrestrial in nature not only due to the already plentiful terrestrial species to deal with, but also due to the notion that water pollution is by practice already covered adequately in aquatic toxicology and to some extent also in environmental toxicology.

Although perhaps not as commonly utilized as aquatic toxicology, wildlife toxicology tends to offer a more conceivable real-life situation for human health than would any other form of non-human models on chemical exposure or toxicity analysis. It has been argued that *in situ* exposures of pesticides to indicator species under semi-controlled, real-life conditions would offer a more realistic evaluation of effects by linking laboratory studies to observed conditions in the field (Grue *et al.*, 1982; Steffeck, 1994). Yet it seems unfortunate that much desire for investigation into the adverse effects of environmental contaminants in real-life situations is disregarded just because this type of studies is exceptionally cumbersome and time-consuming to carry out with any due rigor (McBee and Lochmiller, 1996). Otherwise, as McBee and Lochmiller (1996) put it, field studies on wildlife and their ecosystems would offer far greater human health implications than much of the efforts would that have gone into similar analyses with laboratory models.

22.1.3. Relevance of Hazardous Waste Toxicology

Hazardous waste is defined as any *discarded* material harmful or potentially harmful to humans or the environment. It can be a cleaning agent, fuel product, pesticide, or by-product of an industrial process. Hazardous waste thus can be in the form of a gas, liquid, solid, or sludge. The levels of various toxic wastes have been on the rise for many years, amidst the public's rising concern that individuals and industries continue to ignore this major global environmental pollution issue. Many residents and industries simply do not make a true effort to reduce the generation of hazardous waste materials or to mitigate their environmental impacts.

The reality is that many consumers tend to get rid of stuff without realizing that these waste materials would end up in a landfill or a dumpsite, and that through evaporation or leaching they could eventually come back to the residents as well as to the local or even global environment. Industries likewise often want to lower the high costs for the disposal of their hazardous and other wastes. Accordingly, they prefer to have their waste materials either removed by another party at the lowest cost possible or buried in landfills that they have built on site.

In any event, thousands of persistent toxic metals and chemicals can be found in hazardous waste materials. These substances can be harmful or even lethal when absorbed or ingested. When hazardous waste is landfilled, the contaminated liquid may leach and pollute groundwater used for human consumption. The human health implications are therefore much more apparent and direct with hazardous waste toxicology or waste pollution than with the other two subdivisions. In the United States, the Love Canal disaster is one of the most appalling environmental tragedies in the nation's history, and is regarded as the most tragic environmental disaster in the nation's history of toxic site contamination. That infamous tragedy involved the burial and subsequent discovery of some 20,000 tons of toxic waste beneath the neighborhood of Love Canal located near Niagara Falls, New York. As noted in Chapter 2, some 80 different substances were contained in that pile of toxic waste, of which a handful were already known or suspected as human carcinogens.

22.2. Aquatic Toxicology and Human Health

As defined more specifically in some literature (e.g., Rand and Petrocelli, 1985; Rand *et al.*, 1995), aquatic toxicology is the qualitative as well as quantitative study of the adverse effects of contaminants on aquatic organisms. The toxic effects of concern involve lethality and sublethal toxicity. Examples of sublethal toxicity include adverse modifications in development, growth, reproduction, behavior, toxic response, and the related biochemical, physiological, or pathological functions. These detrimental effects may be expressed by quantifiable criteria such as number of organisms affected, percent of eggs hatched, percent of enzyme inhibition, change in body weight or length, incidence in skeletal abnormalities, and incidence in tumor development. In short, these adverse effects and their expressions are similar in principle to those observed and analyzed for wildlife and human health. Aquatic toxicology is also concerned with the concentrations and quantities of toxicants that occur or will occur in aquatic systems. Accordingly, the field necessarily includes the study of transport, distribution, biotransformation, and ultimate fate of contaminants in the aquatic environment. A historical account of aquatic toxicology can be found in the chapter by Nikinmaa (2014) or the paper by Pritchard (1993).

22.2.1. The Basic Aquatic Environment

Some knowledge about the characteristics of the particular ecological niche which a specific aquatic species occupies in its environment is a prerequisite to studying aquatic toxicology (or to wildlife toxicology in general). Such knowledge should begin with some understanding of the world's (aquatic) biomes, defined as the Earth's major (aquatic) communities classified according to the predominant plants and animal species that have adapted to exist in.

The aquatic environment is complex and diverse. The two principal types of aquatic ecosystems are marine and freshwater, each with its own kind of biomes. Within each of these biomes, many different biotic (living) and abiotic (nonliving) components co-subsist.

Marine biomes, and hence their ecosystems as well, each consist of largely the open ocean, coral reefs, and estuaries. They each also include salt marshes, lagoons, mangroves, the deep sea, and many other components, though most of which receiving comparatively less academic emphasis and interest. Collectively, these components cover roughly 70% of the Earth's surface (e.g., Crowe *et al.*, 2015), provide over 97% of its water (e.g., UNEP, 2002), and generate about 45% of its net primary production (e.g., Geider *et al.*, 2001). The ocean region, which is the largest section of a marine biome, can be subdivided into separate zones including *oceanic* (the relatively shallow part of the ocean that lies over the continental shelf), *intertidal* (the area where the ocean meets the land), *pelagic* (where the water in the open ocean is farther from the land), *benthic* (the part below the pelagic zone), and *abyssal* (the ocean bottom). Coral reefs are regarded as the rainforests of an ocean in that corals consist of predominately algae (e.g., zooxanthellae) which via photosynthesis provide a huge supply of the basic nutrients and energy for other marine lives in the food web. Estuaries are areas where freshwater streams or rivers merge with the ocean. This mixing of waters with different salt and mineral contents offers a unique aquatic ecosystem to support a highly diverse fauna, including a variety of oysters, turtles, fishes, and waterfowls.

The marine biome is home to a myriad of numerous various species ranging from microscopic planktonic organisms (e.g., phytoplankton and zooplankton), which comprise the base of the marine food chains, to large marine mammals such as whales, dolphins, and seals. Thousands of fish species reside in this biome, including angelfish, eel, flounder, mackerel, scup, seabass, squid, and thousands more. Coastal birds are likewise plentiful, including gulls, loons, pelicans, shorebirds, terns, and hundreds or thousands more. Marine ecosystems are distinct from freshwater ecosystems due to the presence of different amounts and types of dissolved materials, especially salts, in the water and accordingly the different types of aquatic species. Over 80% of the dissolved materials in seawater are sodium (Na) and chlorine (Cl) molecules.

Freshwater ecosystems collectively cover less than 1% of the Earth's surface (e.g., Likens, 1973), provide about 0.01% of its water supply or about 2.5% of its water in the form of permanent ice or snow (e.g., UNEP, 2002), and generate a negligible amount of its net primary production compared to the marine and terrestrial ecosystems (e.g., Geider *et al.*, 2001). The freshwater biome is likewise home to thousands of the Earth's known fish species. There are three basic subtypes of freshwater biomes or ecosystems: *lentic* (with slowly-moving water, including ponds and lakes); *lotic* (with rapidly-moving water, including streams and rivers); and *wetlands* (where the soil is inundated for at least part of the time).

In both kinds of biomes, the biotic components consist of myriads of microorganisms, plants, and animals co-inhabiting particular niches. Also co-subsisting within each niche are abiotic components, which include the physical environment (e.g., water flow, temperature, salinity). Each aquatic niche thus represents a dynamic set of complex interactions of biotic and abiotic components. The biological activities of contaminants and their impacts can be affected profoundly by such complex compositions and dynamic interactions within each niche.

The complex, dynamic, and highly interactive nature of aquatic ecosystems makes it difficult for any study to analyze the toxic responses of these systems unless the underlying interactions have been defined and understood to some extent. As Rand and Petrocelli (1985) put it, such an analysis is (further) complicated by the various adaptability and the species diversity of the biotic components in aquatic ecosystems, as well as by the substantial variations in structural and functional responses among the biotic components.

22.2.2. Aquatic Toxicity Tests

To study the adverse responses involved in aquatic ecosystems, certain toxicity tests need to be performed. These toxicity tests are analytical tools used to quantify the toxicant amount and the exposure duration required to yield a critical or criterion effect. Due to substantial species difference, toxicity tests employed in aquatic toxicology necessarily differ from those developed for wildlife or human health.

Algae, macroinvertebrates (e.g., clams, shrimp, oysters), and fishes are the three main groups of test organisms commonly employed in aquatic toxicity tests to represent the wide range of freshwater and saltwater species that would be studied. The treated and untreated aquatic organisms can be exposed to the test water solutions and the untreated water (respectively) in a laboratory and sometimes in a field setting, by applying one or more of the four basic testing techniques (e.g., Rand and Petrocelli, 1985; Rand et al., 1995) listed below:

- *Static test* – This assay involves the use of *still* water where the test organisms are (and where the controls are not) exposed to the test material for a fixed duration.

- *Re-circulation test* – In this assay, the test and control solutions are pumped or filtered through an apparatus to uphold the water quality and the concentration of the test material; it is similar to the static test in all other aspects.

- *Renewal test* – This assay is also similar to the static test assay in all aspects except for the test and control solutions being renewed periodically (typically every 24 hours) by removing the test and control organisms into chambers filled with new test and control solutions.

- *Flow-through test* – In this assay, the test and the control solution flow into and out of their respective chambers housing the test subjects and the controls. The flow-through cycle can be continuous or intermittent.

In keeping with a sound application of the above aquatic toxicity testing techniques, protocols have been standardized by a number of public and non-profit organizations. These include the American Public Health Association, the American Society for Testing and Materials, U.S. EPA, the International Standardization Organization, and the Organization for Economic Cooperation and Development. The testing protocols that these organizations have standardized may be categorized according to the length of exposure and the organisms to be tested. Aquatic toxicity tests thus may be separated into those with fishes, macroinvertebrates, and phytoplankton (e.g., Rand and Petrocelli, 1985; Rand et al., 1995). With phytoplankton, the test assay is typically for a one-time event. With macroinvertebrates (e.g., *Daphnia sp.*, *Acartia sp.*, *Mysidopsis sp.*, oysters, crabs), the test assay is typically for acute or long-term exposure. With fishes, the various toxicity tests employed are typically for bioaccumulation potential as well as for acute, early-life stage, partial chronic, or complete chronic exposure. A graphic example of the early-life stage test in fish is given in Figure 22.1. Note that the test exposure period for the newborn fish in an early-life stage test is species-dependent, as per testing guidelines set forth by U.S. EPA (1996).

The testing protocols and techniques highlighted above have been utilized to establish the water quality criteria (WQC) recommended by U.S. EPA for some 100 water contaminants. Pursuant to Section 304 of the U.S. Clean Water Act, the WQC are updated periodically by U.S. EPA (2015) to provide guidance for states, tribes, and even other nations to apply for water quality standards. Note that these protocols and techniques have been utilized to establish not only the WQC kind for human health but also the criteria and standards for aquatic or other biological life.

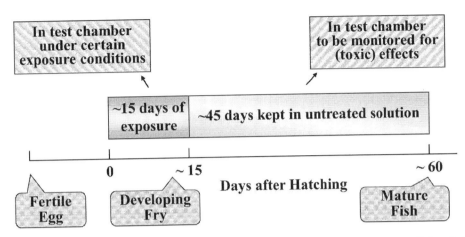

Figure 22.1. A Schematic of Early-Life Stage Aquatic Toxicity Test on Zebrafish

22.2.3. Regulatory Efforts for Water Quality

It is not surprising that in certain places such as near industrial discharges, water pollution can degrade ground or surface water quality so drastically that the water there is no longer safe for drinking, swimming, crop irrigation, and other water-borne activities. In the United States, this kind of health concerns has led to several regulatory efforts made to protect water quality for the public, in addition to the establishment of WQC. In particular, under the authority of the U.S. Clean Water Act, U.S. EPA has established the *National Pollutant Discharge Elimination System* (NPDES) permit program, which mitigates water pollution by regulating point sources that discharge contaminants directly into aquatic systems. Point sources of pollution are defined as discrete conveyances, such as pipes or human-made ditches. In most cases, the NPDES permit program is administered by authorized states. Since its inception in 1972, the NPDES permit program has contributed many significant improvements to the nation's water quality.

Another related regulatory establishment that U.S. EPA is likewise obligated to implement is the *Total Maximum Daily Load* (TMDL) program, which aims to attain ambient water quality standards through the control of both point and non-point sources of pollution. Although the TMDL program also originated from the U.S. Clean Water Act, it was largely overlooked during the 1970s and early 1980s. The overlook was largely due to the circumstance that in those years the states were very busy bringing point sources of pollution into compliance under the NPDES permit program. Several citizen lawsuits were launched in the 1980s to eventually direct U.S. EPA into developing guidance for the TMDL program, which is now regarded as equally effective in achieving the nation's water quality goals.

22.3. Wildlife Toxicology and Human Health

Wildlife toxicology has its root in the late 1800s, when ingestion of spent lead pellets from hunting was first noticed as a mortality factor in waterfowls (e.g., Calvert, 1876; Holland, 1882). Over the years, the field has evolved from numerous pollution-related tragedies and episodes that undermined human health. In the United States, earlier forms of wildlife toxicology arose by many of the concerns raised on pesticide toxicity from the 1950s to 1960s, including those publicized in the then widely read *Silent Spring* (Carson, 1962). Recently, the nation's concerns with wildlife toxicology have expanded to include critically imperiled species (e.g., bison, wild pigeon) from extinction, as protected under the Endangered Species Act of 1973, and the devastating effects of oil pollution, as evidenced from passage of the Oil Pollution Act in 1990.

The world has encountered numerous major oil spills over the past 50 some years, including the Deepwater Horizon BP Oil Spill in the Gulf of Mexico in 2010 and the equally largest, devastating Gulf War Oil Spill in Persian Gulf back in 1991. For the United States, it has estimated (U.S. EPA, 2017) that between 10 to 25 million gallons of oil are spilled into the environment each year, an estimate presumably including the amount from the annual incidences of 2,700 to 6,000 spills documented under the U.S. Coast Guard's jurisdiction (CRS, 2017). Due to these spills, birds and other small wildlife species are often found getting killed in oily sludges and liquids. Such small creatures can get trapped by oil tank leaks, oil tank loading spills, and soils contaminated with oily liquids, frequently to the extent that they will ultimately die from suffocation. Incubating embryos too can be killed by oil transferred to eggs via the mother bird's contaminated feathers. Under the Resource Conservation & Recovery Act (RCRA) of 1976, U.S. EPA has the federal authority to force the cleanup by the responsible party for this form of soil contaminations.

While studies are still sparse concerning the health problems among the general public and among workers engaging in the cleanups, there is certainly a potential for human hazard from oil spills. The pressing issue involved is that some substances contained in crude oil have been found highly toxic to human health, such as benzene which is a known human carcinogen (Chapter 13) and mercury which is highly toxic to the human central nervous system (Chapter 14).

22.3.1. Scope and History of Wildlife Toxicology

There are tremendous difficulties in studying wildlife toxicity, as many as those encountered in studying aquatic toxicity if not more. These difficulties revolve around the enormous complexities in determining the various key variables in play: definition of wildlife; species interactions; species responses; environmental components in wildlife ecosystems; and sources of stressors. It is also a difficult task in dealing with a huge diversity of species in wildlife ecosystems. Regardless, both the scope and the history of wildlife toxicology warrant further discussion here, as there is a misconception that human health implications are less relevant from wildlife toxicology than from the other two subdivisions of ecotoxicology covered in this chapter.

It should be pointed out here that the issues raised in *Silent Spring* concerning the health impacts of pesticides on the environment became not only the centerpiece of today's environmental health movement but also the momentum that helped launch the Wildlife Toxicology Working Group, a functional unit of The Wildlife Society (TWS). Since its foundation in 1937, TWS has maintained a mission to foster greater awareness and understanding of the adverse effects of environmental contaminants on wildlife. TWS is a non-profit, international professional association with a commitment to excellence in wildlife stewardship through science and education. Many past and current issues highly relevant to wildlife toxicology have been reflected in the numerous various presentations given in each year's workshops and special sessions sponsored by TWS.

Two case examples that come to mind are the utilization of feathers as temporal bioindicators of PCB (polychlorinated biphenyl) exposure in Clapper Rails (Summers *et al.*, 2008), and the application of coastal birds as bioindicators of plastic marine debris (Nevins *et al.*, 2009).

Special concerns and interests in wildlife toxicology can also be reflected in research programs sponsored by other organizations. Three cases in point are the three related studies sponsored by the Contaminant Biology Program at the U.S. Geological Survey. As a series, these three studies (Johnson *et al.*, 2009; Rattner *et al.*, 2004; Toschik *et al.*, 2005) assessed the contaminant exposure and potential reproductive effects in ospreys nesting in three separate localities in the United States. Other similar program studies included the investigation into: the effects of sublethal dietary methylmercury exposure on American kestrels (Albers *et al.*, 2007); the levels of toxic metal and organochlorine pesticide residues in the eggs of wading birds at the Salton Sea (Henny *et al.*, 2008); and the effects of PAHs (polycyclic aromatic hydrocarbons) on marine birds, mammals, and reptiles (Albers and Loughlin, 2003).

Meanwhile, since a decade or two ago, the levels of brominated flame retardants like HBCD (hexabromocyclododecane) and PBDEs (polybrominated diphenyl ethers) in bird eggs reportedly have doubled every few years. More specifically, in his review paper addressing the history of wildlife toxicology, Rattner (2009) postulated that the field had been driven considerably and inevitably by such pollution-related tragedies and events compromising human health. The reviewer further proposed that current challenges should embrace the desire to assess more thoroughly the toxic effects of chemical-related human activities on both the wildlife and their supporting habitat. Such current challenges are by and large consistent with the perspectives on and the future trends of the field wildlife toxicology reflected in the book by Kendall *et al.* (2010) and in the review article by Kendall (2016). In particular, the Kendall article points out that *"Wildlife toxicology now has more access to sophisticated technologies than were available 30 years ago, when the field really began to emerge as a dynamic area of toxicology research."*

22.3.2. The Basic Wildlife Terrestrial Environment

The terrestrial environment where a particular non-aquatic wildlife species inhabits is similar to the aquatic environment in principle, but different in scope and content. In both cases, the biotic and abiotic components within their niches interrelate as well as interact constantly to form a biophysical habitat (i.e., ecosystem) in dynamic equilibrium with its inputs and surroundings. In that sense, ecosystems tend to support higher biodiversity than what the human urban environments would, inasmuch as ecosystems involve greater numbers of plant and animal species.

In addition to the aquatic systems made up of essentially oceans and freshwater bodies, wildlife ecosystems take into account a number of undomesticated terrestrial environments. For environmental toxicologists, the various terrestrial environments may be subsumed under five broad geographic categories as follows (e.g., Daugherty, 1998):

- *Tundra* or *Arctic plain* – This region (biome) covers much of the Earth's surface north of the coniferous forest belt. It refers to an area where the tree growth is retarded by extremely cold temperatures.

- *Taiga* – This biome is a vast belt of coniferous forests consisting mostly of larches, pines, and spruces, extending in a broad band across North America, Europe, and Asia to the southern border of the arctic tundra.

- *Desert* – This is a region receiving very little precipitation (e.g., <10 inches or 25.4 centimeters of annual rainfall), typically with a high average temperature.

- *Chaparral* – This is a shrub or heathland plant biome dominated by evergreen type vegetation with small leaves. The region has a Mediterranean-like climate of a wet, warm winter and a dry, long summer.

- *Forests* – These are subregions each having a high density of trees and other woody vegetation. Collectively, they have occupied an extensive portion of the Earth's terrestrial surface.

In more specific terms, a tundra region has extremely cold climate with dead organic materials for energy and nutrients. It has short seasons for growth and reproduction, low or limited drainage, simple vegetation structure, low biodiversity, as well as large population fluctuations.

Taiga is the world's *largest* terrestrial biome covering most of inland Alaska, Canada, Finland, Sweden, and parts of the northern continental United States. The region has a harsh continental climate with young and nutrient-poor soils. It is home to a number of large herbivorous mammals and small-size rodents.

In contrast, chaparral is the world's *smallest* terrestrial biome found in a small bit of most continents. Its weather is mild and moist in the winter, and dry and hot in the summer. With this type of weather, some of the plant species grown in this region are likely French broom, Lebanon cedar, blue oak, and olive tree. The animal inhabitants are largely grassland and desert types that can adapt to hot and dry weather, such as jackrabbits, mule deer, coyotes, horned toads, alligator lizards, and ladybugs.

In spite of the notorious hot and dry weather that deserts are known for, many still have fairly impressive quantities of specialized vegetation, vertebrates, and invertebrates. There are expectedly fewer large mammals found in the deserts because most large-size animals are not capable of withstanding the heat or storing sufficient water in their body. The desert biome can be separated into four general subtypes based on various meteorological and geographic features involved: *cold deserts*; *hot and dry deserts*; *semi-arid deserts*; and *coastal deserts*. Examples of cold deserts are those found in Greenland, Antarctic, and the Nearctic realm, with jackrabbits, kangaroo rats, and grasshoppers being some of the dominant inhabitants. Examples of hot and dry deserts include those located in the southern Asian realm, Australia, Ethiopia (Africa), Neotropical region (South and Central America), and the United States (e.g., Sonoran, Mojave), with burrowers and kangaroo rats being the dominant animals. Some of the semi-arid deserts are located in the United States, Newfoundland, Russia, Europe, and northern Asia, with skunks, lizards, grasshoppers, kangaroo rats, and snakes being some of the dominant inhabitants. For coastal deserts, some of them can be found in the Atacama of Chile and the Neotropical realm, with golden eagles, lizards, snakes, and amphibians being some of the dominant animals.

For forests, they can be classified into at least six general subtypes according to the major kinds of climates and tree species present: *temperate coniferous*; *temperate deciduous*; *sparse trees and parkland area*; *tropical moist*; *tropical dry*; and *forest plantations*. In all cases, the wildlife and the forests where they inhabit are linked closely together. Forests harbor much of the planet's biodiversity by providing it with abundant and crucial natural resources from timber to medicinal plants. In the recent decades, forests have occupied approximately one-third of all land areas on the Earth (Schmidt and Harbert, 2004).

In some literature (e.g., Urry *et al.*, 2017) or for certain interests, grassland is also considered as one of the major terrestrial biomes, with its predominant vegetation naturally consisting of grasses (and some shrubs). Grassland biome has been further divided into savanna biome (that scattered with shrubs and isolated trees) and temperate grassland biome (that with almost no trees or large shrubs). In any event, the world's biomes, large or small and aquatic or terrestrial, have changed their ecological characteristics numerous times since there was life on the planet, partly as a result of human activities.

22.3.3. Ecological Risk Assessment

Any in-depth characterization of a contaminant's adverse effects on wildlife requires more than an understanding of the (terrestrial) environment involved. It necessitates some form of ecological risk assessment, which is a tool as well as a construct used to develop, organize, and provide scientific information relevant to decisions given for the ecological impacts under assessment. The first influential reference on this type of impact assessment process was seemingly the guidance document *Framework for Ecological Risk Assessment* published by U.S. EPA (1992). This guidance document was updated in the agency's *Guidelines for Ecological Risk Assessment* published six years later (U.S. EPA, 1998). The two versions of the U.S EPA framework remained essentially the same, although the specific assessment steps involved were somewhat different due to subsequent refinement. In both framework documents, the emphasis was on wildlife being the ecological entities of concern.

The assessment framework developed by U.S. EPA was largely an outgrowth of the human health-based risk assessment paradigm introduced in Chapter 1 and revisited more extensively in the next, final chapter. U.S. EPA's framework focuses on the evaluation of pollution impacts on wildlife (including fishes and plants) and their ecosystems, not on human health. During the 1980s, the framework emerged as a prominent tool to guide policy and regulatory decision-making on ecological impacts. Its application progressed rather slowly throughout the 1980s, as evident from the slow-paced regulations of certain pesticides (e.g., diazinon, malathion) concerning potential impacts on bird populations. Despite such a slow progression, the framework has gained a fair amount of global acceptance (e.g., UNEP/IPCS, 1999) since its second release.

The ecological risk approach is distinct from the approach used for assessing human health risk mainly in three specific aspects of its emphases. First, the ecological risk approach may consider adverse effects (i.e., assessment endpoints) beyond the individual or species level to the level of an entire community or ecosystem, despite the fact that data on ecological effects are generally more limited compared to those on human health endpoints. Second, the ecological values (i.e., entities and ecosystem characteristics) to be protected or upheld are selected from a wider range of possibilities based on scientific and policy concerns. Third, an ecological risk assessment may consider the effects of stressors (e.g., chemical, biological, or physical agents) on the ecological environment, not just on the wildlife species of concern (U.S. EPA, 1998). Accordingly, some knowledge of comparative physiology on wildlife along with the unique habitats for them becomes beneficial and useful, as more than one wildlife species niched in its own ecosystem is likely involved in most any ecological risk assessment. To this end, the *Wildlife Exposure Factors Handbook* published by U.S. EPA (1993) can serve as a quick and handy reference. In that handbook, exposure profiles are provided for select (representative) species of birds, mammals, amphibians, reptiles, and more, along with a brief characterization of their natural histories and ecosystems.

U.S. EPA's framework as well as process for ecological risk assessment involves four basic analytical steps or components: (1) problem formulation; (2) exposure analysis; (3) effects analysis; and (4) risk characterization. In practice, the four steps are intended to be carried out in three phases, as depicted in Figure 22.2, with exposure analysis and effects analysis being performed in tandem through frequent exchange of information between the two analytical components.

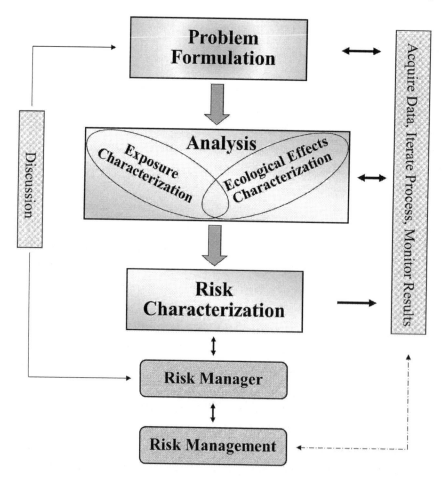

Figure 22.2. General Framework and Process for Ecological Risk Assessment
(*modified from public domain image Figure 1 in U.S. EPA [1992]*)

The framework's *problem formulation* phase involves the tasks of defining assessment goals, selecting endpoints, proposing a conceptual model, and developing an analysis plan. Assessment endpoints are each supposedly an explicit expression of the ecological values (e.g., species, ecological resource, habitat type) to be protected or preserved. These endpoints are only considered useful if they can define the ecological entity and attributes of the entity to be protected or preserved (e.g., reproductive success, age-class structure). The conceptual model describes a series of risk hypotheses used to test how the exposures to stressors may be related to the assessment endpoints. The analysis plan entails a delineation of the assessment design, measures, methods, and data needs for performing the analysis phase of the risk assessment.

The overall (combined) *analysis* phase engages in the generation of profiles used to characterize the exposure of ecological receptors (e.g., certain wildlife species) to stressors (e.g., pollutants) and the relationships between stressor levels and ecological effects. In *exposure* analysis, the modes or mechanisms of contact between stressor(s) and receptor(s) are characterized; and the magnitude as well as the frequency of contact is assessed. For many ecological risk assessments, exposure characterization includes a spatially-explicit type evaluation, for which some knowledge of the wildlife terrestrial environment is essential. In *effects* characterization, the adverse effects of stressors on receptors are determined, usually based on such endpoints as toxicity thresholds or exposure-response relationships. The output of effects characterization is a quantitative estimate of the severity of the harm that might occur. This part (subphase) of the entire analysis step is similar in task to the toxicity analysis phase for human health discussed in Chapter 23.

Risk characterization is the final phase of the ecological risk assessment, in which the effects and exposure analyses are integrated to obtain a *risk* estimate for making decisions on the ecological impacts assessed. This phase should also include assessment of the uncertainty and confidence in the results, the ecological significance of any risk estimated, and the data needs for future assessment. Ecological (as well as human health) risk is technically defined as the probability of an adverse effect on the receptor. In practice, it may be expressed in a number of ways from a simple scientific judgment to a more concrete estimate such as a *hazard quotient*. A simple hazard quotient may be estimated and interpreted as depicted in Box 22.1. Note that the effect concentration or effect dose (e.g., LD_{50}, LC_{50}, RfD) is frequently adjusted downward for the appropriate uncertainty and safety factors added due to data sparsity, interspecies variation, and such. And the site-specific exposure to the stressor is a concentration or dose typically estimated using a set of conservative assumptions to likewise err on the side of ecological protection.

The close relationship between human health and ecological risk assessments has become more apparent since the World Health Organization (IPCS, 2001) developed a perspective for performing risk analyses that should integrate the two assessment frameworks. The WHO perspective was founded on the notion that many national and international entities expressed a need or an urge for a holistic approach to risk analysis capable of addressing real life complex exposure situations, in which multi-chemicals, multi-media, multi-routes, and multi-species are inevitably involved. Supports for such a holistic approach have since emerged in numerous places, such as in the journal *Human and Ecological Risk Assessment*, in the book with a similar title edited by Paustenbach (2002), in the journal paper by Suter *et al.* (2005) on integration of the two frameworks, and in a number of risk assessment projects carried out by the U.S. Department of Agriculture (e.g., USDA, 2006) as well as by its contractors (e.g., SERA, 2008) that have entailed the two frameworks.

Box 22.1. Simplified Computation and Interpretation of Hazard Quotient as Devised for Ecological Risk Assessment

$$\text{Hazard Quotient} = \frac{\text{Exposure Concentration (or Dose)}}{\text{Effect Concentration (or Dose)}}$$

Hazard Quotient	Occurrence of Effect (Risk)
> 1	high
~ 1	potential
< 1	low

22.4. Hazardous Wastes of U.S. and Global Concerns

As introduced earlier, hazardous waste is any *discarded* material harmful to human health or the environment when improperly disposed of. Materials of this kind are generated from many sources such as consumer products, industrial processes (e.g., electroplating, petroleum refining), and small business entities which are in greater numbers (e.g., dry cleaners, automobile repair shops, exterminators). Hazardous waste pollution, along with water pollution and air pollution, is regarded as among the most serious environmental health problems affecting the planet today. In the United States, each year the nation generates over 40 million tons of hazardous waste. Many European nations including Spain, Scotland, and England are also major generators of hazardous waste. They are dumping substantial amounts of their trash in landfills which are already near their full capacity. In particular, 10.2 million tons of waste materials were generated in 2014 in Scotland, of which 4.3 million tons were disposed of (SEPA, 2017a). Yet less than 20% of the 313 disposal sites registered in Scotland were operational during the same year (SEPA, 2017b).

The global concerns on hazardous waste pollution actually have reached a high point for some time, likely since the 1992 ratification of the global treaty nicknamed the Basel Convention. The official name of this treaty is *Basel Convention on the Control and Transboundary Movements of Hazardous Wastes and Their Disposal*, which is regarded as the most comprehensive global environmental treaty on toxic and other wastes. This Convention, having over 170 parties, aims to protect human health and the environment against those harmful effects resulting from the generation, management, transboundary movements, and disposal of various (types of) hazardous wastes.

In the United States, hazardous waste pollution is regulated by a number of federal legislations including the Comprehensive Environmental Response, Compensation, & Liability Act (CERCLA) of 1980, the RCRA of 1976, the Toxic Substances Control Act of 1976, and a number of environmental health regulations pertaining to water or air quality. Both the RCRA and its close legislative cousin CERCLA are directed specifically toward toxic waste pollution and are thus further discussed below with the aim to exemplify the complexities involved across the world.

22.4.1. The RCRA Definition and Implications

In the United States, federal regulations of various (types of) hazardous wastes began with the Solid Waste Disposal Act of 1965, which was amended in 1976 to become what is now known as RCRA (Resource Conservation & Recovery Act). The main contribution of RCRA is its mandate that the generating and operating facilities create a "cradle to grave" system of recordkeeping for all relevant hazardous wastes. In this recordkeeping system, all relevant hazardous wastes need to be tracked from the onset of their generation until their final disposition; that is, the system calls for monitoring every aspect of every relevant waste material's fate and transport over its life cycle. As empowered by the act, U.S. EPA has established a list of more than 500 specific types or species of hazardous wastes. Currently, the agency coordinates closely with business entities and the state as well as local authorities for strategies and programs that can ensure the proper treatment and disposal of the various waste materials specified on the RCRA list.

Under RCRA, which can be found in Title 40 of the *U.S. Code of Federal Regulations* (40 *CFR*) Parts 260 through 280, a discarded material must first be a *solid* waste to qualify as hazardous. The various specific types of RCRA hazardous wastes are thereby subcategories of solid waste. As misleading as the term might seem to be, a solid waste by RCRA's definition can be a liquid or gas as it only needs to be *tangible*. Then for an RCRA waste to be treated as *hazardous*, it must be one that is classifiable as a "listed" or a "characteristics" waste. A characteristics waste is one that exhibits one or more of the following characteristics factors: *ignitability* (e.g., a flammable liquid or gas); *corrosivity* (e.g., a strong acid or alkali); *reactivity* (e.g., a strong oxidizing agent); and *toxicity* (e.g., a pesticide with low LD_{50}). In contrast, a listed waste is one that by default is treated as hazardous owing to its generation by a certain common or specific industry or process. This type is based on solely the process or industry generating it, irrespective of any of the above characteristics factors that the waste may or may not possess. Examples of U.S. EPA's listed hazardous wastes include: certain sludge leftovers from electroplating processes; certain wastes from steel and iron manufacturing; solvent wastes from certain cleaning or degreasing processes; and certain discarded pesticides or pharmaceutical products in a *used* form.

The *listed* hazardous wastes determined by U.S. EPA, as authorized by RCRA of 1976, are organized into four specific (sub)lists under three source categories as follows:

- *The F-list (nonspecific source wastes)* – This group includes wastes from *common* industrial or manufacturing processes such as cleaning or degreasing operations. Because these processes are not specific to any particular sector of industry, wastes on this list are also called "*nonspecific source wastes*". Wastes included on the F-list can be found in the regulations at 40 *CFR* §261.31. Examples of this type include spent degreasing solvents such as tetrachloroethylene (PCE) and trichloroethylene (TCE).

- *The K-list (source-specific wastes)* – This group includes wastes generated from *specific* industries or processes. As such, they are also commonly referred to as "*source-specific wastes*". Wastes included on this list can be found in the regulations at 40 *CFR* §261.32. To be qualified as a K-list waste, the waste must be generated from one of the following industries or sources: organic chemicals; petroleum refining; wood preservation; pesticides; veterinary pharmaceuticals; inorganic chemicals; coking; ink formulation; inorganic pigments; secondary lead; iron and steel; primary aluminum; and explosives. As an example, wastewater treatment sludge from the production of zinc yellow pigments is qualified as a K-list waste generated from the inorganic pigment industry. Another example is distillation bottoms from the production of acetaldehyde (C_2H_4O) with another organic such as ethylene (C_2H_4), which is qualified as from the organic chemical industry.

- *The P-list and the U-list (discarded commercial chemical products)* – These two sub-lists include specific *discarded* commercial chemical products in an *unused* form, and are hence also known as "*discarded commercial chemical products*". Wastes on the "P" (sub)list are knowingly fatal or irreversibly damaging to humans and animals at low doses. Those on the "U" list pose a lesser hazard to humans or the environment when improperly handled. Pesticides and pharmaceuticals are included on both of these lists. Wastes included in this category can be found in the regulations at 40 *CFR* §261.33. Specific examples include aldicarb, parathion, and nitric oxide on the P-list, and acetone, diethylstilbestrol (DES), formaldehyde, and Kepone on the U-list.

In addition to the characteristics and listed wastes, The RCRA of 1976 authorizes U.S. EPA to regulate a fourth source categorized as "universal wastes". This category currently includes pesticides, batteries, mercury-containing equipment (e.g., thermostat) and mercury lamps, that all have been *used*. The regulations (at 40 *CFR* §273) set for this fourth category are directed toward explicitly the retail stores, certain commercial sectors, and implicitly household consumers.

22.4.2. The Superfund Law and Program

CERCLA (Comprehensive Environmental Response, Compensation, & Liability Act) was enacted in 1980 in the United States initially to address the appalling tragedy of Love Canal. It authorizes U.S. EPA to compel responsible parties to clean up the toxic waste sites and, where a responsible party cannot be located, to clean up the site on the agency's own effort using a special trust fund now nicknamed "Superfund". CERCLA is hence commonly known as the Superfund law or program. Prior to the passage of this act, toxic wastes were disposed of in regular landfills until there was evidence showing that the hazardous materials in the landfills could or would seep deep into the ground either to contaminate the soils occupied atop by animals and crops or to reach down the water table to make groundwater there unsafe to consume.

In a nutshell, RCRA and CERCLA both deal specifically with hazardous waste pollution in the United States. Their main difference lies in the release source that they are responsible for. RCRA protects the nation's human health and the environment by setting out a comprehensive regulatory framework for investigating and addressing releases of hazardous wastes at *present* and in some cases *future* storage, treatment, and disposal facilities. In contrast, CERCLA protects the nation's human health and the environment by establishing a similar regulatory framework for investigating and remediating uncontrolled releases of hazardous substances, but at *past* facilities instead. CERCLA has two distinct provisions for the federal government: (1) a tax on the petroleum and chemical industries as sources for the trust fund (i.e., Superfund); and (2) broad federal authority to respond directly to actual or threatened releases of toxic substances at past facilities that may endanger the nation's human health or the environment. The Superfund law (i.e., CERCLA) further authorizes U.S. EPA to take the two types of response actions listed below:

- *Short-term removals* – Regulatory actions of this type should be carried out to address actual or threatened releases of toxic wastes requiring *prompt* response.

- *Long-term remedial responses* – Regulatory actions of this type involve permanent or significant remedial reduction of the hazards associated with the (threat of) releases of toxic wastes that are deemed serious, but not immediately life-threatening. This type of regulatory actions may be implemented only at toxic sites already included on U.S. EPA's National Priorities List (NPL).

Both types of response actions listed above may take place at the same Superfund toxic site, as evident in the case study presented in the next subsection. This case study, as briefly introduced in Section 4.2.3C and serving to illustrate the complexities involved, is concerned with the uncontrolled releases of pesticide residues at the United Heckathorn (UH) Superfund toxic site.

22.4.3. The United Heckathorn Toxic Site (A Case Study)

The UH Superfund toxic site experience is selected as the case study in part because it is a relatively recent toxic site disaster and in part because the cleanup involves many years of endurance. In line with its general theme, this subsection has its focus primarily on activities and events occurring at the site that are deemed pertinent to the Superfund response actions or to the health implications involved.

The UH Superfund toxic site is located in Richmond Harbor, Contra Costa County, California (Figure 22.3). The harbor is in an industrial area dominated by petroleum and shipping terminals. The toxic site was a place used to formulate and package pesticides from 1947 to 1966, and now becomes a major source of DDT and other pesticide wastes contaminating the San Francisco Bay estuary partly bounded by and south(west) of the harbor. In March 1982, the UH site was designated as a state hazardous waste site due to the high levels of pesticide contamination found in its soils. As authorized under CERCLA, U.S. EPA placed the toxic site on its NPL in March 1990, and five months later took over the investigation and cleanup commitments from California.

444 An Introduction to Environmental Toxicology

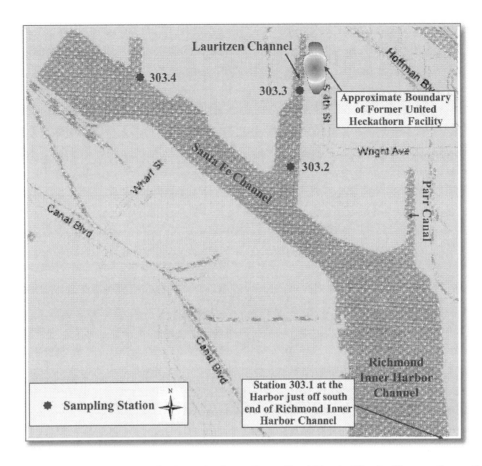

Figure 22.3. Location of the United Heckathorn Superfund Toxic Site in Contra Costa County, California, USA (*map image per se from maps.google.com*)

Chronologically and more specifically, from 1947 through 1966 the toxic site was used for formulating and packaging pesticides by UH and four other minor operators, with DDT accounting for approximately 95% of all pesticides handled on that site at that time. Buildings on the site were demolished from 1966 through 1970. Between 1970 and 1980, the UH site was utilized primarily for bulk storage. In 1981, Levin Metals Corp purchased the property for use as bulk shipping facilities.

U.S. EPA's efforts in cleaning up the UH Superfund toxic site proceeded in two technical steps followed by three phases of investigation on release source. During the 1980s and the early 1990s, U.S. EPA and the state of California, together with the new property owner, removed more than 3,500 cubic yards of the most highly contaminated soils, or the so-called "hot spots", from the UH toxic site. The actual sediment remediation did not begin until 1996, three years after completion of the *immediate* removal actions of cleaning up the hot spots.

The cleanup activity ended in 1997 after dredging the Lauritzen Channel and the Parr Canal, which are located at the harbor's north end (Figure 22.3). Approximately 107,000 tons of sediments were removed from the waterways to designated disposal facilities. Afterwards, soil samples were collected in the area to confirm the remedial results and efforts.

Step II involved setting up a drainage system to collect the potentially contaminated surface runoff, as well as capping approximately 4.5 acres of land to prevent erosion and exposure to residual levels of pesticides in the soils. The capping was achieved by a concrete cover shielding over the area where the pesticide processing facilities had been located. The capping construction began in July 1998 and ended a year later.

After completion of the cleanup activity in July 1997, U.S. EPA began monitoring the pesticide residues in the marine waters nearby. Water samples and mussels were collected in each monitoring year for analysis of pesticide levels. Mussels were the test organisms used to account for the amounts of pesticides bioaccumulating in the living organisms. According to the second Five-Year Review Report (U.S. EPA, 2006), the 2001 monitoring data continued to show unacceptable levels of DDT and dieldrin in sediments around an area excavated in the 1990s. The 2001 results (Table 22.1) triggered U.S. EPA to undertake further investigations to supplement data gaps as well as to determine the potential extent and sources of recontamination of the site. The series of investigations involved a Phase I Source Investigation in 2001, a Phase II Source Investigation in 2002, and a Phase III Fluid Mud/Water Quality Investigation in 2004 (U.S. EPA, 2006).

Table 22.1. Summary of Post-Remediation Concentrations (ng/L) of ΣDDTs and Dieldrin in Water Samples from around the United Heckathorn Superfund Toxic Site[a]

Location[b]	Pre-Remediation	Post-Remediation					
		1998 (Yr 1)	1999 (Yr 2)	2000 (Yr 3)	2001 (Yr 4)	2002 (Yr 5)	2003 (Yr 6)
ΣDDTs							
Richmond	1	0.65	14.4	2.56	0.06	0.66	0.52
Lauritzen/Mouth	NS	42.6	4.61	27.9	2.88	1.70	0.65
Lauritzen/End	50	103	62.3	1,773A	142	18.4	396
Santa Fe/End	8.6	11	19.2	3.70	2.51	0.60	0.67
Parr Canal	NS	NS	NS	NS	NS	2.57	1.8
Seep Outfall	NS	NS	NS	NS	NS	4,455	8,990
Dieldrin							
Richmond	<1	0.65	0.62	1.57	0.08	0.16	0.21
Lauritzen/Mouth	NS	8.18	0.48	8.96	0.46	0.43	0.22
Lauritzen/End	18	18	12.5	625A	8.49	2.08	15
Santa Fe/End	1.8	2.47	0.37	2.11	0.46	0.20	0.17
Parr Canal	NS	NS	NS	NS	NS	0.98	0.88
Seep Outfall	NS	NS	NS	NS	NS	2,520	3,000

[a] modified and adapted from Table 6.1 in the second Five-Year Review Report prepared by U.S. EPA (2006); the remediation goals were 0.59 and 0.14 ng/L, respectively, for the organochlorine pesticides ΣDDTs (i.e., total including all the various isomers of dichlorodiphenyltrichloroethane and of its metabolites) and dieldrin; A ≡ averaged over all replicates (including an outlier replicate); NS ≡ not sampled; Yr ≡ year (of post-remediation).

[b] Richmond ≡ Richmond Inner Harbor (Station 303.1, just off the south end of Richmond Inner Harbor Channel, see Figure 22.3); Lauritzen/End ≡ around the end of Lauritzen Channel (Station 303.3); Lauritzen/Mouth ≡ around the mouth of Lauritzen Channel (Station 303.2); Santa Fe/End ≡ around the end of Santa Fe Channel (Station 303.4); Seep Outfall ≡ a broken concrete outfall, located around and north of Station 303.3.

It should be pointed out that for cleanups of Superfund toxic sites in the United States, a five-year review of the efforts is mandated by statute first within five years of the remedial action and then every five years thereafter to ensure that the levels of hazardous wastes are below the remediation goals (i.e., levels allowing for unlimited exposure). In summer 2008, U.S. EPA specifically collected fish samples of various species (including California halibut, starry flounder, anchovy, and walleyed perch) with the aim to supplement and update the baseline information for human health and ecological risk assessments. The highest tissue residue levels found in the fish samples were in those caught around the north end of Lauritzen Channel, ranging from 28 to 11,000 µg/kg for ΣDDTs and 10 to 550 µg/kg for dieldrin (U.S. EPA, 2008). The third and the fourth Five-Year Review Report for the UH toxic site were released on 21 September 2011 and 8 August 2016 (respectively). Their overall findings (U.S. EPA, 2011, 2016) were similar, both pointing to the conclusion that the levels of total DDTs measured in the sediment, water, and fish tissue samples from the Lauritzen Channel marine area remained high enough to pose a potential exposure risk to the local community and the environment within the vicinity.

References

Albers PH, Loughlin TR, 2003. Effects of PAHs on Marine Birds, Mammals and Reptiles. In *PAHs: An Ecotoxicological Perspective* (Douben PET, Ed.). West Sussex, England: John Wiley & Sons, Chapter 13.

Albers PH, Koterba MT, Rossmann R, Link WA, French JB, Bennett RS, Bauer WC, 2007. Effects of Methylmercury on Reproduction in American Kestrels. *Environ. Toxicol. Chem.* 26:1856-1866.

Calvert HS, 1876. Pheasants Poisoned by Swallowing Shot. *The Field* 47:189.

Carson LR, 1962. *Silent Spring*. Boston, Massachusetts, USA: Houghton Mifflin.

Crowe T, Austen M, Frid C, 2015. Introduction. In *Marine Ecosystems – Human Impacts on Biodiversity, Functioning and Services* (Crowe T, Frid CLJ, Eds.). Cambridge, UK: Oxford University Press, Chapter 1.

Daugherty J, 1998. *Assessment of Chemical Exposures: Calculation Methods for Environmental Professionals*. Boca Raton, Florida, USA: Lewis Publishers, Chapter 5.

Geider RJ, DeLucia EH, Falkowski PG, Finzi AC, Grime JP, Grace J, Kana TM, LaRoche J, Long SP, Osborne BA, *et al.*, 2001. Primary Productivity of Planet Earth: Biological Determinants and Physical Constraints in Terrestrial and Aquatic Habitats. *Global Change Biol.* 7:849-882.

Grue CE, Powell GVN, Gorsuch CH, 1982. Assessing Effects of Organophosphates on Songbirds: Comparison of a Captive and a Free-Living Population. *J. Wildlife Magnt.* 46:766-768.

Henny CJ, Anderson T, Crayon J, 2008. Organochlorine Pesticides, Polychlorinated Biphenyls, Metals, and Trace Elements in Waterbird Eggs, Salton Sea, California, 2004. *Hydrobiologia* 604:137-149.

Holland G, 1882. Pheasant Poisoning by Swallowing Shot. *The Field* 59:232.

IPCS (International Programme on Chemical Safety), 2001. Integrated Risk Assessment. WHO/IPCS/IRA/01/12. IPCS, World Health Organization, Geneva, Switzerland.

Johnson BL, Henny CJ, Kaiser JL, Davis JW, Schulz EP, 2009. Assessment of Contaminant Exposure and Effects on Ospreys Nesting along the Lower Duwamish River, Washington, 2006-07. U.S. Geological Survey Open-File Report 2009-1255. U.S. Geological Survey, Reston, Virginia, USA.

Kendall RJ, 2016. Wildlife Toxicology: Where We Have Been and Where We Are Going. *Environ. Anal. Toxicol.* 6:348 (online journal).

Kendall RJ, Lacher TE, Cobb GC, Cox SB (Eds.), 2010. *Wildlife Toxicology: Emerging Contaminant and Biodiversity Issues*. Boca Raton, Florida, USA: CRC Press.

Likens GE, 1973. Primary Production: Freshwater Ecosystems. *Hum. Ecol.* 1:347-356.

McBee K, Lochmiller RL, 1996. Wildlife Toxicology in Biomonitoring and Bioremediation: Implications for Human Health. In *Ecotoxicity and Human Health: A Biological Approach to Environmental Remediation* (de Serres FJ, Bloom AD, Eds.). Boca Raton, Florida, USA: CRC Press, Chapter 6.

Nevins H, Donnelly E, Hester M, Hyrenbach D, 2009. Seabirds as Bioindicators of Plastic Marine Debris. Session 22 (Symposium): Diseases and Toxicants Affecting Marine Wildlife: Causes, Conflicts, Solutions. The Wildlife Society 16th Annual Conference, Monterey, California, USA, 20-24 September.

Nikinmaa M, 2014. *An Introduction to Aquatic Toxicology*, 1st Edition. Cambridge, Massachusetts, USA: Academic Press (Elsevier), Chapter 1.

NMFS (U.S. National Marine Fisheries Service), 2015. Fisheries of the United States, 2014. U.S. Department of Commerce, NOAA Current Fishery Statistics No. 2014. NMFS, National Oceanic and Atmospheric Administration, Silver Spring, Maryland, USA.

NRS (U.S. Congressional Research Service), 2017. Oil Spills: Background and Governance (reported by J. L. Ramseur, dated 15 September). CRS Report for Congress RL33705. Library of Congress, Washington DC, USA.

Paustenbach DJ (Ed.), 2002. *Human and Ecological Risk Assessment: Theory and Practice*. New York, New York, USA: John Wiley & Sons.

Pritchard JB, 1993. Aquatic Toxicology: Past, Present, and Prospects. *Environ. Health Perspect.* 100:249-257.

Rand GM, Petrocelli SR, 1985. Introduction. In *Fundamentals of Aquatic Toxicology: Methods and Applications* (Rand GM, Petrocelli SR, Eds.). Washington DC, USA: Hemisphere Publishing, Chapter 1.

Rand GM, Wells PG, McCarty LS, 1995. Introduction to Aquatic Toxicology. In *Fundamentals of Aquatic Toxicology: Effects, Environmental Fate, and Risk Assessment* (Rand GM, Ed.), 2nd Edition. Philadelphia, Pennsylvania, USA: Taylor & Francis, Chapter 1.

Rattner BA, 2009. History of Wildlife Toxicology. *Ecotoxicology* 18:773-783.

Rattner BA, McGowan PC, Golden NH, Hatfield JS, Toschik PC, Lukei RF Jr, Hale RC, Schmitz-Afonso I, Rice CP, 2004. Contaminant Exposure and Reproductive Success of Ospreys (*Pandion haliaetus*) Nesting in Chesapeake Bay Regions of Concern. *Arch. Environ. Contam. Toxicol.* 47:126-140.

Schmidt V, Harbert W, 2004. Planet Earth and the New Geoscience. Pittsburgh, Pennsylvania, USA: Metropolitan Pittsburgh Public Broadcasting, Unit 16.

SEPA (Scottish Environmental Protection Agency), 2017a. Waste Data for Scotland – Waste from All Sources Summary Document and Commentary Text, 2014 (waste data available in PDF file). https://www.sepa.org.uk/environment/waste/waste-data/waste-data-reporting/waste-data-for-scotland/ (retrieved 9 July 2017).

SEPA (Scottish Environmental Protection Agency), 2017b. List of Landfill Sites and Capacities in Scotland, 2014 (site list data available in Microsoft Excel® spreadsheets). https://www.sepa.org.uk/environment/waste/waste-data/waste-data-reporting/waste-site-information/waste-sites-and-capacity-excel/ (retrieved 9 July 2017).

SERA (Syracuse Environmental Risk Assessment), 2008. Malathion Human Health and Ecological Risk Assessment (Final Report). SERA TR-052-02-02c. USDA Forest Service Contract: AG-3187-C-06-0010. SERA, 5100 Highbridge Street, 42C, Fayetteville, New York, USA.

Steffeck DW, 1994. The Role of Monitoring in Assessing Pesticide Effects on Avian Species and Their Habitats. In *Wildlife Toxicology and Modeling: Integrative Studies of Agroecosystems* (Kendall RJ, Lacher TE, Jr, Eds.). Boca Raton, Florida, USA: CRC Press, Chapter 28.

Summers JW, Gaines KF, Garvin N, Mills GL, 2008. The Use of Feathers as Temporal Bioindicators of PCB Exposure in Clapper Rails. The Wildlife Society 15th Annual Conference, Miami, Florida, USA, 8-12 November.

Suter GW 2nd, Vermeire T, Munns WR Jr, Sekizawa J, 2005. An Integrated Framework for Health and Ecological Risk Assessment. *Toxicol. Appl. Pharmacol.* 207(Suppl):611-616.

Toschik PC, Rattner BA, McGowan PC, Christman MC, Carter DB, Hale RC, Matson CW, Ottinger MA, 2005. Effects of Contaminant Exposure on Reproductive Success of Ospreys (*Pandion haliaetus*) Nesting in Delaware River and Bay, USA. *Environ. Toxicol. Chem.* 24:617-628.

UNEP (United Nations Environment Programme), 2002. *Global Environment Outlook 3: Past, Present, and Future Perspectives.* London, UK: Earthscan Publications.

UNEP/IPCS (United Nations Environment Programme/International Programme on Chemical Safety), 1999. Training Module No. 3: Chemical Risk Assessment – Human Risk Assessment, Environmental Risk Assessment and Ecological Risk Assessment. WHO/PCS/99.2. Geneva, Switzerland.

Urry LA, Cain ML, Wasserman SA, Minorsky PV, Reece JB, 2017. *Campbell Biology*, 11th Edition. London, UK: Pearson, Chapter 52.

USDA (U.S. Department of Agriculture), 2006. 2,4-D Human Health and Ecological Risk Assessment (Final Report). US Forest Service, Arlington, Virginia, USA.

U.S. EPA (U.S. Environmental Protection Agency), 1992. Framework for Ecological Risk Assessment. EPA/630/R-92/001. Risk Forum, Washington DC, USA.

U.S. EPA (U.S. Environmental Protection Agency), 1993. Wildlife Exposure Factors Handbook. EPA/600/R-93/187. Office of Research and Development, Washington DC, USA.

U.S. EPA (U.S. Environmental Protection Agency), 1996. Ecological Effects Test Guidelines: OPPTS 850.1400 – Fish Early-Life Stage Toxicity Test. EPA 712-C-96-121. Office of Prevention, Pesticides, and Toxic Substances, Washington DC, USA.

U.S. EPA (U.S. Environmental Protection Agency), 1998. Guidelines for Ecological Risk Assessment. *Federal Register* 63:26846-26924.

U.S. EPA (U.S. Environmental Protection Agency), 2006. Second Five-Year Review Report for United Heckathorn Superfund Site, Richmond, California. Contract No. 68-W-98-225/WA No. 214-FRFE-09R3. U.S. EPA Region 9, San Francisco, California, USA.

U.S. EPA (U.S. Environmental Protection Agency), 2008. Summary of Fish Tissue Sampling and Analysis, United Heckathorn Superfund Site, Richmond, California, May – June, 2008. Project No. 340138.FI.02. U.S. EPA Region 9, San Francisco, California, USA.

U.S. EPA (U.S. Environmental Protection Agency), 2011. Third Five-Year Review Report for United Heckathorn Superfund Site, Richmond, California. Contract No. EP-S9-08-04/WA No. 214-FRFE-09R3. U.S. EPA Region 9, San Francisco, California, USA.

U.S. EPA (U.S. Environmental Protection Agency), 2015. Final Updated Ambient Water Quality Criteria for the Protection of Human Health. *Federal Register* 80:36986-36989.

U.S. EPA (U.S. Environmental Protection Agency), 2016. Fourth Five-Year Review Report for United Heckathorn Superfund Site, Richmond, Contra Costa County, California (prepared by the U.S. Army Corps of Engineers). U.S. EPA Region 9, San Francisco, California, USA.

U.S. EPA (U.S. Environmental Protection Agency), 2017. Oil Spills Research (webpage updated 18 September 2017). https://www.epa.gov/land-research/oil-spill-research (retrieved 23 November 2017).

Review Questions

1. Briefly highlight the relevance of aquatic toxicology, of wildlife toxicology, and of hazardous waste toxicology to human health.
2. Name the two largest oil spills in the world's history. And briefly explain how oil spills in general are harmful to wildlife.
3. What are the two main types of aquatic environment? And briefly explain why coral reefs are regarded as the rainforests of an ocean region.
4. Which of the following aquatic toxicity test types requires the filtration of both the control and the test solution through an apparatus to maintain the water quality and the concentration of the test material? a) static; b) re-circulation; c) renewal; d) flow-through.
5. Name and give one example for *each* of the three basic types of freshwater ecosystems.
6. In a *typical* early-life stage test, how long should the newborn fish be exposed to a test material? a) 5 days; b) 10 days; c) 15 days; d) species-dependent; e) for the entire study period.
7. What are the main differences between U.S. EPA's NPDES (National Pollutant Discharge Elimination System) permit program and the agency's TMDL (Total Maximum Daily Load) program?
8. Which of the following pairs includes both the largest and the smallest type of terrestrial biomes in the world? a) tundra and chaparral; b) desert and forest; c) taiga and tundra; d) taiga and chaparral; e) desert and chaparral.
9. In what ways was (still is) Carson's *Silent Spring* relevant to the mission and functions of The Wildlife Society's Wildlife Toxicology Working Group?
10. Which of the following wildlife species is *not* specifically mentioned in this chapter in relation to wildlife toxicology issues? a) kestrels; b) clapper rails; c) loons; d) ospreys.
11. Name three animal species that can adapt to the climate in a chaparral, and three that can adapt to the climate in a coastal desert.
12. What are the four general analytical components included in a typical ecological risk assessment? And why in practice they are intended to be carried out in three phases?
13. Briefly describe the *analysis* phase included as a key step in a typical ecological risk assessment. And how is it relevant to the *risk characterization* phase?
14. Define the terms *conceptual model*, *stressor*, *receptor*, and *assessment endpoint*, as used in the U.S. EPA framework for ecological risk assessment.
15. Give the general algorithm for deriving a simple hazard quotient (HQ). And what would be the risk implication if this calculated HQ were close to unity (e.g., 0.95 or 1.03)?
16. Which of the following is regarded as the most comprehensive global environmental agreement on hazardous and other wastes? a) Basel Convention; b) Stockholm Convention; c) Vienna Convention; d) Montreal Convention.
17. What are the main differences between the two U.S. hazardous waste pollution legislations *RCRA of 1976* and *CERCLA of 1980*, in terms of their regulatory jurisdictions and authorities?
18. Briefly describe the distinction between short-term removal actions and long-term remedial responses that U.S. EPA may carry out as authorized under Superfund.

19. Match each example of hazardous waste given in the left column to the specific type in the right column that the waste belongs to, as classified by U.S. EPA.

    (1) unused DES (diethylstilbestrol)   (a) the P-list
    (2) unused parathion   (b) the U-list
    (3) used TCE (trichloroethylene)   (c) universal wastes
    (4) acetaldehyde-based distillation bottoms (d) the F-list
    (5) used batteries   (e) the K-list

20. Which of the following was the United Heckathorn Superfund toxic site used for in 1981? a) packaging of pesticides; b) bulk shipping facilities; c) bulk storage; d) bulk fishery facilities.

21. Briefly describe the two technical steps used in cleaning up the United Heckathorn Superfund toxic site during the 1990s.

22. Which of the following were used in 2001 or 2008 as test organisms in monitoring the tissue levels of dieldrin and total DDTs around the United Heckathorn Superfund toxic site? a) oysters, mussels; b) oysters, fish; c) clams, shrimp; d) mussels, fish.

23. In which years were the three phases of investigation on release source carried out by U.S. EPA for the United Heckathorn Superfund toxic site?

24. Which specific location at or around the United Heckathorn Superfund toxic site had the highest water concentrations of dieldrin and total DDTs measured in 2002?

25. What and where was the highest fish tissue concentration of total DDTs measured around the United Heckathorn Superfund toxic site in 2008?

CHAPTER 23

Environmental Health Risk Assessment

23.1. Introduction

More than three decades ago, U.S. National Research Council (NRC, 1983) published a human health-based risk assessment paradigm which now has become a classic framework referenced or applied by many regulatory entities. Since the publication of this framework, numerous volumes of textbooks, guidance documents, and other reference materials have been written to extend or advocate its application. One volume noteworthy is the training manual *Chemical Risk Assessment* prepared jointly by the United Nations Environment Programme and the International Programme on Chemical Safety (UNEP/IPCS, 1999). This manual represents the joint effort by the two organizations in advancing the three separate frameworks that they have advocated for *human* risk assessment, *environmental* risk assessment, and *ecological* risk assessment.

The UNEP/IPCS framework for *human* risk assessment includes an analytical component focusing on workers, consumers, and the general public exposed to environmental pollutants as the receptors of concern. That framework is largely comparable to those adopted by many other entities for human health-based risk assessment, including the several by U.S. EPA (1986, 1991, 1996, 1998a, 2005) and the exceptional one with detailed guidelines by Environmental Health Australia (EHA, 2012). Nonetheless, the exposure analysis component in the UNEP/IPCS framework for *environmental* risk assessment has a somewhat confusing or overlapping theme not easy to follow. That framework considers not only the exposures of humans and other mammals from drinking water polluted by chemical substances, but also those of aquatic organisms to the pollutants in surface waters. Given that the exposures of people and aquatic organisms to water pollutants can be covered in the human and the ecological risk assessment, respectively, the UNEP/IPCS framework for environmental risk assessment may not have a focus as specific as should be.

Amidst the confusion led to by UNEP/IPCS, *environmental health* risk assessment is synonymous with *human health* risk assessment within the realm of environmental toxicology, at least in terms of principle and process. The former is used as this chapter's title and implicit throughout this book largely because it has a nicer ring to environmental toxicology. Regardless, to ease the writing in this chapter, much of the time either term has been shortened to *health risk assessment*.

23.1.1. Health Risk Assessment Activities

A reality with (environmental) health risk assessment is that its framework and activities are not only subject to social values and public concerns. And in practice, its activities tend to be carried out in fragments at some government levels or within some nongovernment organizations, inasmuch as most of these entities have limited resources and special agenda. It is due to this kind of fragmentation that environmental toxicology, environmental epidemiology, and other relevant sciences (e.g., public health) cannot always play a more important role in health risk assessment to promote public or environmental health.

Yet in spite of such hurdles, many health risk assessment activities continue to expand substantially and are performed in many places everywhere every day, especially by government health agencies in the advanced countries. For simplicity, these assessment activities can be subsumed under four major (health) risk categories as follows.

The first category involves those health risks that rely on either an individual's self-initiative or a health organization's effort for exposure prevention and mitigation, rather than on some government interventions. In the United States, this type is considered and assessed mostly by the U.S. Department of Health and Human Services, by its National Institutes of Health, and by its Centers for Disease Control and Prevention (CDC). A familiar case analysis under this health risk category is CDC's health risk assessment or analysis for the tampon-toxic shock syndrome and its episode reported in 1980 (Section 3.2).

The second category deals with those health risks subject to regulatory control and mitigation of exposure. This type is mostly associated with environmental pollution and product use. As implicit in Figure 1.1 and noted by Thongsinthusak and Dong (2010), although exposure mitigation is a crucial component of health risk *management*, the necessity of its implementation is contingent on the outcomes of a health risk assessment performed under a structured framework. In the United States, health risks under this category are assessed mostly by U.S. EPA. Other government regulatory agencies under this category include FDA (U.S. Food and Drug Administration) and CPSC (U.S. Consumer Product Safety Commission). In terms of health risk assessment activities, CPSC has been less involved in federal efforts to regulate toxic substances, in part due to its small size and limited operating budget. Yet owing to the unique provisions contained in the older version of the Federal Hazardous Substances Act, CPSC is among the forefronts in providing criteria for toxicity tests, especially those related to acute toxicity in animals (e.g., the primary irritation assay in rabbits). Otherwise, CPSC obtains much of its health risk assessment information from other sources, including predominantly U.S. EPA and FDA.

The third category differs from the second above only in that the health risks involved are those due to exposures occurring in workplaces. In the United States, health risks in this category are regulated by OSHA (U.S. Occupational Safety and Health Administration). OSHA's most controversial health and safety standards have been exposure limits for hazards present in workplaces. In its early years, OSHA rejected the use of health risk assessment for occupational carcinogens and other toxic agents under the presumption that its statute would not permit the use of such a quantitative process. However, one key impetus to the adoption of health risk assessment as a decision-making tool by all the U.S. federal health regulatory agencies today (i.e., including OSHA) was the U.S. Supreme Court's decision on the OSHA standard for worker exposure to benzene (NRC, 1994). That court decision argued for some form of health risk assessment as a prelude to the determination whether a health risk is high enough to merit regulatory action.

The fourth category includes all environmental-relevant health risks generated or aggravated by the so-termed (mostly economic) development policies and programs (DPP), particularly in or for the developing regions. DPP can be broadly subsumed under five subgroups leading to five different sources for potential adverse impacts: (1) agricultural growth and food supply; (2) macroeconomic growth; (3) energy; (4) housing; and (5) industrialization. Health risk assessment's connection with DPP, unlike with public health, is more subtle but at times equally relevant and forceful. One general step included in an environmental health impact assessment (EHIA), which is an integral part of most if not all of the DPP-associated actions and activities, is the analysis of potential health and environmental impacts. It is for this analysis step that some form of health risk assessment is required to complete an EHIA for many of these development projects.

In the United States, the Affordable Care Act was passed in 2010 with the basic intent to reduce the number of American people without health insurance. In that sense, the goal as well as the intent of that federal healthcare act is at least for more Americans to have access to healthcare and thereby partially related to the nation's economic growth. The act mandates that a health risk assessment be included in analyzing the annual wellness visit benefit authorized for Medicare beneficiaries (i.e., those adults aged 65 or older receiving benefits under the federal health insurance program). In response to this mandate, CDC (2011a) has provided policymakers, researchers, and the general stakeholders with an evidence-informed framework for patient-centered health risk assessments. A health risk assessment framework of this type has yet to be fully comprehended first, a reservation well reflected in the public comments and insights compiled by CDC (2011b) for the framework's development. In essence, this type of health risk assessment either should have a risk category on its own, as for lack of its full appreciation, or for convenience sake may be subsumed under DPP's subgroup of macroeconomic growth.

23.1.2. Subtle Aspects of Health Risk Assessment

In many ways and particularly in concept and principle, the basic analytical process of ecological impact (or risk) assessment discussed in Section 22.3.3 is similar to the one involved with the health-based paradigm. As briefly introduced in Chapter 1 without much discussion, and depicted schematically below in Figure 23.1, four key analytical components are also inherent in NRC's human health-based risk assessment paradigm. In the present and final chapter, further elaborations are given on these four components in an attempt to bring the book to a closure, with the aim as well as intent to integrate as many as practical the concepts and issues presented in the other chapters.

As a prelude to the elaborations, one subtlety worth reminding here is that health risk characterization, as reflected in Figure 23.1, is the final phase in the health risk assessment paradigm. Literally, this phase is the final analytical step in which the potential health risk of concern is assessed as well as *characterized*, utilizing all the relevant information gathered from hazard identification, dose-response assessment, and human exposure assessment. Given that a health risk cannot be characterized until it has been *assessed* at least qualitatively, health risk assessment as a *quantitation* process or task, instead of being treated as a framework, construct, or discipline, can be regarded as a subpart of health risk characterization.

Another subtlety noteworthy here is that over two decades ago, NRC (1994) revised its initial paradigm to (attempt to) combine hazard identification and dose-response assessment into a single phase termed *toxicity assessment* or *analysis* (Figure 23.1). NRC based its revision on the notion that the data and tasks required for the two uniting phases are practically inseparable.

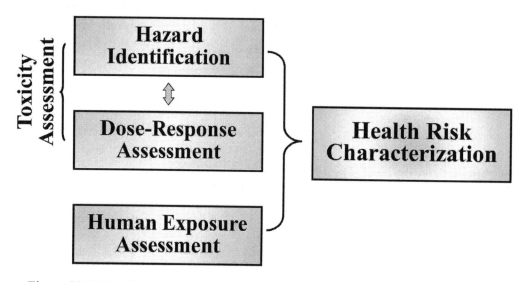

Figure 23.1. Key Components/Phases of (Environmental) Health Risk Assessment

23.2. Toxicity Assessment

Unlike ecological risk assessment (Section 22.3.3), health risk assessment generally does not proceed with *problem formulation* as a formal first step. Instead, it generally begins with hazard identification (HI), the phase that involves the determination of potential adverse health effects from exposure to a biological, physical, or chemical agent of concern. Problem formulation is almost not needed in performing health risk assessment because the justification, the conceptual model, and the action plan involved are comparatively more straightforward. Many substances under health risk assessment either are active ingredients in products that are subjected to safety evaluation prior to registration or re-registration for use, or are those suspected to cause environmental health hazard. In practice, the main task of HI is to first analyze all potential *toxic* endpoints identified and then to determine the one(s) *of critical concern*, mostly in terms of severity, toxic effect type, or both. In contrast, the output of the problem formulation phase in ecological risk assessment will include a set of *assessment* endpoints that, while reflecting the ecosystem, are determined to be both measurable and affected by the stressor(s) in question.

More specifically, an assessment endpoint in ecological risk assessment is generally defined as an explicit expression of the ecological value to be protected or upheld (U.S. EPA, 1998b). The ecological attributes for the value to be protected and thereby to be assessed can be as broad as maintaining a balanced indigenous population in waters receiving radioactive plumes from a nuclear power plant, as stipulated by Section 316(b) of the U.S. Clean Water Act. In contrast, when performing the health risk assessment for a particular (toxic) substance, the practice in the HI phase has been to let the available toxicity test results define the toxic endpoints (e.g., Suter and Barnthouse, 1993).

23.2.1. Hazard (Endpoint) Identification

Conceptually, the task of hazard (endpoint) identification (HI) need not be initiated with the application of chemical-specific animal or human toxicity data. However, for health risk assessment purposes, the use of well-conducted chemical-specific animal toxicity studies is not only encouraged but in most cases also warranted. This is because strong evidence is required to ensure or reassure that the toxic effect is caused by the suspect agent or activity involved. More so than ecological risk assessment, health risk assessment by law often requires such strong evidence because there is more at stake with the suspect agent's *legal* use and the activity involved.

Naturally, the most convincing evidence for a strong causal relationship is supposedly from a well-conducted epidemiological study in which a positive association has been observed between exposure and adverse effect in human subjects, since human data offer evidence that is most direct. Yet well-conducted human or epidemiological studies are hard to come by, as it is unethical to deliberately subject humans to doses sufficient to cause them bodily harm. The use of animal data from well-designed experiments thus becomes a crucial part of the HI task. At the least, the dose given to the test animals is more controllable, compared to human exposure. Regardless, the main problem with utilizing animal toxicity results is that the test agent could induce a toxic effect in animals very different from that observed or anticipated in humans. After all, the rodent and human bodies are anatomically (and in many cases physiologically) very different.

Other types of toxicity studies used for or in the HI phase include short-term tests ranging from bacterial mutation assays performed entirely *in vitro* to more elaborate short-term bioassays such as skin-painting studies in rodents. Suffice to say, a test agent's physicochemical properties also play a significant role in providing crucial information on its toxic effects in humans.

23.2.2. Animal Toxicity Studies and Test Guidelines

The assessment of a toxic agent's adverse health effects in animals normally examines most, if not all, of the eight general toxicity categories listed in Table 23.1 below for one or more of the three common routes of exposure: oral (by ingestion); inhalation; and dermal (by absorption via the skin). For illustration purposes, also included in the table are select testing guidelines (a.k.a. test guidelines) published by U.S. EPA for the eight toxicity categories listed.

Table 23.1. General Categories of Health Effects and Their Select Test Guidelines as Considered and Used (by U.S. EPA) in a Typical Health Risk Assessment

Category of Health Effects	Select Guidelines Published by U.S. EPA
Acute toxicity	Acute Oral Toxicity (2002)
Subchronic toxicity	Ninety-Day Inhalation (1998c)
Chronic toxicity	Chronic Toxicity (1998d)
Genetic toxicity	Bacterial Reverse Mutation (1998e)
Neurotoxicity	Neurotoxicity Screening Battery (1998f)
Carcinogenicity	Carcinogenicity (1998g)
Immunotoxicity	Immunotoxicity (1998h)
Reproductive/Developmental toxicity	Reproduction/Developmental Screening (2000a)

The health effects test guidelines issued by U.S. EPA total to about 50. This is not the only set made available for use as study protocols in testing the safety of pesticides, food additives, industrial chemicals, and pharmaceuticals. Comparable test guidelines have been made available to the public by other organizations, including prominently the Organization for Economic Cooperation and Development (OECD) and the International Conference on Harmonization (ICH). The OECD guidelines represent a collection of some 100 most relevant testing protocols used by governments, the industry, and independent laboratories to identify and characterize potential hazards of new and existing chemical substances in all categories. These OECD guidelines, of which most are currently accessible online at the organization's website, are regularly updated with the assistance of thousands of scientific experts from its some 30 member countries (e.g., Australia, Chile, France, Japan, Korea, Mexico, Norway, Spain, United Kingdom, United States). The ICH guidelines, currently available online at the FDA website, are intended for pharmaceutical products only. They represent the joint effort of the six founding members from the United States, the European Union, and Japan, with one regulatory authority and one pharmaceutical manufacturers association serving for each jurisdiction. As expected, FDA is the regulatory authority representing the United States. In addition to a group of regulatory members (e.g., Health Canada), ICH currently has a sizable pool of observers including notably the World Health Organization (WHO).

At times, the potential health effects of a toxic agent may also be conveniently categorized into the following three groups or six subgroups for exposure assessment purposes: acute *vs.* chronic effects; local *vs.* systemic effects; and reversible *vs.* irreversible effects (as defined in Table 9.1). Regardless of the categorization scheme used, in practice the toxic endpoints of concern are quantified primarily in terms of NO[A]EL (i.e., the no observed *adverse* effect level NO*A*EL or the no observed effect level NOEL) for all types of health effects subject to health risk analysis, except for cancer and acute toxicity. Acute toxicity is one that manifests shortly after a single exposure and is typically expressed as LD_{50} or LC_{50}, which is the dose or concentration (respectively) required to kill half of the test population. For cancer, the effect unit of concern generally is the so-termed *cancer potency factor* (*CPF*), which in many cases is expressed as the slope of the dose-response curve generated for the toxic agent at issue. The rationale and justification for the utilization of CPF is discussed in the next subsection on dose-response assessment, which is concerned with how health effects can be quantified and reassured.

23.2.3. Dose-Response Assessment

Once the toxic endpoints of concern are identified, the next crucial step is to determine the highest dose at which biologically and statistically no significant adverse effect is expected to occur relative to the control group. This highest dose is generally referred to as NO[A]EL, the dosage ideally *just* below the lowest observed [adverse] effect level (LO[A]EL) which ideally *just* begins to show noticeable increase in the observed effect. The difference between NO*A*EL and NOEL rests on the definition of *adverse* effect (NRC, 1994). As inferred to in Section 23.1.2, most toxicity studies are conducted not only for HI purposes, but also for dose-response assessment (DRA). It is for this reason that NRC (1994) made an effort to revise its initial health risk assessment paradigm to combine HI and DRA into a single phase termed *toxicity assessment*.

One crucial function of DRA is to ascertain the reasonable lowest dose to be employed as the LO[A]EL, or the reasonable highest dose utilized as the NO[A]EL. Oftentimes, there are merely three or four dose levels and a very limited number of animals used per level in a toxicity study, primarily because any type of animal toxicity studies is expensive to be carried out costing easily over $500,000 each (e.g., Klaassen and Eaton, 1991, in present value). The resultant LO[A]EL or NO[A]EL thus generally turns out to be less appreciable particularly when a statistically acceptable dose-response curve cannot be constructed from the very few responses observed. As a point for argument here, if the intermediate dose of a threesome yielded the highest response (e.g., that having most test animals with the effects), the lower or negative response from the lowest dose tested could be construed as an artifact, or due to chance. In any case, if a dose-response curve could be constructed (*see*, e.g., Figure 23.2) with some level of confidence showing a very steep slope, then the response would be treated as highly sensitive to dose level with the implication that the NO[A]EL is (fairly or very) close to the LO[A]EL. Conversely, if the slope appeared less steep, the response would be treated as less dose-sensitive. The use of NO[A]EL or LO[A]EL in health risk assessment is typically based on the notion that the exposure has to reach a threshold before any (non-cancer) adverse health effects can occur.

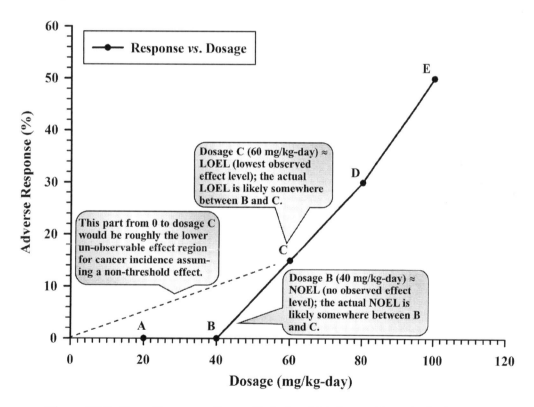

Figure 23.2. Dose-Response Curve (Relationship) from a Hypothetical Study Having Five Dosage Points A, B, C, D, and E

DRA plays a relatively more prominent role where the adverse health effect of concern is cancer, for which no threshold is generally presumed. Because the general presumption or tendency is

458 An Introduction to Environmental Toxicology

that human doses are typically lower than the experimental LO[A]EL derived from animal studies, there are many uncertainties and interests about how a human dose behaves biologically in the *unobservable* region below the experimental LO[A]EL, especially when a no threshold effect is assumed. The general practice has been to extrapolate from responses at (all or most of) the experimental doses down to the region below the LO[A]EL (as illustrated in Figure 23.2) by means of a theorized mechanistic model such as a linearized multistage or a low-dose linear model (e.g., EHA, 2012; U.S. EPA, 2005). This type of extrapolation is part of the DRA task.

The slope extrapolated from such theorized models is known as cancer slope factor (CSF) or CPF (cancer potency factor), expressed typically in units of $(mg/kg\text{-}day)^{-1}$. This slope is basically a rate constant implicating or asserting that the magnitude or level of the response is (linearly) proportional to the exposure level (again, typically in units of mg carcinogen per kg body weight per day). As hinted earlier, the steeper the slope, the more potent each dosage is implicated for cancer risk since it takes less exposure to induce the same level of cancer response (risk). As further elaborated on in Section 23.4.1, excess (lifetime) cancer risk can be quantified by multiplying an estimated dose or dosage of concern by the associated (i.e., predetermined) CPF.

23.3. Human Exposure Assessment

In this crucial phase of the health risk assessment process, assessors responsible for the task will often face chemical, physical, or biological contaminants that are less concrete than desired, especially in terms of exposure level. The perspectives that follow explain to some extent why health scientists with sufficient knowledge in epidemiology tend to have a better edge in assessing human exposure to environmental toxicants. The exposure sources and pathways in Figure 23.3 are depicted to reflect the complexity as well as the general scheme involved in performing this difficult task known as human exposure assessment or human exposure analysis.

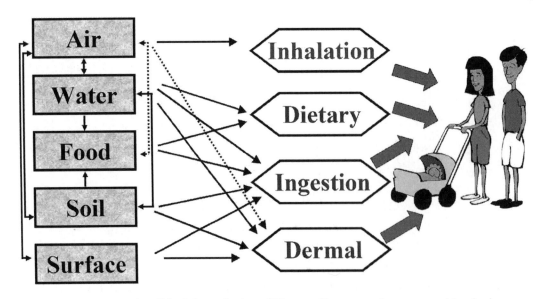

Figure 23.3. Simplified Complexity of Human Exposure Assessment/Analysis

In essence, human exposure to environmental toxicants can occur via dermal contact, inhalation, ingestion, and dietary intake. Throughout this book, ingestion and dietary intake are treated as different although in both cases the route of exposure is oral. Dietary intake involves the exposure from daily food consumption, frequently including drinking water. In contrast, ingestion generally refers to any other oral intake, such as from hand-to-mouth by a toddler after crawling on a carpet treated with a flea killer fogger. Figure 23.3 also suggests that in addition to the common environmental media such as air, soils, foods, and drinking water, the contaminant may be present on foliar or other structural surfaces. Moreover, for some contaminants, certain exposure sources and pathways play a more prominent role than others do. For instance, compared to dermal contact, inhalation generally is a route more critical for soil fumigants due to their high volatility.

23.3.1. Past and Current Perspectives

Several definitions have been given for human exposure assessment. To some scholars, there may need to be a distinction between the terms *human exposure measurement* and *human exposure assessment*. The former generally is limited to the quantitation of human exposure, whereas the latter extends to considering the implication or impact of the exposure level measured. In this chapter, however, the term *exposure analysis* is used much of the time for no reasons other than to avoid such a distinction as well as to ease the writing somewhat.

Exposure analysis rests on the widely accepted toxicological concept that the magnitude, the frequency, and the route of dosing or exposure all have a significant impact on the nature, the severity, and the potential of an adverse effect to be induced. Oftentimes, repeated exposures at a lower dosage are assumed to have the same (or at least similar) toxic effect(s) induced by a single exposure at a proportionated higher dosage (*see*, Section 10.2.2A).

As pointed out in the guidelines published by U.S. EPA (1992), exposure analysis in various forms dates back at least to the early 20th century, particularly in the field of epidemiology and those dealing with occupational exposure. U.S. EPA defines exposure as the contact between an agent and a human body's outer boundary (e.g., the skin, lungs, gastrointestinal tract). In contrast, applied dose refers to the amount of a substance placed at or around one or more of these outer boundaries which act as absorption barriers. The term *dosage* differs from *dose* only in the former referring to an amount that is relative to a physiological parameter (e.g., per kg of body weight) and/or to a time interval (e.g., per day). As also introduced in Section 1.2.1, another closely related term is internal dose, which is the amount of a substance that has been absorbed via all body barriers plus the portion produced or left in the body, if any. This is simply the total amount available for biological interaction with receptors located in any body tissue.

Despite the supposition that (human) exposure analysis is important to toxicologists engaging in health risk assessment, documentation of this subject matter in toxicology textbooks is incomplete and fragmented. To date, most toxicology textbooks and references have offered only a few sections on exposure analysis, usually as part of a chapter addressing some form of health risk assessment or analysis. Many toxicologists do not find exposure analysis appealing in part because they are better trained to use animal models or bioassays as investigation tools. Another subtle reason is that health risk assessment, of which exposure analysis is a key part, is still a young field.

There are undoubtedly toxicologists measuring exposure levels for pathological examination, forensic investigation, and the kind. Yet measurements of such are on single individuals typically without the immediate intent of protecting public health on a large scale.

In any event, it is somewhat a relief now to find that more toxicologists have been willingly and constantly working with or for epidemiologists and other health scientists in performing exposure analysis. For instance, some toxicologists have been performing animal (and at times human) studies to determine the dermal or inhalation absorption of chemical substances. These absorption studies will enable exposure assessors to estimate the internal dose from dermal or inhalation exposure to the substance in test animals (i.e., by utilizing the estimate obtained as surrogate for human value). Food toxicologists and nutritional epidemiologists are also frequently seen working together in assessing dietary intakes. Furthermore, many more environmental toxicologists now have acquired a fair amount of knowledge about the air, water, and soil concentrations of certain contaminants in various parts of a country and the world.

For different objectives, exposure analysis for environmental (including occupational) hazards is covered more fully and more frequently in epidemiology textbooks. Despite such coverage and efforts, there are still reasons why some epidemiologists too may find exposure analysis not appealing. First, the efforts by many epidemiologists to associate human exposures to health outcomes are primarily for etiology testing, not so much for (environmental) health risk assessment. Second, exposure analyses for environmental hazards are performed mainly for chemical, physical, or biological contaminants present in the environment. Yet epidemiologists outside of the environmental health discipline usually face different issues or agenda whenever they assess human exposures to or for certain intrinsic factors. Third, as noted earlier, health risk assessment as a scientific discipline is at best in its adolescence, if not still in its infancy.

Epidemiologists who are less concerned with exposure analysis for environmental hazards are those dealing with either intangible exposures or those of more concrete levels, not in-between. For instance, when conducting a clinical trial, most epidemiologists already have a good idea on the dose or treatment levels at which the patients or volunteers are being or to be exposed. And for psychosocial epidemiologists, they tend to work with personal trait, lifestyle, or socioeconomic status as some form of exposure in the name of risk factors. These factors are intrinsic as well as intangible, as their measurements rely on the use of more quantifiable but less relevant determinants as surrogates, such as through work histories, observed behaviors, and surveys.

23.3.2. Direct and Indirect Measurements

There are essentially two approaches to estimating human exposure to most any environmental toxicant (or hazard). One approach is to first identify the major exposure sources or pathways involved (e.g., inhalation, dermal, dietary, ingestion, onsite, indoor). The exposures from, to, or with these environmental components are then assess separately and indirectly. In most instances, indirect exposure measurements are performed by means of the toxicant's (or the hazard's) quantities in one or more appropriate media (e.g., air, soils, water, foods, foliage).

Most, if not all, indirect measurement methods available to date are still built on the well received, yet not fully validated, simple algorithm presented in Box 23.1 below:

Box 23.1. Basic Algorithm for Calculation of Human Environmental Exposure

Human Exposure
≈ [*Environmental Quantity of Toxicant or Hazard*] x [*Human Contact*]

It is intuitive that the reverse implication of the premise in Box 23.1 is always true. That is, no human exposure would occur if there were no human contact with the toxicant or hazard whether directly or indirectly. Nor would there be any such human exposure if the toxicant or hazard were not present in the person's environment.

Another approach to measuring human exposure is to estimate the person's (e.g., daily) dosage directly through biomonitoring (as defined in Section 20.3.2). Biomonitoring of human exposure generally involves the measurement of an internal dose. Yet in reality, the biomonitoring approach does not truly offer a direct measurement method. This is because technically the dose or dosage so measured is still via some form of indirect estimation. In practice, the internal dose so derived is almost always based on the amounts of the toxicant measured in only a couple of biological media such as blood, expired air, or urine. More bluntly, the amounts estimated for other body tissues need to be inferred or accounted for indirectly. If a metabolite were monitored instead, which is not uncommon, then additional correction or back-calculation would be needed to account for the portion of the parent compound that had been biotransformed to the metabolite, so that the total amount of human exposure to the parent compound (which is usually the chemical species of regulatory concern per health risk assessment) could be fully determined.

For a comprehensive exposure analysis, the calculations of *aggregate* and *cumulative* doses (or exposures) are warranted. Aggregate dose is defined as that level accumulated from multiple exposure pathways and media, whereas cumulative dose refers to an aggregate dose that accounts for the additional exposures to (all) relevant chemicals sharing a crucial mechanism of toxicity in common. The advantage of using biomonitoring data to estimate exposure is thus manifold. Because biomonitoring integrates the exposures supposedly by all routes of entry, this type of exposure monitoring should help reduce the concern with exposure events that may occur concurrently. In addition, the application of aggregate or cumulative dose derived from well-designed biomonitoring studies would reduce the uncertainties inherent in animal dermal absorption or other similar types of extrapolation (Dong and Ross, 2001; Ross *et al.*, 2000).

Unfortunately, the limitations of using biomonitoring data are likewise numerous (*see* Section 20.3.2). In particular, the total body burden derived from this type of data is not route-specific, unless further efforts are made such as collecting air samples on the side to account for the dose from inhalation exposure alone. To put it another way, for risk mitigation purposes, it is important to know which route of entry is the principal exposure pathway. For instance, if exposure via dermal route turns out to be much more crucial than from inhalation, then the workers will be required to wear adequate protective coveralls instead of an approved respirator.

In human exposure assessment, the indirect measurement method currently is more popular compared to biomonitoring. This is because the indirect approach is still considered more practical and economical. Another important reason is that knowledge of a substance's toxicokinetics is a prerequisite for the application of human monitoring and for the interpretation of its results on the substance. Yet frequently, such knowledge is not available or attainable. Furthermore, collection of body fluids, including urine, from human subjects is considered an unpleasant or invasive ordeal to many people.

23.3.3. Aggregate and Cumulative Exposures

In performing a comprehensive human exposure analysis, estimation of aggregate exposure is apparently needed when relying on the indirect measurement method over biomonitoring. The hypothetical exposure scenario depicted in Figure 23.4 below may serve to illustrate the complexity involved. This scenario highlights the multiple exposure pathways via multiple media for children spending some time at a playground in which the playset structures had been treated with a wood preservative of health concern, such as chromated copper arsenate (CCA). In performing a comprehensive analysis of the children's daily or seasonal exposure to one or more of the three metallic (chromium, copper, arsenic) ingredients in the CCA residues, it is necessary for the assessor to consider at least the four common routes of exposure outlined graphically in Figure 23.4.

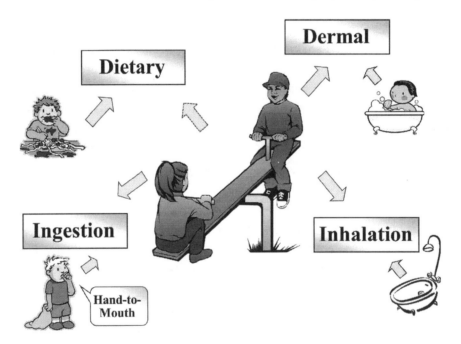

Figure 23.4. Potential Routes for Aggregate Exposure of Children to Pesticide Residues
(e.g., as to Residues of Pressure-Treated Wood Preservative Used in Playground Structures)

In reality, it is not improbable for a young child to be exposed to the CCA residues via dermal contact with the contaminated soils around the treated playset structures. The child's clothing and skin could also come in contact with the residues (long) deposited on/in the old playset structures, and potentially with the indoor surface residues that had been translocated over via the contaminated outdoor air and soils. Another source of dermal uptake could be the shower or bath water whose supply line had been contaminated at a site even far away from the playground. The child could inhale one or more of the metals evaporated off the shower or bath water. Both the indoor and the outdoor air could also be sources for inhalation exposure. In addition to drinking water and foods found with one or more of the metals at considerable levels, the child could ingest the CCA residues on/in the playset structures or soils via hand/object-to-mouth exposure.

Note that in performing a comprehensive exposure analysis as part of a health risk assessment, the background level from sources other than the treated or contaminated site is as critical or crucial. This is because the adverse health effect, if any, is to be induced by the *total* effective amount of the target substance in or on the body. Furthermore, there is often the legally or scientifically probable situation in which one or more other relevant substances share a common mechanism of toxicity at issue and are reachable to the child's local environment at considerable levels. In that case, the child's exposures from many or all of the aforesaid pathways and sources need to be estimated for these other substances in the same manner as for the target substance, and then to be added to his or her total exposure for the day, the month, and/or the year.

Both the analysis and the estimation of aggregate and cumulative exposures for the above or similar exposure scenarios are often complex. Many presumptions and assumptions are required to deal with the exposure nature and duration range for each of the pathways involved. The concentration range for each of the environmental exposure media is needed as well. All of these parameters and their practical value ranges are subject to challenge by the stakeholders, the scientific sector, and the higher or other regulatory entities. For cumulative exposure, there is an additional need for defending the decision made that the other relevant substances share a critical common mechanism of toxicity with the target substance. U.S. EPA (2003, 2007a) has published a resource guide and a framework document that together offer the much needed concepts, methods, and data sources to assist in the performance of multi-exposure, multi-chemical, and population-focused cumulative risk assessments.

23.4. Environmental Health Risk Characterization

According to U.S. EPA's *Risk Characterization Handbook* (2000b), risk characterization is *"the final, integrative step of risk assessment"* that *"conveys the risk assessor's judgment as to the nature and existence (or the lack) of human health or ecological risks."* That handbook reiterates NRC's paradigm, asserting that hazard (endpoint) identification, dose-response assessment, human exposure assessment, and (environmental) health risk characterization are the key steps in the analysis of health risk. In that sense, risk characterization can be regarded as a major part of the newly emerging discipline known as (environmental) health risk assessment.

However, in a narrower context, health risk characterization can be treated as a simple quantitation process involving the *comparison* of one or more estimated exposure levels of concern *to* a benchmark (level) at or below which the estimated exposure is accepted as insignificant by regulatory standards. The health risk is assumed to be proportionally greater if the exposure level is increased farther (though within a reasonable range) beyond the benchmark. In many instances, the benchmark so adopted for is expressed as, or derived from, one of the health risk measures described in the next subsection.

23.4.1. Health Risk Measures

Over the years, there have been a dozen or so quantitative measures employed to account for, directly or indirectly, the significance of a health risk assessed. These risk measures, more commonly known by their acronyms, include: ADI, RfD, RfC, CPF, ECR, NO[A]EL, LO[A]EL, PEL, TWA, STEL, BMD, BMC, and MCL. Of these, the first three (ADI, RfD, RfC) typically have their values already built in with a safety margin. Closely related to these dozen measures are the likewise commonly employed MOE and HQ in certain regulatory sectors.

ADI (*acceptable daily intake*) is the predetermined daily dosage (e.g., mg per kg body weight) of a toxic substance (e.g., pesticide, food additive, metal) that presumably may be *ingested* daily by people over their entire lifetime without causing any significant adverse health effect. This dosage is determined by dividing the NO[A]EL by a set of safety factors (SFs), typically of multiples of 10, to account for *intra*species sensitivity, *inter*species variation, and other uncertainties of concern (e.g. low quality or quantity of toxicity data available for use). The definitions of NO[A]EL and LO[A]EL are given in Section 23.2.3. The term *ADI* was first employed in 1961 by the Food and Agriculture Organization of the United Nations/World Health Organization Expert Committee on Food Additives. Now it is also utilized extensively by FDA in the United States.

RfD (*reference dose*), employed by many programs within U.S. EPA, is derived similarly. The potential difference between RfD and ADI is the possibly different SFs (safety factors) and toxicity studies used by the different agencies. RfC (*reference concentration*) is likewise determined and applied similarly by U.S. EPA. It differs from RfD only in that air, water, or soil *concentration*, instead of the actual (human) exposure (dose), is used.

PEL (*permissible exposure limit*) and the kind, such as STEL (*short-term exposure limit*) and TWA (*time-weighted average*), are the maximum environmental levels of a toxicant that workers (or sometimes a community) presumably can be exposed to within a given time interval without causing any significant adverse health effect (Chapter 20). In the United States, worker exposure limits of this type are employed mainly by OSHA. On the other hand, as utilized mostly by U.S. EPA, MCL is the *maximum contaminant level* of a substance in a water system that is considered as harmless to consumers.

BMD (*benchmark dose*) can be determined and used to represent the lower confidence limit on a dose that produces an acceptable small percentage (e.g., 5%) increase in a particular adverse effect. It is thus supposed to be a more accurately quantified as well as a more realistic LO[A]EL for assessors to use. BMC (*benchmark concentration*) differs from BMD in that it deals with the substance's concentration to be exposed to, instead of its dose to be received.

For carcinogenicity, excess (lifetime) risk is generally calculated by multiplying an estimated dose of concern by the associated CPF (*cancer potency factor*). This mathematical product represents an upper bound on the probability of having *excess cancer risk* (ECR) from lifetime or long-term exposure to a carcinogen. The probability is expressed as a population risk, such as 1×10^{-6} meaning that 1 in 1 million exposed people is estimated or expected to have the cancer. As ECR = dose × CPF, it follows that dose = ECR ÷ CPF. Therefore, the exposure dose considered as safe (say denoted by $dose_{al}$) for the cancer risk at issue can be estimated in terms of CPF alone, as long as an *ac*ceptable *l*evel of ECR, say ECR_{al} (e.g., 1×10^{-6}), has been predetermined.

Those measures utilized to characterize health risk *indirectly* include ADI, RfD, RfC, PEL, CPF, and the kind. They are regarded as *indirect* health risk measures in that their (predetermined) values must be checked against the calculated exposure dose at issue before their risk implications can be appreciated. For instance, a higher (i.e., less potent) ADI value for toxicant A might turn out to implicate a higher health risk than would a lower (more potent) ADI value for toxicant B, if the same person were exposed to a much higher level of toxicant A than of toxicant B.

ECR is considered a *direct* health risk measure in that *its estimated value* can be readily appreciated by direct comparison to the preset dose$_{al}$ value (as defined and denoted earlier). For noncarcinogenic adverse effects, the direct risk measures commonly employed by regulatory agencies are MOE (*margin of exposure*), HQ (*hazard quotient*), and some variants of the two.

Until recently, MOE was used interchangeably with MOS (*margin of safety*). This measure is typically determined by dividing the NO[A]EL (or its equivalent) by the estimated exposure dose of concern. HQ is the ratio of the estimated exposure dose or concentration to an effect dose (e.g., RfD) or concentration (e.g., RfC), respectively (Box 22.1). The main difference between MOE and HQ is that the latter can be used as is, as one or more SFs have been incorporated to derive the RfD or RfC. Accordingly, an HQ value *much* less than 1 is treated as having a low or negligible ecological (or health) risk. In contrast, an acceptable (i.e., the benchmark) MOE is typically 100 or greater to account for at least an uncertainty factor of 10 for interspecies variation and another 10 for intraspecies sensitivity. Note that MOE is mathematically related to HQ by the latter's (set of) SF_{HQ} used (which may not be the same as the former's SF_{MOE} used); that is, $MOE \approx SF_{HQ} \div HQ$.

23.4.2. Uncertainty and Safety Factors

From the discussion given thus far in this chapter, it is apparent that health risk assessment is inadequate without at least some consideration of how the uncertainty and safety factors are analyzed and treated. Their impacts on health risk implication are substantial, in that they are deliberately incorporated into some health risk measures (e.g., RfD, RfC, ADI). It is intuitive that the uncertainties of concern involved here can be broadly subsumed under the two key analytical components with which they tend to associate: (1) toxicity assessment (analysis); and (2) human exposure assessment (analysis). Despite such triviality, any fair account of the uncertainties involved in most any health risk assessment would require volumes of discussion, for which this chapter as well as this book is not the appropriate place. In this subsection, only certain uncertainties that are deemed having the (more) common impacts on health risk assessment are highlighted, all in an effort to illustrate the complexity and dynamics involved. In fact, it is due to the difficult, lengthy process of resolving many of the uncertainties involved that sometimes it can take years to finalize a full-scale health risk assessment as well as its documentation.

One of the major uncertainty issues frequently encountered with toxicity assessment is that many toxicants can each be found to cause more than one type of adverse health effects, depending on the species tested and on the route, the amount, as well as the duration of dosing used. Where two or more types of effects were observed, they might not have been caused by exposures at the same level or via the same route. It is therefore important for the risk assessor to analyze and determine which observed adverse effect(s) should be treated as the toxic endpoint(s) *of critical concern*. The health effects test guidelines such as those listed in Table 23.1 have been made available partly with the intent to help minimize this type of uncertainties.

More specifically, the main issues with hazard (endpoint) identification are the interpretation of toxicity data and the concerns with strength- and weight-of-evidence. For instance, the toxic effect could show up in a study with dogs as the test animals, but not one with rats. Does this mean that the dog species is more sensitive to the toxicant? Or that only the dog study was conducted properly? More concrete examples can be found in Chapter 10 concerning species and other biological traits being cofactors (hence as well as confounders) that can seriously affect toxicity.

The various types of adverse health effects listed in Table 23.1 are also problematic in terms of their actual applications. For instance, *acute* toxicity involves an adverse effect that by definition manifests within a short time interval following dosing. However, the upper end of this interval is not always well defined or agreed upon. That is, should it be 3, 24, 47.5, or 79 hours (in the animal study)? Another issue is that much implication of mutagenesis for carcinogenesis has not been fully resolved. Still another issue is that irritation scores given in a skin sensitization test are based on some degree of human subjective evaluation. This type of evaluation can make skin sensitization less accepted as a primary adverse effect even when compared to decrease in body weight gain. This is not so much that the former effect is treated as less detrimental, but only because it is less quantifiable compared to some endpoints like body weight gain or loss.

Another limitation or concern with toxicity assessment is that the toxic endpoint with the *lowest* NO[A]EL observed among studies may not always be the best candidate in that such a more health protective endpoint value is credible only if it is derived from good data, which however is a criterion not for any assessor to deal with in a manner fair enough to *all* sectors. Moreover, the adverse effects observed via different exposure routes might not come out to be even similar. Oftentimes the toxic endpoints of regulatory concern do not represent the most severe effects, but are those with a low enough NO[A]EL to call for exposure mitigation. The notion here is that when the *lower* critical exposure (or dose) required for inducing the (oftentimes less severe) adverse health effect under regulatory concern were adequately mitigated, so would the *higher* critical exposures (or doses) required for inducing other (even more severe) toxic effects.

The uncertainty with animal-to-human extrapolation is one of the most concerning and troublesome issues in toxicity assessment. Contrary to general brief, when an adverse health effect is observed in an animal study, the first thing that will come to the risk assessor's mind is not always the question whether the same health effect would occur in humans. Frequently, the first question is whether the same effect would occur in other strains of the test species or in another animal species. This is because while knowing that human data are hard to come by, the strength- and the weight-of-evidence would have to rest on animal data alone or mostly. And such evidence would increase if the same effect could be reproduced in another strain or in another animal species. Rats are commonly used as a test model largely because they are relatively inexpensive and inbred to reduce variability (Ross *et al.*, 2000). Yet certain chemicals or drugs, such as the notorious teratogen thalidomide, are highly species-specific or highly sensitive to time of exposure.

The uncertainty issues associated with human exposure analysis are likewise enormous and in many situations even more overwhelming. Exposure analysis is often thought to be more dynamic and more complicated than toxicity assessment. Such a notion is based on the general observation that overall, both the framework and the process for toxicity assessment are more solid and controllable compared to those for (human) exposure assessment. To put it another way, relatively fewer assumptions and presumptions are needed in toxicity analysis while at the same time animal toxicity studies in general are or can be better designed compared to exposure monitoring studies and the kind.

Human contact, being a behavioral as well as a physiological variable, is often more difficult to be defined, quantified, and thus defended or justified for. For instance, inhalation exposure is a function of a person's respiration rate and of the toxicant's air concentration within that person's breathing zone. Yet respiration rate is not only gender- and age-specific, but also a function of human activity which cannot be quantified easily. Moreover, the toxicant's concentration in the air is not only a source-dependent but also a temporal as well as a spatial variable. It is fair to say that the toxicant's actual concentration in a specific space and time period at best can only be approximated with some level of uncertainty.

Another important lingering uncertainty with exposure analysis is how to determine fairly, if not accurately, the duration and frequency for chronic (and sometimes even acute) exposure. It is not easy to give a fair account of all the potential human exposure events for an average day or month. It is even harder or more complicated to determine the number of times a person is exposed to a toxicant in a season, a year, or a lifetime. The uncertainty and complexity with the determination of exposure duration or frequency may be best appreciated in terms of the following analogies or challenges: Would the (health) effect on a person be the same between the person taking 1 (e.g., vitamin) pill daily for one year *vs.* the same person taking 2 pills a day for 182 days (i.e., 1 year ≈ 182 days x 2)? Or would the effect be the same between the person taking 2 pills daily for 182 *consecutive* days *vs.* the same person taking 2 pills daily *intermittently* for 182 days over the year? If the effects from these various dosage schemes cannot be the same, then how should they be normalized in order to proceed with the health risk analysis?

Moreover, values used for many exposure parameters or variables are generally based on policy defaults, professional judgment, or more ideally empirical data. Yet it is important to realize that nearly all of such empirical data available to date were derived from small, unrepresentative grab or spot samples. By spot samples, it means that the sample size is less than adequate while at the same time the measurements involved are less than complete or representative. Grab samples are those in which the test subjects or observation units were not randomly selected or assigned. These are simply opportunistic samples. Therefore, any conclusion or assertion made that spot or grab samples would give a fair account about the target population's exposure-related activities or routines is an intention at best.

For instance, the Nationwide Food Consumption Survey conducted every ten years or so by the U.S. Department of Agriculture covers all ages, genders, and regions in the United States. Yet even with a survey so complexly as well as so comprehensively large, there is still a missing link between people living in regions with known food residue levels and their consumption rates. That is, there is still a lack of correlation between where exactly a contaminant concentrates its residues and what the dietary patterns are for residents living in that contaminated region.

There can also be uncertainties with the default values used as exposure factors, such as for rate of soil ingestion by children in recreational areas where playground structures were treated with a wood preservative (e.g., Figure 23.4). Two- or three-year-olds might not stay and play in the sandbox for longer time than older children would. The hand-to-mouth movements of the younger children could be more or less frequent. And how well or how frequent their hands would be cleaned during playtime or shortly afterwards depends on how health conscious these children and their parents are. The *Exposure Factors Handbook* published by U.S. EPA (2011) provides the percentiles and other statistics on soil ingestion rate, body weight, and many other factors by age and gender intended for the *general* population. It is debatable whether or not these default values should be used to represent the distributions of body weight, soil ingestion rate, and the kind for children under assessment whose physical build might be different.

To date, most regulatory agencies still apply an uncertainty factor (UF) or SF (safety factor) of 10 for interspecies extrapolation, thinking that humans can be up to 10 times more susceptible than the test species used in an animal study. Yet there is no sound justification for the *adequacy* of this UF of 10, other than perhaps the account by Dourson and Stara (1983). Before such an uncertainty can be truly accounted for, the equivalence of animal to human dosage must be resolved first. For example, would or should 1 unit of dose given daily to a test animal exactly equal to 1 unit of dose received daily by a human, even after normalization for body weight? Is it not possible that the test animal (e.g., the rat) would detoxify or bioactivate the same amount of the substance faster or slower than a human would? And to what extent or in what manner?

Another UF or SF commonly applied in health risk assessment is the 10-fold factor for intraspecies sensitivity which also has a direct impact on the derivation of RfD or ADI. Where the human exposure was calculated for populations other than workers, should this UF be greater than 10 to account for the lack of healthy worker effect? Or should this UF be less than 10 when occupational exposure is considered? By healthy worker effect (e.g., Li and Sung, 1999; Shah, 2009), it means that workers on the whole are apparently healthier and thereby likely to be less susceptible to toxic insults compared to those of the same age group that are too ill to work or do not have to work. In essence, there seems to be always the uncertainty about the extent to which the factor of 10 should be applied for intraspecies, interspecies, or other uncertainties.

23.4.3. Health Risk Perception

As noted in Section 23.1.1, health risk assessment activities are partly bound by social values and public concerns. Such a constraint conceives the notion that health risk perception plays a key role in the performance of (environmental) health risk assessment. The society's risk perception certainly has much to say and do with how health risk assessment is actually or may be performed, as readily demonstrated by the tampon-toxic shock story highlighted in Section 3.2. Health risk perception on this level may also be translated into practice via health regulations and will eventually complicate the health risk characterization as well as the assessment process. For instance, largely due to the public's rising concerns and accordingly via the U.S. Food Quality Protection Act of 1996, the U.S. federal government is now mandated to take into serious consideration the assessment of aggregate as well as cumulative exposure (Section 23.3.3) for children's health.

The centerpiece of risk perception is subjective or perceived risk which can be defined as the *sum* of objective risk (or hazard) *and* outrage (Beecher *et al.*, 2005; Covello and Sandman, 2001; Sandman, 1987). As stated in Section 22.3.3, ecological or health risk can be technically defined as the probability of an adverse effect on the receptor. More broadly, it is about the likelihood that a dangerous event would occur. Yet the outrage of a stakeholder (an individual with an interest in the matter) is influenced by a number of perception factors including dread, control, nature of the hazard, familiarity, trust, and more (Covello and Sandman, 2001; U.S. EPA, 2007b). Fortunately, as pointed out by U. S. EPA (2007b), even when a subjective risk takes much more into account, with the proper perspective it is as manageable as an objective risk.

Any appreciation of health risk assessment therefore should also rest on the public's health and risk perceptions of the hazard at issue. Risk perception and health perception each have strong impacts on the populace's value choices of public health agenda and are basic elements to health risk assessment movement. They rest on mostly the two key human behavioral factors *controllability* and *familiarity* with the hazard of concern. Stakeholders tend to accept higher risks linked to voluntary activities than to those imposed on them without their consent. On the other hand, shock, horror, and fear to people tend to multiply when the event is unexpected or sudden, or when the nature of the hazard is complex.

The public sectors react differently to most misfortunes, as do many organizations and professional groups including regulatory toxicologists. By definition, health risk perception starts with health effects that people perceive. Inasmuch as health effects may be determined by various types of toxicity tests, interpretations of test results are not always consistent among regulatory agencies. Such differences in health risk perception help explain why FDA, U.S. EPA, and some other entities in and outside of the United States apply different terminology to safe human dose for exposure hazards in their health risk analysis. As noted in Section 23.4.1, U.S. EPA prefers to use RfD for benchmark human exposure level in their analysis. In contrast, FDA opts to use ADI instead. ADI values are also used by WHO to define lifetime allowable daily intake of pesticide and food additive residues. Differences between RfD and ADI rest on the manner in which the NO[A]EL and the uncertainty factors are treated, and sometimes on the choice of toxicity data as well.

23.4.4. Health Risk Communication

In all cases, health risk assessment should never end with just the completion of a (health) risk characterization or its document. Risk assessment as a process is merely a regulatory or scientific tool, not an end in itself. The entity that has performed the human health or the ecological risk assessment is obligated to relate the outcomes to its stakeholders and other audiences. In the past (or in some cases even today), the conventional way in which many government agencies dealt (deal) with the public on regulatory decisions is the *decide-announce-defend* or *"DAD"* approach (e.g., Beecher *et al.*, 2005; Scherer and Juanillo, 2003). This classic approach was (is) built on the notion that the decisions that the experts make are sound and fair, and defend their decisions only when they are challenged. However, in recent years, many public sectors (e.g., parents, patients, news media, labor union) are seen to increasingly challenge regulatory decisions and demand active involvement in the decision-making process, especially those decisions involving health risks.

More now than before, many people in the public sectors perceive the experts as those not always able to assess environmental health risks accurately or fairly.

In response to this new trend for greater participation by the public sectors, many health regulatory entities begin to appreciate the need for taking (health) risk communication into fuller consideration in their health risk assessment agenda. As NRC (1989) puts it, the health risk characterization process can be treated as successful only if it "*satisfies those involved that they are adequately informed within the limits of available knowledge.*" The U.S. Agency for Toxic Substances and Disease Registry (ATSDR, 1994) further contends that "*Merely disseminating the outcome information without regard for communicating the complexities and uncertainties of risk does not ensure necessarily effective risk communication.*" It is therefore important that any productive risk characterization must rest on how health risk assessors can treat the uncertainties involved professionally and then address them effectively to stakeholders and other audiences.

According to NRC (1989), "*(Health) risk communication is an interactive process of exchange of information and opinions among individuals, groups, and institutions. It often involves multiple messages about the nature of the risk or expressing concerns, opinions, or reactions to risk messages or to the legal and institutional arrangements for risk management.*" U.S. EPA (2007b) refines this concept to suggest that any ideal risk communication process would put a risk into proper perspective, would make contrasts with other risks, and would advocate a fruitful dialogue between those that deliver and those that receive the risk assessment outcome(s). In that same document, U.S. EPA reiterates the seven cardinal rules (e.g., Covello and Allen, 1988) for the practice of (health) risk communication. Those cardinal rules are reproduced in Box 23.2 below.

Box 23.2. Cardinal Rules for Risk Communication (e.g., Covello and Allen, 1988)

- Accept and involve the public as a partner.
- Listen to the public's specific concerns.
- Be honest, frank, and open.
- Work with other credible sources.
- Meet the needs of the media.
- Speak clearly and with compassion.
- Plan carefully and evaluate the communication effort.

In addition to the seven cardinal rules, U.S. EPA (2007b) highlights the four theories below for a sound risk communication practice: (1) the trust determination theory; (2) the negative dominance theory; (3) the mental noise theory; and (4) the risk perception theory. In essence, the trust determination theory hypothesizes that when people are upset or under stress, they easily do not trust that other people are listening, caring, competent, empathetic, or committed. The negative dominance theory suggests that when people are upset or under stress, they focus more on the negative than on the positive aspects of a situation. The mental noise theory contends that when people are upset or under stress, they have difficulty listening, understanding, and remembering relevant information. The risk perception theory postulates that when people are upset or under stress, their concerns and perceptions of threat differ from those of experts. Overall, these risk communication theories all revolve around the message receiver's state of mind, and collectively lend strong support for the cardinal rules listed in Box 23.2.

In closing, it should be pointed out that public sectors are not the only audiences to a health or an ecological risk assessment. At the professional or legal end, risk assessors must realize that concerns with adverse effects vary substantially among health statutes and thus among regulatory agencies. Such variations need to become explicit in the risk characterization document, so that the variations in health risk perception and risk prevention goal can be kept to a minimum among stakeholders and other audiences. As a point for further clarification on such a concern, the U.S. Clean Water Act allows primarily the *best available technology* approach for regulatory abatement, whereas the U.S. Clean Air Act promulgates largely *risk-based standards*.

In the United States, the best available technology approach is used mainly to limit discharges of water contaminants by use of technologically feasible abatement principles and strategies. Similar terms for the best available technology approach include *best available techniques*, *best practicable means*, and *best practicable environmental option*. In contrast, the risk-based approach requires that, for example, the ambient air quality for certain pollutants be upheld in terms of a set of air quality standards, such as the NAAQS (National Ambient Air Quality Standards) referred to in Chapter 11. For certain specific types of air pollutants, the U.S. Clean Air Act also allows the use of the *best available control technology* approach to limit their emissions. In all cases, these and similar regulatory abatement criteria need to be effectively communicated in the risk characterization document, whether explicitly or implicitly, not only to the peer reviewers but also to the public sectors as well as to all other audiences.

References

ATSDR (U.S. Agency for Toxic Substances and Disease Registry), 1994. A Primer on Health Risk Communication Principles and Practices. U.S. Department of Health and Human Services, Atlanta, Georgia, USA.

Beecher N, Harrison E, Goldstein N, McDaniel M, Field P, Susskind L, 2005. Risk Perception, Risk Communication, and Stakeholder Involvement for Biosolids Management and Research. *J. Environ. Qual.* 34:122-128.

CDC (U.S. Centers for Disease Control and Prevention), 2011a. A Framework for Patient-Centered Health Risk Assessments – Providing Health Promotion and Disease Prevention Services to Medicare Beneficiaries. U.S. Department of Health and Human Services, Atlanta, Georgia, USA.

CDC (U.S. Centers for Disease Control and Prevention), 2011b. Comments Requested in the Federal Register for the Development of Guidance for Health Risk Assessments (HRSs). U.S. Department of Health and Human Services, Atlanta, Georgia, USA.

Covello V, Allen F, 1988. Seven Cardinal Rules of Risk Communication. OPA-87-020 (leaflet). Office of Policy Analysis, Washington DC, USA.

Covello VT, Sandman PM, 2001. Risk Communication: Evolution and Revolutions. In *Solutions to an Environment in Peril* (Wolbarst AB, Ed.). Baltimore, Maryland, USA: Johns Hopkins University Press, Chapter 15.

Dong MH, Ross JH, 2001. Coping with Aggregate Pesticide Exposure Assessment: An Integration Approach. In *Hayes' Handbook of Pesticide Toxicology* (Krieger R, Ed.), 2nd Edition. San Diego, California, USA: Academic Press, Chapter 19.

Dourson ML, Stara JF, 1983. Regulatory History and Experimental Support of Uncertainty (Safety) Factors. *Regul. Toxicol. Pharmacol.* 3:224-238.

EHA (Environmental Health Australia, Ltd.), 2012. Environmental Health Risk Assessment – Guidelines for Assessing Human Health Risks from Environmental Hazards. PO Box 2222, Fortitude Valley BC, Queensland, 4006, Australia.

Klaassen CD, Eaton DL, 1991. Principles of Toxicology. In *Casarett and Doull's Toxicology: The Basic Science of Poisons* (Amdur MO, Doull J, Klaassen CD, Eds.), 4th Edition. New York, New York, USA: Pergamon Press, Chapter 2.

Li CY, Sung FC, 1999. A Review of the Healthy Worker Effect in Occupational Epidemiology. *Occup. Med. (Lond.)* 49:225-229.

NRC (U.S. National Research Council), 1983. *Risk Assessment in the Federal Government: Managing the Process.* Washington DC, USA: National Academic Press.

NRC (U.S. National Research Council), 1989. *Improving Risk Communication.* Washington DC, USA: National Academy Press.

NRC (U.S. National Research Council), 1994. *Science and Judgment in Risk Assessment.* Washington DC, USA: National Academy Press.

Ross JH, Dong MH, Krieger RI, 2000. Conservatism in Pesticide Exposure Assessment. *Regul. Toxicol. Pharmacol.* 31:53-58.

Sandman PM, 1987. Communicating Risk: Some Basics. *Health Environ. Digest* 1:3-4.

Scherer CW, Juanillo NK Jr, 2003. The Continuing Challenge of Community Health Risk Management and Communication. In *Handbook of Health Communication* (Thompson TL, Dorsey AM, Miller KL, Parrott R, Eds.). Mahwah, New Jersey, USA: Lawrence Erlbaum Associate, Chapter 11.

Shah D, 2009. Healthy Worker Effect Phenomenon. *Indian J. Occup. Environ. Med.* 13:77-79.

Suter GW II, Barnthouse LW, 1993. Assessment Concepts. In *Ecological Risk Assessment* (Suter GW II, Ed.). Boca Raton, Florida, USA: CRC Press, Chapter 2.

Thongsinthusak T, Dong MH, 2010. Mitigation Measures for Exposure to Pesticides. In *Hayes' Handbook of Pesticide Toxicology* (Krieger R, Ed.), 3rd Edition. San Diego, California, USA: Academic Press, Chapter 54.

UNEP/IPCS (United Nations Environment Programme/International Programme on Chemical Safety), 1999. Training Module No. 3 – Chemical Risk Assessment: Human Risk Assessment, Environmental Risk Assessment and Ecological Risk Assessment. WHO/PCS/99.2. World Health Organization, Geneva, Switzerland.

U.S. EPA (U.S. Environmental Protection Agency), 1986. Guidelines for Mutagenicity Risk Assessment. *Federal Register* 51:34006-34012.

U.S. EPA (U.S. Environmental Protection Agency), 1991. Guidelines for Developmental Toxicity Risk Assessment. *Federal Register* 56:63798-63826.

U.S. EPA (U.S. Environmental Protection Agency), 1992. Guidelines for Exposure Assessment. *Federal Register* 57:22888-22938.

U.S. EPA (U.S. Environmental Protection Agency), 1996. Guidelines for Reproductive Toxicity Assessment. *Federal Register* 61:56274-56322.

U.S. EPA (U.S. Environmental Protection Agency), 1998a. Guidelines for Neurotoxicity Risk Assessment. *Federal Register* 63:26926-26954.

U.S. EPA (U.S. Environmental Protection Agency), 1998b. Guidelines for Ecological Risk Assessment. *Federal Register* 63:26846-26924.

U.S. EPA (U.S. Environmental Protection Agency), 1998c. Health Effects Test Guidelines: OPPTS 870.3465 – 90-Day Inhalation Toxicity. EPA 712-C-98-204. Office of Prevention, Pesticides, and Toxic Substances, Washington DC, USA.

U.S. EPA (U.S. Environmental Protection Agency), 1998d. Health Effects Test Guidelines: OPPTS 870.4100 – Chronic Toxicity. EPA 712-C-98-210. Office of Prevention, Pesticides, and Toxic Substances, Washington DC, USA.

U.S. EPA (U.S. Environmental Protection Agency), 1998e. Health Effects Test Guidelines: OPPTS 870.5100 – Bacterial Reverse Mutation Test. EPA 712-C-98-247. Office of Prevention, Pesticides, and Toxic Substances, Washington DC, USA.

U.S. EPA (U.S. Environmental Protection Agency), 1998f. Health Effects Test Guidelines: OPPTS 870.6200 – Neurotoxicity Screening Battery. EPA 712-C-98-238. Office of Prevention, Pesticides, and Toxic Substances, Washington DC, USA.

U.S. EPA (U.S. Environmental Protection Agency), 1998g. Health Effects Test Guidelines: OPPTS 870.4200 – Carcinogenicity. EPA 712-C-98-211. Office of Prevention, Pesticides, and Toxic Substances, Washington DC, USA.

U.S. EPA (U.S. Environmental Protection Agency), 1998h. Health Effects Test Guidelines: OPPTS 870.7800 – Immunotoxicity. EPA 712-C-98-351. Office of Prevention, Pesticides, and Toxic Substances, Washington DC, USA.

U.S. EPA (U.S. Environmental Protection Agency), 2000a. Health Effects Test Guidelines: OPPTS 870.3550 – Reproduction/Developmental Toxicity Screening Test. EPA 712-C-00-367. Office of Prevention, Pesticides, and Toxic Substances, Washington DC, USA.

U.S. EPA (U.S. Environmental Protection Agency), 2000b. Risk Characterization Handbook. EPA 100-B-00-002. Science Policy Council, Washington, DC, USA.

U.S. EPA (U.S. Environmental Protection Agency), 2002. Health Effects Test Guidelines: OPPTS 870.1100 – Acute Oral Toxicity. EPA 712-C-02-190. Office of Prevention, Pesticides, and Toxic Substances, Washington DC, USA.

U.S. EPA (U.S. Environmental Protection Agency), 2003. Framework for Cumulative Risk. EPA/630/P-02/001F. Risk Assessment Forum, Washington DC, USA.

U.S. EPA (U.S. Environmental Protection Agency), 2005. Guidelines for Carcinogen Risk Assessment. EPA/630/P-03/001F. Risk Assessment Forum, Washington DC, USA.

U.S. EPA (U.S. Environmental Protection Agency), 2007a. Concepts, Methods, and Data Sources for Cumulative Health Risk Assessment of Multiple Chemicals, Exposures and Effects: A Resource Document. EPA/600/013F. Office Research and Development, Cincinnati, Ohio, USA.

U.S. EPA (U.S. Environmental Protection Agency), 2007b. Risk Communication in Action: The Risk Communication Workbook. EPA/625/R-025/003. Office Research and Development, Cincinnati, Ohio, USA.

U.S. EPA (U.S. Environmental Protection Agency), 2011. Exposure Factors Handbook 2011 Edition (Final). EPA/600/R-09/052F. National Center for Environmental Assessment, Washington DC, USA.

Review Questions

1. What are the four key components (steps) of human health-based risk assessment?
2. What are the main differences between the hazard (endpoint) identification phase in health risk assessment and the problem formulation phase in ecological risk assessment?
3. What is the main objective of hazard (endpoint) identification, and its overall task?
4. List the types (categories) of adverse health effects commonly considered in a health risk assessment.
5. Name three organizations that help harmonize the health effects test guidelines utilized by government agencies, laboratories, and the industry.
6. What is the crucial function (or task) of dose-response assessment in health risk analysis?
7. What is the implication for effect response when the dose-response slope is very steep?
8. What does (or should) the term *toxicity assessment* refer to in health risk assessment?
9. What are the (subtle) differences among exposure, applied dose, dosage, and internal dose?
10. Briefly explain why compared to environmental toxicologists, environmental epidemiologists tend to be more ready or willing to assess human exposure to environmental toxicants.
11. What is the widely received, yet not fully validated, simple algorithm for the determination of human exposure?
12. Briefly distinguish the direct and indirect measurement methods generally applied for human exposure assessment.
13. In their simplest terms, what are aggregate and cumulative exposure assessments?
14. In their simplest terms, what are health risk characterization and health risk assessment?
15. Why or how does it become a crucial uncertainty issue when the upper end of the exposure interval is not well defined for an acute toxicity test?
16. When an adverse health effect is observed in an animal study, what is likely the first thing that will come to the health risk assessor's mind in performing a toxicity assessment?
17. Match each of the health risk measures in the left column to its definition, characteristics, or application in the right column.

    (1) PEL   (a) [NOEL in concentration] ÷ [Safety Factor]
    (2) RfC   (b) direct risk measure for carcinogenic effects
    (3) BMD   (c) direct risk measure for non-cancer effects
    (4) MOE   (d) likely a more accurately quantified LO[A]EL
    (5) CPF   (e) cancer slope factor
    (6) ECR   (f) primarily used by FDA for intake of food additives
    (7) ADI   (g) primarily used by OSHA
    (8) HQ   (h) frequently used in ecological risk assessment

18. Match each of the U.S. federal agencies (left column) to the type of health risk assessment activities that it engages in (right column).

    (1) OSHA   (a) replying on self for exposure mitigation
    (2) CDC   (b) relying on regulation for exposure mitigation
    (3) U.S. EPA   (c) involving health risks in a workplace

19. What is the basic definition of perceived (subjective) risk?

20. With the proper perspective, subjective risk is as manageable as objective risk: a) TRUE; b) FALSE.
21. What appears to be the major issue with using the empirical data available to date to set values for the exposure parameters used in human exposure analysis?
22. Briefly explain why health risk assessors might need to take into account the healthy worker effect when applying the safety factor for intraspecies variation.
23. Which of the following was the classic "*DAD*" approach that many government agencies used in the past in dealing with the general public on regulatory decisions? a) define-announce-decide; b) decide-announce-defend; c) define-announce-defend; d) define-anticipate-defend.
24. List the seven cardinal rules for (health) risk communication. And briefly explain how they are related to the risk communication theories mentioned in this chapter.
25. Briefly describe the main differences between the risk-based approach and the best practical means approach in regulating environmental health hazards.

INDEX

(Acronyms are cross-referenced here only if they have been actively used in the text; otherwise, they are included here in parentheses merely to signify their common recognition/usage.)

γ-HCH (γ-hexachlorocyclohexane). *See* lindane (γ-HCH)

1

1,2-dibromo-3-chloropropane (DBCP), 26, 149, 379
1,3-dimethylol-5,5-dimethylhydantoin
   as formaldehyde-releasing ingredient, 416
1,4-dioxane, 415

2

2,3,7,8-TCDD, 58, 75, 77, 85, 87, 88, 139, 151, 275, 276, 308, 309, 310, 355, 372
2,3,7,8-tetrachlorodibenzo-*p(ara)*-dioxin. *See* 2,3,7,8-TCDD
2,4,5-T, 275, 276, 307
2,4,5-trichlorophenoxyacetic acid. *See* 2,4,5-T
2,4-D, 275, 276, 307, 393
2,4-dichlorophenoxyacetic acid. *See* 2,4-D

4

4,4′-methylenedianiline, 151

7

7-ethoxyresorufin-*o*-deethylase (EROD), 126

A

abiotic transformation. *See* transformation: chemical (abiotic)
acceptable daily intake (ADI), 407, 409, 410, 464, 465, 468, 469
acephate, 271
acetaminophen, 61, 418, 419
acetyl CoA, 121, 246
acetylation, 119, 121
acetylcholinesterase (AChE), 121, 145, 269, 270, 271, 272, 334, 391
ACGIH®. *See* American Conference of Industrial Hygienists (ACGIH®)
AChE. *See* acetylcholinesterase (AChE)
Acid Deposition Act, U.S., 182
acid rain, 20, 34, 39, 58, 59, 69, 71, 105, 162, 180, 181, 182, 184, 185
   formation of, 71

active transport. *See* toxicants: mechanisms of entry
acute beryllium disease, 248
acute respiratory distress syndrome, 280
acyl-CoA amino acid:*N*-acyltransferase, 125
additivity. *See* interaction, chemical: additivity
ADI. *See* acceptable daily intake (ADI)
advection (of environmental toxicants), 66, 69
aerodynamic diameter
   definition of, 198
aerosol(s), 196
   atmospheric, 196
   bioaerosol(s), 206, *See also* Kosa bioaerosol
   forms of, 196
Affordable Care Act, U.S., 453
aflatoxicol, 327
aflatoxin(s), 27, 60, 150, 151, 325, 328, 355, 412
   B_1, 27, 122, 141, 164, 318, 325, 327, 328, 347, 348, 349, 355
   B_2, 327, 328, 355
   G_1, 327, 328, 355
   G_2, 327, 328, 355
   M_1, 327
   M_2, 327
Agent Orange, 275, 276
aggregate dose. *See* aggregate exposure(s)
aggregate exposure(s), 161, 462, 463, 468, *See also* health risk assessment: aggregate exposure(s)
   definition of, 461
Ah hydroxylase, 307
AhR (Ah receptor). *See* receptors (proteinaceous): aryl hydrocarbon receptor (AhR)
AIDS (acquired immune deficiency syndrome), 321, 322, 323
air pollutants
   criteria air pollutants, U.S., 56, 57, 61, 177, 196, 240
   direct deposition. *See* air pollutants: dry deposition *or* wet deposition
   dry deposition, 69, 200, 211
   fate of, 67, 68, 69, 70, 71
   indirect deposition, 69
   transport of, 67, 68, 69, 70, 71
   wet deposition, 69, 181, 211, 246

air pollution, 20, 22, 33, 34, 35, 39, 45, 61, 66, 67, 137, 157, 159, 178, 182, 185, 188, 196, 203, 204, 207, 208, 209, 211, 289, 414, 440
    definition of, 20
air toxics. *See* hazardous air pollutants
airborne microbes, 205
ALAD (δ-ALAD). *See* *delta*-aminolevulinic acid dehydratase (δ-ALAD)
alanycarb, 272
aldehyde oxidase, 165
aldicarb, 272, 375, 442
aldrin, 29, 61, 85, 91, 92, 266, 267, 290, 375, 392, 393
alkaloid(s), 270, 278, 331
    batrachotoxins, 336
    epibatidines, 336
    ergot, 328
    from toads, 336
    histrionicotoxins, 336
    indolizidine, 331
    pumiliotoxins, 336
    pyrrolizidine, 331
    taxine, 331
allergic reaction(s)/effect(s). *See also* allergic response
allergic response, 141, 147, 330, *See also* toxicants: mechanism(s) of (toxic) action: adverse (indirect *or* secondary) actions
    histamine, 141
allura red AC. *See* FD&C red No. 40: food colorant
alpha (α) particle (α radiation), 253, 255
alpha cells, 369
alpha$_{2\mu}$-globulin nephropathy, 169
Alternaria, 58
aluminum (Al), 200, 211, 245, 253, 408, 409, 442
Alzheimer's disease, 18, 90, 145, 210, 245, 246, 251, 271, 408
American Conference of Industrial Hygienists (ACGIH®), 390, 391, 392
American Lung Association, 26, 416
American Public Health Association, 432
American Society for Testing and Materials, 432
Ames test, 349
amino acid conjugation(s), 121, 125
ammonia (NH_3), 178, 197, 221, 417
amygdalin, 331
An Inconvenient Truth, 40
anabolism. *See* toxicants: metabolism
androgen(s), 26, 369, 370
    adrenal, 369
anesthetic effects. *See* toxicants: toxicodynamics
aneuploidy. *See* chromosome aberration: aneuploidy

aniline, 121, 224
animal migration. *See* biotransport (animal migration)
ankylosing spondylitis, 254
antagonism. *See* interaction, chemical: antagonism
anticoagulant(s), 143, 168, 264, 278, 279, 335
    poisoning, 278
antioxidant enzyme(s), 118, 124, 125, 127
antioxidant(s), 28, 60, 118, 124, 125, 126, 127, 137, 169, 178, 348, 406
apoptosis, 148, 280, 326, 350
aquatic environment, 75, 86, 430, 435
aquatic toxicity tests, 428, 431, 432, 433
    early-life stage, 432, 433
aquatic toxicology, 428, 429, 430
    relevance to human health, 428, 430
Arctic Ocean, 289
Arctic, the, 94, 289, 299, 300, 304
Aroclor. *See* polychlorinated biphenyls (PCBs)
aromatase, 277
arsenic (As), 1, 3, 6, 55, 60, 72, 127, 150, 151, 157, 158, 238, 239, 245, 246, 247, 375, 393, 462
    arsenate reductase, 246
    arsenate(s), 55, 246
    arsenides, 246
    arsenite(s), 246
    arsenobetaine, 246
    arsine, 151, 247
    glutaredoxin. *See* arsenic (As): arsenate reductase
    lead arsenate, 246
    monosodium methyl arsenate, 246
    pentoxide, 246
    the Borgias family, 247
    trioxide, 167
aryl hydrocarbon receptor (AhR). *See* receptors (proteinaceous): aryl hydrocarbon receptor (AhR)
asbestos, 27, 57, 58, 167, 177, 347, 355, 388, 390, 393, 396, 397, 398
    actinolite, 58
    anthophyllite, 58
    chrysotile, 57, 397
    crocidolite, 58, 397
    mesothelioma, 58
    tremolite, 58
Aspergillus, 58, 322, 325, 328, 348
    flavus, 60, 325, 328, 412
    parasiticus, 325, 328, 412
asphyxiation. *See* toxicants: toxicodynamics
assessment endpoint(s), 437, 439, 454
asthma, 13, 23, 26, 56, 57, 58, 59, 60, 150, 184, 187, 208, 209, 222, 252, 337, 413, 416
asthma triggers, 60

atrazine, 79, 276, 277, 278, 373, 375
atropine, 270, 329
ATSDR. *See* U.S. Agency for Toxic Substances and Disease Registry (ATSDR)
attention deficit hyperactivity disorder (ADHD), 271
Aum Shinrikyo cult, 271, *See also* sarin: Aum Shinrikyo cult
Australia Department of the Environment and Energy (ADEE), 44, 45
autosomal dominant disorders
   definition of, 345
azinphos-methyl, 271

B

BAF. *See* bioaccumulation factor (BAF)
BAL. *See* British anti-Lewisite (BAL)
ban on artificial food dyes, 409
ban on plastic bags, 53
ban on trans fats, 49, 52, 161, 407
ban on triclosan, 422
Bangkok Fashion City Area, Thailand, 206
base excision repair (BER). *See* DNA (deoxyribonucleic acid): repair
Basel Convention, 44, 291, 440
Basel Convention on the Control of Transboundary Movements of Hazardous Wastes and Their Disposal. *See* Basel Convention
BCF. *See* bioconcentration factor (BCF)
beauvericins, 327, 328
bee sting, 333
Beijing (China), 20, 182, 203, 204
BEIVs. *See* biological exposure index values (BEIVs)
benchmark concentration (BMC), 464
benchmark dose (BMD), 464
benzaldehyde
   direct food additive, 409
benzene (C_6H_6), 55, 60, 62, 119, 150, 151, 189, 218, 219, 223, 224, 225, 229, 266, 268, 275, 276, 292, 302, 306, 395, 396, 410, 419, 434, 452
   exposures and toxic effects, 224
   sources and use, 223
benzene hexachloride (BHC). *See* hexachlorobenzene (HCB)
benzo[α]pyrene (BαP), 122, 347, 348, 349, 355, 375, 379
berylliosis, 248
beryllium (Be), 245, 247, 248, 394, 395
best available technology, 471
beta (β) particle (β radiation), 253
beta cells, 369
beta-bungarotoxin (β-bungarotoxin), 335

beta-glucosidase, 331
BHA. *See* butylated hydroxyanisole (BHA)
BHT. *See* butylated hydroxytoluene (BHT)
bioaccumulation, 67, 82, 83, 84, 86, 87, 89, 90, 92, 93, 95, 161, 241, 287, 288, 289, 294, 299, 432
   (environmental) mobility, 93, 94
   bioavailability, 93
   cases (studies), 87
   dynamic equilibrium effect, 95
   exposure hazard assessment, 84
   food chain(s)/web(s), 82
   influencing factors, 92, 93, 94, 95
   lipophilicity, 93
   metabolic potential, 93
bioaccumulation factor (BAF), 89, 288
bioconcentration, 67, 82, 84, 86, 92, 288
bioconcentration factor (BCF), 73, 84, 85, 86, 288, 305
biodegradation, 72, 75, 76, 77, 78, 294
   co-metabolism, 76
biological (biotic) transformation, 66, 72, 75, 76, *See also* transformation: biological (biotic)
biological (toxic) agents, 7, 11, 24, 48, 210, 318, 353, 355, 356, 405, *See also* (workplace) biological hazards
biological exposure index values (BEIVs), 391
biological hazards, 398
biological monitoring. *See* biomonitoring (biological monitoring)
biomagnification, 67, 82, 86, 87, 88, 89, 95, 161, 305
   cases (studies), 87
biomagnification factor (BMF), 89
biomembrane(s), 101, 102, 106, 117
   glycolipids, 102
   integral proteins, 102
   peripheral proteins, 102
   sphingolipids, 102
   structure of, 101, 102
biomonitoring (biological monitoring), 225, 391, 392, 461, 462
Bioterrorism Act, U.S., 42
biotic transformation. *See* transformation: biological (biotic)
biotransformation (of toxicants/xenobiotics). *See* toxicants: biotransformation (of xenobiotics)
biotransport (animal migration), 66, 94
birth defect(s), 6, 13, 23, 24, 25, 26, 28, 62, 148, 149, 275, 277, 362, 363, 374, 376, 377, 378, 413
   average national annual prevalence, U.S., 376
   definition of, 25, 363
   impacts and causes, 363

major structural types of, 376
metabolic disorders, 377
bisphenol A (BPA), 49, 50, 51, 59, 375, 410, 411, 419
black (soot) carbon particulate matter. *See* particulate matter (PM): of diesel
Blastomyces dermatitidis, 322
bloodborne pathogens (BBP) standard. *See* U.S. Occupational Safety and Health Administration (OSHA): bloodborne pathogens (BBP) standard
blood-brain barrier, 150, 168
BMF. *See* biomagnification factor (BMF)
bone diseases
industrial disease, 25
botulin, 325, 326
botulinum, 2, 60, 325, 326
botulinum toxin, 2, 142, *See also* botulin
botulism, 320, 325, 326
bovine spongiform encephalopathy (BSE), 11, 12, 320
brevetoxin, 21, 324, 329
Karenia brevis, 21
brilliant blue. *See* FD&C blue No. 1: food colorant
British anti-Lewisite (BAL), 247
brominated flame retardants (BFRs), 59, 298, 300, 435
brompheniramine (antihistamine), 418
Brown Cloud, 212
Brownian diffusional force, 198
BSE. *See* bovine spongiform encephalopathy (BSE)
BTEX, 419
Burkitt's lymphoma, 347
Bush, George W (former U.S. President), 290
butylated hydroxyanisole (BHA), 60, 375, 409
butylated hydroxytoluene (BHT), 60, 409

C

cadmium (Cd), 21, 28, 54, 55, 72, 79, 143, 145, 157, 158, 163, 170, 200, 201, 239, 242, 243, 244, 375, 379, 393, 394, 395
cigarette (tobacco) smoke, 243
heavy metal, 242
itai-itai, 243, 244
calcitonin, 369
calcium (Ca), 139, 143, 151, 165, 168, 182, 239, 249, 369, 408
California (USA)
ban on plastic bags, 53
ban on trans fats, 52, 161
bioaccumulation study, 88
BSE (new) case, 12
healthcare cost for asthma, 23
pesticide usage, 263, 264

Proposition 65 list, 24, 277
standards on VOCs, 219
Superfund toxic site
United Heckathorn, 54, 443, 444
triazines, 277
use of lindane, 268
wolf spiders, 333
California Department of Pesticide Regulation, 263
California disease, 323
California Environmental Protection Agency, 38
California newts, 335
Campylobacter, 320
Canadian Arctic, 87
Canadian Environmental Protection Act (CEPA), 288
cancer
characteristics of, 345
childhood type, 23
definition of, 25
epidemiology, 10
incidence in California, 24
leading cause of death, 18
metastatic (secondary), 353
of the bladder, 122, 247
of the bone, 255
of the breast, 26, 374
of the cervix, 149, 378
of the colorectum, 415
of the gastrointestinal tract, 308
of the head, 255
of the liver, 59, 122, 150, 247, 327, 331
of the lung, 26, 58, 127, 150, 160, 167, 187, 244, 247, 248, 253, 255, 397
of the nasal passage (the nose), 222, 255
of the prostate, 379
of the scrotum, 9, 25, 384
of the skin, 151
of the testicle, 26, 277
of the vagina, 378, *See also* cancer: vaginal clear cell carcinoma
of the vascular system, 272
risk, 2, 251
vaginal clear cell carcinoma, 364
cancer potency factor (CPF), 456, 458, 464, 465
cancer slope factor (CSF). *See* cancer potency factor (CPF)
Candida, 322
capsaicin, 418
carbamate(s) [CB(s)], 145, 150, 269, 271, 272
carbaryl, 271, 272, 375, 393
carbofuran, 272
carbon dioxide (CO_2), 20, 22, 55, 56, 69, 71, 112, 177,

179, 186, 190, 191, 226, 407, 415
carbon disulfide, 151, 223, 379
carbon monoxide (CO), 20, 55, 56, 123, 136, 140, 141, 148, 149, 151, 162, 168, 177, 178, 186, 188, 189, 190, 191, 203, 337
   characteristics of, 189
   effects on humans and animals, 190
   effects on plants, 191
   poisoning, 162, 168, 228
   sources of pollution, 188
   toxic effects and advisories, 190
carbon tetrachloride (CCl_4), 122, 138, 150, 151, 167, 218, 227, 305, 410
carbonyl reductase, 124
carbosulfan, 272
carboxylesterase, 124
carcinogen(s)
   definition of, 342
   environmental, 353
   vs. mutagen(s), 342
carcinogenesis, 28, 122, 148, 342, 350, 351, 354, 466
   concepts of, 350
   in relation to cell cycle, 349
   induced by free radicals, 28, 61
   mechanism of, 122, 270, 351, 352, 353
carcinogenic effects. *See* toxicants: toxicodynamics
carcinogenicity
   definition of, 342
   potential for humans, 353
cardiac glycosides. *See* glycoside(s): cardiac
Carson, Rachel, 8, 23, 33, 36, 37, 38, 261, *See also Silent Spring*
catabolism. *See* toxicants: metabolism
catalase (CAT), 118, 125
catalytic converter(s), 189, 250
   requirement, 189
cataract(s), 151, 254, 399
CEC. *See* Commission for Environmental Cooperation, the trinational (CEC)
cell cycle, 326, 349, 350, 351, 356
   checkpoints, 350, 356
   interphase, 349
cell differentiation. *See* developmental-reproductive process: cell differentiation
cell migration. *See* developmental-reproductive process: cell migration
cell proliferation, 142, 148, 350, 351, 365, *See also* developmental-reproductive process: cell proliferation
CEQ. *See* U.S. Council of Environmental Quality (CEQ)

CERCLA. *See* Comprehensive Environmental Response, Compensation, & Libility Act, U.S. (CERCLA)
cervical stenosis, 149
cetirizine (antihistamine), 418
chaparral. *See* wildlife terrestrial environment: chaparral
Charcot-Marie-Tooth neuropathy. *See* chromosome aberration: Charcot-Marie-Tooth neuropathy
chelation, 141, 142, *See also* toxicants: mechanism(s) of (toxic) action: adverse (indirect *or* secondary) actions
   therapy, 142, 167, 251
chemical (abiotic) transformation, 66, 69, 72, *See also* transformation: chemical (abiotic)
chemical biotransformation. *See* toxicants: biotransformation (of xenobiotics)
chemical disposition. *See* toxicants: disposition (of xenobiotics)
chemical persistence, 287, 288
chemical pneumonitis, 248
Chemical Risk Assessment, 451
Chernobyl nuclear explosion, Ukraine, 336
chloracne, 59, 151, 275, 303, 304, 308
chlordane, 29, 61, 91, 266, 267, 290, 375
chlordecone. *See* Kepone (chlordecone)
chlorobenzene, 395
chlorobenzilate, 265
chlorofluorocarbons, 20, 69, 70, 395
chloroform ($CHCl_3$), 151, 218, 223, 227, 230, 410
chlorosis
   of plants, 100, 137
chlorpyrifos, 270, 271
cholestasis, 150
chromated copper arsenate (CCA), 55, 246, 462, 463
chromium (Cr), 20, 28, 55, 56, 60, 166, 239, 249, 250, 251, 252, 393, 394, 411, 462
chromosome aberration, 345, 346, 347
   aneuploidy, 346
   Charcot-Marie-Tooth neuropathy, 347
   clastogenicity, 346
   cri du chat syndrome, 346
   deletion, 346
   Down syndrome, 25, 346, 376, 377
   duplication, 347
   inversion, 347
   Pick complex diseases, 347
   translocation, 347
   Turner syndrome, 346
chromosome deletion. *See* chromosome aberration: deletion

chromosome duplication. *See* chromosome aberration: duplication
chromosome inversion. *See* chromosome aberration: inversion
chromosome translocation. *See* chromosome aberration: translocation
chromosome(s), 344
    autosomes, 344
    chromatids, 344
    chromatin, 344
    definition of, 344
chronic glomerulonephritis, 396
chronic obstructive pulmonary disease (COPD), 26, 208, 209
chrysotile. *See* asbestos: chrysotile
cigarette (tobacco) smoke, 22, 25, 26, 28, 55, 122, 123, 129, 149, 183, 197, 210, 219, 221, 223, 224, 243, 348, 351, 379
cigarette (tobacco) smoking, 58, 159, 160, 167, 252, 255
    lung cancer mortality, 159
ciguatera, 330
ciguatoxin, 27, 319, 329, 330, 413
    produced by *Gambierdiscus toxicus*, 329
cilantro, 142
cisplatin, 348, 356
citric acid cycle. *See* Krebs cycle
Cladosporium, 58
clastogenicity. *See* chromosome aberration: clastogenicity
Clean Air Act, U.S., 38, 39, 43, 177, 471
Clean Water Act, U.S., 38, 39, 42, 43, 432, 433, 454, 471
cleft lip, 25, 376, 377
cleft palate, 376, 377, 378
Clostridium, 2, 60, 325, 326, 412
    botulinum, 2, 325
CMEP. *See* Ministry of Environmental Protection, China (CMEP)
coagulation (of $PM_{0.1}$). *See* particulate matter (PM): $PM_{0.1}$ (nano- and ultrafine particles): coagulation
cobalt (Co), 149, 150, 165, 204, 249, 394
cocamide DEA, 413, 415
cocamide diethanolamine. *See* cocamide DEA
Coccidioides
    immitis, 323
    posadasii, 323
codon(s)
    definition of, 344
coenzymes (of enzymes). *See* enzymes: coenzymes
cofactors (of enzymes). *See* enzymes: cofactors

colony collapse disorder, 279
Commission for Environmental Cooperation, the trinational (CEC), 44, 45
Compound 1080. *See* rodenticides: Compound 1080
Comprehensive Environmental Response, Compensation, & Liability Act, U.S. (CERCLA), 42, 43, 54, 441, 442, 443
    Superfund, 39
condensation (of $PM_{0.1}$). *See* particulate matter (PM): $PM_{0.1}$ (nano- and ultrafine particles): condensation
Consumer Product Safety Act (CPSA), U.S., 41, 43, 405
Conventional Reduced Risk Program, 279
COPD. *See* chronic obstructive pulmonary disease (COPD)
copper (Cu), 55, 62, 125, 129, 151, 165, 168, 178, 180, 182, 200, 204, 239, 244, 246, 247, 249, 250, 251, 252, 262, 395, 462
    IUDs (intrauterine devices), 251
    Menkes syndrome, 250
    oral contraceptives, 251
    Wilson's disease, 251
corrosive effects. *See* toxicants: toxicodynamics
corticosteroids, 369
Corynebacteria, 332
Cosmetic Ingredient Review, 415
coumarin(s), 274, 278, 279
    3,4-coumarin epoxide, 278
CPSA. *See* Cosumer Product Safety Act (CPSA), U.S.
CPSC. *See* U.S. Consumer Product Safety Commission (CPSC)
Creutzfeldt-Jakob disease (CJD), 11
cri du chat syndrome. *See* chromosome aberration: *cri du chat* syndrome
Crigler-Nijar syndrome, 124
criteria air pollutants. *See* air pollutants: criteria air pollutants, U.S.
crocidolite. *See* asbestos: crocidolite
Cryptosporidium, 323
CS syndrome
    effect of Type II pyrethroids, 272
cumulative dose. *See* cumulative exposure(s)
cumulative exposure(s), 161, 166, 262, 463, 468, *See also* health risk assessment: cumulative exposure(s)
    definition of, 461
cumulative risk assessment
    for atrazine, simazine, and propazine, 276
cumulative risk(s), 166
cyanuric acid, 52
cyclodiene(s), 268
CYP1A1, 124, 126, 129, 165

CYP1A2, 129, 165
CYP2D6, 127, 129, 169, 170
CYP2E1, 129, 164, 165
CYP3A4, 123, 129, 165, 169
cytochrome *c* oxidase, 140
cytochrome P450, 120, 122, 123, 124, 127, 129, 164, 165, 169, 170
    activities and locations, 123
    characteristics of, 123
    families of, 123
cytokinesis
    definition of, 350

D

DBCP. *See* 1,2-dibromo-3-chloropropane (DBCP)
DDD (dichlorodiphenyldichloroethane), 87, 265, 266
DDE (dichlorodiphenyldichloroethylene), 87, 266, 374
DDT (dichlorodiphenyltrichloroethane), 29, 36, 37, 54, 62, 85, 87, 88, 89, 91, 92, 94, 109, 265, 266, 272, 290, 374, 375, 379, 392, 393, 443, 444, 445, 446
    analogues, 373
DDTs (ΣDDTs). *See* DDT (dichlorodiphenyltrichloroethane)
*deca*brominated biphenyl (*deca*BB), 297, *See also* polybrominated biphenyls (PBBs)
*deca*brominated diphenyl ether (*deca*BDE), 59, 298, 299, 300, *See also* polybrominated diphenyl ethers (PBDEs)
decide-announce-defend (DAD) approach, 469
Deepwater Horizon BP Oil Spill of 2010, 434
deforestation, 18, 19, 22, 56
    source for carbon dioxide, 56
degradation half-life, 287, 289
    of environmental health concern, 288
delayed neuropathy, 270
Delhi (India), 182, 212, 262
delta-aminolevulinic acid dehydratase (δ-ALAD), 145, 240, 241
dengue fever, 332
dermal absorption/penetration. *See* toxicants: uptake of, by humans
dermophyte, 322
desert. *See* wildlife terrestrial environment: desert
development policies and programs (DPP), 452, 453
developmental toxicants
    definition of, 374
developmental-reproductive cycle, 362, 365, *See also* developmental-reproductive process
    for humans, 365, 366
developmental-reproductive effects, 374

developmental-reproductive process, 362, 366, *See also* developmental-reproductive cycle
    cell differentiation, 365
    cell migration, 365
    cell proliferation, 365
    organogenesis, 365, 366
    predifferential period, 365, 366
developmental-reproductive system, 362, *See also* developmental-reproductive progress *or* cycle
dextromethorphan (DXM), 141
diabetes (mellitus), 13, 18, 57, 151, 369, 380
dialkylpiperidine hemolytic factors, 334
diazinon, 270, 271, 355, 393, 437
dichlorodiphenyldichloroethane. *See* DDD (dichlorodiphenyldichloroethane)
dichlorodiphenyldichloroethylene. *See* DDE (dichlorodiphenyldichloroethylene)
dichlorodiphenyltrichloroethane. *See* DDT (dichlorodiphenyltrichloroethane)
dichloromethane (DCM). *See* methylene chloride (MC)
dichlorvos, 270, 271
dicofol, 265, 375
dieldrin, 27, 29, 54, 62, 85, 91, 92, 266, 267, 290, 374, 375, 393, 445, 446
diesel, 178, 189, 197
    exhaust fumes, 207, 210
    fuel, 59, 60, 200
    particulate matter, 210
Dietary Supplement Health and Education Act, U.S. (DSHEA), 408
dietary supplements, 408, 409
    definition of, 408
diethylstilbestrol (DES), 26, 60, 355, 364, 370, 373, 375, 377, 378, 442
diffusion (of environmental toxicants), 66, 69, 72, 75
Digitalis purpurea, 330
dioxins. *See* polychlorinated dibenzo-*p(ara)*-dioxins (PCDDs)
diphenylhydantoin, 378
direct chemical reversal. *See* DNA (deoxyribonucleic acid): repair
distal (convoluted) tubule, 111
DNA (deoxyribonucleic acid), 2, 122, 123, 140, 141, 148, 149, 224, 225, 269, 321, 326, 342, 344, 345, 346, 347, 349, 357
    damage, 136, 348, 350, 351, 354, 356, 357, 358
    definition of, 342
    hotspots on, 345
    metabolism, 357
    repair, 350, 351, 354, 357

structure of, 343
transcription, 373
DNA adduct(s), 122, 141, 225, 348, 349
DNA AP endonuclease. *See* DNA (deoxyribonucleic acid): repair
DNA damage tolerance mechanism. *See* DNA (deoxyribonucleic acid): repair
DNA glycosylase. *See* DNA (deoxyribonucleic acid): repair
DNA ligase. *See* DNA (deoxyribonucleic acid): repair
DNA polymerase. *See* DNA (deoxyribonucleic acid): repair
DNA repair mechanism. *See* DNA (deoxyribonucleic acid): repair
DNA TLS (translesion synthesis) polymerases. *See* DNA (deoxyribonucleic acid): repair
DNA topoisomerases. *See* DNA (deoxyribonucleic acid): repair
DNA translesion synthesis. *See* DNA (deoxyribonucleic acid): repair
domoic acid, 324, 329, 413
Donora, Pennsylvania (USA), 137, 178, 207
dose-response assessment, 457, 463, *See also* health risk assessment: dose-response assessment
dose-response curve, 456
dose-response relationship, 1, 3, 5, 146, 147, 156, *See also* health risk assessment: dose-response relationship
DOT. *See* U.S. Department of Transportation (DOT)
Down syndrome. *See* chromosome aberration: Down syndrome
doxylamine (antihistamine), 418
drinking water contaminants, 49, 59, 60
Drosophila (flies), 125
drug (chemical) interaction, 405, 409, 418, 419
dry deposition. *See* air pollutants: dry deposition
DSHEA. *See* Dietary Supplement Health and Education Act, U.S. (DSHEA)
dumb cane (*Dieffenbachia*), 331
dust storm(s)
in Beijing (China), 204
in Sydney (Australia), 204
north Africa, 206
dysplastic phase. *See* carcinogenesis: mechanism of

E

Eastern red-spotted newts, 335
Ebola (virus), 11, 13, 48, 400
Filoviridae, 11
occupational disease, 400
ecological risk assessment, 82, 84, 437, 438, 440, 446, 451, 453, 454, 455
assessment endpoint(s), 454
effects analysis, 439
exposure analysis, 438, 439
framework of, 438, 451
hazard quotient (HQ), 440
problem formulation, 438, 439, 454
risk characterization, 438, 439
ecological toxicology. *See* ecotoxicology
ecotoxicology, 3, 7, 8, 9, 10, 17, 100, 428
definition of, 3, 8
human health aspects, 428
vs. environmental toxicology, 8, 100
ECR. *See* excess cancer risk (ECR)
ED (erectile dysfunction). *See* reproductive damage (disorders): ED (erectile dysfunction)
EDCs. *See* endocrine-disrupting chemicals (EDCs)
edetate disodium. *See* EDTA (ethylenediaminetetraacetate)
EDTA (ethylenediaminetetraacetate), 142
EEA. *See* European Environmental Agency (EEA)
EEDs. *See* environmental endocrine disruptors (EEDs)
EHIA. *See* environmental health impact assessment (EHIA)
electronic waste. *See* e-waste
elimination rate constant. *See* toxicants: toxicokinetics
emphysema, 26, 27, 187, 243
Employee Right-To-Know Act, U.S., 398
encephalitis, 321, 322, 363
Japanese, 322
rabies, 322
St. Louis, 322
Endangered Species Act, U.S., 434
endocrinal effects
examples of, 375
endocrine disruption, 135, 362, 364, 370, 372, 373, 374, 421
concepts, 364
mechanisms, 372
modes, 372
neuoendocrine disruption, 278
endocrine system (network), 29, 61, 362, 366
endocrine-disrupting chemicals (EDCs), 362, 364, 372, 373, 374
examples of, 375
types of, 373
endocrine-reproductive system, 362, 365
endocytosis. *See* toxicants: mechanisms of entry
endosulfan, 266, 290, 375, 379
endotoxins, 142, 324

endrin, 29, 163, 266, 290
Entamoeba histolytica, 323
Enterobius follicularis, 323
enterohepatic circulation, 107, 111
environmental carcinogenesis, 349
environmental carcinogens, 19, 49, 353
   examples of, 355
environmental change(s), 17, 18, 19, 22, 34
environmental contaminants, 10, 22, 23, 34, 44, 45, 48, 49, 80, 99, 116, 429, 434
   definition of, 50
   grouping of, 49, 50
environmental disease(s)
   concerns, 17, 19, 23, 24
   costs, 11, 23
   definition of, 22
   grouping of, 25, 28
   incidence and spectrum, 11, 19, 22, 23
environmental endocrine disruptors (EEDs), 49, 59, 60, 362
environmental health, 9, 11, 17, 18, 19, 36, 40, 41, 42, 44, 45, 48, 49, 150, 156, 168, 198, 202, 217, 218, 239, 249, 318, 336, 372, 440, 441, 452, 454
   definition of, 40
   discipline/science of, 17
   world's (WHO's) perspective, 19
environmental health impact assessment (EHIA), 453
environmental health laws, 40
   in the United States, 42, 43
   international, 44, 46
environmental health risk assessment, 10, 319, 451, 463, *See also* health risk assessment
environmental justice
   definition of, 38
environmental movement(s), 36, 37, 38, 39, 385, 413
environmental mutagenesis, 342, 345
environmental mutagens, 345, 347
   examples of, 348
environmental persistence, 287, 288, 289
environmental pollutants. *See* environmental contaminants
environmental pollution, 9, 11, 13, 17, 33, 34, 35, 36, 38, 45, 267, 337, 405, 413, 429, 452
   concerns, 36, 38, 429
   costs in China, 34
   definition of, 33, 36
   impacts, 34, 35, 38
   perceptions, 35
   sources of, 218
   U.S. EPA's responsibility, 38
environmental reproductive toxicants, 377

environmental risk assessment
   framework of, 451
environmental sciences, 8
   definition of, 17
environmental teratogen(s), 49, 365, 374, 376
environmental toxicants, 48
   concerns, 11, 54
environmental toxicology, 3, 17, 35, 48, 49, 50, 55, 77, 100, 155, 156, 239, 244, 245, 264, 281, 306, 318, 319, 385, 428, 429, 451
   ally with epidemiology, 9
   definition of, 3, 11
   importance, 10, 19, 24
   knowledge for/of. *See* environmental toxicology: principles for/of
   principles for/of, 3, 4, 5, 6, 7
   scope, 1, 11
   vs. ecotoxicology, 8, 100
   with pesticide residues, 261
enzymatic activities, 136
   disruption, 143, 144
enzymes
   characteristics of, 118
   coenzyme(s), 118, 119, 121, 127, 128, 130, 143, 164
   coenzymes
      inhibition of, 143
   cofactor(s), 118, 125, 126, 127, 128, 129, 143, 164, 165
   cofactors
      inhibition of, 143
   inducers of, 128, 129
   inhibitors of, 128, 129, 145, 333
ephedrine (decongestant), 418
epidemiology, 2, 7, 9, 17, 388, 460
   analytical, 9
   definition of, 9
   descriptive, 9
   environmental, 10
   exposure analysis, 458, 459, 460
   human exposure assessment, 10, *See also* health risk assessment: exposure analysis
   occupational, 10
epigenetic carcinogen(s)
   definition of, 351
epinephrine, 230, 232, 369, 370, 371
epoxide hydrolase, 124
EPSP synthase, 280
erectile dysfunction (ED). *See* reproductive damage (disorders): ED (erectile dysfunction)
ergotism, 328

Erin Brockovich, 20, 28, 250
Escherichia coli (E. coli), 60, 320, 326
estradiol, 370, 371, 373, 380
estrogen(s), 25, 26, 51, 277, 303, 364, 369, 370, 372, 373, 374
    functions of, 370
ethiofencarb, 272
ethion, 271
ethylan, 265
ethylene dibromide, 26
ethylene glycol, 6
ethylene oxide, 379, 415
ethylenediaminetetraacetate. *See* EDTA (ethylenediaminetetraacetate)
EU. *See* European Union (EU)
European Commission (EC), 288
European Environmental Agency (EEA), 44, 45
European Union (EU), 45, 218, 222, 276, 299, 385, 409, 456
    Framework Directive, 386
eutrophication, 185
e-waste, 18, 21, 49, 50, 54, 297, 298, 299, 302
    recycling, 89, 379
excess cancer risk (ECR), 458, 464, 465
excess lifetime cancer risk. *See* excess cancer risk (ECR)
exotoxin(s), 60, 142, 324, 326, 412
Exposure Factors Handbook, 468
exposure limit values, 390
    PEAK, 391
    STEL, 391, 464
    TWA, 390, 391, 392, 393, 464
Exxon Valdez
    oil pollution incident, 42

F

facilitated diffusion. *See* toxicants: mechanisms of entry
FD&C Act. *See* Federal Food, Drug, and Cosmetic Act (FD&C Act), U.S.
FD&C blue No. 1
    food colorant, 409
FD&C red No. 40
    food colorant, 409
FD&C yellow No. 5
    food colorant, 409
FDA. *See* U.S. Food and Drug Administration (FDA)
fecal excretion. *See* toxicants: excretion/elimination (of xenobiotics)
Federal Employers Liability Act, U.S., 385
Federal Environment(al) Agency, Germany (UBA), 44, 45
Federal Food, Drug, and Cosmetic Act (FD&C Act), U.S., 42, 43, 261, 404
Federal Hazardous Substances Act, U.S. (FHSA), 42, 43, 452
Federal Insecticide, Fungicide, and Rodenticide Act, U.S. (FIFRA), 38, 39, 42, 43, 261, 423
fenthion, 271
Fenton reaction, 137, 138
FHSA. *See* Federal Hazardous Substances Act, U.S. (FHSA)
fiberglass. *See* synthetic mineral fibers (SMFs)
fibrogenic dust, 397
Fick's law of diffusion, 103
    rate of diffusion, 103
FIFRA. *See* Federal Insecticide, Fungicide, and Rodenticide Act, U.S. (FIFRA)
filtration. *See* toxicants: mechanisms of entry
fine particles. *See* particulate matter (PM): $PM_{0.1-2.5}$ (fine particles)
first-pass effect, 109
flow-through test. *See* aquatic toxicity tests
fluoroacetate, 281, *See also* rodenticides: Compound 1080
fluorocitrate, 144
fluorosis
    dental, 408
    skeletal, 408
follicle-stimulating hormone (FSH), 367, 369
fonofos, 271
food (toxicants)
    additives, 6, 18, 41, 60, 245, 410
    concerns, 404
    contaminants, 60, 404, 405, 406, 412, 413
    direct additives, 60, 404, 405, 406
        anticaking agents, 406, 407, 408
        antioxidants, 407, 409
        colorants, 406, 407, 409, 416
        dietary supplements, 408, 409
        emulsifiers, 406, 407, 408
        flavoring agents, 406, 407, 409
        leavening agents, 409
        preservatives, 60, 178, 348, 406, 407, 409
        stabilizers, 406, 407, 408
        thickeners, 406, 407
        vitamins and minerals, 406, 407
    indirect additives, 404, 405, 406, 410
        agrochemicals, 411, 412
    mitigation and prevention, 422, 423
    persistent toxic substances in seafood, 420
    pesticides, 413

source categories, 406
toxic metals, 413
toxins, 412
food additives, 6, 18, 22, 245, 404, 405, 406, 410, 415, 456, 464, 469
    definition of, 404
    functions of, 60
food allergies, 407
Food and Agriculture Organization of the United Nations (FAO), 22, 90, 464
food chain(s). *See* food chain(s)/web(s)
food chain(s)/web(s), 3, 12, 29, 67, 82, 83, 84, 86, 248, 252, 265, 301, 413, 431
    prey-predator relationships, 82, 83
    trophic level, 83
food infection
    definition of, 412
food intoxication, 423
    definition of, 412
food poisoning(s), 242, 320, 321, 325, 326, 329, 405, 412, 423
    definition of, 412
    scombrotoxic, 330
    seafood, 330
    Staphylococcal, 325
Food Quality Protection Act, U.S. (FQPA), 42, 43, 161, 166, 261, 262, 275, 404, 468
food web(s). *See* food chain(s)/web(s)
foodborne illness(es), 320, 326, 330, 404, 412, 413
forests. *See also* wildlife terrestrial environment: forests
    environmental importance, 22
formaldehyde (CH_2O), 55, 56, 60, 218, 219, 220, 221, 222, 223, 355, 393, 416, 417, 442
    exposures and toxic effects, 222
    sources and use, 220
FQPA. *See* Food Quality Protection Act, U.S. (FQPA)
fragrances, 53, 414, 415, 416
    sick building syndrome, 416, *See also* sick building syndrome
    toxic household products, 416
frameshift mutation, 346
Framework for Ecological Risk Assessment, 437
free radical(s), 28, 59, 61, 122, 125, 135, 136, 137, 138
    scavengers, 125
free radical-mediated cellular damage, 127, *See also* toxicants: mechanism(s) of (toxic) action: free radical-mediated actions
freshwater biome(s), 431
    lentic, 431
    lotic, 431
    wetlands, 431
FSH. *See* follicle-stimulating hormone (FSH)
Fukushima nuclear crisis (in Japan), 336
fumonisin(s), 325, 327, 328
    B_1, 327
    B_2, 327

G

gametogenesis, 365
gamma (γ) particle (γ radiation), 253
gamma-aminobutyric acid (γ-GABA), 266, 267, 272
    neurotransmitter, 266, 268
    receptor, 266, 268
gastrointestinal absorption. *See* toxicants: uptake of, by humans
gene mutation. *See* point mutation *or* intragenic mutation
gene(s), 12, 123, 139, 170, 346, 347, 350, 351
    definition of, 344
    DNA repair genes, 351
    expression, 124, 139, 169, 372, 375
    oncogene(s), 344, 351
    proto-oncogene(s), 344, 351
    tumor suppressor genes, 351
General Industry Air Contaminants Standard, U.S., 389
generally recognized as safe (GRAS), 406, 407
genetic polymorphism, 123, 127
genome
    definition of, 344
genotoxic carcinogen(s). *See* ultimate carcinogen(s)
germinal stage (germinal period). *See* developmental-reproductive process: predifferentiation period
Giardia lamblia, 323
Gilbert's syndrome, 124
ginger Jake paralysis, 270
global cooling effect, 197
global warming, 19, 40, 56, 70
glomerular filtration, 110, 111
glucagon, 369, 371
glucuronidation, 119, 121, 122
glucuronosyltransferase (UGT), 129
glutathione (GSH), 119, 121, 130
    conjugation, 121
    peroxidase (GPx), 125, 126, 127
    S-transferase (GST), 127, 128, 165
glycol ether(s), 26, 379
glycoside(s), 278, 329, 330, 331
    cardiac, 62, 330
    cyanogenic, 331

glycosylphosphatidylinositol. *See* malaria
glyphosate, 277, 279, 280
Gore, Al (former U.S. Vice-President), 40, 364
GRAS. *See* generally recognized as safe (GRAS)
grasshopper effect, 68, 288
Great Lakes basin, U.S., 289
greenhouse effect, 20, 56, 69, 70
greenhouse gases, 19, 20, 69
Guidelines for Ecological Risk Assessment, 437
Guillain-Barré syndrome, 13
guinea worm (*Dracunculus medinensis*), 318, 323
Gulf War Oil Spill of 1991, 434
Guyana
    health concerns, 23

H

H1N1 (virus), 11, 12, 13, 36, 48, 205
HAB (harmful algal bloom). *See* red tide pollution
Haber's law, 160
Haemophilus influenzae, 320
Harbin (China)
    chemical explosion, 224
harmful physical agents. *See* physical hazards
Hazard Communication Standard, 398, 413, *See also*
    U.S. Occupational Safety and Health
    Administration (OSHA): Hazard Communication
    Standard
hazard identification. *See* health risk assessment:
    hazard (endpoint) identification
hazard quotient (HQ), 439, 440, 464, 465
    computation and interpretation, 440
hazardous air pollutants, 177
hazardous waste pollution, 440, 441, 443, *See also*
    hazardous waste toxicology
    relevance to human health, 429
hazardous waste toxicology, 428, 429, *See also*
    hazardous waste pollution
hazardous waste(s), 21, 42, 43, 54, 62, 218, 245, 248,
    250, 291, 429, 440, 441, 442, 443, 446
    characteristics waste, 441
    definition of, 440
    F-list, 441
    K-list, 442
    listed (hazardous) waste, 441, 442
    P-list, 442
    U-list, 442
    universal wastes, 442
HBCD. *See hexa*bromocyclododecane (HBCD)
HCBD. *See hexa*chlorobutadiene (HCBD)
Health Canada, 44, 45, 294, 456
health effects tests
    categories of, 455
    guidelines, 455, 456
health risk
    definition of, 439, 469
health risk assessment, 3, 7, 10, 84, 146, 156, 166, 281,
    319, 407, 451, 452, 453, 454, 455, 456, 457, 458,
    459, 460, 461, 463, 465, 468, 469, 470
    activities, 7, 451, 452, 468
    aggregate exposure(s), 468
    assessment endpoint(s), 454
    categories of animal toxicity studies, 455
    components, 454
    cumulative exposure(s), 468
    dose-response assessment, 7, 453, 456
    dose-response curve, 457
    dose-response relationship, 3, 457
    exposure analysis, 453, 458, 459, 460, 461, 462,
        463, 466, 467
        aggregate and cumulative exposures, 462
        basic algorithm, 461
        direct and indirect measurements, 460
        past and current perspectives, 459
    exposure assessment, 7, *See also* health risk
        assessment: exposure analysis
    framework of, 7, 451
    hazard (endpoint) identification, 7, 10, 453, 454,
        455, 466
    health risk characterization, 3, 7, 453, 454, 463,
        469, 470, 471
    health risk communication, 469, 470
    health risk measures, 463, 464, 465
    health risk perception, 468, 469, 471
    role of epidemiology, 10
    subtle aspects, 453
    toxicity assessment, 439, 454, 456, 465, 466, 467
    uncertainty and safety factors, 465, 466, 468
health risk characterization. *See* health risk
    assessment: health risk characterization
health risk communication. *See* health risk assessment:
    health risk communication
health risk measures. *See* health risk assessment:
    health risk measures
health risk perception, 35, *See also* health risk
    assessment: health risk perception
    definition of, 469
healthy worker effect, 468
heavy metal(s), 28, 157, 170, 239, 244, 248, 391
    definition of, 239
    secondary (pseudo), 244, 245
helminthes. *See* pathogenic (microbial) agents:
    parasites

Henle-Koch postulates, 320
hepatic excretion. *See* toxicants: excretion/elimination (of xenobiotics)
heptachlor, 29, 75, 85, 266, 267, 290, 375
*hexa*brominated biphenyl (*hexa*BB), 290, 295, 297, 298, *See also* polybrominated biphenyls (PBBs)
*hexa*bromocyclododecane (HBCD), 290, 300, 301, 435, *See also* polybrominated cyclododecanes (PBCDs)
   characteristics, uses, and sources, 300
   environmental health concerns, 301
hexachlorobenzene (HCB), 29, 85, 91, 268, 269, 290
*hexa*chlorobutadiene (HCBD), 290, 305, 306, *See also* polychlorinated butadienes (PCBDs)
   characteristics, uses, and sources, 305
   environmental health concerns, 306
hexachlorocyclohexane (HCH), 163, 268, 269, 290
Himalayan rhubarb, 330
histones, 344
Histoplasma capsulatum, 323
HIV (human immunodeficiency virus), 151, 320, 321, 355
holoenzyme(s), 128, 129
honey bee depopulation syndrome. *See* colony collapse disorder
hormonal disruption. *See* endocrine disruption
hormone(s), 53, 60, 104, 136, 139, 151, 163, 351, 362, 364, 365, 367, 369, 370, 372, 373, 412
   amine, 370
   peptide, 370
   sex, 26, 51, 122, 277, 364, 368, 369, 370, 380
   steroid, 139, 370, 373
hornet stings, 333
household (toxic) substances, 61, *See also* toxic household products
HQ. *See* hazard quotient (HQ)
Human and Ecological Risk Assessment, 439
human endocrine system
   location of glands, 368
human exposure assessment. *See* health risk assessment: exposure analysis
human herpesviruses (HHVs), 322
human papillomavirus(es), 149, 348, 355
human risk assessment
   framework of, 451
humidity, 161, 162, 206, 392
   effects of, 162
hyaluronidases, 334, 335
hydrogen cyanide (HCN), 140, 148, 151, 264
hydrogen fluoride (HF), 100, 136, 178, 179
hydrogen sulfide (H_2S), 178, 179
hydroxyl radical (HO·), 28, 70, 71, 137, 180, 183, 184, 186, 217, 221, 228, 229, 231, 356
Hypericum, 331
   perforatum (H. perforatum), 331
hyperplastic phase. *See* carcinogenesis: mechanism of
hypersensitivity. *See* toxicants: toxicodynamics
hypervitaminosis A, 28

I

IARC. *See* International Agency for Research on Cancer (IARC)
idiosyncratic reaction(s)/effect(s), 5, 146
imidacloprid, 279
imidazolidinyl urea
   as formaldehyde-releasing ingredient, 416
impotence. *See* reproductive damage (disorders): ED (erectile dysfunction)
incidence (of disease)
   definition of, 9
indandione(s), 278, 279
indoleacetic acid, 275
indoxacarb, 272
industrial diseases
   classic, 384
Industrial Revolution Period, 384
industrialization, 19, 23, 307, 453
infection
   definition of, 319
   vs. infectious disease, 319
infectious disease
   definition of, 319
   vs. infection, 319
infertility. *See* reproductive damage (disorders): infertility
inhalable [coarse] particles. *See* particulate matter (PM): PM_{10} (inhalable [coarse] particles)
inhalable [fine] particles. *See* particulate matter (PM): $PM_{2.5}$ (inhalable [fine] particles)
inhalable coarse particles. *See* particulate matter (PM): $PM_{2.5-10}$ (inhalable coarse particles)
initiation phase. *See* carcinogenesis: mechanism of
insulin, 369, 370, 371
integral proteins. *See* biomembrane(s): integral proteins
interaction, chemical
   additivity, 6, 146, 166, 167
   antagonism, 6, 146, 166, 167, 168
   potentiation, 6, 146, 166, 167
   synergism, 6, 146, 166, 167
Intergovernmental Panel on Climate Change (IPCC), 19, 38, 40

International Agency for Research on Cancer (IARC), 222, 225, 227, 228, 230, 232, 241, 242, 244, 246, 247, 248, 250, 251, 253, 255, 266, 267, 268, 269, 272, 274, 276, 277, 278, 280, 294, 297, 299, 301, 305, 306, 308, 353, 354, 355, 397
    classification of carcinogenicity potential, 354
    examples of human carcinogenicity potential, 355
    objectives of, 353
International Conference on Harmonization (ICH), 456
International Programme on Chemical Safety (IPCS), 302, 304, 306, 310, 451
International Standardization Organization, 432
International Union of Pure and Applied Chemistry (IUPAC), 229, 230
INTER-NOISE Congresses, 338
interphase, 349, 350, *See also* cell cycle: interphase
interstrand crosslink. *See* DNA (deoxyribonucleic acid): damage
intestinal excretion. *See* toxicants: excretion/elimination (of xenobiotics)
intragenic mutation, 345, 346
intrastrand crosslink. *See* DNA (deoxyribonucleic acid): damage
IPCS. *See* International Programme on Chemical Safety (IPCS)
iron (Fe), 140, 165, 204, 239, 249, 250, 251, 252, 395, 408, 441, 442
    deficiency, 249
    overdose, 249
    titanium, 200
irritation. *See* toxicants: toxicodynamics
Irving Selikoff
    on environmental disease, 23
islets of Langerhans, 369
itai-itai (byo), 56, 243, *See also* cadmium (Cd): *itai-itai*
IUPAC. *See* International Union of Pure and Applied Chemistry (IUPAC)

J

Jack Lewis
    The Birth of EPA, 38
James River (pollution), 267
Jinzū River basin, Japan, 243
JMOE. *See* Ministry of the Environment, Japan (JMOE)

K

Kepone (chlordecone), 26, 128, 129, 266, 267, 268, 290, 375, 379, 442

Kosa bioaerosol, 207
K_{ow}. *See* octanol-water partition coefficient (K_{ow})
Krebs cycle, 144, 151, 246, 281

L

lactic acidosis, 409
LC_{50} (median lethal concentration), 2, 158, 161, 306, 439, 456
LD_{50} (median lethal dose), 2, 161, 169, 439, 441, 456
lead (Pb), 1, 3, 20, 21, 26, 50, 51, 54, 55, 56, 57, 109, 145, 168, 177, 200, 239, 240, 241, 245, 246, 248, 251, 375, 384, 391, 393, 394, 419, 420, 421, 442
    acetate, 241
    acute poisoning, 240
    biological exposure index value, 391
    classic industrial disease, 384
    compounds, 26, 177, 200, 240, 241, 379
    criteria air pollutant, U.S., 177
    endocrine disruptor, 375
    glazes
        classic industrial disease, 25, 384
    heavy metal, 240
    on children's jewelry and toys, 51, 161, 240, 420
    on paint, 379
    phosphate, 241
    poisoning (plumbism), 23, 240, 241, 384, 420, 421
    pollution, 145
    reproductive effects, 240
    spent (lead) shot, 433
    systemic poison, 240
    tetraethyl, 223
leaf
    internal anatomy, 104
lecithin, 407, 408
lectin, 330
Legionella pneumophila, 384, 399
legionellosis, 384, 399
Legionnaires' disease, 205, 384, 399
    Norway incidence, 399
    Philadelphia (Pennsylvania, USA) incidence, 384, 399
leukemia, 151, 167, 222, 224, 225, 230, 275, 344, 378, 396
    acute nonlymphocytic, 225
    chronic lymphocytic, 275
    chronic myeloid, 127
lily of the valley (*Convallaria majalis*), 330
lindane (γ-HCH), 27, 62, 85, 268, 269, 290, 373, 375, 393
linoleic acid, 164
lipid peroxidation, 122, 137, 165, 304

lipophilicity, 72, 82, 93, 95, 163, 265, 395, 422
lizards, 334, 335, 436
    alligator, 436
    Gila monster (*Heloderma suspectum*), 335
    Komodo dragons, 335
    Mexican beaded (*Heloderma horridum*), 335
LO[A]EL. *See* lowest observed [adverse] effect level (LO[A]EL)
London (UK), 20, 157, 178, 183, 203, 207
    cancer of the scrotum, 384
London fog of 1952, 18, 20, 137, 157, 178
long-range transport (LRT), 29, 67, 94, 186, 288, 289, 290, 294, 300
loratadine (antihistamine), 418
Los Angeles (USA), 20, 182, 188, 203, 210, 211
Love Canal (tragedy), 18, 21, 39, 42, 54, 429, 430, 442
lowest observed [adverse] effect level (LO[A]EL), 5, 456, 457, 458, 464
lung cancer mortality. *See* cigarette (tobacco) smoking *or* (exposure to) radium (Ra)
luteinizing hormone (LH), 367, 368, 369, 380

M

MAC. *See* maximum allowable concentration (MAC)
mad-cow disease. *See* bovine spongiform encephalopathy (BSE)
magnesium (Mg), 143, 165, 168, 239, 249
    oxide, 297, 395
    stearates, 407
malaria, 23, 37, 318, 323, 324, 332
    glycosylphosphatidylinositol (the toxin), 324
    Plasmodium falciparum (producing the toxin), 324
malathion, 27, 270, 271, 375, 393, 437
malnutrition, 163, 164
manganese (Mn), 125, 200, 249, 252, 389, 395
man-made mineral fibers (MMMFs). *See* synthetic mineral fibers (SMFs)
Mantle cell lymphoma, 347
margin of exposure (MOE), 464, 465
marine biome(s), 430, 431
    abyssal, 430
    coral reefs, 430
    ocean regions, 430
    oceanic, 430
    pelagic, 430
mastitis, 321
Material Safety Data Sheet (MSDS), 161, 413, 415
maximum allowable concentration (MAC), 390
maximum contaminant level (MCL), 218, 277, 464
MCL. *See* maximum contaminant level (MCL)

mechanism(s) of (toxic) action. *See* toxicants: mechanism(s) of (toxic) action
median lethal concentration. *See* LC_{50} *(median lethal concentration)*
medications
    side effects, 141
meiosis, 346, 350
    definition of, 350
melamine, 51, 52, 221
    dinnerware, 49, 52
melatonin, 162, 163, 368, 370, 371
Menkes syndrome, 250, *See also* copper (Cu): Menkes syndrome
Merck Veterinary Manual, 24
mercury (Hg), 1, 2, 21, 49, 51, 52, 53, 55, 57, 67, 68, 72, 77, 78, 82, 142, 145, 149, 150, 151, 239, 241, 242, 243, 262, 318, 375, 378, 391, 393, 395, 413, 434, 442
    biological exposure index value, 391
    heavy metal, 241
    level in tuna, 49, 52
    methylmercury, 82, 241, 242, 377, 378, 435
    Minamata syndrome, 57, 242
    poisoning (mercurialism), 242
MERS (Middle East respiratory syndrome), 12, 48
mesothelioma. *See* asbestos: mesothelioma
MET. *See* methyltransferase (MET)
metabolism, 25, 56, 60, 88, 112, 118, 151, 249, 281, 357, 362, 363, 367, 372, 373, 399, 408, *See also* toxicants: metabolism
    cellular (as in Krebs cycle), 281
    co-metabolism (type of biodegradation), 76
    DNA, 357
    metabolic disorders (birth defects), 363
    oxidative, 169
metal fume fever, 395
metal(s)
    definition of, 238
    environmental health concerns, 239
    heavy metals, 239
    periodic table, 238
    radioactive metals, 253
    secondary (pseudo) heavy metals, 244
    toxic trace metals, 248
metalloid(s), 55, 238, 246, 247
    definition of, 238
metallothionein (MT), 244
    Cd-MT binding, 244
metastasis, 345, 353, *See also* carcinogenesis: mechanism of
methane (CH_4), 20, 69, 221

met-hemoglobin (metHb), 151
methlochlor, 265
methomyl, 272
methoxychlor, 128, 129, 265, 375, 379, 393, 417
methyl bromide, 177, 262
methyl methanesulfonate, 379
methyl *tert(iary)*-butyl ether (MTBE), 60, 218, 225, 226, 227
    exposures and toxic effects, 226
    sources and use, 225
methylation, 119, 121
methylene chloride (MC), 218, 219, 227, 228, 230, 231, 393, 395, 410, 419
    exposures and toxic effects, 228
    sources and use, 227
methylmercury. *See* mercury (Hg): methylmercury
methyltransferase (MET), 121, 125
MGK-264, 273
microbic (microbial) invasion, 141, 142, 319
microcephaly, 13, 346, 377, 378, 421
Middle East respiratory syndrome. *See* MERS (Middle East respiratory syndrome)
Minamata syndrome. *See* mercury (Hg): Minamata syndrome
Mine Safety and Health Act, U.S., 388
mineral
    definition of, 239
mineral wool. *See* synthetic mineral fibers (SMFs)
Ministry of Environmental Protection, China (CMEP), 44, 45
Ministry of the Environment, Japan (JMOE), 44, 45
mirex, 29, 62, 94, 123, 128, 129, 266, 267, 290, 375
mismatch repair. *See* DNA (deoxyribonucleic acid): repair
mitosis, 349, 350, 351, 352, 365
    definition of, 350
mobility of toxicant. *See* toxicants: (environmental) mobility
MOE. *See* margin of exposure (MOE)
molecular complexation. *See* chelation
molybdenum (Mo), 165, 249
monosodium glutamate (MSG)
    direct food additive, 409
Montevideo (Latin America)
    PM_{10} levels, 204
Montreal Protocol, 44, 262
Montreal Protocol on Substances That Deplete the Ozone Layer. *See* Montreal Protocol
MOS (margin of safety). *See* margin of exposure (MOE)
MSDS. *See* Material Safety Data Sheet (MSDS)
MSHA. *See* U.S. Mine Safety and Health Administration (MSHA)
MT. *See* metallothionein (MT)
MTBE. *See* methyl *tert(iary)*-butyl ether (MTBE)
Mumbai (India), 203
mushroom poisoning (mycetism), 325
mutagen(s), 342, 345, 347, 349
    categories of, 349
    definition of, 342
    environmental, 347
    examples of, 348
    vs. carcinogen(s), 342
mutagenesis, 148, 342, 345, 348, 354, 466
    concepts, 345
mutagenicity, 122, 345, 349, 407
    definition of, 342
mycetism. *See* mushroom poisoning (mycetism)
Mycobacterium tuberculosis. *See* tuberculosis: *Mycobacterium tuberculosis*
mycotoxin(s), 27, 60, 122, 151, 325, 327, 328, 412
    major groups, 328

N

NAAQS. *See* National Ambient Air Quality Standard, U.S. (NAAQS)
N-acetyltransferase (NAT), 121, 125
nano-particles. *See* particulate matter (PM): $PM_{0.1}$ (nano- and ultrafine particles)
narcotic effects. *See* toxicants: toxicodynamics
NAT. *See* *N*-acetyltransferase (NAT)
National Ambient Air Quality Standard, U.S. (NAAQS), 177, 180, 184, 187, 190, 201, 205, 471
National Environmental Policy Act, U.S. (NEPA), 33, 37, 38, 41, 43
National Health and Nutrition Examination Survey, U.S. (NHANES), 23, 299
National Pollutant Discharge Elimination System, U.S. (NPDES), 433
National Priorities List, U.S. (NPL), 443
National Research Council. *See* U.S. National Research Council (NRC)
Nationwide Food Consumption Survey, U.S., 467
necrosis, 228
    hepatic, 251
    in umbilical, embryonic, placental cells, 280
    of plants, 100, 137
    of the jaw, 254, 384
    of the tissue, 319
neem, 262
neonicotinoid(s), 279
neoplasm. *See* cancer

nephron, 110, 111
    (proximal) tubular reabsorption, 110, 111
    distal (convoluted) tubule, 110
    glomerulus, 110, 111
    proximal (convoluted) tubule, 110
    the functional unit (of the kidney), 110
nervous system
    components of, 149, 150
    functions of, 366, 367
neurological diseases (disorders), 25, 27, 347, 384
neurotoxic esterase (NTE), 270
    inhibition of, 270
neurotoxin(s), 2, 21, 27, 325, 326, 329, 330, 331, 333, 335, 405
New York (USA), 20, 188, 203, 207, 211, 219, 329
    air pollution, 188
    Love Canal (tragedy), 21, 430
    Mount Sinai School of Medicine, 23
NHANES. *See* National Health and Nutrition Examination Survey, U.S. (NHANES)
nickel (Ni), 125, 150, 151, 200, 249, 251, 252, 253, 393, 395
    carbonyl, 253, 393, 395
    carbonyl poisoning, 253
nickel-cadmium batteries, 55
nicotine, 62, 264, 279, 372, 379
NIH. *See* U.S. National Institutes of Health (NIH)
NIOSH, 389, *See also* U.S. National Institute for Occupational Safety and Health (NIOSH)
    Criteria Documents, 389
    Pocket Guide to Chemical Hazards, 389, 393
    recommended exposure limit/limits (REL), 389, 390, 392, 393
nitric acid (HNO_3), 71, 183, 184, 185, 196, 200
nitric oxide (NO), 58, 67, 70, 71, 149, 182, 183, 184, 186, 187, 221, 442
    synthase, 127
nitrobenzene, 121, 224, 417
nitrogen dioxide (NO_2), 58, 67, 70, 71, 100, 121, 136, 182, 183, 184, 185, 186, 187, 221
    characteristics of, 183
    effects on humans and animals, 184
    effects on plants, 185
    sources of pollution, 183
    toxic effects and advisories, 184
nitrogen fixation, 183
nitrogen mustard(s), 347, 348, 355, 356, 372, 379
nitrogen oxides (NO_x), 20, 57, 58, 60, 177, 178, 182, 183, 184, 186, 196, 200, 203, 217, 337
nitrous oxide (N_2O), 20, 69
Nixon, Richard (former U.S. President), 37, 38, 281, 385
no observed [adverse] effect level (NO[A]EL), 2, 407, 456, 457, 464, 465, 466, 469
NO[A]EL. *See* no observed [adverse] effect level (NO[A]EL)
Noise Control Act, U.S., 338, *See also* U.S. Environmental Protection Agency (U.S. EPA): Noise Control Act, U.S.
noise pollution, 34, 45, 49, 318, 336, 337, 338
    control measures, 338
    mortality among animal species, 338
non-inhalable coarse particles. *See* particulate matter (PM): PM_{10+} (non-inhalable coarse particles)
North American Agreement on Environmental Cooperation, 45
NPDES. *See* National Pollutant Discharge Elimination System, U.S. (NPDES)
NPL. *See* National Priorities List, U.S. (NPL)
NRC. *See* U.S. National Research Council (NRC)
NTE. *See* neurotoxic esterase (NTE)
nucleation (of $PM_{0.1}$). *See* particulate matter (PM): $PM_{0.1}$ (nano- and ultrafine particles): nucleation
nucleotide excision repair. *See* DNA (deoxyribonucleic acid): repair
nuisance dust (particles), 393, 397
nutrient(s), 22, 52, 56, 73, 78, 90, 118, 128, 150, 163, 164, 182, 185, 197, 205, 349, 353, 408, 436
    definition of, 408
    depletion of, 22
    essential, 28, 249, 250, 251
    loading, 21
    macronutrients, 118, 164, 408
    metabolism, 118
    micronutrients, 163, 164, 165
    overload of, 22
    toxicities of, 409
    uptake by plants, 104, 105, 211
nutrition
    definition of, 163
nutritional biochemistry, 118
nutritional deficiencies, 24, 330, 408
nutritional factors, 117, 155, 163, 164
nutritional metabolism. *See* nutrient(s): metabolosim
nutritional status
    anorexia nervosa, 163
    fasting, 163
    malnutrition, 163
    nutritional disorders, 163
    obesity, 163
    starvation, 163
nutritional toxicology

definition of, 163

O

Occupational Disease Control Act, China, 385
occupational diseases, 25, 384, 385
    definition of, 384
occupational health (and safety), 336, 385, 386, 389, 395, 398
    hazards, 10, *See also* workplace biological *or* physical hazards
    laws, 385
    legislation for, 386
    U.S. legislation for, 386
Occupational Health and Safety Act, South Africa, 385
Occupational Health, Safety and Welfare Act, South Australia, 385
Occupational Safety and Health Act (OSH Act), U.S., 41, 43, 385, 386, 387, 388
occupational toxicants
    biological (toxic) agents. *See* workplace biological hazards
    examples of, 393
    fibers/dusts, 392, 396
    metals, 392, 394
    metalworking fluids, 398
    organic solvents, 392, 395
    pesticides, 392, 394
        acute poisoning, 392
    physical (toxic) agents. *See* workplace physical hazards
occupational toxicology, 8, 224, 336, 384, 387
    basic principles of, 385
    relevant concepts of, 390
*octa*brominated diphenyl ether (*octa*BDE), 59, 290, 297, 298, *See also* polybrominated diphenyl ethers (PBDEs)
*o*ctanol-*w*ater partition coefficient (K_{ow}), 73, 74, 84, 85, 288, 300, 310
OECD. *See* Organization for Economic Cooperation and Development (OECD)
OH-PCBs. *See* polychlorinated biphenyls (PCBs): OH-PCBs
Oil Pollution Act, U.S. (OPA), 42, 43, 434
oil spills, 43, 434
    concerns, 24
omega-3 fatty acids, 90
    ALA (alpha-linolenic acid), 90
    DHA (docosahexaenoic acid), 90
    DPA (docosapentaenoic acid), 90
    EPA (eicosapentaenoic acid), 90

one-compartment model. *See* toxicants: toxicokinetics
oogenesis, 365
OPA. *See* Oil Pollution Act, U.S. (OPA)
OPIDN. *See* organophosphate-induced delayed neuropathy (OPIDN)
Orfila, Mathieu, 1
organic matter(s), 73, 74, 79, 197, 251, 310
organic solvents, 27, 223, 225, 227, 229, 230, 390, 392, 395, 396, 419
Organization for Economic Cooperation and Development (OECD), 86, 432, 456
    Test Guidelines 305, 86
organochlorines (OCs, OC pesticides), 27, 29, 49, 76, 91, 128, 150, 262, 264, 265, 266, 267, 269, 290, 445
    cyclodiene-related, 265, 266, 267, 268, 272
    cyclohexane-related, 265, 268
    dichlorodiphenylethane-related, 265, 266
organogenesis. *See* developmental-reproductive process: organogenesis
organophosphate-induced delayed neuropathy (OPIDN), 270
organophosphates (OPs, OP pesticides), 27, 49, 106, 121, 145, 150, 166, 262, 264, 269, 270, 271
    acetylcholinesterase inhibitors, 270, 271
    delayed neurotoxic agents, 270
    poisoning, 270
    SLUDGE, 271
OSH Act (USA). *See* Occupational Safety and Health Act (OSH Act), U.S.
OSHA. *See* U.S. Occupational Safety and Health Administration (OSHA)
Our Stolen Future, 364, 373
OurStolenFuture.org, 373, 375
ovarian cysts, 26, 363, 378, 379, *See also* reproductive damage (disorders): ovarian cysts
over-the-counter (OTC) medicines, 53, *See also* toxic household products: over-the-counter (OTC) medicines
oxalate, 331
oxidative phosphorylation, 151, 278, 279
oxidative stress, 28, 100, 125, 126, 137, 169, 301, 304
oxygen free radicals. *See* reactive oxygen species (ROS)
ozone (O_3), 19, 20, 44, 55, 57, 67, 69, 70, 100, 136, 150, 167, 177, 179, 182, 184, 185, 186, 187, 188, 203, 217, 219, 221, 262
    characteristics of, 186, 187
    effects on humans and animals, 187
    effects on plants, 188
    smog, 190

sources of pollution, 186
stratospheric, 187, 262
toxic effects and advisories, 187, 188

P

p53 (protein), 350
PAHs. *See* polycyclic aromatic hydrocarbons (PAHs)
PAN. *See* peroxyacetylnitrate (PAN)
Paracelsus (Philippus von Hohenheim), 1, 156
Paracoccidioides brasiliensis, 323
paraquat, 151, 279, 280
parathion, 27, 106, 269, 270, 393, 442
parathyroid hormone, 369
Paris Basin (France), 203
particulate matter (PM), 59, 61, 67, 89, 94, 150, 177, 183, 196, 197, 198, 199, 203, 204, 210, 217, 245
   airborne microbes. *See* airborne microbes
   characteristics of, 197
   composition of, 196, 200
   criteria air pollutant, U.S., 196
   definition of, 196
   effects on cardiovascular system, 209
   effects on respiratory tract, 208
   effects/impacts on the environment, 211
   episodes of particulate pollution, 203
   fine *vs.* coarse particulates, 200
   formation of, 200
   half-life, 200
   issues on urban particulate pollution, 202
   monitoring of, 204
   motions of, 198, 199
   of diesel, 210
   other serious health effects, 210
   $PM_{0.1}$ (nano- and ultrafine particles), 198, 199, 200, 202
      coagulation, 200, 201
      condensation, 200, 201
      nucleation, 200, 201, 202
   $PM_{0.1-2.5}$ (fine particles), 199, 200, 201, 204
   PM_{10} (inhalable [coarse] particles), 198, 199, 201, 202, 203, 204, 206, 207, 208, 209, 211
   PM_{10+} (non-inhalable coarse particles), 198, 199
   $PM_{2.5}$ (inhalable [fine] particles), 159, 198, 200, 202, 207, 208, 209, 210, 211
   $PM_{2.5-10}$ (inhalable coarse particles), 198, 199, 200, 201, 204, 210
   secondary organic matter, 217
   sizes of, 197
   sizes of regulatory importance, 198
   sources of, 200
   toxic effects, 207
   travel distance, 200
   urban particulate pollution, 202
passive diffusion. *See* toxicants: mechanisms of entry
pathogenic (microbial) agents, 319
   bacteria, 320
   fungi, 322
   parasites, 323
   viruses, 321
PBBs. *See* polybrominated biphenyls (PBBs)
PBDEs. *See* polybrominated diphenyl ethers (PBDEs)
PB-PK (physiologically-based pharmacokinetics) model/modeling, 113, 232
PB-TK (physiologically-based toxicokinetics) model/modeling. *See* PB-PK (physiologically-based pharmacokinetics) model/modeling
PBTs (persistent, bioaccumulative, and toxic substances), 84, 289, 298, *See also* persistent toxic substances (PTS)
PCBs. *See* polychlorinated biphenyls (PCBs)
PCDDs. *See* polychlorinated dibenzo-*p(ara)*-dioxins (PCDDs)
PCDEs. *See* polychlorinated diphenyl ethers (PCDEs)
PCDFs. *See* polychlorinated dibenzofurans (PCDFs)
PCE (PERC). *See* tetrachloroethylene (PCE/PERC)
PCNs. *See* polychlorinated naphthalenes (PCNs)
PEAK. *See* exposure limit values: PEAK
Pearl River Delta (Urban Agglomeration), China, 92, 206
Penicillium, 58, 328
*penta*brominated diphenyl ether (*penta*BDE), 59, 290, 298, *See also* polybrominated diphenyl ethers (PBDEs)
pentachlorobenzene (PeCB), 269, 290
pentachlorophenol (PCP), 75, 77, 78, 85, 290, 411
perfluorooctane sulfonate (PFOS), 60, 290, 291, 292, 293, 294, 295, 375
   characteristics, uses, and sources, 292
   environmental health concerns, 294
perfluorooctane sulfonic acid. *See* perfluorooctane sulfonate (PFOS)
perfluorooctane sulfonyl fluoride (PFOS-F), 290, 291, 292, 293, 295
   characteristics, uses, and sources, 292
   environmental health concerns, 294
perfluorooctanoic acid (PFOA), 59, 60, 294, 295, 355, 411
peripheral proteins. *See* biomembrane(s): peripheral proteins
permethrin, 27, 151, 273, 274, 375
permissible exposure limit/limits (PEL), 218, 224, 387, 388, 389, 390, 391, 392, 393, 398, 464

peroxyacetylnitrate (PAN), 70, 182, 184, 185
persistence criteria (numerical), 288
persistent organic pollutants (POPs), 28, 29, 38, 39, 44, 48, 62, 86, 94, 151, 275, 289, 290, 291, 292, 293, 294, 297, 298, 299, 300, 303, 305
    the dirty dozen, 29, 44, 290, 392
persistent organochlorine compounds (POCs), 29, 49, 57, 58, 62, 72, 73, 74, 75, 76, 77, 82, 83, 84, 85, 86, 87, 89, 90, 91, 92, 93, 94, 95, 413, 420, 423
    bioaccumulation in seafood, 90
    fate and transport in water, 72
        key (environmental) variables, 73
persistent toxic substances (PTS), 84, 287, 289, 290, 419, 420
pesticide residues. *See* pesticides: residues
pesticides, 261
    definition of, 61, 261
    economic poisons, 18
    health impacts and concerns, 261
    neurotoxic agents, 27
    of environmental health concern, 61
    residues, 20, 42, 43, 49, 60, 100, 261
        as pollutants, 262
        definition of, 261
    select novel/specialty pesticides, 279
    Silent Spring (by Rachel Carson), 36
    usage and classification, 262
        classification, 264
        usage, 262, 263
PFOA. *See* perfluorooctanoic acid (PFOA)
PFOS. *See* perfluorooctane sulfonate (PFOS)
PFOS-F. *See* perfluorooctane sulfonyl fluoride (PFOS-F)
phagocytosis. *See* toxicants: mechanisms of entry
pharmaceutical waste, 49, 53, 54
Phase I (enzymatic) reactions, 118, 119, 120, 121, 122, 127
Phase I enzymes. *See* cytochrome 450 *or* Phase I (enzymatic) reactions
Phase II (enzymatic) reactions, 118, 119, 120, 121, 122, 123, 124
Phase II enzymes, 124, *See also* Phase II (enzymatic) reactions
phase-transfer (of environmental toxicants)
    (ad)sorption, 72, 73, 74, 75, 79
    atmospheric deposition, 69, 75
    desorption, 75
    dissolution, 72, 73, 75
    precipitation, 75
    sedimentation, 75
    volatilization of, 66, 72, 74, 75, 77

phenol (C_6H_5-OH), 119, 221, 224, 417
phenoxy pesticides, 274
phenylketonuria (PKU), 377, 378
phosphodiesterases, 334, 335
phospholipases, 334, 335
    phospholipases-A_2, 334, 335
phossy jaw. *See also* necrosis: of the jaw
    classic industrial disease, 25, 384
photochemical reaction, 70, 221
photochemical smog reaction, 180, 182
photodecomposition. *See* photochemical reaction
photodissociation. *See* photochemical reaction
photosynthesis, 56, 71, 76, 104, 137, 185, 191, 208, 211, 276, 280, 431
phthalates, 375, 410, 411
physical (toxic) agents, 11, 24, 318, 336, 354, 386, 388, 390, 438, *See also* (workplace) physical hazards
physical hazards, 318, 336, 363, 398
    underrated, 318, 336
physiological toxicology, 147
physiologically-based pharmacokinetics model. *See* PB-PK (physiologically-based pharmacokinetics): model/modeling
phytochemical(s), 129, 268, 356, 357
    antioxidants, 125
    enzyme inhibitors, 128
phytoremediation, 105
Pick complex diseases. *See* chromosome aberration: Pick complex diseases
picrotoxin, 268
pinocytosis. *See* toxicants: mechanisms of entry
piperonyl butoxide, 273
pirimicarb, 272
PKU. *See* phenylketonuria (PKU)
plant toxicants, 59, 62, *See also* toxins: from plants
Plasmodium falciparum, 324, 332
plastic marine pollution, 49, 53
    plastic bags, 53
plastics (polymers), 411
    e-waste, 21
    high-density polyethylene, 411
    low-density polyethylene, 411
    polycarbonate, 51
    polypropylene, 411
    polystyrene, 224, 298, 411
    thermoplastics, 221
$PM_{[10]}$. *See* particulate matter (PM): PM_{10} (inhalable [coarse] particles)
$PM_{0.1}$. *See* particulate matter (PM): $PM_{0.1}$ (nano- and ultrafine particles)

PM$_{0.1-2.5}$. *See* particulate matter (PM): PM$_{0.1-2.5}$ (fine particles)
PM$_{1.0}$, 208
PM$_{10-}$, 199
PM$_{10+}$ (non-inhalable coarse particles). *See* particulate matter (PM): PM$_{10+}$ (non-inhalable coarse particles)
PM$_{2.5-}$, 199
PM$_{2.5-10}$. *See* particulate matter (PM): PM$_{2.5-10}$ (inhalable coarse particles)
PM$_{nano}$, 198, *See also* particulate matter (PM): PM$_{0.1}$
pneumoconiosis, 27, 384, 388, 398
POCs. *See* persistent organochlorine compounds (POCs)
point mutation, 345, 346, 357
poison dart frogs, 336
poison ivy, 27, 331
poison oak, 27
poison sumac, 27, 331
poisonous plants, 1, 24, 329
   health effects, 329
polybrominated biphenyls (PBBs), 291, 293, 295, 296, 297, 298, 299, 301, 302, 306, 375
   characteristics, uses, and sources, 295
   contamination incident in Michigan (USA), 297
   environmental health concerns, 297
polybrominated cyclododecanes (PBCDs), 291, 293, 300
   characteristics, uses, and sources, 300
   environmental health concerns, 301
polybrominated diphenyl ethers (PBDEs), 54, 57, 59, 60, 89, 290, 291, 293, 296, 298, 299, 301, 306, 375, 435
   characteristics, uses, and sources, 298
   environmental health concerns, 299
polybromobiphenyls (PBBs). *See* polybrominated biphenyls (PBBs)
polychlorinated biphenyls (PCBs), 21, 26, 29, 54, 58, 59, 60, 68, 76, 87, 88, 89, 90, 91, 92, 94, 109, 126, 140, 151, 158, 160, 223, 289, 290, 291, 293, 296, 301, 302, 303, 306, 308, 309, 355, 374, 375, 379, 420
   Aroclor compound(s), 158, 161, 302
   characteristics, uses, and sources, 301
   dioxin-like, 87, 88, 89, 302, 306, 307, 308, 309, 310
   environmental health concerns, 302
   OH-PCBs, 87, 303, 375
polychlorinated butadienes (PCBDs), 291, 292, 293, 305
   characteristics, uses, and sources, 305
   environmental health concerns, 306

polychlorinated dibenzofurans (PCDFs), 29, 58, 59, 87, 92, 290, 291, 293, 302, 306, 307, 309, 375
   characteristics, uses, and sources, 307
   environmental health concerns, 307
polychlorinated dibenzo-*p(ara)*-dioxins (PCDDs), 50, 58, 60, 68, 76, 87, 88, 89, 92, 109, 126, 140, 151, 290, 291, 293, 302, 306, 307, 308, 309, 310, 422
   characteristics, uses, and sources, 307
   environmental health concerns, 307
polychlorinated diphenyl ethers (PCDEs), 88
polychlorinated naphthalenes (PCNs), 290, 291, 293, 303, 304, 306, 308
   characteristics, uses, and sources, 304
   environmental health concerns, 304
polycyclic aromatic hydrocarbons (PAHs), 123, 126, 129, 140, 201, 223, 415, 435
polyethylene glycol (PEG), 411, 415
polyethylene terephthalate, 411
polyhalogenated aromatic hydrocarbons (PHAHs), 292
polymers. *See* plastics (polymers)
polynuclear aromatic hydrocarbons. *See* polycyclic aromatic hydrocarbons (PAHs)
polystyrene. *See* plastics (polymers): polystyrene
polytetrafluoroethylene (PTFE), 411
POPs. *See* persistent organic pollutants (POPs)
porphyria cutanea tarda, 268
portal venous system, 107, 108, 109
potentiation. *See* interaction, chemical: potentiation
potter's disease. *See* lead (Pb) *or* silicosis: classic industrial disease
pralidoxime, 270
prevalence (of disease)
   definition of, 9
   U.S. national annual on birth defects, 376
prion(s), 11, 319, 320
procarcinogens
   definition of, 351
progesterone, 369, 370, 371, 373, 375, 380
   functions of, 370
progestogens, 370
progression phase. *See* carcinogenesis: mechanism of
promotion phase. *See* carcinogenesis: mechanism of
Prop 65. *See* Proposition 65 (California, USA)
propargite, 27, 100, 151
propargyl bromide, 78
propazine, 276, 277, 278
Proposition 65 (California, USA), 24, 277, *See also* California (USA): Proposition 65 list
propoxur, 272
propyl gallate, 375, 409

propylene glycol (PG), 415
proteases, 334, 335
protozoa. *See* pathogenic (microbial) agents: parasites
pseudoephedrine (decongestant), 418
Pseudomonas, 320
psoralen, 356
PTS. *See* persistent toxic substances (PTS)
pulmonary excretion. *See* toxicants:
    excretion/elimination (of xenobiotics)
pyrethrins (pyrethrin pesticides), 93, 272, 273, 274, 331
    allergic contact dermatitis, 274
    Pyrethrins I, 273
        cinerin I, 273
        jasmolin I, 273
        pyrethrins I, 273
    Pyrethrins II, 273
        cinerin II, 273
        jasmolin II, 273
        pyrethrins II, 273
pyrethroids (pyrethroid pesticides), 27, 272, 273, 274
    CS syndrome, 272
    paresthesia, 274
    T syndrome, 272
    Type I, 272
    Type II, 272
pyrethrum, 62, 272, 393
pyruvate dehydrogenase, 246

Q

Quieting the World's Cities, 338

R

radioactive wastes, 59, 62, 320
radium (Ra), 60, 254, 255
    lung cancer, 255
radon (Rn), 55, 57, 60, 197, 205, 254, 255
rate of diffusion. *See* toxicants: mechanisms of entry
rBST. *See* recombinant bovine somatotropin (rBST)
RCRA. *See* Resource Conservation & Recovery Act, U.S. (RCRA)
reactive oxygen species (ROS), 28, 61, 136, 169, 251, 356
receptors (proteinaceous)
    γ-GABA receptor, 266, 268
    antagonism, 168
    aryl hydrocarbon receptor (AhR), 126, 139, 140, 302, 306, 307, 308, 310, 372
    defintion, 136
    enzyme (catalytic) receptor, 118
    estrogen receptor, 372
    G protein-coupled receptor, 139
    hormone receptor, 303, 370, 372, 373
    integral protein receptor, 139
    intracellular, 139
    ionotropic, 139
    metabotropic, 139
    modulation of functions, 135, 136, 138, 373
    nicotinic acetylcholine receptor, 279
re-circulation test. *See* aquatic toxicity tests
recombinant bovine somatotropin (rBST), 412
recommended exposure limit/limits (REL). *See*
    NIOSH: recommended exposure limit/limits (REL)
red tide pollution, 21, 39
    Solutions to Avoid Red Tide (START), 39
reference concentration (RfC), 464, 465
reference dose (RfD), 439, 464, 465, 468, 469
refractory ceramic fibers. *See* synthetic mineral fibers (SMFs)
renal excretion. *See* toxicants: excretion/elimination (of xenobiotics)
renewal test. *See* aquatic toxicity tests
reproductive damage (disorders), 26, 29, 362, 363, 377, 380
    concerns, 363
    definition of, 26
    ED (erectile dysfunction), 363, 364, 375, 377, 379, 380
    infertility, 26, 149, 185, 299, 327, 328, 363, 374, 375, 377, 379
    ovarian cysts, 26, 363, 364, 375, 378, 379
reproductive system
    human female, 380
    human male, 380
reproductive toxicants, 362
    definition of, 374
    sources for exposure, 374
Resource Conservation & Recovery Act, U.S. (RCRA), 43, 434, 441, 442, 443
    definition and implications, 441
respiratory diseases (disorders)
    chronic lower, 18
    definition of, 26
    exposure to PM_{10}, 208, 209
    exposure to $PM_{2.5}$, 208
    exposure to toxic metals, 395
    types of, 150
respiratory uptake. *See* toxicants: uptake of, by humans
retro-transposons, 345
RfC. *See* reference concentration (RfC)
RfD. *See* reference dose (RfD)

Rhamnus purshiana, 330
Rhus, 331
ricin, 330
ringworm(s), 322
Risk Characterization Handbook, 463
risk communication, 470, 471
    cardinal rules, 470, 471
    mental noise theory, 470
    negative dominance theory, 470
    risk perception theory, 470, 471
    trust determination theory, 470
risk perception, 35, 468
    definition of, 469
risk-based standards, 471
RNA (ribonucleic acid)
    definition of, 342
    double-stranded RNA (dsRNA), 324
    mRNA (messenger RNA), 139, 140, 169, 344, 350
    viruses, 348
rodenticides, 61, 264, 278, 279, 281, 392
    bromethalin, 278
    Compound 1080, 144, 279, 280, 281, 393
    coumarin-based, 278
    DDT, 278
    red squill, 278
    strychnine, 278
    thallium sulfate, 278
    zinc phosphide, 278
ROS. *See* reactive oxygen species (ROS)
rotenone, 62, 262, 264
Rotterdam Convention, 276
Rotterdam Convention on the Prior Informed Consent Procedure for Certain Hazardous Chemicals and Pesticides in International Trade. See Rotterdam Convention
Roundup®. *See* glyphosate

S

safety factors. *See* health risk assessment: uncertainty and safety factors
Salmonella, 320, 321, 326, 342, 349, 412
    typhimurium, 349
Salmonella assay, 342, 349, *See also* Ames test
sarin, 269, 271
    Aum Shinrikyo cult, 271
    chemical weapons attack allegedly in Syria, 271
SARS (severe acute respiratory syndrome), 12, 48, 205, 399, 400
    occupational disease, 399
saxitoxin, 324, 329, 413
scombrotoxin, 329, 330, 413

scorpions, 332, 333
    Centruroides exilicauda, 333
    chlorotoxin, 333
    deathstalker, 333
seasonal affective disorder syndrome (SADS), 368
selenium (Se), 28, 125, 126, 142, 165, 393
Sentinel Event Notification System for Occupational Risks (SENSOR)-Pesticides program, 394
serotonin (syndrome), 141
SETAC. *See* Society of Environmental Toxicology and Chemistry (SETAC)
severe acute respiratory syndrome. *See* SARS (severe acute respiratory syndrome)
Seveso (Italy), 308
Seveso dioxin, 308, *See also* 2,3,7,8-TCDD
Sevin. *See* carbaryl
shellfish poisoning, 324, 329
sick building syndrome, 416, *See also* fragrances: sick building syndrome
sickle-cell anemia, 345, 346
Silent Spring, 8, 23, 36, 37, 38, 261, 413, 434, *See also* Carson, Rachel
silicosis, 25, 384, 398
    classic industrial disease, 25, 384
    in China, 398
    in the United States, 398
    one form of pneumoconiosis, 398
simazine, 79, 276, 277, 278
site of (toxic) action
    definition of, 135
skin absorption/penetration. *See* toxicants: uptake of, by humans
skin disorders (diseases), 27, 303, 398, 415
    dermatitis, 27, 151
    irritation, 21, 50, 142, 151, 222, 230, 415
SMFs. *See* synthetic mineral fibers (SMFs)
snakes, 62, 333, 334, 335, 436, *See also* venoms: from snakes
    Elapidae family, 334
    Viperidae family, 334
Society of Environmental Toxicology and Chemistry (SETAC), 17
sodium (mono)fluoroacetate, 279, 280, 393, *See also* rodenticides: Compound 1080
sodium laureth sulfate (SLeS), 415
sodium lauryl sulfate (SLS), 415
sodium nitrate
    direct food additive, 409
sodium nitrite
    direct food additive, 409
soil contaminants, 20, 49, 67, 77, 78, 104, 105, 230

degradation of, 77, 78
erosion and runoff of, 77, 78
fate of, 77
leaching of, 77, 78
transport of, 77
uptake via plant roots, 105
volatilization of, 77, 78
soil contamination, 20, 224, 434
Solanum nigrum, 157, 158
solar radiation
absorption and release, 69
Solid Waste Disposal Act, U.S., 441
soman, 271
soot
particles, 207, 210
pollution, 210
sorbitan monostearate
stabilizer (food additive), 408
sorbitan tristearate
stabilizer (food additive), 408
sorption potential, 74
spermatogenesis, 365, 377
sphingomyelinase D, 332
spiders, 332, 333
black widow species (*Latrodectus*), 332
brown recluse species (*Loxosceles*), 332
jumping species (*Phidippus*), 332, 333
wolf species (*Pardosa*), 332, 333
yellow sac species (*Chiranthium*), 332, 333
squill (*Urginea maritima*), 278, 330
St. Anthony's Fire. *See* ergotism
St. John's wort. *See Hypericum: perforatum (H. perforatum)*
Staphylococcus(ci), 320, 321, 326, 412
aureus, 321, 326
methicillin-resistant (MRSA), 321
State Environmental Protection Administration, China (CSEPA), 45
static test. *See* aquatic toxicity tests
steatosis, 150
STEL. *See* exposure limit values: STEL
Stockholm Convention, 29, 38, 39, 44, 289, 290, 291, 292, 293, 295, 297, 300, 301, 303, 305, 392
aims and actions, 291
persistent pollutants of concern, 290
Stockholm Convention on Persistent Organic Compounds (POPs) of 2001, 44, *See also* Stockholm Convention
stomata, 100, 105, 181
functions of, 105
strength-of-evidence, 466

Streptococcus(ci), 36, 320, 326
aureus, 36
pyogenes, 326
Strychnos nux vomica, 278
sudden infant death syndrome (SIDS), 185, 207, 210, 211
sulfanilamide, 404
sulfation, 119, 121, 122
sulf-hemoglobin (sulfHb), 151
sulfhydryl (thiol) group(s), 121, 145, 239, 240, 244, 246
sulfite oxidase, 165
sulfosate, 280
sulfotransferase (SULT), 121, 124
sulfur dioxide (SO_2), 59, 67, 71, 100, 136, 157, 162, 167, 168, 177, 178, 179, 180, 181, 183, 184, 185, 188, 200, 203
effects of acid rain, 181
effects on humans and animals, 180
effects on plants, 181
sources of pollution, 178
toxic effects and advisories, 180
sulfur oxides (SO_x), 20, 57, 59, 178, 196
sulfur trioxide (SO_3), 71, 178, 180
sulfuric acid (H_2SO_4), 59, 71, 162, 178, 180, 181, 182, 183, 189, 190, 196, 207
SULT. *See* sulfotransferase (SULT)
Superfund (law and program). *See* Comprehensive Environmental Response, Compensation, & Libility Act, U.S. (CERCLA)
superoxide dismutase (SOD), 125, 127
superoxide radical, 28, 137
Swainsonine. *See* alkaloid(s): indolizidine
synergism. *See* interaction, chemical: synergism
synergistic effect (damage), 167, 185
among NO_2, O_3, and SO_2, 185
between asbestos and cigarette smoking, 167
between O_3 and SO_2, 167, 188
synthetic mineral fibers (SMFs), 393, 396, 397

T

T syndrome
effect of Type I pyrethroids, 272
tabun, 271
tartrazine. *See* FD&C yellow No. 5: food colorant
taxol, 331
Tay-Sachs disease (TSD), 377
TCDD. *See* 2,3,7,8-TCDD
TCE. *See* trichloroethylene (TCE)
TDE. *See* DDD (dichlorodiphenyldichloroethane)
TEF. *See* toxic equivalency factor/factors (TEF)

Teflon®. *See* polytetrafluoroethylene (PTFE)
Tegucigalpa (Latin America)
    PM_{10} levels, 204
TEPP. *See* tetraethyl pyrophosphate (TEPP)
TEQ. *See* toxic equivalency (TEQ)
teratogenic effects. *See* toxicants: toxicodynamics
teratogens, 148, 149, 362, 366, 374, 378
    definition of, 148, 362
    effects, 149, 365, 366, 374, 377, 378
    environmental, 49
    examples of, 378
terbufos, 271
testosterone, 122, 277, 369, 370, 371, 373, 375, 380
    functions of, 369
tetanus, 320, 325
    (tetanus) toxin, 325
    Clostridium tetani (the bacterial agent), 325, 326
tetrachloroethylene (PCE/PERC), 218, 219, 229, 230, 231, 232, 417, 442
    exposures and toxic effects, 230
    sources and use, 229
tetraethyl pyrophosphate (TEPP), 270
tetrodotoxin, 27, 319, 329, 330, 335, 413
thalidomide, 6, 26, 378, 466
the Arctic. *See* Arctic, the
The New York Times
    reforestation, 39
The Safe Drinking Water and Toxic Enforcement Act of 1986 (California, USA). *See* Proposition 65 (California, USA)
The Wildlife Society, 434
thiol group. *See* sulfhydryl (thiol) group(s)
thiourea, 169
thorium (Th), 254, 255
threshold limit values (TLV®s), 390
Threshold of Regulation program. *See* U.S. Food and Drug Administration (FDA): Threshold of Regulation program
thyroxine, 369, 370, 371
Time (magazine)
    on environmental disease, 23
TMDL. *See* Total Maximum Daily Load, U.S. (TMDL)
TNF. *See* tumor necrosis factor (TNF)
TOCP. *See* tri-*ortho*-cresyl phosphate (TOCP)
Tokyo (Japan), 203, 271
    Aum Shinrikyo cult (with sarin), 271
toluene, 149, 218, 223, 224, 411, 419
Total Maximum Daily Load, U.S. (TMDL), 433
total suspended particles (TSP), 199, 202, 205, 206
toxaphene, 29, 62, 266, 290, 375

toxic consumer (food and household) products
    didactic cases, 419
    mitigation and prevention, 422
toxic effects
    on target organs/systems. *See* toxicants: toxicodynamics
toxic equivalency (TEQ), 87, 89, 92, 308, 310
    in bioaccumulation, 87
toxic equivalency factor/factors (TEF), 87, 166, 303, 308, 309, 310
    application of, 310
toxic household products, 413, 414
    cleaning agents, 414, 416
    fragrance-free policy, 416
    gasoline, 419
    lead on children's jewelry and toys, 420
    mitigation and prevention, 422
    other organic compounds, 414, 419
    over-the-counter (OTC) medicines, 405, 414, 417
        (understated) health concerns, 405
        antihistamines, 418
        cold medicines, 418
        decongestants, 418
        pain relievers, 418
        side effects, 418, 419
    personal care products, 414
    pesticide products, 419
    source categories, 414
    statistics on poisoning, 404
    toxic substances, 413
    triclosan in antibacterial products, 421
toxic response
    definition of, 135
toxic shock syndrome (TSS), 36, 326, 452
    tampon-toxic shock scare, 35, 36, 452, 468
Toxic Substances Control Act, U.S. (TSCA), 43, 304, 441
toxicant clearance. *See* toxicants: toxicokinetics: (toxicant) clearance
toxicants
    (environmental) mobility, 93
    bioactivation (of xenobiotics), 119, 122, 164
    biotransformation (of xenobiotics), 93, 95, 101, 117, 118, 119
        affecting factors, 126
        definition of, 117
        general processes, 118, 119
        other processes, 122
    definition of, 2
    detoxification (of xenobiotics), 122, 123, 124, 125, 135, 164, 186

disposition (of xenobiotics), 5, 100, 101, 112, 113, 115, 136, 155, 168, 428, *See also* toxicants: toxicokinetics
distribution (of xenobiotics), 67, 95, 101, 106, 107, 109, 112, 113, 114, 115, 150, 151, 430, *See also* toxicants: toxicokinetics
excretion/elimination (of xenobiotics), 109, 119
mechanism(s) of (toxic) action, 135, 136, 137, 147, 306, 372
    adverse indirect actions, 136, 141
    adverse secondary actions, 136, 141
    and toxicodynamics, 135, 145
    binding with a cell's constituent, 136, 140
    common action for AhR activation, 306
    definition of, 135
    direct damage, 135, 136, 137, 211, 318
    disruption of enzymatic activities, 136, 143, 145
    endocrine disruption, 372
    free radical-mediated actions, 136
    mechanism-based adverse effects, 147
    mediated toxic actions, 136, 137
    modulation of receptor functions, 135, 138
    primary toxic actions, 136
mechanisms of entry, 101, 103
metabolism, 5, 93, 95, 101, 109, 117, 127, 150, 169
metabolism *vs.* biotransformation, 117
non-systemic effects, 100, 391
systemic, 100
systemic effects, 5, 100, 101, 147, 150, 151, 247, 391, 415, 456
toxicodynamics, 135, 136, 145, 146, 147, 148, 149, 151, 428
    and mechanisms of toxic action, 135
    basic types of toxic effects, 146
    definition of, 136, 145
    mechanism-based adverse effects, 147
toxicokinetics, 112, 113, 115, 136, 146, 232, 407, 428, 461
    (toxicant) clearance, 114
    area under the curve, 115
    definition of, 112
    elimination rate constant, 114
    mathematical principles, 113
    numerical example, 115
    one-compartment model, 113
    PB-PK (PB-TK) model/modeling, 113
    two-compartment model, 113
    volume of distribution, 114
uptake (and absorption) of, 100, 103
uptake of, by humans, 106
uptake of, by plants, 104

toxicity
    definition of, 155
toxicity affecting factors, 155
    biological (co)factors, 156, 168
    environmental factors, 155, 156
    extrinsic factors, 155
    intrinsic factors, 155
    nutritional factors, 155, 163
    physicochemical factors, 155, 166
toxicity assessment, 456, *See also* health risk assessment: toxicity assessment
toxicokinetics. *See* toxicants: toxicokinetics
toxicologists
    activities for, 7
toxicology
    definition of, 1
    historical development, 1
    terminology, 2, 3
toxin K1, 324
toxin K2, 324
toxin K28, 324
toxins
    as food contaminants (from bacteria or animals), 60
    definition (per U.S. Code), 2, 318
    from bacteria, 324, 326
    from fishes, 329
    from fungi, 325, 328
    from microorganisms, 324
    from mushrooms, 325
    from plants, 329
    from viruses, 324
Toxoplasma gondii, 323
traffic congestion, 49, 182, 189, 318, 336
trans fats, 48, 51, 52, 53, 161, 407
transformation
    biological (biotic), 72, 75
    chemical (abiotic), 72, 75
transposons, 345
triazine (pesticides), 274, 276
trichloroethylene (TCE), 218, 219, 229, 230, 231, 232, 393, 395, 410, 442
    exposures and toxic effects, 231
    sources and use, 230
trichloromethyl free radical, 122, 138
trichothecenes, 325, 327, 328
triclosan, 50, 51, 59, 419, 421, 422
triiodothyronine, 369, 370, 371
trimethadione, 378
tri-*ortho*-cresyl phosphate (TOCP), 270
triphenylmethyl radical, 28
trophic level. *See* food chain(s)/web(s)

TSP. *See* total suspended particles (TSP)
tuberculosis, 18, 255, 320
   Mycobacterium tuberculosis, 320
tubular reabsorption. *See* nephron: (proximal) tubular reabsorption
tumor. *See* cancer
tumor necrosis factor (TNF), 324
tumorigenesis. *See* carcinogenesis
tundra. *See* wildlife terrestrial environment: tundra
Turner syndrome. *See* chromosome aberration: Turner syndrome
TWA. *See* exposure limit values: TWA
two-compartment model. *See* toxicants: toxicokinetics
Type I hypersensitivity. *See* toxicants: toxicodynamics
Type II hypersensitivity. *See* toxicants: toxicodynamics
Type III hypersensitivity. *See* toxicants: toxicodynamics
Type IV hypersensitivity. *See* toxicants: toxicodynamics

U

U.K. Department for Environmental, Food, and Rural Affairs (U.K. DEFRA), 288
U.S. Agency for Toxic Substances and Disease Registry (ATSDR), 42, 50, 181, 220, 225, 226, 230, 231, 254, 296, 305, 379, 470
   creation of, 42
U.S. Bureau of Mines, 385
U.S. Centers for Disease Control and Prevention (CDC), 25, 36, 376, 386, 404
   Affordable Care Act (ACA), 453
   annual prevalence of birth defects, 25, 376
   foodborne illnesses, 404
   health risk assessment activities, 452
   major groups of birth defects, 376
   toxic shock syndrome, 36, 452
U.S. Clean Air Act. *See* Clean Air Act, U.S.
U.S. Clean Water Act. *See* Clean Water Act, U.S.
U.S. Coast Guard (USCG), 434
   areas of regulatory concern, 43
U.S. Code of Federal Regulations (CFR), 386, 389, 410, 411, 413, 441, 442
U.S. Consumer Product Safety Commission (CPSC), 6, 41, 42, 43, 45, 404, 419, 422, 452
   areas of regulatory concern, 43
   concerns with toxic household products, 405
   functions of, 41
   health risk assessment activities, 452
   investigation on lead poisoning, 420
   pediactric poisonings at homes, 404
   poisoning from toxic household products, 404
   prevention tips for toxic household products, 422
U.S. Council of Environmental Quality (CEQ), 37, 38
U.S. Department of Agriculture (USDA), 440, 467
U.S. Department of Health and Human Services (DHHS), 41, 386, 452
U.S. Department of Labor (DOL), 41, 386
U.S. Department of Transportation (DOT), 41, 42, 43
   areas of regulatory concern, 43
   functions of, 41
U.S. Environmental Protection Agency (U.S. EPA), 6, 37, 38, 39, 41, 42, 43, 45, 52, 53, 54, 55, 60, 61, 85, 86, 90, 92, 161, 177, 180, 184, 196, 198, 199, 200, 210, 217, 219, 220, 224, 227, 228, 241, 244, 247, 248, 250, 251, 253, 261, 262, 263, 264, 272, 274, 276, 277, 279, 280, 288, 294, 304, 306, 310, 338, 354, 373, 375, 394, 397, 414, 419, 420, 423, 432, 433, 437, 438, 441, 442, 443, 444, 445, 446, 451, 452, 455, 456, 459, 463, 468, 469, 470
   (aquatic) early-life stage test, 432
   (drinking) water contaminants, 60, 432
   (health) risk communication, 470
   (health) risk perception, 469
   advisory on tuna consumption, 52
   air pollutants, 177
   air toxics (hazardous air pollutants), 177
   areas of regulatory concern, 43
   categories and guidelines of health effects tests, 455, 456
   CERCLA (for toxic wastes), 42, 54, 442, 443
   classification of carcinogenicity potential, 354
   cleanup efforts/actions for Superfund sites, 442, 443, 444, 445, 446
   Conventional Reduced Risk Program, 279
   cumulative (and aggregate) risk assessment, 463
   cumulative risk assessment for atrazine-like, 276
   definition and concept of (human) exposure, 459
   ecological risk assessment, 437
   Exposure Factor Handbook, 468
   functions of, 41
   guidelines for estimation of bioconcentration factors, 86
   health risk assessment activities, 451, 452
   health risk characterization, 463
   household (toxic) substances, 61
   limits on VOC content, 219
   list of (potential) endocrine disruptors, 375
   list of toxic wastes, 441
   maximum contaminant level (MCL), 464

National Priorities List, U.S. (NPL), 443
Noise Control Act, U.S., 338
NPDES (for water quality), 433
on sizes of particulate matter (PM), 198, 199, 200
persistence criteria (numerical), 288
proposal on waste pharmaceuticals, 53, 54
RCRA (for toxic wastes), 441
reference dose (RfD), 464, 469
responsibilities and early efforts, 38
screening values (of public health concern), 90, 92, 420
Superfund (law and program). *See* U.S. Environmental Protection Agency (U.S. EPA): CERCLA (for toxic wastes)
The Birth of EPA, 38
TMDL (for water quality), 433
United Heckathorn (Superfund toxic site), 54, 443, 444, 445, 446
usage data on pesticides, 263, 264
water quality criteria (WQC), 432
U.S. EPA. *See* U.S. Environmental Protection Agency (U.S. EPA)
U.S. Federal Emergency Management Agency, 61, 222
U.S. Food and Drug Administration (FDA), 6, 41, 42, 43, 45, 51, 52, 404, 406, 407, 410, 416, 422, 452, 456, 464, 469
acceptable daily intake (ADI), 464, 469
action level for mercury in tuna, 52
advisory on tuna consumption, 52
approval of new food additives, 407
areas of regulatory concern, 43
ban on trans fats, 407
ban on triclosan, 422
concerns with food toxicants, 404
functions of, 41
health risk assessment activities, 452
Threshold of Regulation program, 410
toxic household cosmetic products, 416
toxicity testing, 456
U.S. Geological Survey, 53, 435
U.S. Mine Safety and Health Administration (MSHA), 199, 388, 390, 397
U.S. National Center for Environmental Health (NCEH), 55
U.S. National Environmental Policy Act. *See* National Environmental Policy Act, U.S. (NEPA)
U.S. National Institute for Occupational Safety and Health (NIOSH), 386, 388, 389, 390, 392, 393, 394, 395, 396, *See also* NIOSH
structure and functions of, 388

U.S. National Institute on Deafness and Other Communication Disorders, 337
U.S. National Institutes of Health (NIH), 2, 3, 452
U.S. National Library of Medicine (NLM), 55
U.S. National Oceanic and Atmospheric Administration (NOAA), 89
U.S. National Research Council (NRC), 3, 7, 342, 411, 412, 451, 453, 454, 456, 463, 470
U.S. Occupational Safety and Health Administration (OSHA), 7, 41, 43, 45, 199, 218, 224, 386, 387, 388, 389, 390, 393, 397, 398, 452, 464
areas of regulatory concern, 43
bloodborne pathogens (BBP) standard, 387, 399
exposure to asbestos standard, 388
functions of, 41
Hazard Communication Standard, 398
health risk assessment activities, 452, 464
permissible exposure limits (PELs), 387, 390
personal protective equipment (PPE) requirements, 387
right-to-know standard, 387
synthetic mineral fibers (SMFs), 397
U.S. Personal Care Products Council, 415
UBA. *See* Federal Environment(al) Agency, Germany (UBA)
UDP-glucuronosyltransferase (UGT), 119, 121, 124
UGT. *See* UDP-glucuronosyltransferase (UGT)
ultimate carcinogen(s), 122
definition of, 351
ultrafine particles. *See* particulate matter (PM): $PM_{0.1}$ (nano- and ultrafine particles)
uncertainty factors. *See* health risk assessment: uncertainty and safety factors
UNECE. *See* United Nations Economic Commission for Europe (UNECE)
UNEP. *See* United Nations Environment Programme (UNEP)
United Heckathorn (Superfund toxic site), 49, 54, 443, 444, 445
as a case study, 443
United Nations Economic Commission for Europe (UNECE), 288, 289
United Nations Environment Programme (UNEP), 44, 288, 290, 294, 298, 304, 305, 306, 364, 373, 375, 451
Universal Waste Rule, U.S., 53
uptake (and absorption) of toxicants. *See* toxicants: uptake (and absorption) of
uranium (U), 57, 254, 255, 347, 348, 399
urban particulate pollution, 202, 203, 204, 205
airborne microbes. *See* airborne microbes

episodes, 203
lignite mining operations, 204
monitoring issues, 204
urbanization, 17, 19, 22
Urginea maritima, 278, *See also* squill (*Urginea maritima*)
USCG. *See* U.S. Coast Guard (USCG)

V

valproic acid, 378
vapor migration (vapor intrusion), 231
venoms
    definition of, 318
    from amphibians, 334, 335
    from arachnids, 332
    from arthropods, 331
    from insects, 333
    from lizards, 335
    from reptiles, 334
    from scorpions, 333, *See also* venoms: from arachnids
    from snakes, 318, 334
    from spiders, 332, *See also* venoms: from arachnids
vinyl chloride, 62, 150, 218, 229, 347, 348, 355, 379
viral gastroenteritis, 240, 321, 420, 421
viral toxin. *See* toxins: from viruses
virion(s), 142, 143, 321
viroids, 319, 320
virus L-A, 324
vitamin A (e.g., retinol, retinal), 28, 125, 164, 165, 374, 378, 407, 408
vitamin B group, 165
    B_1 (thiamine), 165
    B_{12} (cobalamin), 165
    B_2 (riboflavin), 130, 165
    B_3 (niacin), 130
    B_5 (pantothenic acid), 130
vitamin C (ascorbic acid), 28, 125, 127, 130, 165, 167, 408
vitamin D (e.g., D_3, cholecalciferol), 165, 407, 408
vitamin E (tocopherol and tocotrienol), 125, 127, 408
vitamin H (B_7 or biotin), 130
vitamin K (2-methyl-1,4-naphthoquinone), 143, 165, 278, 355
vitellogenin (VTG), 303
    gene, 303
VOCs. *See* volatile organic compounds (VOCs)
volatile organic compounds (VOCs)
    chlorinated solvents, 218
    definition of, 62, 217
    environmental health concerns, 218, 219
    fuel components, 218
    precursors of ozone, 217
    precursors of particulate matter, 217
    sources of pollution, 218
    use standards, 218
volume of distribution. *See* toxicants: toxicokinetics
VX, 271

W

warfarin, 143, 168, 278
wasp sting, 333
water contaminants, 49, 59, 60, 71, 76, 77, 432, 471
    fate of, 72, 73, 74, 75, 76, 77
    transport of, 72, 73, 74, 75, 76, 77
water pollution, 19, 20, 22, 24, 33, 34, 35, 41, 45, 78, 429, 433, 440
    definition of, 20
water quality, 41, 43, 428, 432
    criteria (WQC), U.S., 432, 433
    regulatory efforts for, U.S., 433
weight-of-evidence, 241, 466
WELs. *See* workplace exposure limits (WELs)
WES. *See* workplace exposure standard
West Nile virus, 270
wet deposition. *See* air pollutants: wet deposition
WHO (World Health Organization), 11, 12, 13, 19, 40, 44, 87, 156, 166, 168, 180, 184, 187, 190, 200, 201, 202, 203, 204, 209, 220, 222, 228, 232, 241, 261, 266, 294, 308, 309, 310, 320, 349, 353, 364, 373, 375, 398, 400, 439, 456, 464, 469
    IARC's classification of carcinogenicity potential, 354
    Public Health Emergency of International Concern, 13
Wildlife Exposure Factors Handbook, 438
wildlife terrestrial environment, 435, 439
    chaparral, 436
    desert, 436
    forests, 436, 437
    taiga, 436
    tundra, 435, 436
wildlife toxicology, 428, 429, 430, 433, 434, 435
    relevance to human health, 429, 433
    scope and history, 434
Wildlife Toxicology Working Group, 434
Wilson's disease, 251, *See also* copper (Cu): Wilson's disease
Wingspread Conference Center, Wisconsin (USA)
    endocrine disruption, 364
worker (employee) right-to-know laws, 336

worker right-to-know movement, 398
workplace biological hazards, 398
    Ebola, 400
    infectious agents, 399
    occupational diseases, 400
    SARS, 399, 400
workplace exposure limits (WELs), 390
workplace exposure standard (WES), 390, 392, 393
workplace physical hazards, 398
    cold, 399
    heat, 399
    ionizing radiation, 399
    noise, 399
    non-ionizing radiation, 399
    vibration, 399
WorkSafe New Zealand (WSNZ), 392, 393
World Health Day, 11
World Health Organization. *See* WHO (World Health Organization)

X

xanthine oxidase, 165
xenobiotics. *See* toxicology: terminology
xylene(s), 218, 223, 355, 393, 395, 419

Z

zearalenones, 325, 327, 328
Zika (virus), 11, 13, 48, 377, 378
    Flaviviridae, 11
    microcephaly cases, 13
Zikv. *See* Zika (virus)
zinc (Zn), 28, 125, 142, 165, 190, 200, 239, 243, 244, 249, 250, 251, 252, 395, 408, 442
    deficiency, 165
    oxide, 395
    phosphide, 278
zygocin, 324

Made in the USA
Columbia, SC
18 January 2021